1998
YEAR BOOK OF
ORTHOPEDICS®

Statement of Purpose

The YEAR BOOK Service

The YEAR BOOK series was devised in 1901 by practicing health professionals who observed that the literature of medicine and related disciplines had become so voluminous that no one individual could read and place in perspective every potential advance in a major specialty. In the final decade of the 20th century, this recognition is more acutely true than it was in 1901.

More than merely a series of books, YEAR BOOK volumes are the tangible results of a unique service designed to accomplish the following:

- to *survey* a wide range of journals of proven value
- to *select* from those journals papers representing significant advances and statements of important clinical principles
- to provide *abstracts* of those articles that are readable, convenient summaries of their key points
- to provide *commentary* about those articles to place them in perspective

These publications grow out of a unique process that calls on the talents of outstanding authorities in clinical and fundamental disciplines, trained literature specialists, and professional writers, all supported by the resources of Mosby, the world's preeminent publisher for the health professions.

The Literature Base

Mosby and its editors survey approximately 500 journals published worldwide, covering the full range of the health professions. On an annual basis, the publisher examines usage patterns and polls its expert authorities to add new journals to the literature base and to delete journals that are no longer useful as potential YEAR BOOK sources.

The Literature Survey

The publisher's team of literature specialists, all of whom are trained and experienced health professionals, examines every original, peer-reviewed article in each journal issue. More than 250,000 articles per year are scanned systematically, including title, text, illustrations, tables, and references. Each scan is compared, article by article, to the search strategies that the publisher has developed in consultation with the 270 outside experts who form the pool of YEAR BOOK editors. A given article may be reviewed by any number of editors, from one to a dozen or more, regardless of the discipline for which the paper was originally published. In turn, each editor who receives the article reviews it to determine whether the article should be included in the YEAR BOOK. This decision is based on the article's inherent quality, its probable usefulness to readers of that YEAR BOOK, and the editor's goal to represent a balanced picture of a given field in each volume of the YEAR BOOK. In addition, the editor indicates when to include figures and tables from the article to help the YEAR BOOK reader better understand the information.

Of the quarter million articles scanned each year, only 5% are selected for detailed analysis within the YEAR BOOK series, thereby assuring readers of the high value of every selection.

The Abstract

The publisher's abstracting staff is headed by a seasoned medical professional and includes individuals with training in the life sciences, medicine, and other areas, plus extensive experience in writing for the health professions and related industries. Each selected article is assigned to a specific writer on this abstracting staff. The abstracter, guided in many cases by notations supplied by the expert editor, writes a structured, condensed summary designed so that the reader can rapidly acquire the essential information contained in the article.

The Commentary

The YEAR BOOK editorial boards, sometimes assisted by guest commentators, write comments that place each article in perspective for the reader. This provides the reader with the equivalent of a personal consultation with a leading international authority—an opportunity to better understand the value of the article and to benefit from the authority's thought processes in assessing the article.

Additional Editorial Features

The editorial boards of each YEAR BOOK organize the abstracts and comments to provide a logical and satisfying sequence of information. To enhance the organization, editors also provide introductions to sections or individual chapters, comments linking a number of abstracts, citations to additional literature, and other features.

The published YEAR BOOK contains enhanced bibliographic citations for each selected article, including extended listings of multiple authors and identification of author affiliations. Each YEAR BOOK contains a Table of Contents specific to that year's volume. From year to year, the Table of Contents for a given YEAR BOOK will vary depending on developments within the field.

Every YEAR BOOK contains a list of the journals from which papers have been selected. This list represents a subset of approximately 500 journals surveyed by the publisher and occasionally reflects a particularly pertinent article from a journal that is not surveyed on a routine basis.

Finally, each volume contains a comprehensive subject index and an index to authors of each selected paper.

The 1998 Year Book Series

Year Book of Allergy, Asthma, and Clinical Immunology: Drs. Rosenwasser, Borish, Boguniewicz, Nelson, Routes, and Spahn

Year Book of Anesthesiology and Pain Management®: Drs. Tinker, Abram, Chestnut, Roizen, Rothenberg, and Wood

Year Book of Cardiology®: Drs. Schlant, Collins, Gersh, Graham, Kaplan, and Waldo

Year Book of Chiropractic®: Dr. Lawrence

Year Book of Critical Care Medicine®: Drs. Parrillo, Balk, Calvin, Franklin, and Shapiro

Year Book of Dentistry®: Drs. Meskin, Berry, Jeffcoat, Leinfelder, Roser, Summitt, and Zakariasen

Year Book of Dermatologic Surgery®: Drs. Greenway, Barrett, Papadopoulos, and Whitaker

Year Book of Dermatology and Dermatologic Surgery™: Drs. Thiers and Lang

Year Book of Diagnostic Radiology®: Drs. Osborn, Groskin, Dalinka, Maynard, Pentecost, Rebner, Ros, Smirniotopoulos, and Young

Year Book of Drug Therapy®: Drs. Lasagna and Weintraub

Year Book of Emergency Medicine®: Drs. Wagner, Dronen, Davidson, King, Niemann, and Roberts

Year Book of Endocrinology®: Drs. Bagdade, Braverman, Horton, Kannan, Landsberg, Molitch, Morley, Nathan, Odell, Poehlman, Rogol, and Ryan

Year Book of Family Practice®: Drs. Berg, Bowman, Davidson, Dexter, and Scherger

Year Book of Gastroenterology®: Drs. Aliperti and Fleshman

Year Book of Geriatrics and Gerontology®: Drs. Burton, Beck, Ostwald, Rabins, Reuben, Roth, Shapiro, and Whitehouse

Year Book of Hand Surgery®: Drs. Amadio and Hentz

Year Book of Hematology®: Drs. Spivak, Bell, Ness, Quesenberry, Wiernik, and Horowitz

Year Book of Infectious Diseases: Drs. Keusch, Barza, Bennish, Poutsiaka, Skolnik, and Snydman

Year Book of Medicine®: Drs. Cline, Frishman, Jett, Klahr, Malawista, Mandell, McCallum, and Utiger

Year Book of Neonatal and Perinatal Medicine®: Drs. Fanaroff, Maisels, and Stevenson

Year Book of Nephrology, Hypertension, and Mineral Metabolism: Drs. Schwab, Bennett, Emmett, Hostetter, Kumar, and Toto

Year Book of Neurology and Neurosurgery®: Drs. Bradley and Gibbs

Year Book of Nuclear Medicine®: Drs. Gottschalk, Blaufox, Neumann, Strauss, and Zubal

Year Book of Obstetrics, Gynecology, and Women's Health: Drs. Mishell, Herbst, and Kirschbaum

Year Book of Occupational and Environmental Medicine®: Drs. Emmett, Frank, Gochfeld, and Hessl

Year Book of Oncology®: Drs. Ozols, Eisenberg, Glatstein, Loehrer, and Tallman

Year Book of Ophthalmology®: Drs. Wilson, Augsburger, Cohen, Eagle, Grossman, Laibson, Maguire, Nelson, Penne, Rapuano, Sergott, Spaeth, Tipperman, Ms. Gosfield, and Ms. Salmon

Year Book of Orthopedics®: Drs. Morrey, Beauchamp, Currier, Tolo, Trigg, and Swiontkowski

Year Book of Otolaryngology–Head and Neck Surgery®: Drs. Paparella and Holt

Year Book of Pathology and Laboratory Medicine®: Drs. Raab, Cohen, Olson, Sirgi, and Stanley

Year Book of Pediatrics®: Dr. Stockman

Year Book of Plastic, Reconstructive, and Aesthetic Surgery®: Drs. Miller, Bartlett, Garner, McKinney, Ruberg, Salisbury, and Smith

Year Book of Psychiatry and Applied Mental Health®: Drs. Talbott, Ballenger, Frances, Lydiard, Meltzer, Schowalter, and Tasman

Year Book of Pulmonary Disease®: Drs. Jett, Maurer, Ryu, Strollo, and Wenzel

Year Book of Rheumatology®: Drs. Panush, Hadler, LeRoy, Liang, Reichlin, Simon, and Weinblatt

Year Book of Sports Medicine®: Drs. Shephard, Drinkwater, Eichner, Torg, Alexander, and Mr. George

Year Book of Surgery®: Drs. Copeland, Bland, Deitch, Eberlein, Howard, Luce, Seeger, Souba, and Sugarbaker

Year Book of Thoracic and Cardiovascular Surgery®: Drs. Ginsberg, Wechsler, and Williams

Year Book of Urology®: Drs. Andriole and Coplen

Year Book of Vascular Surgery®: Dr. Porter

1998

The Year Book of ORTHOPEDICS®

Editor-in-Chief
Bernard F. Morrey, M.D.
Professor of Orthopedics, Mayo Medical School; Emeritus Chairman, Consultant, Department of Orthopedics, Mayo Clinic, Rochester, Minnesota

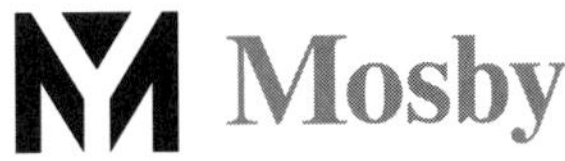

St. Louis Baltimore Boston Carlsbad Naples New York Philadelphia Portland London
Madrid Mexico City Singapore Sydney Tokyo Toronto Wiesbaden

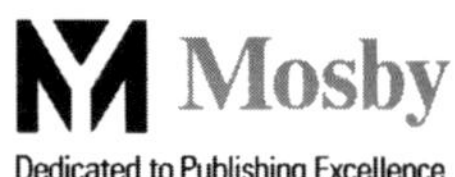

Dedicated to Publishing Excellence

Publisher: Theresa Van Schaik
Developmental Editor: Jaime Pendill
Manager, Periodical Editing: Kirk Swearingen
Production Editor: Stephanie M. Geels
Project Supervisor, Production: Joy Moore
Production Assistant: Karie House
Manager, Literature Services: Idelle L. Winer
Illustrations and Permissions Coordinator: Phyllis K. Thompson

Printed in the United States of America
Composition by Reed Technology and Information Services, Inc.
Printing/binding by Maple-Vail

Editorial Office:
Mosby, Inc.
11830 Westline Industrial Drive
St. Louis, MO 63146

International Standard Serial Number: 0276-1092
International Standard Book Number: 0-8151-9716-0

Table of Contents

Journals Represented xv

Publisher's Preface xvii

1. Basic Science 1

    Introduction 1

2. Pediatrics 17

    Introduction 17

    Fractures 17

    Scoliosis 26

    Congenital Hip Disorders 31

    Congenital Hand and Foot Disorders 34

    Gait Analysis 37

    Genetic Disorders 42

    Sports Injury 45

    Juvenile Arthritis 46

    Miscellaneous 48

3. Topics of General Orthopedic Interest 57

    Introduction 57

4. Trauma and Amputation Surgery 77

    Introduction 77

    Amputation Surgery 78

    Musculoskeletal Trauma 85

    Open Fractures 88

    Compartmental Syndrome 93

    Adult Respiratory Distress Syndrome 94

    Pelvic Fractures 99

    Hip Fractures 101

    Femur 104

    Tibia 108

    Miscellaneous 117

5. Forearm, Wrist, and Hand 121

    Introduction 121

    Evaluation and Diagnosis 122

Wrist 128

Forearm 143

Hand 146

Neurovascular 154

6. Elbow 161

Introduction 161

Tennis Elbow 161

Synovectomy 164

Trauma 168

Miscellaneous 172

7. Shoulder 177

Introduction 177

Cuff 177

Instability 185

Miscellaneous 193

8. Hip Reconstruction 203

Introduction 203

Primary Total Hip Arthroplasty 203

Femoral Revision 212

Acetabular Revision and Issues 216

Complications 222

Avascular Necrosis 227

9. Knee 231

Introduction 231

Reconstruction/Arthritis 231

Outcomes 231

Total Knee Arthroplasty 234

Complications and Related Issues 239

Sports 242

Arthroscopy 242

Anterior Cruciate Ligament 246

Arthritis 251

Patella 257

10. Complications 261

    Introduction 261

11. Foot and Ankle 279

    Introduction 279

    Ligament Injuries 279

    Tendon and Related Injuries 284

    Osseous Injuries 288

    Arthritis/Arthrodesis 292

    Revision 301

    Miscellaneous 304

12. Spine 313

    Introduction 313

    Bone Graft Substitutes 313

    Coding and Documentation 315

    Degenerative Conditions 319

    Infection 324

    Instrumentation 328

    Outcomes of Surgical Management 336

    Pathophysiology of Sciatica 340

    Practice Guidelines 343

    Spinal Cord Injury 344

13. Orthopedic Oncology 347

    Introduction 347

    Chemotherapy 348

    Ewing's Sarcoma 360

    Metastatic Disease 363

    Miscellaneous 376

    Radiology 391

    Reconstruction 399

    Soft Tissue Sarcoma 419

    SUBJECT INDEX. 423

    AUTHOR INDEX 461

Journals Represented

Mosby and its editors subscribe to and survey approximately 500 U.S. and foreign medical and allied health journals. From these journals, the editors select the articles to be abstracted. Journals represented in this YEAR BOOK are listed below.

Acta Anaesthesiologica Scandinavica
Acta Orthopaedica Scandinavica
American Journal of Roentgenology
American Journal of Sports Medicine
American Surgeon
Anesthesia and Analgesia
Annals of Rheumatic Diseases
Annals of Surgical Oncology
Annals of the Royal College of Surgeons of England
Archives of Orthopaedic and Trauma Surgery
Archives of Physical Medicine and Rehabilitation
Arthroscopy
British Journal of Anaesthesia
British Journal of Plastic Surgery
British Journal of Surgery
British Medical Journal
Cancer
Clincial Biomechanics
Clinical Orthopaedics and Related Research
Clinical Radiology
Critical Care Medicine
Diabetes Care
European Journal of Cancer
Foot & Ankle International
Injury
International Journal of Radiation, Oncology, Biology, and Physics
International Orthopaedics
Journal of Arthroplasty
Journal of Bone and Joint Surgery (American Volume)
Journal of Bone and Joint Surgery (British Volume)
Journal of Clinical Investigation
Journal of Clinical Oncology
Journal of Computer Assisted Tomography
Journal of Foot and Ankle Surgery
Journal of General Internal Medicine
Journal of Hand Surgery (American)
Journal of Hand Surgery (British)
Journal of Neurosurgery
Journal of Occupational Rehabilitation
Journal of Orthopaedic Research
Journal of Orthopaedic Trauma
Journal of Orthopaedic and Sports Physical Therapy
Journal of Pediatric Orthopaedics
Journal of Pediatric Orthopaedics Part B
Journal of Pediatrics
Journal of Rheumatology
Journal of Spinal Disorders

Journal of the American Academy of Orthopaedic Surgeons
Journal of the American Geriatrics Society
Journal of the American Medical Association
Journal of the National Cancer Institute
Lancet
Mayo Clinic Proceedings
Medical Journal of Australia
New England Journal of Medicine
Occupational Medicine
Occupational and Environmental Medicine
Orthopedics
Plastic and Reconstructive Surgery
Radiology
Radiotherapy and Oncology
Skeletal Radiology
Southern Medical Journal
Spine
Surgery
Techniques in Hand and Upper Extremity Surgery

STANDARD ABBREVIATIONS

The following terms are abbreviated in this edition: acquired immunodeficiency syndrome (AIDS), cardiopulmonary resuscitation (CPR), central nervous system (CNS), cerebrospinal fluid (CSF), computed tomography (CT), deoxyribonucleic acid (DNA), electrocardiography (ECG), health maintenance organization (HMO), human immunodeficiency virus (HIV), intensive care unit (ICU), intramuscular (IM), intravenous (IV), magnetic resonance (MR) imaging (MRI), and ribonucleic acid (RNA).

NOTE

The YEAR BOOK OF ORTHOPEDICS® is a literature survey service providing abstracts of articles published in the professional literature. Every effort is made to assure the accuracy of the information presented in these pages. Neither the editors nor the publisher of the YEAR BOOK OF ORTHOPEDICS® can be responsible for errors in the original materials. The editors' comments are their own opinions. Mention of specific products within this publication does not constitute endorsement.

To facilitate the use of the YEAR BOOK OF ORTHOPEDICS® as a reference tool, all illustrations and tables included in this publication are now identified as they appear in the original article. This change is meant to help the reader recognize that any illustration or table appearing in the YEAR BOOK OF ORTHOPEDICS® may be only one of many in the original article. For this reason, figure and table numbers will often appear to be out of sequence within the YEAR BOOK OF ORTHOPEDICS®.

Publisher's Preface

The publication of the 1998 YEAR BOOK OF ORTHOPEDICS commences the editorship of Bernard F. Morrey, M.D. He has assembled a distinguished group of colleagues to serve as associate editors: Christopher P. Beauchamp, M.D.; Bradford L. Currier, M.D.; Marc F. Swiontkowski, M.D.; Vernon T. Tolo, M.D.; and Stephen D. Trigg, M.D.

We know you will agree that Dr. Morrey and his editorial board provide our readers with the informative and clinically relevant literature and thought-provoking commentary that they have come to expect from the YEAR BOOK OF ORTHOPEDICS.

1 Basic Science

Introduction

There has been an explosion of information related to the modulation of cellular activity by cytokines. This has a particularly exciting application for patients experiencing the effects of debris particle osteolysis. Clearly there are patients more prone to this problem than others. By understanding the various mechanisms by which it occurs, we can prevent the process from occurring. This, I believe, will have an effect on patient care in the very near future.

I have included two articles dealing with radiation risk for the orthopedic team (Abstracts 1–3 and 1–5); both are must-read articles, especially for resident staff.

Christopher P. Beauchamp, M.D.

The Effects of Particulate Cobalt, Chromium and Cobalt-Chromium Alloy on Human Osteoblast-like Cells In Vitro

Allen MJ, Myer BJ, Millett PJ, et al (Addenbrooke's Hosp, Cambridge, England)
J Bone Joint Surg Br 79-B:475–482, 1997

1–1

Introduction.—In the pathogenesis of a septic loosening of total joint prostheses, particulate wear debris is strongly implicated. The relationship between particulate wear debris, bone resorption, and aseptic loosening has been studied. A number of cytokine and prostanoid inflammatory mediators have been released by cells exposed to particulate debris. In supernatants from cultured explants of interfacial membranes from around loose cemented and cementless prostheses, high levels of these bone-resorbing mediators have been identified. Bone resorption may not be the only factor in periprosthetic bone loss. A balance between bone formation and bone resorption is involved in normal bone turnover, and the result of a reduction in bone formation, with or without a concomitant increase in bone resorption, may be part of the net loss of periprosthetic bone in aseptic loosening. In osteoblast cultures exposed to metallic wear debris, cytotoxicity has been demonstrated. Two human osteoblast-like osteosarcoma cells lines were exposed to particulate cobalt, chromium, and cobalt-chromium alloy to investigate the hypothesis that particulate

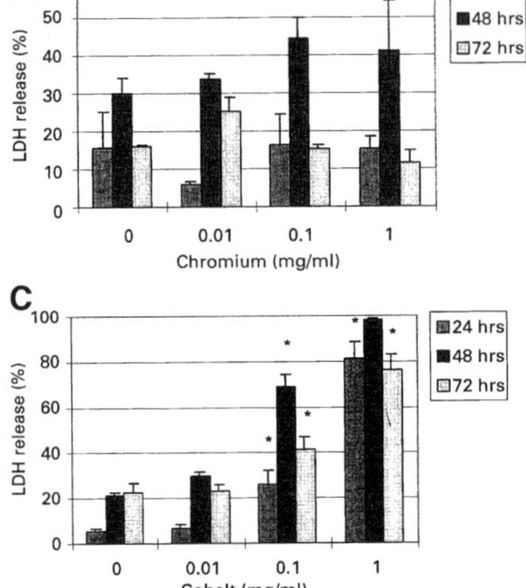

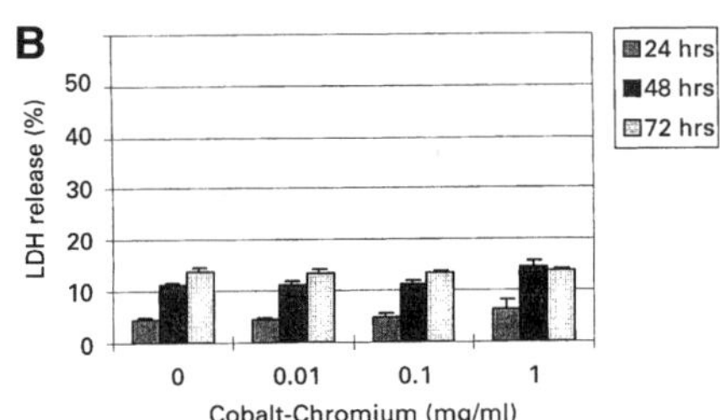

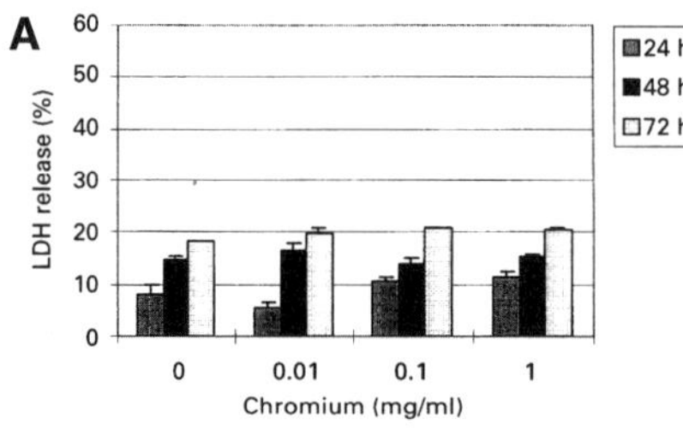

FIGURE 2.—Cytotoxicity of particulate chromium (**A**), cobalt-chromium alloy (**B**), and cobalt (**C**) for SaOS-2 osteoblast-like cells in vitro. The results are expressed as the mean ± SEM for triplicate samples and each experiment was performed in duplicate. *Asterisk* indicates $P < 0.05$. *Abbreviation: LDH*, lactate dehydrogenase. (Courtesy of Allen MJ, Myer BJ, Millet PJ, et al: The effects of particulate cobalt, chromium and cobalt-chromium alloy on human osteoblast-like cells in vitro. *J Bone Joint Surg Br* 79-B:475–482, 1997.)

debris can have a direct effect on the metabolic activity of bone cells in vitro.

Methods.—At concentrations of 0, 0.01, 0.1, and 1.0 mg/mL, 2 human osteoblast-like cell lines were exposed to particulate cobalt, chromium, and cobalt-chromium alloy.

Results.—Cobalt was toxic to both cell lines, and the production of type-I collagen, osteocalcin, and alkaline phosphatase was inhibited. Both cell lines tolerated chromium and cobalt-chromium with no inhibition of type-I collagen synthesis and no cytotoxicity (Figs 2, A and B; 3, A and B). Alkaline phosphatase activity was inhibited by chromium at the highest

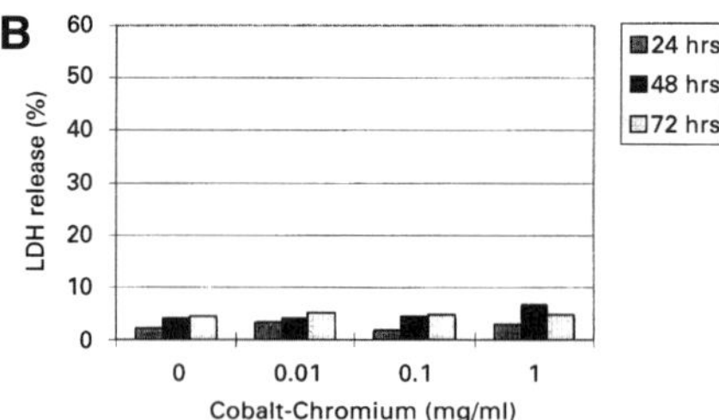

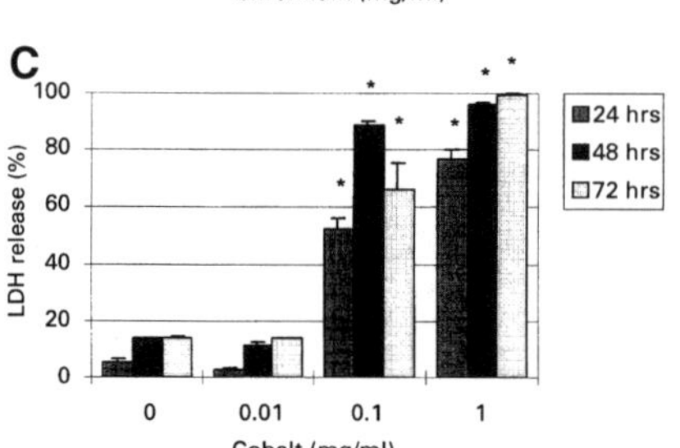

FIGURE 3.—Cytotoxicity of particulate chromium (**A**), cobalt-chromium alloy (**B**), and cobalt (**C**) for MG-63 osteoblast-like cells in vitro. The results are expressed as the mean ± SEM for triplicate samples and each experiment was performed in duplicate. *Asterisk* indicates $P < 0.05$. *Abbreviation: LDH*, lactate dehydrogenase. (Courtesy of Allen MJ, Myer BJ, Millet PJ, et al: The effects of particulate cobalt, chromium and cobalt-chromium alloy on human osteoblast-like cells in vitro. *J Bone Joint Surg Br* 79-B:475–482, 1997.)

concentration tested (1.0 mg/mL). Cobalt caused dose-dependent increases in the release of lactate dehydrogenase (a cytoplasmic enzyme present within all mammalian cells), particularly at concentrations of 0.1 mg/mL in both cell lines (Figs 2, C and 3, C). Osteocalcin expression was inhibited by both chromium and cobalt-chromium alloy.

Conclusions.—The growth and metabolism of osteoblastic cells in vitro can be modulated by particulate metal debris. An important mechanism by which particulate wear debris influences the pathogenesis of aseptic loosening in vivo may be a reduction of osteoblastic activity at the bone-implant interface.

▶ The authors examined the effects of particulate metal debris on the growth and metabolism of osteoblast cells in vitro. They demonstrated clearly that cobalt itself was toxic to cells and resulted in inhibition of collagen production as well as osteocalcin and alkaline phosphatase. Chromium and the alloy cobalt-chromium were much better tolerated by cell lines. As we gain more understanding as to the effects of particulate debris in joint arthroplasty, we may gain an understanding not only of the mechanism by which they act, but also methods by which we may modulate their biological effects.

C.P. Beauchamp, M.D.

Modulation of the Production of Cytokines in Titanium-stimulated Human Peripheral Blood Monocytes by Pharmacological Agents: The Role of cAMP-mediated Signaling Mechanisms

Blaine TA, Pollice PF, Rosier RN, et al (Univ of Rochester, NY)
J Bone Joint Surg Am 79-A:1519–1528, 1997   1–2

Introduction.—Major complications of joint replacement continue to be osteolysis and loosening of prosthetic implants. Osteolysis was found adjacent to 57% of femoral implants within 6 years after surgery in one study. The tissue macrophage is central to this process of response to the phagocytosis of particulate debris with the synthesis and secretion of interleukin-1 (IL-1), IL-6, and tumor necrosis factor-α (TNF-α). The pharmacologic inhibition of activated macrophages is a possible method for preventing aseptic loosening of total joint replacements. In the stimulation of osteolysis associated with prosthetic loosening, TNF-α may play a pivotal role. In titanium particle–stimulated cultures of human peripheral blood monocytes, the mechanism of signal transduction involved in the synthesis of TNF-α was studied. The degree to which TNF-α can be inhibited by pharmacologic agents that affect signal transduction was also examined.

Methods.—In the synthesis of IL-6 and TNF-α, the role of the cAMP–protein kinase A signal transduction pathway was studied. In human peripheral blood monocytes stimulated with titanium particles, the effect of potential pharmacologic regulators of this pathway also was examined.

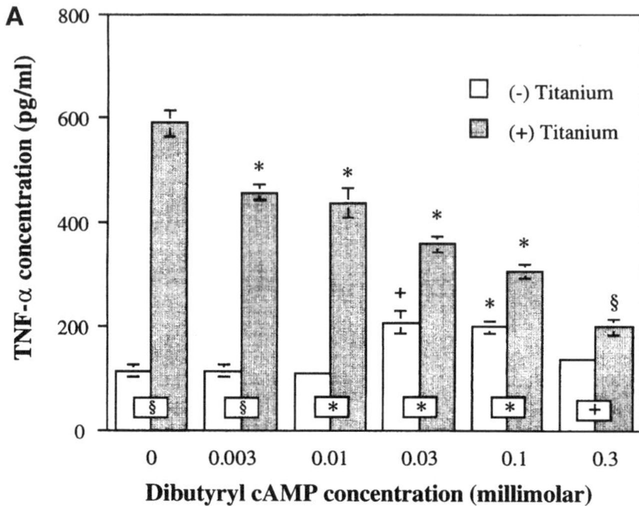

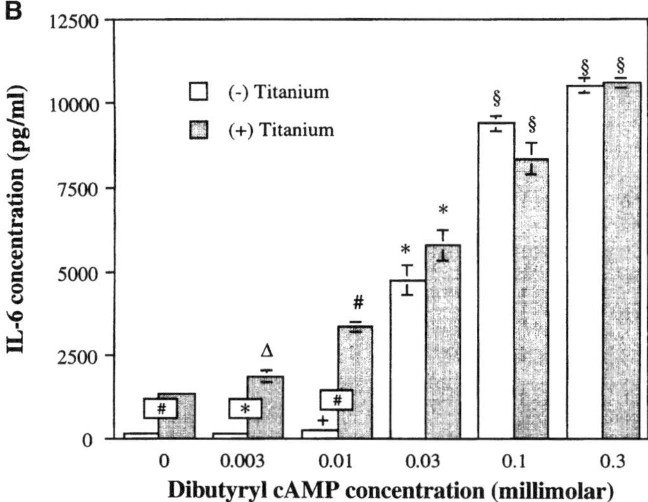

FIGURE 1.—Graphs showing the effect of dibutyryl cAMP on the release of tumor necrosis factor-α (*TNF-α*) (**A**) and interleukin-6 (*IL-6*) (**B**) by human peripheral blood monocytes. Isolated monocytes were treated with various concentrations of dibutyryl cAMP in the presence and absence of titanium particles, and the mean concentration of TNF-α or IL-6 was measured with enzyme-linked immunosorbent assay. The *symbols* at the top of the *bars* denote the *P* value for the comparisons between the titanium-stimulated and titanium-free cultures and the respective dibutyryl cAMP-free controls. The *symbols* in the *boxes* denote the *P* value for the comparisons between the titanium-free cultures and the titanium-stimulated cultures for each dose of dibutyryl cAMP. §, $P < 0.0001$; *, $P < 0.005$; +, $P < 0.01$; #, $P < 0.001$; Δ, $P < 0.05$. The *I-bars* represent the SEM; in some cases, the SE is too small to be observed on the graphs. (Courtesy of Blaine TA, Pollice PF, Rosier RN, et al: Modulation of the production of cytokines in titanium-stimulated human peripheral blood monocytes by pharmacological agents: The role of cAMP-mediated signaling mechanisms. *J Bone Joint Surg Am* 79-A:1519–1528, 1997.)

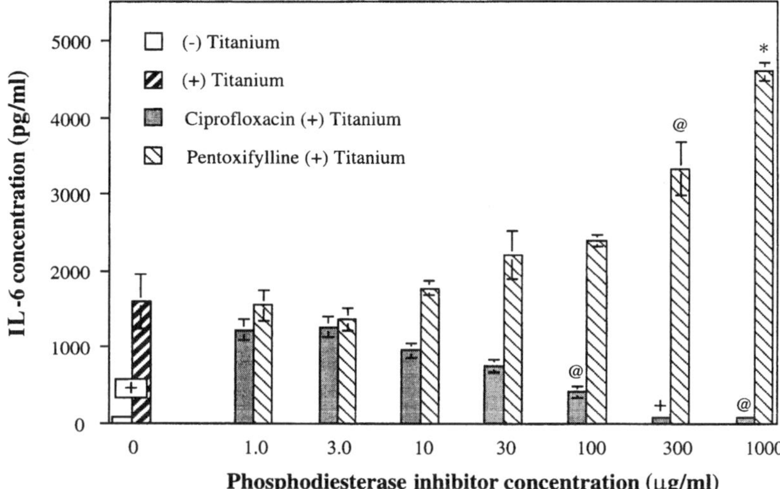

FIGURE 5, B.—Graph showing the effect of ciprofloxacin and pentoxifylline on the release of interleukin-6 (*IL-6*) by human peripheral blood monocytes. Isolated monocytes were treated with various concentrations of ciprofloxacin or pentoxifylline, and the mean concentration of IL-6 was measured. The *symbols* at the top of the *bars* denote the *P* value for the comparisons between the titanium-stimulated cultures and the titanium-stimulated ciprofloxacin or pentoxifylline-free controls. The *symbols* in the *boxes* denote the *P* value for the comparisons between the titanium-free control cultures and the titanium-stimulated control cultures. *, $P < 0.005$; @, $P < 0.025$; +, $P < 0.01$. The *I-bars* represent the SEM; in some cases, the SE is too small to be observed on the graph. (Courtesy of Blaine TA, Pollice PF, Rosier RN, et al: Modulation of the production of cytokines in titanium-stimulated human peripheral blood monocytes by pharmacological agents: The role of cAMP-mediated signaling mechanisms. *J Bone Joint Surg Am* 79-A:1519–1528, 1997.)

To examine effects on the synthesis of cytokines, additional agents that alter the intracellular levels of cAMP were also examined.

Results.—The synthesis of TNF-α was decreased but the synthesis of IL-6 was increased by dibutyryl cAMP, indicating the complexity of the release of cytokines in wear-debris-stimulated monocytes (Fig 1). Potent inhibitors of the synthesis of TNF-α were prostaglandins E_1 and E_2, but they stimulated the synthesis of IL-6. The stimulatory effects of titanium particles on TNF-α were enhanced by indomethacin, resulting in a three-fold increase in the maximum levels of TNF-α. A decrease in the production of TNF-α and an increase in the production of IL-6 were caused by phosphodiesterase inhibitors, such as isobutyryl methylxanthine and pentoxifylline. A dose-dependent inhibition of the synthesis of TNF-α and IL-6 by titanium-stimulated monocytes was caused by the fluoroquinolone antibiotic ciprofloxacin (Fig 5, B).

Conclusions.—Novel therapeutic strategies to prevent the loosening of implants can occur with the use of pharmacologic agents in combination with efforts at reducing the generation of wear debris. These events are regulated by normal physiologic mechanisms in titanium-stimulated human peripheral blood monocytes rather than by an irreversible toxic response, as is evidenced by alteration of the synthesis of cytokines in response to pharmacologic manipulation of cAMP–protein kinase A signaling pathway. Tumor necrosis factor-α and IL-6 have a differential response to agents that alter intracellular levels of cAMP, indicating that these 2 cytokines are independently regulated. Multiple agents to inhibit diverse regulatory pathways may need to be involved in pharmacologic strategies to inhibit the release of cytokines. For the efficient design and selection of inhibitory agents, basic-science studies are essential to the pathways involved in titanium-mediated synthesis of cytokines.

▶ Continued improvements in the design of prostheses remain hampered by the effects of wear-debris-induced osteolysis. This study examines the mechanism by which the cytokines responsible for osteolysis are effected by wear debris and regulated by intracellular mechanisms. The authors have clearly demonstrated that these mediators can be modulated by pharmacologic agents. This provides an exciting possibility in the future for the management of patients with significant osteolysis, as well as for preventing the development of osteolysis. The authors have demonstrated that the mechanism by which this occurs is clearly multifactorial and would likely require treatment with multiple agents to effect biological control of this mechanism. This has positive implications to patients with well-fixed components, minimal polyethylene wear, and massive osteolysis.

C.P. Beauchamp, M.D.

Ionising Radiation: Are Orthopaedic Surgeons' Offspring at Risk?
Zadeh HG, Briggs TWR (Royal Natl Orthopaedic Hosp Trust, Stanmore, Middlesex, England)
Ann R Coll Surg Engl 79:214–220, 1997   1–3

Introduction.—Genetic damage can result from exposure to ionizing radiation, which may manifest in congenital abnormalities or childhood malignancies in the next generation. Orthopedic and trauma surgeons use radiographic imaging often, but previous reports have shown that exposure to X-rays during diagnostic imaging is within the recommended limits. The health of the children in these groups has not been amply studied, however. In a group of orthopedic surgeons, the incidence of congenital abnormalities and childhood malignancies was ascertained and compared with the normal population and a control group of surgeons who do not use x-ray imaging routinely.

Methods.—There were 504 questionnaires sent to orthopedic surgeons and 1,597 questionnaires sent to 1,597 obstetricians and gynecologists. There was a 66% response rate from the orthopedic surgeons and a 62% response rate from the obstetricians and gynecologists. They were asked to report congenital abnormalities of their children.

Results.—In both groups, there was a higher rate of congenital abnormalities when compared with the normal population, but there were no statistically significant differences in the rate of congenital abnormalities between the offspring of orthopedic surgeons, and those of gynecologists

TABLE 3.—Congenital Abnormality Rates and Sex Ratios

	Congenital abnormality rates per 10,000 live/stillbirths	Sex ratio male/female
Population (OPCS 1991) (*10*)	101.5	51%/49%
Orthopaedic surgeons	288.2	47%/53%
Obstetricians and gynaecologists	232.4	49%/51%
Orthopaedic surgeons (corrected)*	190.9	—
Obstetricians and gynaecologists (corrected)*	143.5	—
Male orthopaedic surgeons	269.0	47%/53%
Male obstetricians and gynaecologists	236.6	48%/52%
Female obstetricians and gynaecologists	222.2	51%/49%

*Corrected for the total number of children, assuming there were no further congenital abnormalities in the children of nonresponders.

(Courtesy of Zadeh HG, Briggs TWR: Ionising radiation: Are orthopaedic surgeons' offspring at risk? *Ann R Coll Surg Engl* 79:214–220, 1997.)

and obstetricians (Table 3) (Table 4). Factors other than exposure to X-rays may be involved in the increased rate of congenital abnormalities observed in both groups of physicians. A higher incidence of female children was found among male surgeons when compared with the normal population. The incidence of childhood malignancies was not raised in either group.

Conclusions.—An increased risk of congenital abnormalities or childhood malignancies in their children was not found among orthopedic surgeons exposed to the current levels of occupational exposure to X-rays. Occupational exposure to the operating theater environment may be the main etiologic cause for the increased incidence of congenital abnormalities seen in the children of obstetricians, gynecologists, and orthopedic surgeons.

▶ This paper presents an interesting glimpse at the sequelae of environmental hazards that orthopedic surgeons are exposed to. We are all concerned about our exposure to radiation, anesthetic inhalational agents, and

TABLE 4.—Comparative Analysis for Congenital Abnormalities

Comparative analysis for congenital abnormalities	χ^2	P
Population *vs* orthopaedic surgeons	13.82	0.0002
Population *vs* orthopaedic surgeons (corrected)*	4.55	0.033
Population *vs* obstetricians and gynaecologists	25.00	0.0000006
Population *vs* obstetricians and gynaecologists (corrected)*	3.97	0.046
Male orthopaedic surgeons *vs* male obstetricians and gynaecologists with no history of radiation exposure	0.08	0.78
Male obstetricians and gynaecologists *vs* female obstetricians and gynaecologists	0.09	0.76
Obstetricians and gynaecologists with no history of radiation exposure *vs* obstetricians and gynaecologists with history of radiation exposure	0.00	0.99

*Corrected for the total number of children, assuming there were no further congenital abnormalities in the children of nonresponders.

(Courtesy of Zadeh HG, Briggs TWR: Ionising radiation: Are orthopaedic surgeons' offspring at risk? *Ann R Coll Surg Engl* 79:214–220, 1997.)

methylmethacrylate during surgical procedures; this is in addition to the numerous other biohazards associated with direct patient care. This study demonstrated a disturbingly higher rate of congenital abnormalities in the offspring of orthopedic surgeons and obstetricians and gynecologists compared with the rate found in the normal population. Radiation exposure, however, is not implicated as the cause. Further study needs to be directed toward the previously mentioned risk factors.

C.P. Beauchamp, M.D.

Human Arthroplasty Derived Macrophages Differentiate Into Osteoclastic Bone Resorbing Cells

Sabokbar A, Fujikawa Y, Neale S, et al (Nuffield Orthopaedic Centre, Oxford, England; Univ of Adelaide, Australia)
Ann Rheum Dis 56:414–420, 1997   1–4

Introduction.—The most common cause of late failure of cemented and uncemented joint replacements is aseptic loosening. A prominent foreign body macrophage response to polymeric and metallic wear particles in the pseudocapsule and pseudomembrane surrounding the implant is often associated with aseptic loosening. The cellular mechanisms responsible for this pathologic bone resorption, and the way in which the heavy foreign body macrophage infiltrate in periprosthetic tissues contributes to osteolysis are not known. One theory is that differentiation of cells into bone-resorbing osteoclasts may be the means whereby macrophages could contribute directly to the osteolysis of aseptic loosening. Whether human wear

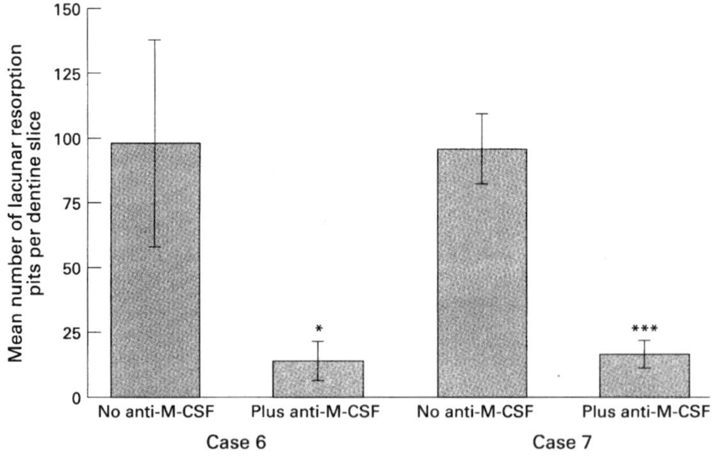

FIGURE 4.—Effect of neutralizing anti–macrophage colony-stimulating factor (anti–M-CSF) antibody on the mean number of lacunar pits formed on dentine slices from co-cultures of arthroplasty-derived macrophages from case numbers 6 and 7. Results are expressed as mean (SD). Levels of significance using Student's paired *t* test: *, $P = 0.024$; †, $P = 0.00092$. (Reprinted with permission of the BMJ Publishing Group, from Sabokbar A, Fujikawa Y, Neale S, et al: Human arthroplasty derived macrophages differentiate into osteoclastic bone resorbing cells. *Ann Rheum Dis 56:414–420, 1997.*)

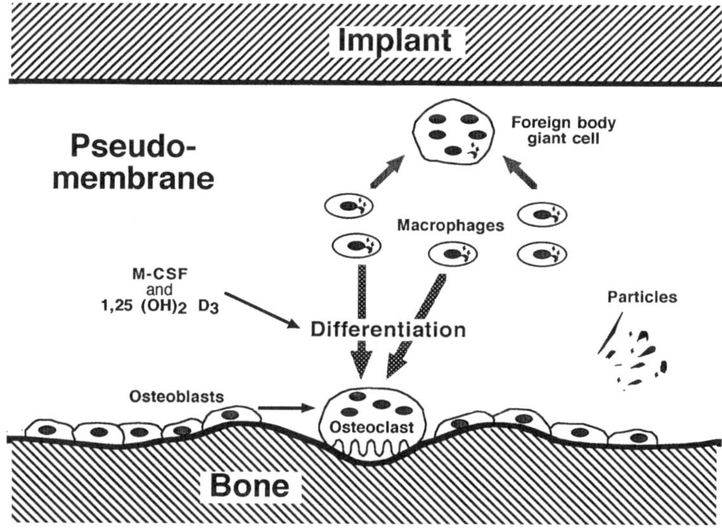

FIGURE 5.—Proposed cellular and humoral mechanism whereby human wear particle induced foreign body macrophages in the periprosthetic tissues differentiate into osteoclastic bone resorbing cells. (Reprinted with permission of the BMJ Publishing Group, from Sabokbar A, Fujikawa Y, Neale S, et al: Human arthroplasty derived macrophages differentiate into osteoclastic bone resorbing cells. *Ann Rheum Dis* 56:414–420, 1997.)

particle–associated macrophages are present in the periprosthetic tissues around loosened osteoclastic bone-resorbing cells was determined, as well as which cellular and humoral conditions are required for this to occur. The role of macrophage colony-stimulating factor was also characterized.

Methods.—The pseudocapsule and pseudomembrane of loose cemented and uncemented hip arthroplasties were used to isolated macrophages. This was performed at the time of revision surgery and was co-cultured on glass cover slips and dentine slices with UMR 106 rat osteoblast-like cells in the presence and absence of 1,25 dihydroxyvitamin D_3. As a control group, macrophages were isolated from the synovial membrane of patients with osteoarthritis having hip replacements.

Results.—Macrophage CD11b and CD14 were strongly expressed by most cells isolated from the periprosthetic tissues after 24 hours' incubation, but not osteoclast markers. Numerous multinucleated cells showing the phenotypic features of osteoclasts were found after 14 days' incubation that were formed in co-cultures of arthroplasty-derived macrophages and UMR 106 cells. These were positive for tartrate-resistant acid phosphatase and vitronectin receptor, and were capable of extensive lacunar resorption. Macrophage-osteoclast differentiation was considerably reduced along with the lacunar resorption in these co-cultures by the addition of an antibody to macrophage colony-stimulating factor (Fig 4). But when macrophage colony-stimulating factor was added, there was little or no evidence of macrophage-osteoclast differentiation in osteoarthritis synovial macrophage/UMR 106 co-cultures.

Conclusions.—Human macrophages isolated from periprosthetic tissues surrounding loosened implants can differentiate into multinucleated cells that have functional and cytochemical characteristics of osteoclasts (Fig 5). For this to occur, macrophage colony-stimulating factor is not required. In light of the heavy macrophage response to wear particles in periprosthetic tissues, macrophage-osteoclast differentiation may be an important cellular mechanism by which osteolysis is effected in aseptic loosening.

▶ This paper explores the mechanisms by which macrophages isolated from failed joint arthroplasty differentiate into osteoclasts, contributing to osteolysis and subsequent failure of the implant. The authors have successfully demonstrated that macrophages isolated in the pseudocapsule of failed joint arthroplasty can differentiate into osteoclasts, and that interference with macrophage colony-stimulating factor will reduce this differentiation. Drugs designed to modulate cellular differentiation would be beneficial to arthroplasty patients.

C.P. Beauchamp, M.D.

Radiation Exposure to the Orthopaedic Surgical Team During Fluoroscopy: "How Far Away Is Far Enough?"

Mehlman CT, DiPasquale TG (Univ of Cincinnati, Ohio; Ohio Univ, Athens; Florida Orthopaedic Inst, Tampa)
J Orthop Trauma 11:392–398, 1997   1–5

Introduction.—For the orthopedic surgeon, the fluoroscope is an important tool, but there are concerns about radiation exposure to the surgeon and other members of the surgical team. Few studies have addressed the topic of distance and radiation exposure in the surgical setting. "How far away is far enough" was determined by correlating radiation exposure and distance from a simulated fluoroscopically assisted orthopedic procedure for members of an orthopedic surgical team based on their relative positions.

Methods.—The positions that were studied were those of a surgeon, first assistant, scrub nurse, and an anesthesiologist in this simulated, fluoroscopically assisted, orthopedic procedure in which fluoroscopic units and dosimetry badges were used. The badges measured "eye" (ocular lens), "shallow" (hands/skin), and "deep" (whole-body) radiation exposure. The surgeon was at 12 inches from beam contact, the first assistant at 24 inches, the scrub nurse at 36 inches, and the anesthesiologist at 60 inches. A protocol intended to maximize radiation scattered was used to systemically expose dosimetry badges. Ten minutes was the maximum time for continuous fluoroscope use. Readings of radiation exposure were taken from the dosimetry badges.

Results.—There was about 4,000 mrem/min of radiation exposure. There was 20 mrem/min of deep exposure for the surgeon and 6 mrem/min for the first assistant (Table 3). For the surgeon, superficial exposure was

TABLE 3.—OEC (69 kV/3.3 mA) Deep Exposure Data (Reported in mrem)

	Unprotected surgeon	Protected surgeon	1st assistant	Scrub nurse	Anesthesia
		Neck-level badges			
1 min	0	0	0	0	0
2 min	10	0	0	0	0
3 min	10	0	0	0	0
5 min	40	0	0	0	0
10 min	80	0	20	0	0
		Waist-level badges			
1 min	0	0	0	0	0
2 min	0	0	0	0	0
3 min	20	0	0	0	0
5 min	50	0	0	0	0
10 min	200	0	20	0	0

(Courtesy of Mehlman CT, DiPasquale TG: Radiation exposure to the orthopedic surgical team during fluoroscopy: "How far away is far enough?" *J Orthop Trauma* 11:392–398, 1997.)

29 mrem/min and for the first assistant, it was 10 mrem/min. For the surgeon, eye exposure was 19 mrem/min and for the first assistant, 6 mrem/min. No deep or eye exposure was detected at the scrub nurse position. At the scrub nurse position, 1 positive badge for shallow exposure was noted, reflecting an exposure rate of 2 mrem/min. Hand/skin limit would be reached for a scrub nurse positioned 36 inches away from the x-ray beam after 5,000 cases (Table 10). Badges assigned to the anesthesiologist position never registered any positive readings after 10 minutes of continuous exposure.

Conclusions.—Little or no radiation was measured at the positions of the scrub nurse and anesthesiologist. At the unprotected surgeon and first assistant locations, however, significant amounts of radiation were measured. For individuals working 24 inches or less from a fluoroscopic x-ray beam, the importance of proper personal radiation protection is reinforced. Exposure to the thyroid, hands, and eyes is of particular concern because these areas aren't routinely protected. The routine use of a thyroid shield is recommended for surgeons who frequently perform fluoroscopi-

TABLE 10.—Number of 5-Minute Fluoro Cases Needed to Meet or Exceed Established Occupational Exposure Limits

	Deep (whole body)	Shallow (hands/skin)	Eye (ocular lens)
Surgeon	50	345	300
1st assistant	167	1,000	500
Scrub nurse	?	5,000	?
Anesthesia	?	?	?

Extrapolated data (accepting estimate of 5 minutes of fluoro use per orthopedic case) based on 1993 National Council on Radiation Protection and Measurements (NCRP) recommendations.

(Courtesy of Mehlman CT, DiPasquale TG: Radiation exposure to the orthopedic surgical team during fluoroscopy: "How far away is far enough?" *J Orthop Trauma* 11:392–398, 1997.)

cally assisted procedures during which they are 24 inches or less from the beam. Hands should never enter the fluoroscopic beam.

▶ There have been a number of studies recording exposure rates for the orthopedic surgeon during fluoroscopically assisted surgical procedures. This is the first such study, however, to evaluate the dosages of radiation exposure to other individuals in the operating room. This would be extremely valuable information to other members of the surgical team. As the study results demonstrate, their risk of exposure to radiation is extremely low. It is also very reassuring to note that adequate shielding does provide adequate protection. Good surgical discipline with the 24-inch rule and keeping one's hands away from the field being irradiated should be continuously emphasized, especially to surgeons in training.

C.P. Beauchamp, M.D.

Evaluation of Glucocorticosteroid Injection for the Treatment of Trochanteric Bursitis
Shbeeb MI, O'Duffy JD, Michet CJ Jr, et al (Mayo Clinic and Found, Rochester, Minn; Mayo Clinic and Found, Scottsdale, Ariz; Dept of Health Sciences Research, Rochester, Minn)
J Rheumatol 23:2104–2106, 1996   1–6

Introduction.—Trochanteric bursitis is a common regional pain syndrome, characterized by chronic or intermittent aching pain over the lateral aspect of the hip. There are several favorable reports on the use of corticosteroid injection for treatment of trochanteric bursitis. Few trials have addressed dose and long-term follow-up. The short- and long-term effects of single dose local glucocorticosteroid injection was evaluated in 75 patients with trochanteric bursitis.

Methods.—Patients were randomly assigned to 1 of 3 conventional doses of betamethasone with 1% lidocaine: 6, 12, and 24 mg in 20, 32, and 22 patients. A standardized questionnaire and visual analogue scale were administered at baseline to evaluate pain severity and functional limitations. These were repeated on weeks 1, 6, and 26 to determine patient response to treatment.

Results.—The mean age of 62 women and 13 men was 66.2 years. Most patients reported improvement in pain and functional limitations after a single glucocorticosteroid injection and at each time point (Table 1). Patients receiving higher doses of betamethasone were significantly more likely to get pain relief than patients with lower doses.

Conclusion.—Local corticosteroid and lidocaine injection seem to be effective treatment for trochanteric bursitis. Patients reported protracted pain relief from the injections.

▶ This extremely common musculoskeletal disorder has not received much attention. The study evaluates the long-term results of rather standard

TABLE 1.—Follow-up Response

	Week 1	Week 6	Week 26
Evaluable/total patients (%)	68/75 (90.7)	64/75 (85.3)	62/75 (82.7)
Improvement after injection			
Yes: number/evaluable patients (%)	54/68 (77.1)	44/64 (68.8)	38/62 (61.3)
Not sure: number/evaluable patients (%)	11/68 (15.7)	10/64 (15.6)	13/62 (21)
No: number/evaluable patients (%)	6/68 (7.1)	10/64 (15.6)	11/62 (17.7)
VAS, range (mean)	0.00–75 (37.6)	0.00–75 (32.5)	0.00–80 (32.3)

Abbreviation: VAS, visual analogue scale.

(Courtesy of Shbeeb MI, O'Duffy JD, Michet CJ Jr, et al: Evaluation of glucocorticosteroid injection for the treatment of trochanteric bursitis. *J Rheumatol* 23:2104–2016, 1996.)

treatment. It does confirm other reports in the literature that trochanteric bursitis is effectively treated with glucocorticosteroids, but points out that this is dose dependent. It would be interesting to evaluate those patients who did not respond, as there are a number of other entities that can overlap the symptoms of trochanteric bursitis that have local explanations, such as abductor tendinitis and partial tears of the abductor mechanism, the latter being less responsive to therapy with steroid injections.

C.P. Beauchamp, M.D.

Steroid-induced Adipogenesis in a Pluripotential Cell Line From Bone Marrow

Cui Q, Wang G-J, Balian G (Univ of Virginia, Charlottesville)
J Bone Joint Surg Am 79-A:1054–1063, 1997   1–7

Introduction.—Steroid treatment creates hypertrophy and hyperplasia of marrow fat cells with concomitant increase of pressure in the femoral head and decrease in blood flow, which can result in collapse of the sinusoids in the femoral head. This may contribute to some forms of osteonecrosis. The mechanism of action of dexamethasone on cells in bone and other organs that may contribute to abnormal lipid metabolism is unknown. The effect of steroids on D1, a pluripotential bone-marrow cell line previously cloned from mouse bone-marrow stroma was assessed.

Methods.—Cells were treated with increasing (10^{-9}, 10^{-8}, and 10^{-7}-molar) concentrations of dexamethasone. This was undertaken for increasing durations, ranging from 48 hours to 21 days.

Results.—The appearance of triglyceride vesicles in the cells demonstrated that this treatment had induced the differentiation of the cell into adipocytes. The number of cells containing triglyceride vesicles and the expression of 422(aP2), a fat-cell-specific gene rose with prolonged durations of exposure to (Fig 4) and higher concentrations of dexamethasone (Fig 3). The expression of $\alpha1$ type-I collagen mRNA and osteocalcin mRNA was decreased with dexamethasone treatment. Cells not treated with dexamethasone showed osteogenic properties.

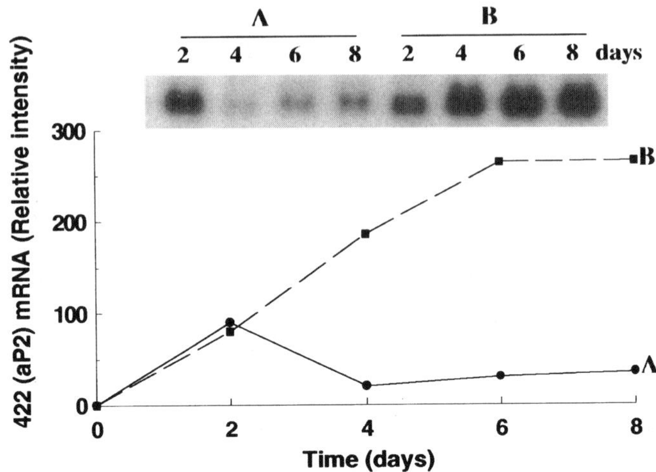

FIGURE 4.—Graphs of the effect of increasing the duration of treatment with dexamethasone on the expression of 422(aP2)mRNA by D1 cells. All of the cells were treated with 10^{-7}-molar dexamethasone for 48 hours. The treatment then either was discontinued (A) or was continued (B) for 8 days with the mRNA measured at 2-day intervals for 8 days. **Inset:** Northern blot of total RNA that was hybridized with 422(aP2)cDNA at 2, 4, 6, and 8 days. (Courtesy of Cui Q, Wang G-J, Balian G: Steroid-induced adipogenesis in a pluripotential cell line from bone marrow. *J Bone Joint Surg Am* 79-A:1054–1063, 1997.)

Conclusion.—Pluripotential mesenchymal cell D1 is osteogenic and differentiates primarily into osteoblasts when not exposed to dexamethasone. Exposure to the steroid diminishes differentiation into osteoblasts and greatly increases differentiation into adipocytes. The rapid appearance of 422(aP2) mRNA after dexamethasone treatment indicates that expression

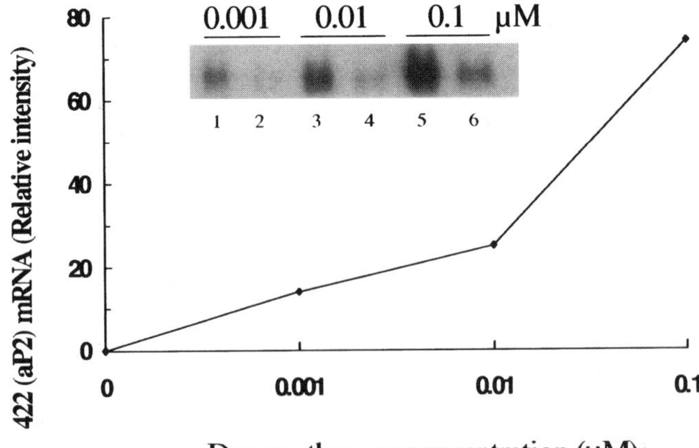

FIGURE 3.—Graph of expression of 422(aP2) mRNA by D1 cells in response to treatment with increasing (10^{-9}, 10^{-8}, and 10^{-7}-molar) concentrations of dexamethasone. **Inset:** Northern blot of total RNA that was hybridized with 422(aP2) cDNA. Lanes 1, 3, and 5 = 40 µg of RNA, and lanes 2, 4, and 6 = 20 µg micrograms of RNA. (Courtesy of Cui Q, Wang G-J, Balian G: Steroid-induced adipogenesis in a pluripotential cell line from bone marrow. *J Bone Joint Surg Am* 79-A:1054–1063, 1997.)

of this gene is followed by accumulation of fat-containing vesicles with increasing duration of treatment. Few adipocytes were detected in cultures not treated with steroids. These findings are in contrast of all previously described preadipose cell lines (3T3-L1 and 3T3-F422A). It seems dexamethasone was needed for the expression of the fat-cell phenotype in the D1-cell line isolated from bone marrow.

▶ This is a very important study on the effect of steroids and the differentiation of pluripotential mesenchymal cells. This has significant implications for our understanding of the process by which steroid-induced osteonecrosis occurs. Fat cell hypertrophy has long been implicated in the development of steroid-induced osteonecrosis and perhaps with alcohol-induced osteonecrosis as well. Not only were the authors able to demonstrate that adipogenesis can occur, but that it is also dose dependent. A better understanding of the mechanisms by which this disabling entity occurs will hopefully give us mechanisms to identify patients who are at risk for its development and therapeutic strategies to limit the differentiation of pluripotential cells.

C.P. Beauchamp, M.D.

2 Pediatrics

Introduction

These are exciting times in pediatric orthopedics. The application of new genetic and molecular biology information is leading to new treatments of inherited musculoskeletal disorders. New knowledge of congenital disorders is appearing. Assessment of pediatric orthopedic care has improved, both with functional outcome assessments more commonly included in clinical studies, as well as with the use of computerized gait analysis to gain a more objective evaluation. In addition, we are becoming more aware of the potential errors in our use of radiographic classification systems that have been used for decades to evaluate our treatment efforts. The whole approach we are taking toward patient care and outcome evaluation is becoming significantly more evidence-based.

Fractures in children continue to be the primary pediatric problem seen by orthopedists everywhere. There has been a significant change in favor of the surgical treatment of isolated pediatric fractures over the past decade, based in part on the surgically aggressive approach used successfully in pediatric polytrauma. The nonoperative treatment of long-bone fractures in children continues to yield excellent results. The time may have come to step back a bit and evaluate whether we have now become too surgically oriented in pediatric fracture care.

The articles selected for this chapter cover these and other topics within pediatric orthopedics and have been chosen to highlight problems unique to children and adolescents. The excitement continues.

Vernon T. Tolo, M.D.

Fractures

External Fixation or Flexible Intramedullary Nailing for Femoral Shaft Fractures in Children

Bar-On E, Sagiv S, Porat S (Hadassah Med Centre, Jerusalem, Israel)
J Bone Joint Surg Br 79-B:975–978, 1997   2–1

Objective.—The use of surgery for children with fractures of the femoral shaft has increased in recent years, including patients with isolated femoral fractures. External fixation (EF) was previously used at the study institution for pediatric femoral fractures requiring surgery, but recently flexible intramedullary nailing (FIN) has been used. These 2 approaches were compared in a randomized trial.

Methods.—The 1-year, prospective study included 20 children aged 5–15 years with fractures of the femoral shaft requiring surgery. They were randomly assigned in equal numbers to undergo EF or FIN. The average follow-up was 14 months.

Results.—Callus formation was significantly less in the EF group than in the FIN group. Average time to full weight-bearing was 10 weeks in the EF group vs. 7 weeks in the FIN group. Time to full range of movement was 16 vs. 9 weeks, and time to return to school was 13 vs. 5 weeks, respectively. All parents of FIN-treated patients said they would choose the same treatment again, whereas 2 of 8 parents in the EF group said they would opt for nonsurgical treatment.

Conclusions.—For children with fractures of the femoral shaft requiring surgery, FIN offers better results in terms of alignment and fewer complications than EF. The authors now use FIN for most such fractures, performing EF only in children with open or severely comminuted fractures.

▶ This randomized, prospective study is small and not statistically tested, but the results reported reflect current practice in much of the world at the present time. The use of operative treatment in pediatric long-bone fractures has escalated in the past decade for several reasons. The success of operative treatment of long-bone fractures, in pediatric patients who have sustained polytrauma led to its use in isolated long-bone fractures, just as new implants for these fractures began coming on the market. In addition, the economic factor of decreasing hospital stay led surgeons and administrators to look favorably on operative treatment of femoral fractures, rather than treating the child in traction in hospital for 3 weeks before spica casting. At the present time, pediatric orthopedists will tend to treat femoral fractures operatively, whereas many general orthopedists in community practice still use traction and casting for the children between 5 and 12 years of age. Those of us using the methods described in this article need to compile our data, both functional and financial, to compare with the excellent results that are almost uniformly obtained with the traditional traction-cast treatment. How these data will shake out remains unsettled for now.

V.T. Tolo, M.D.

Intramedullary Nailing Versus Plate Fixation for Unstable Forearm Fractures in Children
Van der Reis WL, Otsuka NY, Moroz P, et al (Univ of California, San Francisco; McMaster Univ, Hamilton, Ont)
J Pediatr Orthop B 18:9–13, 1998   2–2

Introduction.—In most circumstances, closed reduction and casting are used for treatment of fractures of the diaphysis of the radius and ulna in children. Indications for open reduction of both bones of the forearm include open fractures, irreducible fractures, unstable fractures, pathologic fractures, neurovascular compromise, and malunion fractures. Children younger than 10 years have a greater ability to remodel forearm fractures than children older than 10 years. Diaphyseal fractures are not as capable of remodeling as those of the distal third. Specific angular and rotational criteria are debatable, but consensus seems to be that angular deformity greater than 10 degrees, rotational deformity greater than 45 degrees, or complete displacement is not acceptable. There are no reports comparing outcome of intramedullary nailing vs. plate fixation for unstable diaphyseal fractures of the radius and ulna in children. The clinical and radiographic outcome of plate and screw fixation and intramedullary nailing for unstable fracture of both bones of the forearm were compared in children.

Methods.—Medical records of 91 patients ages 5–15 (average, 10 years) were reviewed. Of 91 patients, 50 underwent closed reduction and cast immobilization, 23 were treated with plate and screw fixation, and 18 were treated with intramedullary nailing. Indications for surgical treatment included open fractures, irreducible fractures, and unstable fractures.

Results.—Fourteen patients (78%) in the plate and screw group had excellent results and 4 (22%) had poor results at an average of 12 months after operation. For 23 patients who had intramedullary nailing, results were excellent in 18 (78%) and poor in 5 (22%). Both groups had similar functional results, rate of union, and rate of complications. Average anesthesia time for plate and screw removal was 1 hour and 35 minutes; for rod removal, it was 35 minutes.

Conclusion.—Intramedullary fixation may be a useful option for treating unstable fractures of the radius and ulna. It can shorten operative time and provide excellent cosmesis, minimal soft-tissue dissection, ease of hardware removal, and early motion after nail removal.

▶ Operative treatment for pediatric fractures previously treated with closed reduction and cast immobilization is much more frequent now than a decade ago. In particular, flexible intramedullary implants have enjoyed a surge of popularity, due largely to the limited incisions needed to insert these implants. In general, pediatric fractures do not require as rigid fixation as is needed in adult long-bone fractures, so the flexible intramedullary implants offer the possibility of lining up the bones that then progress to union. The additional use of a cast for a short time will not lead to adjacent joint stiffness as it does in adults. This article reports equal (78%) excellent results with either plates or intramedullary implants for pediatric forearm fractures. The intramedullary implants took less time to put in and less time to take out, and the skin incisions were smaller. However, functionally there was no difference. Both of these approaches led to 22% poorer results, a higher percentage than expected from closed treatment and casting. It may be time to review our indications for aggressive operative treatment of pediatric forearm fractures: the results without operative treatment were really very good.

V.T. Tolo, M.D.

Management of Pulseless Pink Hand in Pediatric Supracondylar Fractures of Humerus

Sabharwal S, Tredwell SJ, Beauchamp RD, et al (British Columbia's Children's Hosp, Vancouver; Alfred I. Dupont Inst, Wilmington, Del; British Columbia's Children's Hosp, Vancouver)
J Pediatr Orthop B 17:303–310, 1997   2–3

Introduction.—In the presence of a viable pink hand after correction of type 3 supracondylar fractures in children, there is no consensus on the treatment of an absent radial pulse. In a pulseless pink hand, it is thought that the rich collateral circulation around the elbow can sustain the viability of the extremity. There may, however, be migration of a brachial artery thrombus, exercise-induced ischemic symptoms, cold intolerance, or limb-length discrepancy. Even in the presence of a viable pink hand after closed reduction, surgical attempts have often been made to reconstitute brachial artery patency. To determine the clinical outcome and brachial artery patency rates in children who had various procedures to re-establish a radial pulse after type 3 supracondylar fractures of the humerus, noninvasive imaging techniques were used.

Methods.—There were 13 of 419 children (3.2%) who had supracondylar fractures with an absence of a radial pulse in an otherwise well-perfused hand. All of the patients had, displaced, extension-type fractures with 12 closed and 1 open. An initial attempt at closed reduction under general anesthesia was unsuccessful in restoring the radial pulse in the 12 children with closed fractures. On all patients, vascular surgery consultation was obtained. The vascular team with the radiology department decided upon vascular repair or urokinase thrombolysis. The noninvasive techniques used were segmental pressure monitoring, color-flow duplex scanning, and magnetic resonance angiography. A brachial artery lesion, based on angiography or intraoperative findings, occurred in all 13 pa-

TABLE 1.—Procedures Leading to Palpable Pulse

Procedure	Total performed	Palpable pulse
Closed red./splint	4	0
Closed red./pinning	4	1
Closed red./olecranon traction	6	0
ORIF	10	4
Vein-patch angioplasty	4	4*
Open thrombectomy	1	1
End-end anastomosis	1	1
Urokinase	4	3*
Total	34	

*Patient 7 lost radial pulse in recovery room after vein-patch angioplasty and subsequently underwent successful urokinase thrombolysis.

Abbreviation: Red, reduction

(Courtesy of Sabharwal S, Tredwell SJ, Beauchamp RD, et al: Management of pulseless pink hand in pediatric supracondylar fractures of humerus. *J Pediatr Orthop B* 17:303–310, 1997.)

tients. A questionnaire was administered and a physical examination was conducted during follow-up.

Results.—Repeated closed reduction and crossed Kirschner-wire fixation, vascular reconstruction, resection with end-to-end anastomosis, open thrombectomy, intra-arterial thrombolyses with urokinase infusion, and open reduction internal fixation led to restoration of a palpable radial pulse (Table 1). There is a high rate of asymptomatic reocclusion and residual stenoses of the brachial artery with early revascularization of a pulseless, yet otherwise well-perfused hand in children with type 3 supracondylar fractures. Transfemoral brachial artery urokinase thrombolysis was performed if the lesion was a thrombus, avoiding an open vascular procedure. Three of 4 patients who had this procedure had success, but 2 of 3 patients had residual stenoses across the distal brachial artery. Surgical exploration and mobilization of the vessel was done if the angiogram showed entrapment of the brachial artery. At follow-up, 3 of 4 of these patients were normal.

Conclusion.—Before more invasive correction of this problem is contemplated, a period of close observation with frequent neurovascular checks should be completed. Extremes of elbow flexion are avoided with early reduction with internal fixation, which is probably the most important step in the management of these injuries.

▶ Nothing in pediatric fracture care is more perplexing to an orthopaedist than how to deal in the emergency room with a supracondylar humeral fracture in a child with an absent radial and ulnar pulse, yet with a warm hand distal to the fracture. If the radial pulse is lost after fracture reduction or if the pulse is absent with a cold hand, the approach is more direct, with open reduction of the fracture and arterial exploration usually recommended. These authors report their approach and review the multitude of non-invasive methods currently available to assess arterial occlusion or injury that can be associated with this fracture. Those patients with an earlier return of a radial pulse had more normal vascular studies at follow-up, but still some questions exist about how best to achieve this. Vascular repair of intimal injuries was not too effective, with 80% of these children still having compromised vessel patency on follow-up. From these data, if circulation can be restored by fracture reduction and vessel mobilization, the results are superior to those of actual vessel reconstruction. While this article gives us more options to noninvasive testing for arterial flow, remember that fracture reduction may take precedence over exhaustive testing, as reduction may be the key to the most predictable return of blood flow at the elbow fracture.

V.T. Tolo, M.D.

Severely Displaced Proximal Humeral Epiphyseal Fractures: A Follow-up Study

Beringer DC, Weiner DS, Noble JS, et al (Akron Children's Med Ctr, Ohio; Summa Health Systems, Akron, Ohio, Notheastern Ohio Universities College of Medicine, Rootstown, et al)
J Pediatr Orthop B 18:31–37, 1998   2–4

Introduction.—Proximal humeral epiphyseal fractures are relatively uncommon and classified from grades I–IV, with grade I displacement being 5 mm or less of shaft diameter, grade II being to one-third of shaft diameter, grade III being to two-thirds of shaft diameter, and grade IV being greater than two-thirds of shaft diameter. Most experts advise against operative intervention, but there is no consensus regarding treatment for persistent, severely displaced fractures of grades III or IV. The complication rate for operative and nonoperative treatment of severely displaced proximal humeral epiphyseal fractures was documented. Late outcome after nonoperative treatment of these fractures was evaluated.

Methods.—There were 48 children with severely displaced proximal humeral epiphyseal fractures, and of these, 21 were followed for an average of 9 years after injury with radiographs, clinical examinations, and a personal interview. The children had an average age of 14.1 years. There were 31 fractures that were displaced by more than 80%, and initial head-shaft displacement averaged 80%. Attempted closed reduction was performed on all children.

Results.—Displacement was not improved significantly in 26–45 attempted closed reductions. Operative treatment was performed on 9 children and the rest had a closed reduction. In 3 of 9 patients who had operative treatment, complications occurred. In the nonoperative group, no complications occurred. No children seen at late follow-up identified any activity or employment restrictions as a result of the injuries. Humeral shortening or imperfect radiographic remodeling was seen in several patients, but neither correlated with clinical outcome.

Conclusion.—Previous recommendations suggesting the avoidance of operative intervention, with few exceptions, have been confirmed by comparing the operative complications with the excellent late results after nonoperative treatment in this series. Operative treatment is not justified by the magnitude of displacement alone. Only in the operative treatment group did complications occur.

▶ These authors add some useful information about approaching the care of a proximal physeal fracture of the humerus in a teenager. This particular physeal fracture occurs most often in teenagers, with the younger children usually fracturing in the proximal metaphyseal area of the humerus. These childhood fractures never (except in the case of open injury) need operative treatment. Concern over a lack of remodeling potential in the mid- and late teens has led some orthopaedists to openly reduce these severely displaced adolescent fractures. However, this article notes that remodeling can still occur after the age of 15, and that less than anatomic radiograph reduction does not mean a functional impairment will follow. In fact, it is impressive how little this fracture seemed to bother the patients several years after healing. Although the functional results from closed reduction or even from no reduction are good, there may still be times when an open reduction is needed. Examination under fluoroscopy during attempted reduction may demonstrate interposed muscle or impaling of muscle by the distal fragment. In these rare instances, open reduction with percutaneous pinning has been a useful and safe technique to improve fracture alignment in my practice. For the most part, avoid surgery on these fractures.

V.T. Tolo, M.D.

Chronic Physeal Fractures in Myelodysplasia: Magnetic Resonance Analysis, Histologic Description, Treatment, and Outcome
Rodgers WB, Schwend RM, Jaramillo D, et al (Children's Hosp, Boston; Capital Region Orthopaedics and Sports Medicine, Jefferson City, Mo; State University of New York at Buffalo, NY)
J Pediatr Orthop B 17:615–621, 1997   2–5

Introduction.—Patients with myelodysplasia commonly have fractures which involve the metaphysis or diaphysis of the insensate lower extremities. Minimal immobilization can be used to treat these injuries, as they heal quickly with exuberant callous formation. When the physis itself is fractured, the physeal injury can take longer to heal, is susceptible to displacement, and can result in growth arrest. The treatment of patients with myelodysplasia with chronic physeal fractures is reviewed.

Methods.—There were 13 patients with myelodysplasia with 19 chronic physeal fractures who were treated with prolonged immobilization in casts or braces for an average of 5.8 months. Operative fixation to facilitate healing was necessary for 4 of the fractures. At the time of fracture, the average age was 8 years with a range of 1 month to 12.8 years. Patients' level of neurologic function ranged from T5 to L4 and 7 of the patients were ambulatory at the time of injury. Five children were treated initially for presumptive infection of the extremity, and another was scheduled for operative biopsy for the presumptive diagnosis of Ewing's sarcoma. The most commonly injured physis was the distal tibia, accounting for 10 of the fractures. Posterior knee soft-tissue release had been used to treat 6 of the patients previously.

Results.—At 4.8 years follow-up, all children were healed, but the growth plate had closed prematurely in 4 of the fractures. Three distinct zones of physeal pathoanatomy were seen on histologic analysis: a normal zone of proliferation, a vascularized zone of fibrous tissue adjacent to the metaphysis, and a thickened, disorganized zone of hypertrophy. There were thickening of the physis and irregularity of the zone of provisional calcification on magnetic resonance imaging. With gadolinium, the physeal cartilage and the juxtametaphyseal fibrovascular tissue enhanced. Magnetic resonance imaging also showed clefts within the physeal cartilage (Fig 3). A thickened perichondrium and periosteum held together the fragments.

Conclusion.—These findings corroborate earlier mechanistic proposals for treating physeal injury in myelodysplasia. A widened, disorganized physis can result from chronic stress or trauma to the insensate limb, which produces micromotion at the zone of hypertrophy. This can lead to fracture, displacement, and delayed union.

▶ Lower extremity fractures in children with spina bifida and resultant impaired sensation will commonly be mistaken for cellulitis, venous thrombosis, or tumor by primary care physicians, since pain is typically absent. In *all* cases of unexplained swelling of 1 leg in children with spina bifida, x-rays should be obtained to evaluate for a long-bone fracture, by far the most common reason for this clinical presentation. Metaphyseal and diaphyseal fractures are easy to see and heal quickly in this group of patients. However, the physeal fractures may be initially missed if nondisplaced, and care needs to be taken to look for physeal widening at the region of swelling. This article

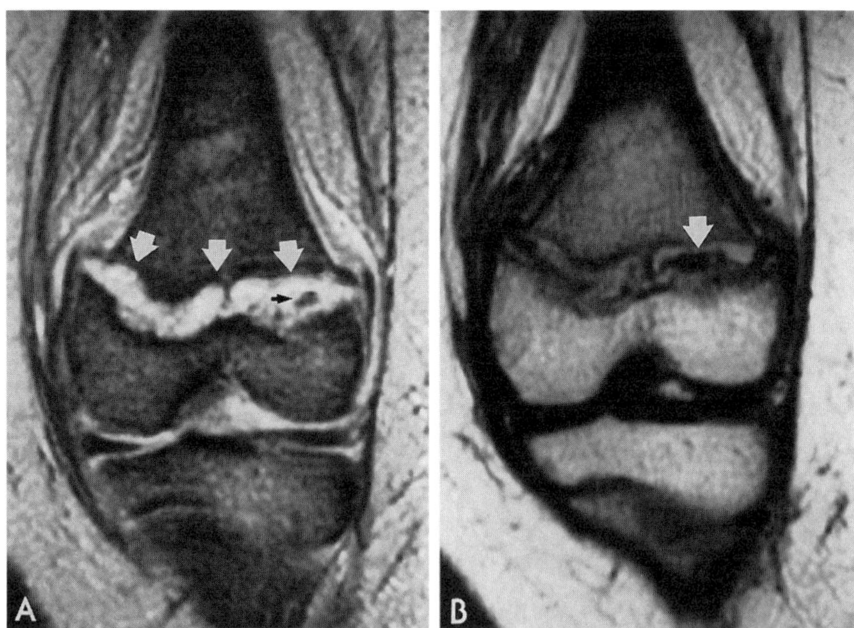

(*Continued*)

FIGURE 3 (cont.)

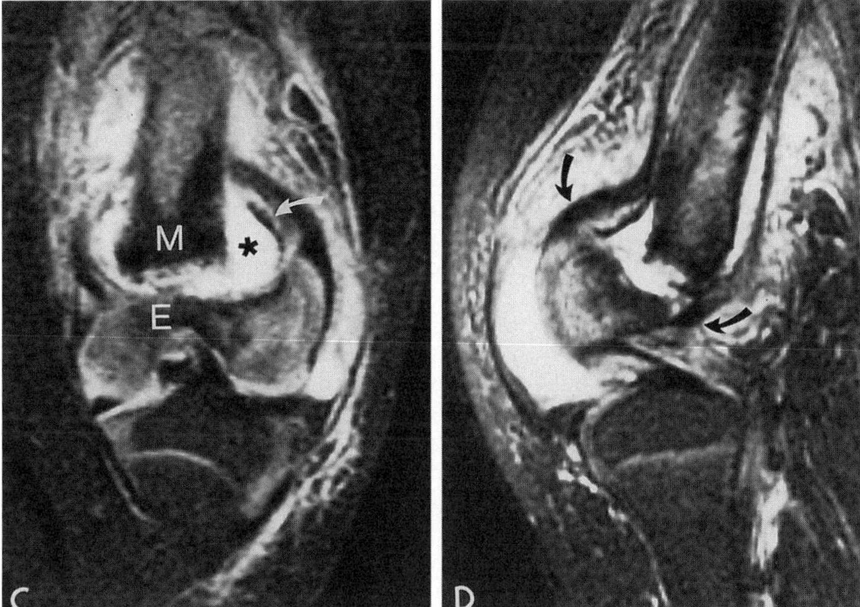

FIGURE 3.—Coronal gradient-recalled echo MRI of the distal femur (patient 13) showing physeal widening (white arrows) with irregularity of the zone of provisional calcification. An area of low signal intensity within the hyperintense cartilage most likely represents an island of calcification (dark arrow). **B,** coronal spin-echo T1-weighted gadolinium-enhanced MRI at the same level (patient 13) shows that there are nonenhancing gaps (arrow) within the wide physis. The juxtaepiphyseal physis and the area adjacent to the metaphysis enhance greatly. **C,** coronal fat-suppressed spin-echo T2-weighted MRI of the distal femur (patient 10) shows separation between the epiphysis (**E**) and metaphysis (**M**). An area of high signal intensity (*) deep to the thick metaphyseal periosteum (arrow) corresponds to the cavity demonstrated on the injection study. **D,** sagittal fat-suppressed spin-echo T2-weighted MRI (patient 10) at the level of the posterior cruciate ligament shows the anterior displacement of the distal fragment. There is marked elevation of the periosteum, which joins the epiphysis at the perichondral attachments (arrows). (Courtesy of Rodgers WB, Schwend RM, Jaramillo D, et al: Chronic physeal fractures in myelodysplasia: Magnetic resonance analysis, histologic description, treatment, and outcome. *J Pediatr Orthop B* 17:615–621, 1997.)

makes a clear case for early and long immobilization of physeal fractures in spina bifida patients, with the histologic and MRI findings well illustrated. An MRI should not be needed to make this diagnosis, but, from this article, it should be obvious why early detection and adequate immobilization treatment of the acute injury is superior to management of a chronic physeal fracture.

V.T. Tolo, M.D.

Scoliosis

A Meta-analysis of the Efficacy of Non-operative Treatments for Idiopathic Scoliosis

Rowe DE, Bernstein SM, Riddick MF, et al (Kalamazoo Ctr for Med Studies, Mich
J Bone Joint Surg Am 79-A:664–674, 1997   2–6

Introduction.—When a lateral spinal curve of at least 11 degrees is observed in a patient between 10 years old and the age of skeletal maturity, the diagnosis is adolescent idiopathic scoliosis, a condition that affects up to 3% of children between the ages of 10 and 16 years. As the degree of curvature increases, the risk of progression increases, and without intervention the curve is likely to progress. Curves more than 30 degrees at the time of diagnosis are usually treated with a brace. For curves of more than 45 degrees, arthrodesis with spinal instrumentation is the treatment of choice. The efficacy of bracing has not been demonstrated definitely or compared with other forms of nonoperative treatment. The results of nonoperative treatment of idiopathic scoliosis were evaluated by meta-analysis.

Methods.—The meta-analysis evaluated 1,910 patients with idiopathic scoliosis who were treated with bracing (1,459), lateral electrical surface stimulation (322), or observation (129). A determination was made on

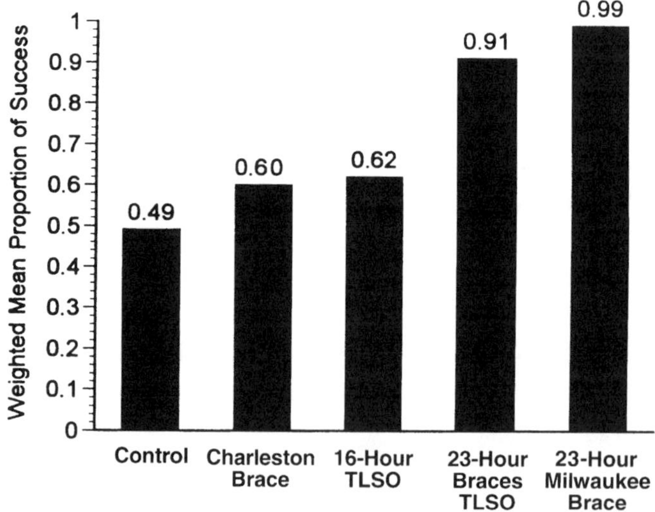

FIGURE 6.—Graph showing the weighted mean proportions of success for the control condition and various bracing regimens. Braces that were worn for 23 hours per day were significantly more effective than all other treatments ($P < 0.0001$). *Abbreviation: TLSO,* thoracolumbosacral orthosis. (Courtesy of Rowe DE, Bernstein SM, Riddick MF, et al: A meta-analysis of the efficacy of non-operative treatments for idiopathic scoliosis. *J Bone Joint Surg Am* 79-A:664–674, 1997.)

which type of treatment, which level of maturity, and which criterion for failure had the greatest impact on outcome. There was also an evaluation of the effects of the type of brace and duration of bracing and the association with success.

Results.—For lateral electrical surface stimulation, the weighted mean proportion of success was 0.39; for observation only, it was 0.49; for bracing 8 hours day, it was 0.60; for bracing 16 hours per day, it was 0.62; and for bracing 23 hours per day, it was 0.93. As the level of maturity increased, curves were generally less likely to progress. The weighted mean proportion of success in the group in which the criterion for failure was 10 degrees was significantly higher than in those with criterion of 3, 5, or 6 degrees. Significantly more success was achieved with the 23-hour brace than with any other treatment (Fig 6). The Milwaukee brace achieved the highest proportion of success.

Conclusion.—For the treatment of idiopathic scoliosis, the effectiveness of bracing has been demonstrated. Progression of the curve was effectively halted with the Milwaukee brace or another thoracolumbosacral orthosis worn for 23 hours a day. A standard protocol needs to be developed, which would include assessment of skeletal age, a description of the curve, and the use of progression of more than 1 degrees from the start of treatment, withdrawal from treatment, or the need for an operation as the only criteria for failure.

▶ This paper has caused a lot of controversy in the community of surgeons who treat adolescent scoliosis. The reports reviewed by this committee of the Scoliosis Research Society included those published up to 1993, so more recent studies of newer brace types are not included. Proponents of the Charleston brace, in particular, believe that the 2 papers regarding this brace that were reviewed for this meta-analysis do not reflect current practice. It is a bit ironic that the Milwaukee brace, shown by this review to be the most successful treatment, seldom is used today and the thoracolumbosacral orthosis remains the mainstay for those who use full-time bracing for idiopathic scoliosis. This paper does, however, point out the importance of wearing the brace nearly all day and night during the treatment period, regardless of the type of brace used. While orthopedists are sometimes cowed by papers using meta-analysis with the statistical methods filling the pages of the reports, this has now become more commonplace as efforts are made to achieve statistical significance from the orthopedic literature in which most studies are retrospective and uncontrolled. It's a lot of work to do a meta-analysis. Despite the detractors of this article, the authors have diligently followed the ground rules for literature survey and have come up with valid findings based on the published information. If we are among the skeptics of this approach, we need to ensure that future studies are prospective with appropriate controls.

V.T. Tolo, M.D.

Anterior Release and Fusion in Pediatric Spinal Deformity: A Comparison of Early Outcome and Cost of Thoracoscopic and Open Thoracotomy Approaches

Newton PO, Wenger DR, Mubarak SJ, et al (Univ of California, San Diego)
Spine 22:1398–1406, 1997   2–7

Introduction.—The most common indication for minimally invasive thoracoscopy of the anterior spine in children is spinal deformity. Anterior release and fusion are used in children with severe rigid scoliosis or kyphosis, or in immature patients with scoliosis who are at risk for development of crankshaft phenomenon after an isolated posterior fusion. The thoracoscopic method is less invasive than an open procedure, but it is technically demanding and has a significant learning curve. Thoracoscopic anterior spinal release and fusion (14 patients) were compared with open throacotomy (18 patients) in a series of pediatric patients with spinal deformity to compare safety, efficacy, total hospital charges, and costs between the two techniques.

Thoracoscopic Technique.—All 14 patients underwent anterior release and fusion with either autograft or allograft bone. Single-lung ventilation was used. After the lung on the operative side was collapsed, the pleura overlying the spine in the area to be released was incised longitudinally and bluntly stripped from the spine and segmental vessels. These vessels were bluntly dissected and ligated. Most of the segmental vessels were divided to allow better visualization of the anterior and opposite side of the disc. The disk excision and release of the spine were performed and the disk spaces were packed with cancellous bone graft. A running closure of the pleura was begun distally and the diaphragm was repaired, if needed.

Outcome.—There were no significant differences in percent curve correction between the thoracoscopic and open procedures: scoliosis 56% and 50%, respectively; and kyphosis, 88% and 94%, respectively. The groups were similar in blood loss and complication rates. Chest tube output was greater in the thoracoscopic group. Length of hospital and ICU stay were similar for both procedures. The thoracoscopic procedure was 29% more costly than the open procedure. The throacoscopic procedure decreased the morbidity of anterior spinal procedure because it avoided cutting the chest-shoulder musculature.

Discussion/Conclusion.—Early results of the thoracoscopic procedure indicate safety and efficacy similar to thoracotomy's in achieving anterior release of the anterior spine. The correction for scoliosis and kyphosis was similar for both procedures. These findings confirm that pediatric spinal deformity correction requiring an anterior thoracic release and fusion is sufficient indication for the thoracoscopic approach. The added cost and effort required for the thoracoscopic approach are justified by the advantages of this muscle-sparing, minimally invasive technique.

▶ Thoracoscopy has been termed minimally invasive surgery, but, once below the skin, the surgery on the spine is fully analogous to what is done with open thoracotomy. The use of video-assisted thoracoscopic surgery is increasing throughout the world as the technology and instrumentation improve to do this safely. The rationale for endoscopic surgery for cholecystectomy, lumbar disc removal, and gynecologic procedures is quite clear: this approach results in less pain and less time in the hospital for the patient. These authors reported the use of video-assisted thoracoscopic surgery in pediatric spinal surgery, for the indications generally accepted as appropriate for anterior discectomy and fusion, prior to same-day posterior spinal fusion and instrumentation, and compared their results with open thoracotomy from the prior year. Results throughout were good, with few complications from both procedures. Costs were 29% less with open thoracotomy than with thoracoscopy. The advantage of avoiding the muscle-splitting with thoracotomy was postulated, but no pain scales or lung tests were used after surgery to determine if this was true. Although thoracoscopic procedures done alone, as with lung biopsy, are clearly beneficial for the patient who otherwise would need a thoracotomy, the advantage is less clear in pediatric spinal deformity, because the child still needs to have the posterior spinal instrumentation and fusion, which is usually the determining factor for how long the hospital stay will be. Video-assisted thoracoscopic surgery will doubtless become more popular and, soon, placement of instrumentation through this approach will be used routinely to correct some spinal deformities. This article, while endorsing the thoracoscopic technique, has cut down on some of the ballyhoo associated with new technology by the authors' honest report of problems as well as good results.

V.T. Tolo, M.D.

Use of Intravenous Premarin to Decrease Postoperative Blood Loss After Pediatric Scoliosis Surgery
McCall RE, Bilderback KK (Shriners Hosps for Children, Shreveport, La)
Spine 22:1394–1397, 1997   2–8

Introduction.—The hemostatic effects of conjugated estrogens (Premarin) in managing uncontrolled bleeding of uterine hemorrhage, duodenal ulcers, and subarachnoid and rectal hemorrhages have been reported. No trials have assessed the effectiveness of Premarin in reducing blood loss in pediatric spinal procedures. Intravenous (IV) Premarin was given immediately after surgery in adolescents undergoing spinal surgery to determine Premarin's effectiveness in reducing Hemovac postoperative drainage.

Methods.—Patients undergoing posterior and anterior/posterior procedures were evaluated prospectively. Thirty-two patients received Premarin

1 mg/kg IV immediately after surgery; 32 patients who did not receive Premarin acted as controls. Hemovac drainage was recorded for 48 hours after surgery.

Results.—There was a prompt and marked (37%) decrease in Hemovac drainage during the first 48 hours after surgery in patients who received IV Premarin during wound closure. This effect was first detected at 8 hours and was significant 16–40 hours after surgery. Patients in both the Premarin and control groups who underwent posterior instrumentation had an increase in drainage at 16 hours, followed by a marked reduction. For patients in both groups who underwent the anterior/posterior procedure, there was a more marked volume of drainage at 8 hours after surgery, and then a subsequent reduction.

Discussion/Conclusion.—The pharmacologic mechanisms of Premarin remain obscure. Theories suggest these estrogens may: (1) act on the capillary apparatus primarily by inducing polymerization in the walls of capillary and arterioles, (2) reduce the permeability of vessel walls, and (3) interfere with coagulation and fibrinolysis by altering Factor V. Administration of Premarin in the immediate postoperative period causes an immediate and marked reduction in Hemovac drainage. The maximum effect occurred 8–16 hours (was significant 16–40 hours) postoperatively. Patients undergoing anterior/posterior procedures initially had a significantly greater postoperative blood loss at 8 hours, compared with a similar finding at 16 hours in the posterior procedure group. Premarin may be recommended for decreasing postoperative blood loss in adolescents undergoing scoliosis surgery.

▶ This article reports another technique to decrease the need for blood transfusion during and after pediatric spinal-deformity surgery. Hypotensive anesthesia, intraoperative blood salvage, autologous donations, and hemostatic agents are routinely used in children and teenagers to eliminate the need for transfusing volunteer-donated blood from the blood bank. These authors do not comment on blood loss during surgery, but noted a 37% reduction in blood loss drainage following surgery when Premarin was administered toward the end of the surgical case. It was not noted whether this 37% reduction in drainage translated into fewer transfusions for the patients, since this difference was only about 4 mL/kg, or a relatively small part of each child's blood volume. While the numbers reported by these authors reached statistical significance, there are other factors that need to be considered in evaluating blood loss during and after surgery. Although hematologic studies were reported in this article to be normal both before and after surgery, this is not always the case with anterior-posterior procedures that last several hours and involve substantial blood replacement, a setting in which more postoperative drainage would be expected. The authors think Premarin can always be beneficial following pediatric spinal surgery, but the study of additional factors that contribute to the presence or absence of bleeding needs to be included to see more clearly where Premarin fits into the big picture of doing all possible to prevent the reliance on bank blood we had in the past.

V.T. Tolo, M.D.

Congenital Hip Disorders

Coxa Vara: Surgical Outcomes of Valgus Osteotomies

Carroll K, Coleman S, Stevens PM (Shriners Hosp, Salt Lake City, Utah)
J Pediatr Orthop B 17:220–224, 1997   2–9

Introduction.—Coxa vara, a condition of a decreased proximal femoral angulation, can be congenital or acquired and has a neck-shaft angle of less than 110 degrees. With an incidence of 1 in 25,000, the deformity is rare. As the physis assumes a more vertical position, coxa vara progresses with resultant forces across the hip, becoming shearing rather than compressive. The bending moment is pathologic to normal continued physeal growth and can recur unless osteotomy normalizes the physeal position. Outcomes of patients who had osteotomies for coxa vara were evaluated.

Methods.—There was a retrospective evaluation of 26 children with 37 affected hips during the past 15 years of surgical experience, and the patients were evaluated for outcome after valgus osteotomy. The study included acquired and congenital types of coxa vara.

Results.—After valgus osteotomy, the overall recurrence rate was 50%. No bearing on recurrence was found with type of surgery, type of implant and etiology, or age at time of surgery. Up to 95% of children had no recurrence of varus if Hilgenreiner's epiphyseal angle was corrected to less than 38 degrees. Head-shaft angle was not a reliable indicator of appropriate correction. There were 83% of children who had excellent acetabular depth, spherical congruency, relief from pain, and correction of Trendelenburg gait if the proximal femur was corrected before age 10.

Conclusion.—The degree of correction determines if correction will be maintained. The shear forces of a varus hip will become compressive with correction of physeal position to a more horizontal position. If repositioned, the physes in the conditions studied can assume normal growth. Even in children with osseous necrosis secondary to infection or developmental dysplasia of the hip, continued proximal femoral growth, implying improved physeal health if normal biomechanics are restored, was seen.

▶ While all the children in this study had a varus deformity of the proximal femur, the causes for this deformity were multiple. Included in this series were 3 children with congenital coxa vara, together with children whose coxa vara was associated with hip dysplasia complications, skeletal dysplasia, rickets, or congenital short femur. This makes it impossible to know if 1 group is a better candidate for valgus osteotomy than another. But despite these varied causes for the coxa vara, the message of this article is clear: full correction is the key to prevention of recurrence. The primary problem at the time of surgery is to obtain and maintain the 50–60 degrees of correction needed to meet the criterion of less than 38 degrees for Hilgenreiner's epiphyseal angle. While these authors used a variety of techniques in their successful cases, 1 method I have found useful to obtain and maintain large corrections involves sharpening an AO dynamic compression plate, using this as a chisel up the femoral neck, and then swinging the femoral neck and head into the corrected position, with the straight plate being used as a side plate for the distal fragment. However you stabilize this valgus osteotomy, don't accept only partial correction, as recurrence will be the norm.

V.T. Tolo, M.D.

Severin Classification System for Evaluation of the Results of Operative Treatment of Congenital Dislocation of the Hip: A Study of Intraobserver and Interobserver Reliability

Ward WT, Vogt M, Grudziak JS, et al (Univ of Pittsburgh, Pa; Bayindir Med Ctr, Ankara, Turkey; Duke Univ, Durham, NC)
J Bone Joint Surg Am 79-A:656–663, 1997   2–10

Introduction.—For the treatment of congenital dislocation of the hip, the Severin classification system is frequently used. To determine the radiographic classification, Severin included no quantitative parameters other than the center-edge angle. Before a classification system is used to promote therapeutic guidelines or to compare results of treatments, it should be validated. The intraobserver and interobserver reliability of the Severin classification was established.

Methods.—The most recent radiographs of 37 children who had medial open reduction for congenital dislocation of the hip an average of 9 years previously (for 56 hips) were evaluated independently by 4 blinded raters and an operating surgeon with the Severin system. Eight weeks later, 3 of the raters evaluated the same radiographs.

Results.—When all Severin classes were analyzed independently, the average kappa coefficient was 0.15 for the 6 pairwise comparisons among the 4 blinded raters. Among the blinded raters and the operating surgeon, the average kappa coefficient for the 4 pairwise comparisons was even lower, at 0.03. For the 3 intraobserver comparisons, the kappa coefficients were 0.20, 0.38, and 0.44, with an average of 0.34. A kappa coefficient that indicated even moderate agreement (of more than 0.50) was not found in any of the comparisons.

Conclusion.—When the Severin system was used to rate the results of operations performed for the treatment of congenital dislocation of the hip, kappa analysis demonstrated variable and low levels of agreement. If this system is to be used for the evaluation of clinical results, the unadjusted kappa coefficient should indicate excellent agreement of more than 0.75. The clinical conclusions of reports in which the Severin system has been used as the basis of proof are called into question by these unacceptably low levels of intraobserver and interobserver reliability.

▶ An increasing number of articles are being published that address interobserver and intraobserver errors in making what seems like a quantitative assessment of a problem or treatment result. Recent examples of this topic include measurement of congenital scoliosis, talocalcaneal angles in club foot, acetabular indices, and evaluation of femoral head involvement in Legg-Perthes. In fact, any radiographic measurement is dependent not only on the measurement but also on the technique with which the radiograph was taken. We are not as good at reproducibly assessing as we thought. This paper cleverly and clearly exposes the weaknesses of the Severin classification for assessing surgical treatment for congenital dislocation of the hip, even among pediatric orthopaedists who have used this classification in practice for some time. The point made needs to be taken seriously: we are making a lot of treatment decisions based on measurements and classifications that may not have been subjected to the rigorous examination reported in this article. Articles such as this make me think, "Are there any clinical measurements that are accurate and reproducible?" Practically speaking, we need to try to continue to measure change, either with or without treatment, but we also need to measure our measurement ability.

V.T. Tolo, M.D.

Long-term Outcome After Open Reduction Through an Anteromedial Approach for Congenital Dislocation of the Hip
Morcuende JA, Meyer MD, Dolan LA, et al (Univ of Iowa, Iowa City)
J Bone Joint Surg Am 79-A:810–817, 1997   2–11

Introduction.—Concentric reduction and maintenance of the reduction to provide the optimum environment for development of the femoral head and the acetabulum are the goals of managing children who have congenital dislocation of the hip. There is controversy over the choice of operative procedure for reducing a congenitally dislocated hip. An anteromedial approach is less invasive and has less stiffness of the joint than an anterolateral approach, but the anteromedial approach also has poor visualization of the acetabulum, associated risk of damage to the medial circumflex vessels, and inability to perform capsulorraphy or concurrent secondary procedures.

Methods.—There were 93 congenitally dislocated hips in 76 children who had open reduction through an anteromedial approach. Adductor and ilipsoas tenotomies were done in all patients, as was arthrography. At the time of reduction, the average age of the children was 14 months and the follow-up time was 11 years. The long-term results after open reduction through an anteriomedial approach were reviewed.

Results.—An excellent or good result was found in 66 hips (71%); a fair result was found in 24 hips (26%); and a poor result was found in 3 hips (3%). Poor roentgenographic results occurred with an inverted neolimbus at the time of the operation and postoperative growth disturbance of the femoral head. There were 22 hips (24%) with type II avascular necrosis, 13 (14%) with type III avascular necrosis, 3 (3%) with type IV avascular necrosis, and 2 (2%) with nonclassifiable lesions. Avascular necrosis was not seen in 53 hips (57%). A higher rate of growth disturbances of the femoral head was associated with a high hip dislocation and an operation after the age of 24 months. There was no association among short-term preoperative traction, type of neolimbus, ligation of the medial circumflex vessel, and the prevalence of growth disturbances. Postoperatively, 2 hips redislocated and transient stiffness was observed in 7 hips.

Conclusion.—In the management of patients with congenital dislocation of the hip who are 24 months old or younger, the anteromedial approach is useful. Direct access to the obstacles to reduction, avoidance of damage of the iliac apophysis and the abductor muscles, minimum blood loss, need for only a single operative session for treatment of both hips, and a cosmetically acceptable scar are the advantages to this type of procedure. There was a greater prevalence of type-II growth disturbances of the femoral head than was expected. Because of the inconsistencies in the literature, the high rates of growth disturbance should not be attributed entirely to an anteromedial approach.

▶ This article reports a frank evaluation of the radiographs of children, an average of 11 years after anteromedial open reduction of a congenitally dislocated hip. Charts were reviewed and they report a nearly normal range of motion of the hips on the latest examination. The avascular necrosis rate was higher than expected, and the authors infer that perhaps other authors are underreporting their rates. Maybe so, but the surgical approach is close to the circumflex vessels, and if the rate of avascular changes is high in the hands of the master of this procedure, should one who uses this approach less often expect even more avascular necrosis? The final results are assessed using the radiographic Severin classification, which has recently been demonstrated to have high inter- and intra-observer error. Would the results be different if functional outcome assessment from the adolescent or the parent were included? The senior author is renowned for his long-term clinical follow-ups and he will likely reassess these patients in another 10 years. I hope he does, with functional assessment included.

V.T. Tolo, M.D.

Congenital Hand and Foot Disorders

Operative Correction of Radial Club Hand: A Long-term Follow-up of Centralization of the Hand on the Ulna
Lamb DW, Scott H, Lam WL, et al (Princess Margaret Rose Orthopaedic Hosp, Edinburgh, Scotland)
J Hand Surg (Br) 22B:533–536, 1997   2–12

Objective.—Whereas centralization is the standard technique for treating radial club hand, there is little information about the long-term outcome of this surgery. A long-term review of 51 patients treated between 1962 and 1975 is presented.

Methods.—Corrective ulnar osteotomy, centralization of the hand on the ulna, and tendon transfer were performed on 43 patients with 79 radial absences. At the time of operation, patients ranged in age from 2 to 13 years. In 34 cases, the records were sufficient for analysis. Thirteen pollicizations were performed. Upper-limb function was assessed using the Moberg "pick up" test and the Jebsen test. Patients filled out a questionnaire about family life, education, employment, recreation, transport, and self-care activities.

Results.—The forearm was between 50% and 66% of normal length. All patients could complete the Moberg and Jebsen tests. Grip strength was significantly diminished in pollicized hands (5.5 kg) and in nonpollicized hands (4.5 kg). The pinch grip test could not be performed. Of the 17 patients who answered the questionnaire, 2 had attended special schools, 17 had been employed full-time but 5 were now considered disabled, 10 were married, 2 were divorced, 5 were single, 16 were driving, all managed self-care activities, all had recreational activities, 8 had occasional pain, and 1 complained of surgical scars.

Conclusion.—Overall function of the hand improved after pollicization, but grip strength was still significantly diminished. A pollicized index finger improved the cosmetic look of the hand.

▶ Lamb is one of the pioneers in the surgical treatment of radial club hand and is one of only a few hand surgeons in the world with the ability to report a long-term follow-up of the surgical treatment of this condition. He should be pleased. Although the tests of upper-extremity function 21–31 years after the surgical correction showed some disability from weakness of grasp, the patients were generally quite pleased with the procedure, as noted in the questionaire administered to the patients. This type of questionaire, similar to what we now refer to as an "outcomes instrument" measures more than the technical result of surgical treatment but provides information on what the treatment did to help the patient. It shows the surgeon what the patient is actually able to do in everyday life as a result of the surgery. It is only with the ongoing use of such functional outcomes assessment that we can determine whether or not what we surgeons *thought* was a successful technical outcome really made a difference in the life and function of the patient.

V.T. Tolo, M.D.

Management of Clubfoot Deformity in Amyoplasia
Niki H, Staheli LT, Mosca VS (Children's Hosp and Med Ctr, Seattle)
J Pediatr Orthop 17:803–807, 1997   2–13

Introduction.—The most common foot deformity in amyoplasia is clubfoot. Rigid and difficult to correct, the amyoplasia clubfoot tends to recur, and management is controversial. The effectiveness of posteromedial release in the management of clubfoot was determined. The value of splinting at night in preventing recurrent deformity was assessed. The usefulness of serial casting in correcting recurrent deformity was evaluated. The practicality of combining posteromedial release, with the operative cor-

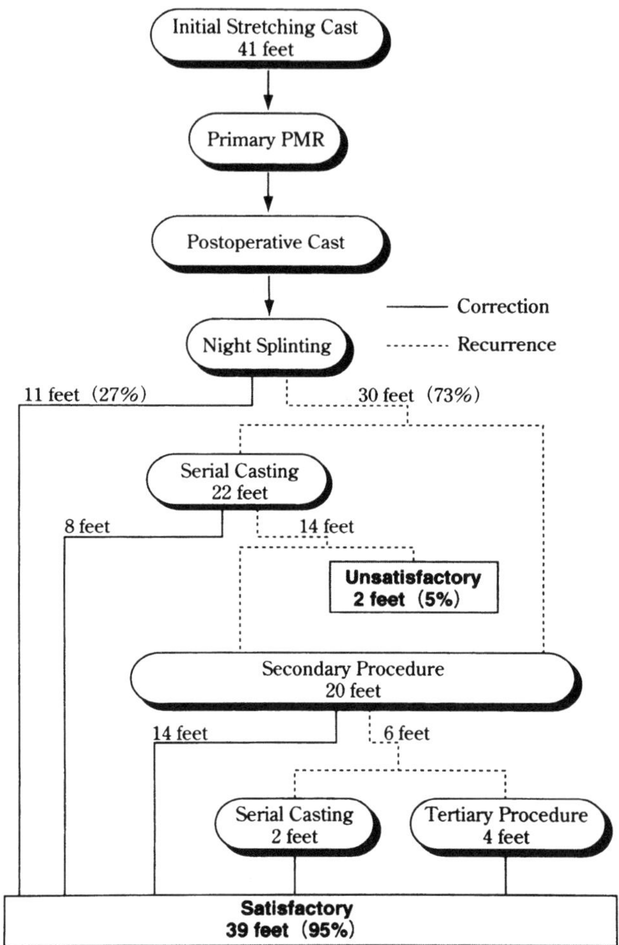

FIGURE 1.—Sequence of management for all patients. (Courtesy of Niki H, Staheli LT, Mosca VS: Management of clubfoot deformity in amyoplasia. *J Pediatr Orthop* 17:803–807, 1997.)

rection of other deformities of the extremities during a single operative session was assessed.

Methods.—A retrospective study was conducted of 22 patients with 41 clubfeet and amyoplasia with a mean duration after surgery of 118 months. Initial stretching casts, posteromedial release, and postoperative splinting at night were the procedures used to manage the clubfeet initially (Fig 1). At the time of surgery, the mean age of patients was 7.3 months.

Results.—In 11 children (27%), the deformity was corrected without recurrence. In 8 feet, serial casting corrected recurrent deformity, and 20 feet required secondary operative procedures. With the serial casting, the casts were changed an average of every 1.5 weeks for a mean of 6 weeks. Two patients required a tertiary operative procedure. The duration of splinting at night after surgery was significantly longer for the feet without recurrence of deformity than for those with recurrence. There were 39 feet (95%) that were plantigrade and considered to be satisfactory at follow-up.

Conclusion.—Posteromedial release can effectively correct most club-feet in amyoplasia, and splinting at night, can reduce recurrence of deformity. Serial cast treatment can often correct recurrence. Talectomy should be regarded as a salvage procedure for recurrent or extremely severe primary deformity. Surgery should be conducted before the child reaches the age of standing.

▶ These authors report excellent final results in a group of patients notorious for clubfoot recurrence (or failure to initially correct) and for complications associated with the foot surgery. Complications are not noted in this article, but the eventual outcome was satisfactory in all but 1 patient after an average of 1.6 operative procedures. The authors' strong recommendation for ongoing splinting of these feet for years after the surgery appears valid, and many physicians who surgically correct clubfoot deformity in this and other "stiff" foot conditions do currently use postcorrection splints for a protracted period to decrease the incidence of recurrence. These authors have a 3-decade experience in the orthopaedic management of all type of arthrogryposis. Their treatment algorithm (Fig 1) deserves close attention, as it is based on practical and first-hand experience.

V.T. Tolo, M.D.

Gait Analysis

The Effect of Limb-length Discrepancy on Gait

Song KM, Halliday SE, Little DG (Children's Hosp and Med Ctr, Seattle; Texas Scottish Rite Hosp for Children, Dallas; New Children's Hosp, Sydney, Australia)

J Bone Joint Surg Am 79-A:1690–1698, 1997   2–14

Introduction.—The degree of limb-length inequality that may cause functional problems and the mechanism by which it impacts gait and stance have not been well-defined. Small discrepancies can alter joint moments and powers and postural sway, but it is not known when treatment is needed to prevent asymmetrical gait. Gait was assessed in 35 neurologically normal children with limb-length discrepancy of the lower extremities of 0.8%–15.8% (0.6–11 cm) of the length of the long extremity.

Methods.—All children had a clinically detectable leg-length discrepancy. Children who were younger than 7 years were excluded to ensure an established pattern of walking. Average patient age was 13 years. Leg-length discrepancy was expressed as the absolute difference in centimeters, measured by an orthoroentgenogram, and as a percentage of the length of the long extremity. A Cybex II was used to test lower-extremity muscle

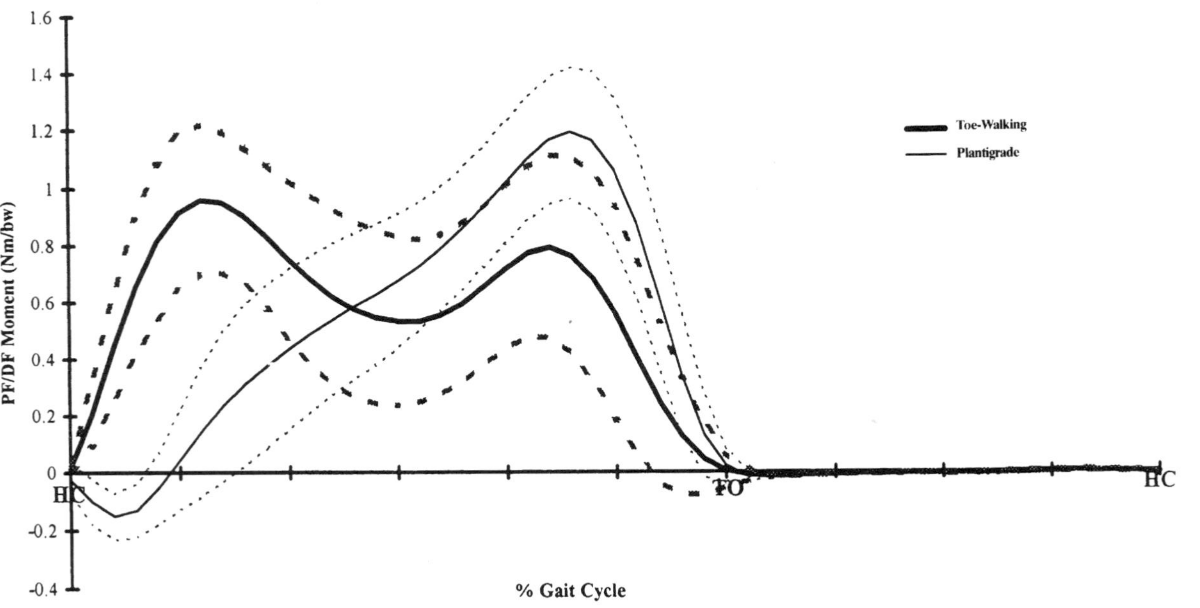

FIGURE 2, A.—Graph of the average kinetic differences between children who used toe-walking as a compensatory strategy and those who walked plantigrade. Children who use toe-walking do not have the normal internal dorsiflexion moment after foot-contact. Because the foot is being forced into dorsiflexion by contact of the toes with the floor, the plantar flexors of the ankle are recruited immediately, resulting in an internal plantar flexion moment (positive numbers on the y axis) during the initial phase of stance. The dotted lines indicate 1 standard deviation. *Abbreviations*: *HC*, heel-contact; *TO*, toe-off; *bw*, body weight; *DF*, dorsiflexion; *PF*, plantar flexion. (Courtesy of Song KM, Halliday SE, Little DG: The effect of limb-length discrepancy on gait. *J Bone Joint Surg Am* 79-A:1690–1698, 1997.)

strength. Gait analysis focused on compensatory strategies of vaulting, toe-walking, circumduction, and persistent flexion of the long limb.

Results.—There was no association between the actual discrepancy or the percent discrepancy and any of the dependent kinematic or kinetic variables, including pelvic obliquity. There was no correlation between discrepancies of less than 3% of the length of the longer extremity and compensatory strategies. Mechanical work was performed by the long extremity and there was a greater vertical displacement of the center of body mass with discrepancies of 5.5% or more. Patients who used toe-walking had more asymmetry and did more total work with the long limb than with the short limb, compared with those patients who walked plantigrade (Fig 2, A). The long limb did more total work in patients with persistent flexion of the long limb. Children with less leg-length discrepancy were able to combine compensatory strategies to normalize the mechanical work of the lower extremities.

Discussion/Conclusion.—There was no association between limb-length discrepancy and pelvic obliquity or abductor-muscle strength. Compensatory strategies for leg-length discrepancies included: equinus positioning of the ankle of the short limb (toe-walking), vaulting over the long limb, increased flexion of the long limb, and circumduction of the long limb. These strategies may shift the timing of kinematic alterations to portions of the gait cycle during which they are not as apparent, dampen oscillations of the center of body mass, and decrease overall energy expenditure during gait. When there is a discrepancy of 5.5% or greater, toe-walking as a compensatory strategy is not able to equalize the work performed by the 2 extremities. These findings may not be applicable to adults with acute acquired limb-length discrepancy.

▶ Much conjecture has been expounded about how great a leg-length difference is significant and when treatment is needed. This article adds science to a topic previously characterized more by smoke and mirrors. Using computerized gait analysis to evaluate children and teenagers with leg-length differences from a variety of causes, these authors characterized compensatory strategies used in this clinical setting. The finding that more total work was needed for the long limb if toe-walking was used with the short leg is important. Even though the authors did not measure oxygen consumption or actual metabolic costs, their data provide excellent guidelines for whom to treat. Now we have a figure to work with—namely, over 5.5% leg-length difference—to help guide our treatment recommendations. In the average patient at maturity, the lower extremity length is usually between 80–90 cm, so this percentage of difference would translate to a difference in leg length of about 4 cm. Current treatment schema usually begin considering treatment at 2 cm difference. This article suggests we can be more conservative in our treatment of differences under 3–4 cm.

V.T. Tolo, M.D.

Comparative Study of Conventional Hip-Knee-Ankle-Foot Orthoses Versus Reciprocating-Gait Orthoses for Children With High-Level Paraparesis

Katz DE, Haideri N, Song K, et al (Texas Scottish Rite Hosp for Children, Dallas)
J Pediatr Orthop 17:377–386, 1997   2–15

Background.—Two different types of orthoses are used for children with high-level paraparesis: hip-knee-ankle-foot orthoses (HKAFO) and reciprocating-gait orthoses (RGO). With the static HKAFO, the child may have either a swing-through or swiveling-type gait pattern. With the RGO, a reciprocal-gait pattern is possible without compromising sagittal-plane stability. A swing-through or swiveling pattern can also be used with the RGO, if desired. The RGO is more expensive and heavier than the statically locked HKAFO. A metabolic comparison of children ambulating with these 2 types of orthoses was conducted.

Methods.—The study included 8 children with thoracic or high lumbar paraparesis. Children with poor upper extremity strength, spasticity, or other involuntary activity of the lower extremities that restricted passive range of motion, or obesity were excluded. Seven children had myelomeningocele; 4 children had no or unilateral hip flexor power, and 4 had bilateral hip flexor power. Each child underwent metabolic studies while ambulating in a custom-fabricated thermoplastic HKAFO and RGO—all children were studied in both devices.

Results.—The average metabolic cost of walking in the orthoses was double that of normal children for the RGO vs. 6 times normal for the HKAFO. For patients with thoracic-level paraparesis, the oxygen cost of ambulation was much higher with the HKAFO. For those with high-lumbar paraparesis, there was no significant metabolic difference (Table 2). Ambulation was faster with the RGO.

Conclusions.—For children with myelomeningocele and thoracic-level paraparesis, ambulation is faster and more energy efficient with an isocentric RGO than with a statically locked HKAFO. The advantages of the RGO justify its greater expense for this group of patients. For patients with high-lumbar paraparesis, the 2 devices are similar in metabolic cost; however, most children prefer the RGO.

TABLE 2.—Averaged Data

	Velocity		HR % increase		O_2 rate		O_2 cost	
	HKAFO	RGO	HKAFO	RGO	HKAFO	RGO	HKAFO	RGO
Group A	6.52	12.70	47.10	38.03	9.15	8.48	1.85	0.72
Group B	17.32	16.37	52.15	33.23	13.48	11.65	1.23	0.75
Normals	70				15.3		0.22	

Abbreviations: HKAFO, hip-knee-ankle-foot orthosis; *RGO,* reciprocating-gait orthosis; *HR,* heart rate.
(Courtesy of Katz DE, Haideri N, Song K, et al: Comparative study of conventional hip-knee-ankle-foot orthoses versus reciprocating-gait orthoses for children with high-level paraparesis. *J Pediatr Orthop* 17:377–386, 1997.)

▶ Each of the children in this interesting study not only had their own HKAFO and RGO, but also had appropriate training periods in each type of brace before the formal testing. These authors clearly showed that if either HKAFO or RGO braces were to be used, the RGO requires less energy with which to walk and is preferred by the users to the HKAFO. In the group of children with thoracic level spina bifida, this would seem to be the brace of choice if the specific qualifying criteria are met. Little difference between these 2 brace types was seen in the children with high-lumbar level paraparesis, so the HKAFO should probably be used here, because it is cheaper and lighter. Practically speaking, most of the children with high-level spina bifida will use wheelchair ambulation primarily by the time they are teenagers. Nonetheless, bracing in the early years does seem to have a positive effect on the involved children and their parents. The guidelines provided by this study are excellent for choosing the right brace for the individual child.

V.T. Tolo, M.D.

Alterations in Surgical Decision Making in Patients With Cerebral Palsy Based on Three-dimensional Gait Analysis
DeLuca PA, Davis RB III, Õunpuu S, et al (Connecticut Children's Med Ctr, Hartford)
J Pediatr Orthop B 17:608–614, 1997   2–16

Introduction.—In the preoperative planning for the child with cerebral palsy, gait analysis has become widely applied. The evaluation of the patient with cerebral palsy was restricted to the physical examination, selected radiographs, and a visual assessment of the patient's gait before the development of 3-dimensional gait-analysis systems. Temporal and stride, 3-dimensional kinematics and kinetics, and electromyographic information is provided by motion-analysis systems. In this patient population, such additional data affect the recommendations made concerning surgical treatment. Recommendations made by pediatric orthopedic surgeons with extensive experience with cerebral palsy and exposure to gait analysis were compared with those made by referring physicians with varying levels of experience in dealing with the cerebral palsy population.

Methods.—There were 91 patients diagnosed with cerebral palsy who were seen in the gait laboratory as part of the surgical decision-making process. For each patient, experienced clinicians reviewed video and clinical examination data and made surgical recommendations. A second set of surgical recommendations was made after joint kinematics and kinetics and electromyography data were reviewed.

Results.—In 52% of the patients, the additional gait-analysis data resulted in changes in surgical recommendations, with an associated reduction in cost of surgery and in the human impact of an inappropriate surgical decision. An increase in surgical recommendations was observed for the gastrocnemius (55%) and rectus femoris (65%), with a decrease in those for the hamstrings (61%), hip adductors (83%), psoas (78%), femur (86%), and tibia (64%).

Conclusion.—With gait analysis, more surgery is recommended for the rectus, tibia, femur, and hamstrings, and less for the adductor, gastrocnemius, and psoas. Compared with the referring physicians' recommendations, there was a net increase (of 8) in the number of procedures recommended, with 114 more procedures recommended and 106 eliminated.

▶ This article reports a 52% change in surgical recommendations subsequent to computerized gait analysis in children with spastic diplegia. In some cases, there were more surgical procedures recommended; in others, less surgery was prescribed. The problem is that it is difficult to know whose recommendation is correct. The authors have a long history of active use of the computerized gait-analysis laboratory and a track record for being relatively aggressive surgically at multiple sites. Compared with referring orthopaedists, the authors recommended more surgery for hamstrings and rectus, as well as for osteotomies of the tibia and femur. However, compared with the authors' initial recommendations from video analysis and physical exam, the authors decreased their number of surgical procedures recommended after the gait data was seen. The increase or decrease in recommendations obviously depends on what the starting point is. Cynics will call this article self-serving—a way to "prove" that computerized gait analysis saves unnecessary surgery and lowers overall cost of care in spastic diplegia. They may be right. While computerized gait analysis has added important capabilities in evaluation of children with cerebral palsy, whether the final recommendations for surgery arrived at by these authors are the correct recommendations for the patients will need to be shown by follow-up gait-analysis and energy-consumption studies.

V.T. Tolo, M.D.

Genetic Disorders

Genetic Correction of Dystrophin Deficiency and Skeletal Muscle Remodeling in Adult *MDX* Mouse via Transplantation of Retroviral Producer Cells
Fassati A, Wells DJ, Sgro Serpente PA, et al (Univ of London; UMDS Guy's Hosp, London; Charing Cross and Westminster Med School, London; et al)
J Clin Invest 100:620–628, 1997   2–17

Introduction.—Patients with the X-linked disease Duchenne muscular dystrophy (DMD) have mutations of the dystrophin gene that cause the absence of dystrophin and related proteins. Retroviral producer cells carrying a therapeutically active dystrophin minigene have been transplanted into adult nude/*mdx* mice, resulting in efficient in vivo infection of activated satellite cells and large numbers of transduced myofibers. Full-length and Becker-type 6.3 kb dystrophin cDNAs can prevent the onset of dystrophy when expressed in *mdx* mouse muscle. The pathologic characteristics of skeletal muscle in these animals are very similar to those seen in very young patients with DMD. The effects of retroviral-mediated transduction of the dystrophin minigene on *mdx* mouse skeletal muscle were analyzed.

Methods and Results.—Mdx mice were transplanted with retroviral producer cells in a single site of the tibialis anterior muscle. This resulted in transduction of 5.5% to 18% of total muscle fibers. The levels of minidystrophin in transduced DMD myotubes were similar to those of endogenous dystrophin. The number of minidystrophin-expressing fibers was similar at 6, 12, and 24 weeks after transplantation. The number of positive fibers was twice as high for mice injected with 3×10^6 producer cells vs. 2.5×10^5 producer cells. Dystrophin gene transfer proceeded just as efficiently in mice with temporary immune suppression after mitomycin C treatment as in nude *mdx* mice. There was evidence of at least partial restoration of the dystrophin with the associated protein complex, which seems to be essential for prevention of muscular dystrophy. From 6 weeks to 12 and 24 weeks after transplantation, the percentage of clustered minidystrophin-positive fibers appears to have increased fivefold.

Conclusions.—These animal studies suggest a promising retroviral-mediated dystrophin gene transfer approach to the treatment of DMD. With temporary immunosuppression and a protocol for mitotic activation of producer cells, it may be possible to control the timing and progression of gene transfer in vivo. The muscle remodeling observed in these experiments may result from degeneration of dystrophin-negative fibers followed by activation, proliferation, and fusion of minidystrophin-positive muscle stem cells transduced in vivo. The process taking place in transduced *mdx* mouse muscle may be similar to the genetic normalization occurring in DMD carriers, which leads to formation of large clusters of dystrophin-positive fibers over time. Dystrophin re-expression probably stabilizes the DAG complex in adult dystrophic muscle, which is probably associated with changes of the extracellular matrix.

▶ As work on the human genome progresses at a rapid rate, an increasing number of gene defects have been described for specific diseases. Some disorders, such as osteogenesis imperfecta, have considerable genetic heterogeneity, but others have a specific genetic defect that is constant among all those affected with that disorder. Such is the case in achondroplasia, with a defect in fibroblast growth factor receptor 3, and in Duchenne muscular dystrophy, with a defect in dystrophin production. It is for these single defect genetic disorders that gene therapy would seem to offer the most hope for families and physicians alike. In this study, the injection of retroviral producer cells allowed release of a vector carrying a dystrophin minigene that led to increased production of dystrophin and an increase in the number of muscle fibers in the mouse model. Although the effective clinical use of gene therapy to reverse the muscle degeneration seen in males with Duchenne muscular dystrophy is still years away, it now appears within reach. How to best accomplish this has yet to be determined, but the methods promulgated in this article will likely play a role. This is exciting stuff.

V.T. Tolo, M.D.

Intravenous Pamidronate Treatment in Osteogenesis Imperfecta

Bembi B, Parma A, Bottega M, et al (Ospedale Civile di Cattinara, Trieste, Italy)

J Pediatr 131:622–625, 1997

2–18

Purpose.—Bisphosphonate drugs, which are synthetic analogues of inorganic pyrophosphate, are inhibitors of osteoclastic bone resorption. Bisphosphonates are widely used in adults, but there have been few reports of their use in children. The use of aminohydroxypropylidene bisphosphonate (pamidronate) to treat osteogenesis imperfecta (OI) in children was evaluated.

Patients.—Three girls, aged 4–9 years, with intermediate or severe OI were treated with cyclic infusions of pamidronate. The starting dosage was 15 or 30 mg IV every 20 days. Treatment also included elemental calcium, 500–1,000 mg/day, and vitamin D, 400 IU/day. Treatment continued for 22–29 months.

Outcomes.—Each of the girls had a sharp drop in the incidence of new fractures and a dramatic improvement in quality of life. Two of the patients had significant increases in bone mineral density. In all 3, linear growth continued along the same percentile as before treatment. All patients had transient fever after their initial infusions, but there were no other adverse effects.

Discussion.—Pamidronate appears to be an effective treatment for OI in children. Bisphosphonates inhibit osteoclastic bone resorption, increasing bone density and reducing fracture risk. Some patients show a progressive increase in bone mineral density, possibly because of reduced ionized calcium activity leading to a parathyroid effect on bone. Because of the long skeletal half-life of bisphosphonates, there is concern that their long-term use could lead to inhibition of bone mineralization and other unfavorable effects.

▶ It has been known for quite some time that the bone mineral density is low in children with OI. Previous trials with supplements, such as fluoride, have shown increased bone density can be achieved, but there has been no effect on the number of fractures these patients with OI sustained. These authors used a bisphosphonate, whose primary effect is to inhibit osteoclast activity, in children with OI and demonstrated an increase in bone density, together with a striking decrease in the number of fractures these treated children had. We have no way to date to treat the underlying type I collagen defect in OI and the orthopedic treatment to date is limited to preventing or treating fractures in this group of children. The promise of an IV medication that assists in the prevention of fractures in children with OI would be welcomed with open arms. Trials are currently in progress to evaluate this, so look for these upcoming results.

V.T. Tolo, M.D.

Sports Injury

Anterior Cruciate Ligament Tears in Children: An Analysis of Operative Versus Nonoperative Treatment
Pressman AE, Letts RM, Jarvis JG (Children's Hosp of Eastern Ont, Ottawa)
J Pediatr Orthop B 17:505–511, 1997   2–19

Introduction.—Management of midsubstance anterior cruciate ligament tears in a child is still puzzling. A significant stress exerted on a child's knee usually results in a physeal injury or subchondral bone avulsion rather than ligamentous injury. However, even the increased healing capacity of children does not result in restoration of the integrity of the ligament when pure ligamentous injuries occur in the anterior cruciate ligament. To return stability to the knee, reconstruction of the ligament appears necessary. However, surgeons hesitate to drill across the physeal plate because of concern in causing physeal arrest. Nonoperative treatment has been sought until physeal closure, but results have been disappointing. For the complete anterior cruciate ligament tear in a child, the optimal management was determined.

Methods.—There were 42 children with arthroscopically confirmed anterior cruciate ligament disruption who were retrospectively reviewed within a 12-year period. The subjective efficacy of treatment was determined. The biomechanical and clinical results of nonoperative and operative management were assessed. The children were between the ages of 5 and 17 years at the time of treatment and were followed up for a mean of 5.3 years. Six injuries were treated by primary repair and 13 were treated nonoperatively. Intra-articular reconstruction employing interosseous tunnels with autologous grafts was used to treat 23 injuries.

Results.—Intra-articular surgical reconstruction was the best treatment for a complete tear of the anterior cruciate ligament. Clinical examination, a composite knee score involving a clinical examination and patient questionnaire, and testing with the KT-1000 arthrometer were used to confirm this result. Patient age or the maturity of the growth plates did not affect the outcome.

Conclusion.—A more stable and functional knee resulted with anterior cruciate reconstruction for complete tears. No deleterious effects of leg-length discrepancy or angular deformities were found. The violation of open tibial and femoral physes was the greatest concern in performing intra-articular repair of the anterior cruciate ligament.

▶ While anterior cruciate ligament (ACL) tears have been successfully treated for years in active adults by patellar tendon or hamstring reconstruction, these procedures have been cautiously used in youngsters with open femoral growth plates, for fear of causing an angular deformity or a leg-length discrepancy. By most criteria, in this article, those patients with ACL reconstruction functioned better than those with nonoperative treatment, and had more stable knees on examination. These authors report no problem with growth disturbance, even in the reconstructions that require drilling through the physis with placement of a tendon graft in the tunnel created. Confirmatory evidence of the safety of this type of reconstruction in those with open physes comes from a recent article[1] in which the authors report no physeal bridging if the physeal drill injury in rabbits was 4% to 5% of the physeal area or if a free tendon graft was left in the drill hole tunnel. While ACL tears in immature patients are still less common than physeal or cartilage injuries, it now appears that, when indicated, adult-type ACL reconstruction is unlikely to lead to growth disturbances, and the presence or absence of an open physis should not be the major consideration in treatment recommendations.

V.T. Tolo, M.D.

Reference

1. Janarv PM, Wikstrom B, Hirsch G: The influence of transphyseal drilling and tendon grafting on bone growth: An experimental study in the rabbit. *J Pediatr Orthop* 18:149–154, 1998.

Juvenile Arthritis

Survivorship of the Charnley Total Hip Arthroplasty in Juvenile Chronic Arthritis: A Follow-up of 186 Cases for 22 Years
Lehtimäki MY, Lehto MUK, Kautiainen H, et al (Tampere Univ Hosp, Finland; Rheumatism Found Hosp, Heinola, Finland; Oulu Univ Hosp, Finland)
J Bone Joint Surg Br 79-B:792–795, 1997   2–20

Introduction.—Patients with juvenile chronic arthritis who have pain, lack of mobility, and radiological evidence of hip involvement have been treated with Charnley low-friction arthroplasty. To clarify the gold-standard status of this operation for juvenile chronic arthritis, a longer-term survivorship analysis was conducted.

Methods.—There were 116 patients with juvenile chronic arthritis who had Charnley low-friction arthroplasty performed on 186 hips in a 20-year period. At operation, the patients had a mean age of 31 years and ranged in age from 14–67 years. There were 47 patients (70 hips) receiving steroids. After surgery, patients were encouraged to walk for 2 months with protected weight-bearing, and if bone grafts had been used, to walk for 6 months with protective weight-bearing. Survival curves were estimated for femoral and acetabular components.

Results.—At 10-year follow-up, overall survival was 91.9%, and at 15-year follow-up, overall survival was 83%. At 10-year follow-up, the femoral component survival was 95.6%, and at 15-year follow-up, it was 91.9%. At 10-year follow-up, the survival of the acetabulum was 95%, and at 15-year follow-up, it 87.8%. Survival was significantly impaired only by the use of steroids (Table 3). Deep infections were found in 2 patients. There was no statistical significance of risk factors such as gender, age, weight, preoperative bleeding, and bone grafting.

TABLE 3.—Patient-related Variables and Survival of the Prosthesis at 5 and 10 Years

	5-year	10-year	p value*
Gender			0.16
Male (n = 22)	100	80 (not calculated)	
Female (n = 164)	97 (93 to 99)	93 (87 to 97)	
Steroids			0.04
Yes (n = 70)	96 (87 to 99)	90 (77 to 96)	
No (n = 116)	98 (94 to 100)	93 (86 to 97)	
Amyloidosis			0.61
Yes (n = 26)	96 (not calculated)	92 (not calculated)	
No (n = 160)	97 (93 to 99)	92 (85 to 96)	
Bone graft			0.94
Yes (n = 13)	100	88 (not calculated)	
No (n = 173)	97 (93 to 99)	92 (86 to 96)	

*Mantel-Cox test for difference in survival curves between groups
(Courtesy of Lehtimäki MY, Lehto MUK, Kautiainen H, et al: Survivorship of the Charnley total hip arthroplasty in juvenile chronic arthritis: A follow-up of 186 cases for 22 years. *J Bone Joint Surg Br* 79-B:792–795, 1997.)

Conclusion.—For patients with juvenile chronic arthritis who require total hip replacement, the use of Charnley low-friction arthroplasty is recommended. Steroids were found to be the main factor for loosening. For hip replacement in juvenile chronic arthritis, Charnley low-friction arthroplasty remains the gold standard.

▶ This is another article that shows just how good the low-friction arthroplasy devised by Sir John Charnley really is. While most series that report on survivorship of total hip arthroplasty in young adults have a sizable revision rate even after 10 years, these authors do much better, probably for 2 reasons: the skill of the surgeon when placing the hip replacement initially and the limited activity many juvenile chronic arthritis patients will have. The fact that 38% of patients were on steroid medication would indicate that the arthritis for the group as a whole was quite advanced and difficult to control, so there was probably less stress put on these prostheses than on those in a more active population. Nonetheless, these results are impressive. Surgeons and orthopaedic implant manufacturers have devised a seemingly endless number of variations on the original Charnley total hip replacement with little or no improvement in long-term results. This article adds further evidence to attest to the brilliance of the ideas and work of Charnley, who has changed orthopaedic care more than any other physician in the past half century. I agree that his arthroplasty remains the "gold standard."

V.T. Tolo, M.D.

Miscellaneous

Intraoperative Latex Anaphylaxis in Children: Classification and Prophylaxis of Patients at Risk
Dormans JP, Templeton J, Schreiner MS, et al (Children's Hosp of Philadelphia, Pa)
J Pediatr Orthop B 17:622–625, 1997   2–21

Background.—Previous reports have described patients with intraoperative anaphylactic reactions to latex. Groups at risk for such reactions have been identified, most of whom had undergone multiple surgical procedures, bladder catheterizations, and radiographic studies. Although approaches to prevent these reactions have been proposed, their efficacy has not been demonstrated. A program for reducing the incidence of intraoperative latex anaphylaxis was developed.

Methods.—In a previously reported, 3-year experience, 21 children with type 1 intraoperative reactions to latex were encountered. The patients were identified from a series of 36,075 general anesthetic procedures. On the basis of this experience, 3 groups of patients at risk for such reactions were identified: high-risk patients, those with a history of systemic anaphylactic reactions to natural rubber or latex; moderate-risk patients, those with a history of nonsystemic allergic reaction to latex; and low-risk patients, those with at-risk diagnoses (i.e., spina bifida or bladder exstrophy) but no history of allergic reaction to latex. The latter group also included children with cerebral palsy, shunts, and multiple previous surgeries. A prospective prophylaxis program, consisting of pharmacologic prophylaxis, was developed for these 3 groups in an attempt to create a latex-free environment.

Results.—After initiation of the prophylaxis program, 34,513 general anesthetic procedures were performed. Eighty-six patients were classified as at-risk: 48% had bladder exstrophy, 43% had myelomeningocele, and 9% had cerebral palsy. There were just 3 cases of suspected intraoperative latex anaphylaxis. Two of these occurred in patients who were not classified as at-risk preoperatively and thus did not receive prophylaxis.

Conclusions.—This study presents a system for classifying risk of intraoperative latex anaphylaxis in children, including prophylactic measures. The risk-to-benefit ratio of preoperative prophylaxis suggests that it should be used on a trial basis. Prevention starts with a careful preoperative history. Patients whose history includes suspected latex sensitivity should undergo preoperative evaluation with latex-specific immunoglobulin E. Performing this test in patients with myelodysplasia, bladder exstrophy, cerebral palsy, shunts, and numerous previous surgeries is recommended.

▶ The incidence of latex allergy in the pediatric population has increased as the awareness of this problem has expanded and the use of latex products in the operating room has continued. This is not simply a theoretical problem, but a problem that all who operate on children with spina bifida, cerebral palsy, muscular dystrophy, and multiple congenital defects will certainly see during their career. In this survey study, the classification of children into potential "at-risk" categories allowed a successful prophylactic program to be put into place. The incidence of latex anaphylaxis during surgery was markedly decreased from a previously reviewed group of about the same size, using the protocol. Although a prospective study would be helpful from the statistical standpoint, the practical approach to improving patient care and safety at once is to use the protocol proposed by these authors right now. There is little risk associated with the prophylactic program outlined and the potential benefits in both patient safety and cost of treatment are great.

V.T. Tolo, M.D.

Sternocleidomastoid Pseudotumor of Infants and Congenital Muscular Torticollis: Fine-structure Research

Tang S, Liu Z, Quan X, et al (Chongqing Univ, China)
J Pediatr Orthop B 18:214–218, 1998   2–22

Introduction.—Despite many previous studies, questions remain about congenital muscular torticollis (CMT) and sternocleidomastoid pseudotumor of infants (SCMPOI). These 2 entities are probably related to each other, but it is unknown whether they represent the same process or why the sequelae of the mass may differ. Changes in the ultrasound findings over time are unrelated to the pathologic findings. The pathologic findings of CMT and SCMPOI were studied to gain insight into the origin and pathogenesis of these conditions.

Methods.—Fifty patients were studied by light and electron microscopy: 16 with SCMPOI and 34 with CMT. The patients were 31 boys and 19 girls, ranging in age from 1 month to 9 years.

Findings.—The proliferation interstitium of SCMPOI showed myoblasts in various stages. Sixteen patients had a mass, showing normal muscles, variously differentiated fibroblasts, and collagen. Younger patients had more myoblasts and fibroblasts in early stages of differentiation and maturation. All patients had varying stages of myoblast and muscular degeneration. All cases of CMT showed varying degrees of decreased myofibrillae. Both SCMPOI and CMT cases showed focal accumulations of inflammatory cells, hemorrhage, edema, muscle infarction, and calcification.

Conclusions.—The clinical manifestations and US findings of the mass in SCMPOI appear to reflect the myoblast-to-fibroblast ratio seen histologically. If myoblast development and differentiation proceed normally, the mass will disappear, resulting in normal sternocleidomastoid muscle. If myoblast degeneration occurs, the fibroblast will produce large amounts of collagen; scarlike contraction of the muscle will occur, resulting in typical torticollis. The findings do not really support the traumatic theory of the origin of SCMPOI and CMT. The myoblasts may arise from remnant mesenchymal cells that remain static during the embryogenesis of the sternocleidomastoid muscle. The cells then differentiate and develop after birth. Myogenesis of myoblasts in the mass determines whether torticollis occurs. The findings may have implications for conservative treatment of the mass: passive stretching of the involved muscles may provide an adaptable stimulation, thus favoring normal myogenesis.

▶ The electron microscopic information reported by these authors provides some new information on congenital muscular torticollis and the presence of a pseudotumor in the sternocleidomastoid in some infants, yet questions remain. Recent reports on the etiology of this condition have focused on intrauterine position, suggesting that neck position leads to a compartment syndrome within the sternocleidomastoid muscle, resulting in fibrosis and pseudotumor formation. However, in this study, nothing in the histologic examination was suggestive of the usual changes seen in muscle affected with a compartment syndrome. These authors provide convincing evidence that myoblasts at various stages are present in this pseudotumor and suggest an intriguing theory that mesenchymal cell remnants in the sternocleidomastoid muscle are stimulated in some unknown way to develop myoblasts, which then develop either normally or form a pseudotumor, depending on unknown external factors. If this is true, the stretching program used in infants to improve neck motion would also theoretically allow myoblastic differentiation into more normal muscle in some cases. This article provides another clue, but the search goes on for why this curious condition occurs in a small number of infants.

V.T. Tolo, M.D.

Incomplete Healing of Simple Bone Cysts After Steroid Injections
Hashemi-Nejad A, Cole WG (Univ of Toronto)
J Bone Joint Surg Br 79-B:727–730, 1997   2–23

Introduction.—Nearly 15% of simple bone cysts heal without treatment during childhood. Most persist or increase in size. The typical treatment of choice is injection into the cyst of a corticosteriod with the patient under general anesthesia. Multiple injections may be required, but the indication for and timing of repeat injections have not been clearly elucidated. The radiologic and symptomatic outcomes of simple bone cysts treated by aspiration, cystography, and injection of corticosteroids were assessed in 32 children.

Methods.—Median age of children was 7 years (range, 4–16 years). Median follow-up from the most recent steroid injection was 5 years (range, 1–10 years). Lesions had the following location: 18 humerus, 11 femur, 2 tibia, and 1 fibula. Cysts that abutted the growth plate were considered active (17 cysts) and the remaining were considered inactive (15 cysts). A median of 3 intralesional injections of 80 mg of methylprednisolone acetate were instilled into each cyst. Clinical outcome was evaluated using the validated Childhood Health Assessment Questionnaire to determine function, pain, and satisfaction.

Results.—Radiologic outcome was not affected by age of the child or activity or size of the cyst. Twenty-four of 32 cysts had satisfactory radiological outcome and 8 were unsatisfactory. Treatment response could not be determined radiologically for a minimum of 3 months. At a median follow-up of 5 years, 4 cysts had healed, 20 cysts were partially visible but sclerotic, 4 remained visible but opaque, and 4 were clearly visible. Cysts that had healed and were partially visible but sclerotic were considered to have satisfactory radiologic healing. This was seen in 14 of 32 cysts after the initial injection, 8 of 21 after the second injection, and in relatively few of the remaining cysts after subsequent injections. All 18 children with humeral cysts, the 1 child with a fibular cyst, and 9 of 13 children (67%) with femoral or tibial lesions had a satisfactory symptomatic outcome, irrespective of radiologic outcome. Five of 8 children (63%) with unsatisfactory radiologic outcome of upper extremity lesions had a satisfactory clinical result. The other 3 children with unsatisfactory results had cysts in the proximal femur that caused pain on exertion and recurrent fractures.

Conclusion.—The response of the cyst to injections could not be reliably determined for 3 months, indicating that further radiographs and treatment should be delayed for at least this peiod. The healing response to intralesional corticosteroids is variable and often incomplete, even with multiple injections. Cysts in non–weight-bearing bones were well tolerated during normal childhood activities, but only 67% of children with cysts of the lower extremity had satisfactory symptomatic outcome. The radiological outcome after corticosteroid injections corresponded to that achieved by multiple drill holes. The therapeutic value of the corticosteroids used is questionable.

▶ For over 20 years, the first line of treatment of presumed unicameral bone cysts in children and teenagers has been the injection of corticosteroid into them. While the patient is under general anesthesia, the cyst has 2 needles placed, with irrigation of the cyst before the steroid injection is done. Why exactly this works has not been well explained—yet it seems to fill in a remarkable number of these cysts eventually. Although these authors conclude that the healing response with corticosteroid injection is unpredictable, all of the upper-extremity lesions stabilized or healed, and it was only the lower-extremity lesions that had problems with pain or recurrent fractures. If these lower extremity lesions don't fill in, it is always possible to do open surgery, though, curiously, open curettage and bone grafting has recurrence rates similar to the injections reviewed here. Allograft paste, bone marrow injections, and even growth factors such as bone morphogenic protein will likely be the injection materials of the future. But for now, as this article reports, the corticosteroid usually works satisfactorily, especially in the upper extremity.

V.T. Tolo, M.D.

Decline of Bone and Joint Infections Attributable to Haemophilus Influenzae Type b

Bowerman SG, Green NE, Mencio GA (Vanderbilt Univ, Nashville, Tenn)
Clin Orthop 341:128–133, 1997   2–24

Objective.—The immunization of children for *Haemophilus influenzae* type b has almost completely eliminated meningitis, pneumonia, and other serious infections caused by this organism. No previous reports have addressed the impact on bone and joint infections, however. The effects of *H. influenzae* type b vaccination on the incidence of septic arthritis and hematogenous osteomyelitis were examined.

Findings.—Records of 165 children with acute hematogenous osteomyelitis or septic arthritis occurring from 1984 to 1996 were analyzed. Cultures were positive in 69% of cases, most of which grew *Staphylocorcus aureus*. Sixteen cultures were positive for *H. influenzae*. Of these, 15 occurred before the advent of effective conjugate vaccines against this organism (Fig 2). Lack of immunization was confirmed in these 15 patients.

Conclusions.—*Haemophilus influenzae* vaccination of children has almost completely eliminated the occurrence of bone and joint infections caused by this organism. The number of cases of acute osteomyelitis and septic arthritis appears to have been unchanged, however. As *H. influenzae* is eliminated as a cause of bone and joint infection, vaccinated children with such infections will no longer need empirical antibiotic coverage for this organism.

▶ Those who do not routinely work with the pediatric population are likely less aware of the tremendous impact the use of vaccinations for *Haemophilus influenzae* has had on all types of infections in infants and toddlers.

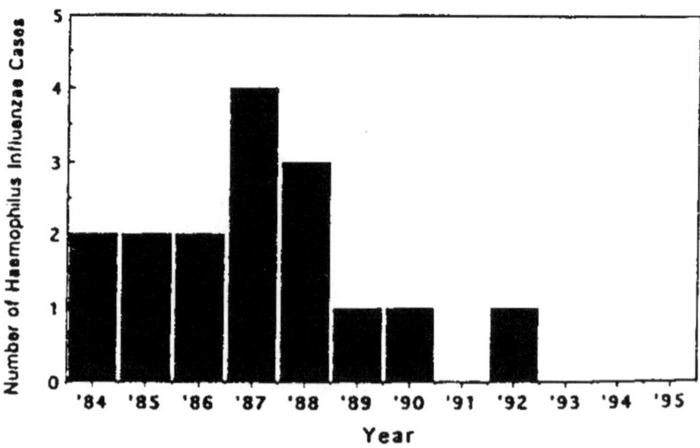

FIGURE 2.—Number of cases per year of acute hematogenous osteomyelitis and septic arthritis attributed to *Haemophilus influenzae*. (Courtesy of Bowerman SG, Green NE, Mencio GA: Decline of bone and joint infections attributable to Haemophilus influenzae type b. *Clin Orthop* 341:128–133, 1997.)

Although, in this retrospective survey, only about 10% of the bone and joint infections were attributable to this organism, essentially all the affected children were unvaccinated. As opposed to the standard practice of only a few years ago, now, in the 3-month to 4-year-old *vaccinated* child with septic arthritis or osteomyelitis, antibiotic coverage for *H. influenzae* is not needed while cultures are pending. On the other hand, particularly in large urban areas or in areas populated by recent immigrants, where vaccinations may not have included *H. influenzae*, preliminary antibiotic coverage for this organism in this age group still is needed until cultures are finalized. Not many orthopedists delve into a detailed immunization history routinely, but in the clinical setting of childhood orthopedic infection, this needs to be done.

V.T. Tolo, M.D.

Brace Treatment of Early Infantile Tibia Vara
Zionts LE, Shean CJ (Univ of Southern California, Los Angeles)
J Pediatr Orthop B 18:102–109, 1998   2–25

Introduction.—The most frequent type of pathologic bowleg is infantile tibia vara or Blount disease, a developmental condition characterized by a varus angulation of the proximal end of the tibia, caused by a disturbance in growth of the proximal medial tibial physis. Treatment of early infantile tibia vara has generated some controversy. Daytime, ambulatory brace treatment was evaluated in the management of children who meet many of the currently accepted diagnostic criteria for early infantile tibia vara.

Methods.—There were 24 children with 42 extremities who had early infantile tibia vara treated with a brace. The children had either a varus deformity that did not improve by age 18–24 months or a persistent varus deformity after 24 months. An above-the-knee brace with a free ankle was prescribed, with a single medial upright with valgus-producing straps. The braces had either a locked hinge joint at the knee or no hinged knee. The children wore the braces during the day and removed them for bedtime. From the initiation of brace treatment, the children were followed up for an average of 27.2 months.

Results.—At follow-up, a good rating was given to 29 extremities (Fig 4), a fair rating to 9 extremities, and a poor rating to 4 extremities. The proximal tibial deformity resolved in 32 extremities at latest follow-up, was unchanged in 8, and decreased 1 grade in 2. None of the deformities progressed to the next Langenskiöld stage. Before treatment, the tibiofemoral angle averaged 24.6 degrees, and at latest follow-up, the angle averaged 1.1 degree of valgus. Before treatment, the proximal tibial metaphyseal-diaphyseal angle averaged 16.4 degrees, and after treatment it averaged 5.7 degrees. Before treatment, the distal femoral metaphyseal-diaphyseal angle averaged 11.1 degrees, and after treatment it averaged 0.2 degrees of valgus.

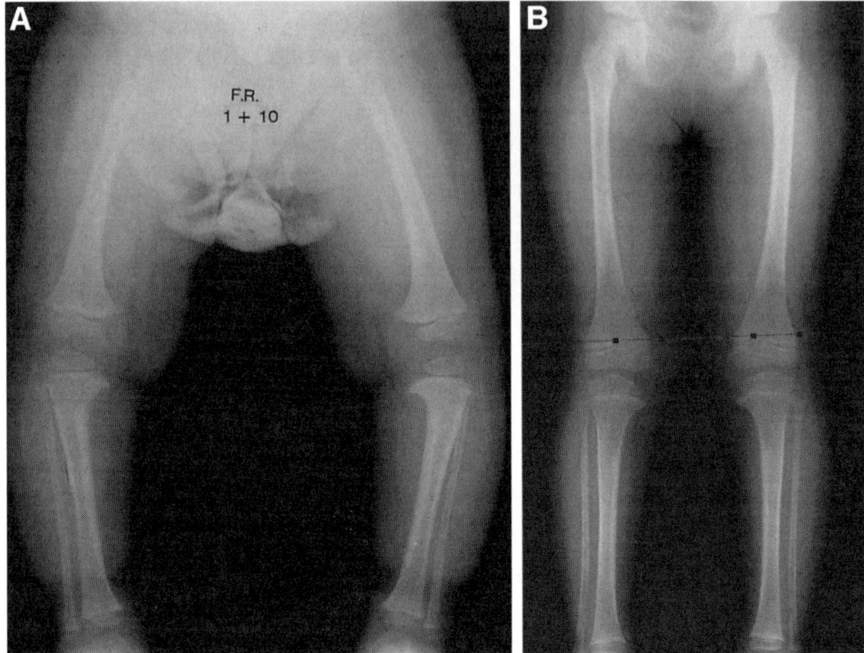

FIGURE 4.—Case 10. **A**, radiograph of a 22-month-old boy who was diagnosed with early bilateral tibia vara. **B**, radiograph taken at latest follow-up (age 4 years). Both extremities were rated good. (Courtesy of Zionts LE, Shean CJ: Brace treatment of early infantile tibia vara. *J Pediatr Orthop B* 18:102–109, 1998.)

Conclusion.—In patients who are younger than 3 years and have Langenskiöld stage I or II deformity, ambulatory brace treatment may favorably alter the natural history of tibia vara. There were 38 of 40 extremities with Langenskiöld stages I and II tibia vara which responded favorably to brace treatment. The 1 patient with stage II disease did not have improvement. Tibial osteotomy may be best reserved for those patients who, despite bracing, do not show satisfactory clinical and radiographic improvement by age 4 years.

▶ Those who have advocated the use of bracing for tibia vara in children between the ages of 2 and 3 have been scoffed at by many, with the explanation for the reported "success" being that the condition treated was really physiologic bowing, which would have improved even without any treatment. These authors have structured their study very well. One type of treatment was used with 1 type of brace used only during daytime hours. The criteria the authors used to diagnose tibia vara from radiographs are all well-accepted measurement criteria, thought by others to be diagnostic of tibia vara and used by those who advocate corrective osteotomy as necessary to allow resolution of the tibia vara. The results reported here are impressive, with over 90% of patients responding favorably to the bracing. Prior skeptics of this treatment should be convinced by the data presented in this article. The avoidance of the surgery (and often complications) of tibial osteotomy in these children benefits not only the patients, but society as well, with the resultant drop in health-care costs. At least in children aged between 2 and 3 years, with radiograph evidence of tibia vara, a brace such as the authors describe should be tried first.

V.T. Tolo, M.D.

3 Topics of General Orthopedic Interest

Introduction

A broad and interesting spectrum of articles that have a general appeal have appeared in this year's literature. The topics range from the value and method of blood salvage to the prognosis of hip fractures in the male population. Basic science contributions to study the effectiveness of the mechanical properties of cement, as well as the density of polyethylene and dissimilar metals, are all useful contributions of clinical relevance. This group of articles offers a high-quality spectrum that have practical value to the clinician as well as providing a scientific basis for the clinical practice.

Bernard F. Morrey, M.D.

Procurement of Bone Graft From the Iliac Crest: An Operative Approach With Decreased Morbidity

Colterjohn NR, Bednar DA (McMaster Univ, Hamilton, Ont)
J Bone Joint Surg Am 79-A:756–759, 1997   3–1

Background.—It has been reported that autogenous bone is more effective than allograft bone for augmenting fusion in spinal arthrodesis. Although the posterior iliac crest is a readily available source of bone graft for posterior spinal arthrodesis, its use often results in infection, hematoma, pain, numbness, and hypersensitivity or irritability of local tissue.

Methods.—In 110 consecutive patients, a comparison was made of the morbidity associated with (1) bone graft taken from the iliac crest through an incision parallel to the superior cluneal nerves and perpendicular to the posterior iliac crest (study group) and (2) from a standard incision parallel to the posterior iliac crest (control group) (Fig 1). At 1 month and 6 months postoperatively, numbness, tenderness, and pain were assessed by an interviewer and by a review of medical records. The interviewer was blinded as to the type of incision.

Results.—Patients in the control group had a greater prevalence of symptoms than patients in the study group. At 1 month, numbness was reported by 44% of patients in the study group and 74% of patients in the

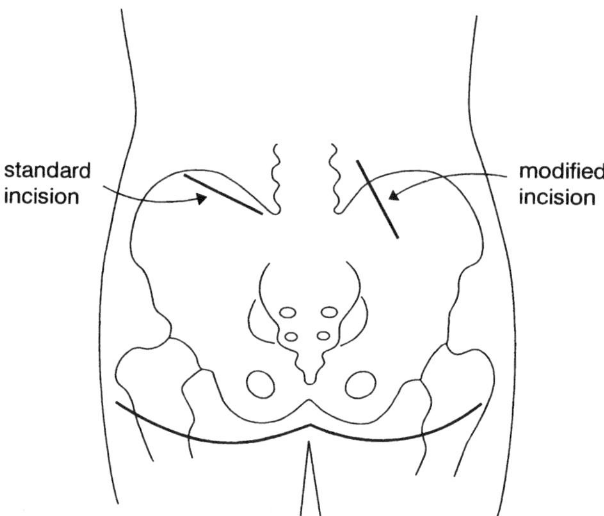

FIGURE 1.—Diagrammatic representation of the standard and modified incisions used to procure bone from the iliac crest. (Courtesy of Colterjohn NR, Bednar DA: Procurement of bone graft from the iliac crest: An operative approach with decreased morbidity. *J Bone Joint Surg (Am)* 79-A:756–759, 1997.)

control group. At 6 months, numbness was reported by 25% of patients in the study group and 58% of those in the control group. At 1 month, tenderness over the incision was reported by 42% of patients in the study group and 68% of patients in the control group. At 6 months, tenderness was reported by 19% of patients in the study group and 51% of those in the control group. At 1 month, deep pain in the region of the iliac crest was reported by 81% of patients in the study group and 75% of patients in the control group. At 6 months, deep pain was reported by 54% of patients in the study group and 60% of patients in the control group. At 1 month, mean analogue scores for pain at the donor site were 6 of 10 points in the study group and 7 of 10 points in the control group. At 6 months, these scores were 2 of 10 points in the study group and 3 of 10 points in the control group.

Discussion.—A review of the anatomy of the iliac crest is necessary for reducing associated morbidity. This modified incision reduces injury to the cluneal nerves by dissection of the subcutaneous tissues in line with the course of the nerves over the iliac crest. Donor site morbidity and pain were not significantly different between groups at 1 month but were significantly different at 6 months. Because deep pain at the donor site associated with actual procurement of bone graft was similar in the 2 groups, the authors believe that the difference in donor site morbidity resulted from the use of the modified incision.

▶ Although the purpose of this paper is to compare exposures to the iliac crest, it provides valuable additional information simply by documenting the incidence of problems associated with the donor site of the bone graft. While these facts are known, the paper does help confirm and reinforce this feature of the procurement. The authors provide data suggesting that the modified or perpendicular incision over the iliac crest does lessen the morbidity associated with harvesting the bone graft, both short term and long term, but particularly the latter.

B.F. Morrey, M.D.

Intra-articular Morphine and Clonidine Produce Comparable Analgesia but the Combination Is Not More Effective

Gentili M, Houssel P, Osman M, et al (Hôpital Tenon, Paris)
Br J Anaesth 79:660–661, 1997   3–2

Introduction.—Intra-articular morphine is commonly used to provide analgesia after arthroscopic knee surgery. Analgesia can also be obtained with intra-articular clonidine. These 2 drugs have synergistic analgesic effects when given intrathecally, but not when given intravenously. Their analgesic effects when given intra-articularly, alone and in combination, were assessed.

Methods.—The prospective, randomized trial included 90 patients undergoing knee arthroscopy with general anesthesia. They were randomized to receive intra-articular injection of 20 mL or isotonic saline solution containing 2 mg of morphine, 150 µg of clonidine, or both. The analgesic effects, including postoperative pain on a visual analog scale and time for rescue medication, were assessed in double-blind fashion.

Results.—The 2 groups had similar pain scores, which decreased over time. There was no significant difference in the number of patients who required additional postoperative analgesia. There were no changes in arterial pressure or heart rate, and no sedation or other side effects.

Conclusions.—For patients undergoing knee arthroscopy, intra-articular morphine and clonidine offer comparable analgesic effects. There is no apparent additive effect when the 2 drugs are used in combination. With either treatment, pain scores are low and the need for rescue medication is limited.

▶ As surgeons continue to explore more efficient means of postoperative analgesia, this controlled study provides some insight with regard to the increasingly popular intra-articular injection of morphine. Since the value of intra-articular morphine appears to be reasonably well established, opportunities to potentiate this mechanism have been sought. Double-blind, prospective studies are particularly effective in helping to resolve this issue. In this particular instance, a carefully performed and designed study failed to demonstrate that the addition of clonidine potentiated the effectiveness of intra-articular morphine. It is hoped that clinical practice will be predicated on the information derived from articles such as this.

B.F. Morrey, M.D.

Tissue Shrinkage With the Holmium:Yttrium Aluminum Garnet Laser: A Postoperative Assessment of Tissue Length, Stiffness, and Structure

Schaefer SL, Ciarelli MJ, Arnoczky SP, et al (Michigan State Univ, East Lansing)

Am J Sports Med 25:841–848, 1997   3–3

Introduction.—The effect of laser energy on joint-associated connective tissue has not been thoroughly assessed. Significant shrinkage of rabbit joint capsular tissue and reduced capsular stiffness have been observed in vitro after application of nonablative laser energy. There are no known in vivo trials evaluating the laser's effect on joint-associated connective tissue. A rabbit patellar tendon model was used to evaluate the effect of laser energy on the length, stiffness, and connective tissue structure.

Methods.—A calculated dose of holmium:yttrium-aluminum garnet laser energy (300 J/cm^2) was delivered to 1 randomly selected patellar tendon in 13 adult New Zealand White rabbits. The contralateral patellar tendon acted as control. Standard lateral radiographs were taken with radiopaque markers placed in the patella and tibial tuberosity to measure patellar tendon length. These measurements were taken before and 4 and 8 weeks after laser application. Limbs were not immobilized after surgery. Tendons were harvested at 0 weeks in 7 rabbits and 8 weeks in 6 rabbits. Tendons were examined for tensile stiffness, cross-sectional area, histologic changes, and electron microscopic appearance.

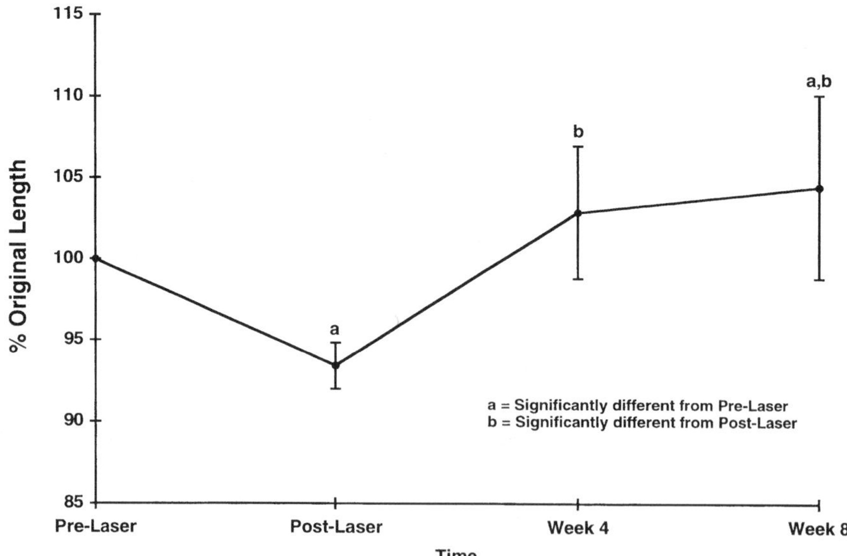

FIGURE 4.—Changes in tendon length immediately after laser application and at 4 and 8 weeks. (Courtesy of Schaefer SL, Ciarelli MJ, Arnosczky SP, et al: Tissue shrinkage with the holmium:yttrium-aluminum garnet laser: A postoperative assessment of tissue length, stiffness, and structure. *Am J Sports Med* 25:841–846, 1997.)

Results.—Significant tendon shrinkage was observed after application of the calculated laser energy dose. Tendon length increased significantly beyond the immediate postlaser length at 4-week follow-up and beyond its original length at 8-week follow-up (Fig 4). The lased tendons were significantly less stiff and had significantly greater cross-sectional areas at 8-week follow-up than controls. A generalized fibroblastic response and marked increase in cellularity was observed throughout the entire lased tendon. The normal bimodal pattern of large- and small-diameter collagen fibers was changed to a unimodal pattern with predominantly small-diameter fibers in the lased tendons.

Conclusion.—The observed tissue alterations in lased tendons indicate that the biologic response of connective tissue to laser energy causes additional compromise in tissue integrity beyond that attributed to the initial physical effects of the laser. Rehabilitative approaches must consider these changes.

▶ This is a most valuable contribution in that it attempts to provide some understanding of the immediate as well as the late-term soft tissue biological response to injury by laser energy. The fact that this experimental study revealed that biological response continues after the initial insult is particularly important. The additional fact that the long-term study showed that the injured lased tendons were significantly less stiff with greater cross-sectional areas prompts one to consider caution in adopting this approach when attempting to stabilize joints by laser treatment.

B.F. Morrey, M.D.

Femoral Lengthening Over an Intramedullary Nail: A Matched-Case Comparison With Ilizarov Femoral Lengthening
Paley D, Herzenberg JE, Paremain G, et al (Maryland Ctr for Limb Lengthening and Reconstruction, Baltimore)
J Bone Joint Surg Am 79-A:1464–1480, 1997   3–4

Objective.—Femoral lengthening by distraction osteogenesis involves protracted use of external fixation. To reduce time for the external fixator to stay in place, an intramedullary nail was inserted concomitantly with the external fixator. At the end of the distraction phase, the nail is locked with screws and the fixator is removed (Fig 4). This new method of lengthening was compared with the Ilizarov method.

Methods.—Between March 1990 and November 1993, 32 femoral lengthenings over an intramedullary nail were performed in 29 patients (12 male), aged 10–53 years. Patients were followed up for an average of 2.8 years. Patients were compared with 31 matched patients (17 male), aged 9–62 years, who had 32 Ilizarov femoral lengthening procedures. Mean duration of follow-up was 3.7 years. Procedures were compared

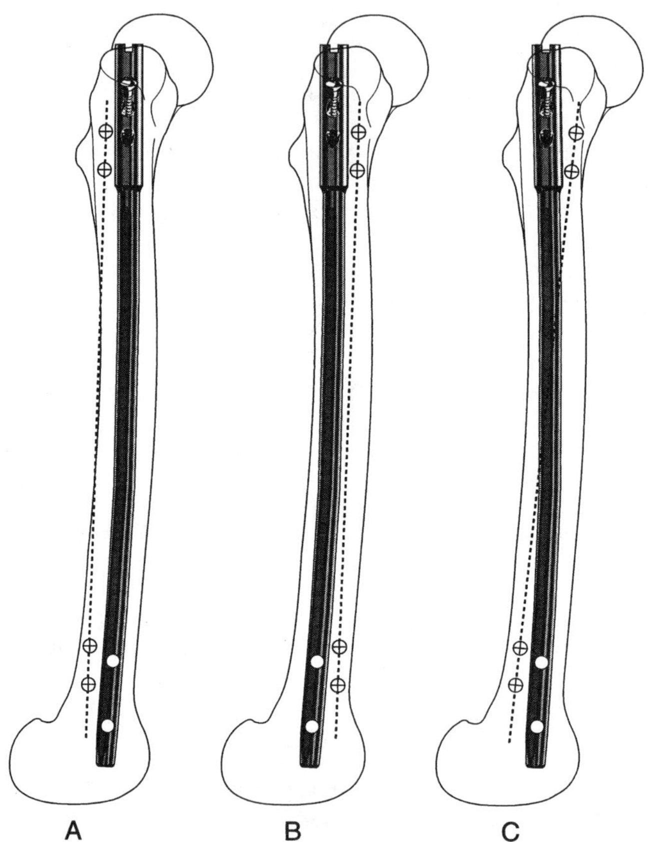

FIGURE 4.—Drawings showing preoperative planning for insertion of the half-pins around a nail during application of a monolateral fixator. With use of the Orthofix apparatus, all 4 half-pins must be inserted in 1 plane (collinear). Depending on the space available after placement of the nail, the 2 pairs of half-pins can be placed posterior to the nail (**A**), the 2 pairs can be placed anterior to the nail (**B**), or 1 pair can be placed posterior and 1 pair can be placed anterior to the nail. (**C**). (Courtesy of Paley D, Herzenberg JE, Paremain G, et al: Femoral lengthening over an intramedullary nail: A matched-case comparison with Ilizarov femoral lengthening. *J Bone Joint Surg Am* 79-A:1464–1480, 1997.)

with regard to the amount of lengthening, age of the patient, etiology of the indication for lengthening, and level of difficulty of the procedure.

Results.—Mean lengthening over an intramedullary nail was 5.8 cm, compared with 5.2 cm in the matched group. Average duration of lengthening over an intramedullary nail was 4 months, compared with 7.5 months in the matched group. The mean external fixation index for lengthening over an intramedullary nail was significantly smaller when compared with the matched group (0.7 vs. 1.7 months/cm). In the group with lengthening over an intramedullary nail, there were 23 excellent, 7 good, and 2 fair results. In the matched group, there were 26 excellent, 4 good, and 2 fair results. Normal knee range of motion returned 2.2 times faster in the group with lengthening over an intramedullary nail than in the matched group. There were 5 refractures in the matched group, and 1 nail failure and 1 locking screw failure in the group with lengthening over an intramedullary nail. The complication rates were 1.4% in the group that had lengthening over an intramedullary nail and 1.9% in the matched group. Lengthening over an intramedullary nail was more expensive and resulted in greater blood loss than the Ilizarov method.

Conclusions.—Despite the increased cost and blood loss, lengthening over an intramedullary nail resulted in a shorter duration of external fixation, a lower refracture rate, and a shorter rehabilitation.

▶ Fortunately, the need to adjust limb length is not common. Femoral shortening over an intramedullary nail is well recognized. The technique presented here combines methodologies, both of which have been previously reported. The one strength of this particular report is the effort to control or compare external fixation over an intramedullary rod with a group receiving lengthening only by an external fixation technique. This fact, along with the relatively large patient sample size, makes this a particularly worthwhile study. The high success rate is impressive, but it should be remembered that this was obtained by a surgeon experienced with both techniques. The complication rate in both groups is significant, and this is in keeping with the rate associated with each of the surgical techniques. The main strength of this report is demonstrating a relatively safe and effective technique. This information will be of value to all orthopedic surgeons, but the procedure itself should be carried out only by those comfortable and familiar with this or a similar technique.

B.F. Morrey, M.D.

Periprosthetic Low-grade Hip Infections: Erythrocyte Sedimentation Rate and C-reactive Protein in 23 Cases
Sanzén L, Sundberg M (Malmö Univ, Sweden)
Acta Orthop Scand 68:461–465, 1997   3–5

Background.—Several studies of the postoperative course of C-reactive protein (CRP) after uncomplicated total hip arthroplasties (THA) have been published. The erythrocyte sedimentation rate (ESR) after uncomplicated as well as infected THA has also been documented. However, the courses of ESR and CRP have not been studied in patients with low-grade infections but no fever, systemic illness, abscesses and fistulas, and with no local clinical signs of inflammation.

Methods and Findings.—Twenty-three patients were followed up from primary THA to revision for bacteriologically proved deep infection with a low virulent organism. Median time to revision was 14 months, with a range of 4–65 months. The median maximum ESR value during this time was 50 mm, and the maximum CRP value was 35 mg/L. Twenty-five of the 98 CRP values were normal, and 22 of 89 ESR values were less than

30 mm/hr. All CRP values were less than 20 mg/L in 6 patients, 5 of whom had an ESR of greater than 30 mm. Before revision, both values were normal in only 1 patient.

Conclusions.—Normal values and slight-to-moderate increases in ESR or CRP are consistent with low-grade periprosthetic hip infection. All patients scheduled for total hip replacement should have baseline ESR values established before surgery.

▶ This is an important topic and issue because low-grade infections, particularly with reoperations, continue to be a major problem for the orthopedic surgeon. Any means to enhance the preoperative suspicion or diagnosis of low-grade infection is of value. The role of the ESR and, even more importantly, the CRP has been somewhat controversial as conflicting reports have shown. The interpretation of the ESR is confounded by its tendency to remain elevated up to 1 year after routine total hip arthroplasty and to be altered by increasing age. Furthermore, the CRP is elevated after routine and noninfected surgical procedures.

This study does confirm that the ESR is more sensitive than the CRP for suggesting the presence of a low-grade infection. Unfortunately, an analysis of sensitivity, specificity, and predictive values were not provided. Although the numbers are probably too small to provide such information, it would have made this study more conclusive.

B.F. Morrey, M.D.

Are Antibiotics Necessary in the Surgical Management of Upper Limb Lacerations?
Cassell OCS, Ion L (Morriston Hosp, Swansea, Wales)
Br J Plast Surg 50:523–529, 1997   3–6

Objective.—Studies have shown no significant effect on wound infection rates of prophylactic administration of antibiotics for clean limb lacerations. Results were presented of a study of infection rates of antibiotic-treated lacerations compared with those untreated. Also investigated were, the overall infection rate when a standardized wound cleaning protocol is used and the wound or management factors likely to increase the risk of infective complications.

Methods.—In a prospective, controlled trial, 137 patients, age 2–84 years, with hand or arm lacerations received no antibiotics, and 113 patients, aged 3–85 years, were given IV co-amoxiclav before tourniquet inflation plus a 5-day oral course. All wounds were scrubbed with a Betadine brush and rinsed with saline, wound edges were excised and irrigated, and cut tendon sheaths were thoroughly washed. Patients were followed up for an average of 14 days. Wounds were assessed, and results were compared statistically.

Results.—A total of 226 patients (100 given antibiotics and 126 controls) were available for review. There were 21 lacerations of the forearm, 35 of the wrist, 118 of the finger, and 1 of the arm. The average laceration length was 33 mm in the antibiotics group and 27 mm in the control group. Time to surgery averaged 14 hours in the control group, significantly longer than the 12.3-hour average in the antibiotics group. Wounds operated on up to 48 hours after injury were included. The overall infection rate was 4%, with the 5% rate in the antibiotics group not significantly different from the 3.2% rate in the control group. Time to surgery and site or extent of injury did not influence infection rate.

Conclusion.—Prophylactic administration of antibiotics for upper limb lacerations does not significantly alter the infection rate if a standardized wound cleaning protocol, including débridement, is adhered to.

▶ This interesting study is strengthened by the fact that it is a prospective, randomized one. Although the study design is not perfect, it does make an effort to control the variables such that the only difference is the presence or absence of antibiotics. It is particularly stimulating in that it does not support the time-honored tradition of the surgeon to use prophylactic antibiotics to avoid infection in the setting of contaminated lacerations. The emphasis on the fact that debridement is the primary barrier or variable relating to avoidance of infection is an important one. It is also important to recognize that other studies support the finding that prophylactic antibiotics are not necessary in the setting described. Whether the recommendations will be followed will depend, to a great extent, on the emotions, as well as the experience, of the surgeon.

B.F. Morrey, M.D.

Quality Assessment of Intraoperative Blood Salvage and Autotransfusion

Spain DA, Miller FB, Bergamini TM, et al (Univ of Louisville, Ky)
Am Surg 63:1059–1064, 1997   3–7

Introduction.—Once little used, intraoperative blood salvage has come into widespread use as a means of reducing exposure to banked blood. Little information is available on the quality of autotransfused blood, which may contain plasma, heparin, and free hemoglobin released from damaged cells. These factors can play a role in the adverse sequelae of autotransfusion. The quality of autotransfused blood was evaluated in patients undergoing various types of surgical procedures.

Methods.—Blood salvaged intraoperatively from 1,593 patients over a 6-year period was tested. Fifty-nine percent of patients were undergoing cardiac procedures, 15% orthopedic procedures, and 13% vascular procedures. A double-lumen catheter anticoagulated with heparin was used to collect the blood, which was then filtered, centrifuged, and washed with saline. Blood quality parameters tested included hematocrit, heparinization, fibrinogen, and free hemoglobin.

Results.—The average yield of salvaged blood was highest for vascular cases and lowest for orthopedic cases, 1,073 vs. 378 mL. Orthopedic cases were also associated with the lowest hematocrit, 39%. Average red cell mass recovered in orthopedic cases was less than 1 U of packed red blood cells, compared with 2.4 U in cardiac cases and 2.9 U in vascular cases. The blood samples showed little residual heparin activity, even when taken from patients undergoing systemic anticoagulation. Free hemoglobin concentration was 476 mg/L in children, lower than in adults undergoing any type of operation. Most specimens had undetectable fibrinogen, measured as a marker of residual plasma.

Conclusions.—Blood salvaged intraoperatively appears to be of high quality, with good hematocrit, low heparin, and minimal plasma. Free hemoglobin levels vary by type of procedure. Further technical advances are needed to address potential concerns about plasma and neutrophil activation.

▶ These investigators demonstrate that the so-called quality of knee intraoperative blood salvaged and retransfused has increased in recent years to provide a very reproducible, high-quality, and effective replacement option. It is of interest to note that of the various surgical procedures in which the technique was employed, including vascular, cardiac, and orthopedic, the volume of salvaged blood and, therefore, the utility of this approach, was less for the orthopedic cases. In our practice, intraoperative salvage and autotransfusion is not used routinely but is reserved for those patients undergoing revision procedures who are thought and known to have a higher volume of loss and, thus, benefit greatest from the technique.

B.F. Morrey, M.D.

Blood Salvage After Total Hip and Total Knee Arthroplasty

Xenakis TA, Malizos KN, Dailiana Z, et al (Univ of Ioannina, Greece)
Acta Orthop Scand 68:135–138, 1997   3–8

Background.—Because of the risk of infectious disease transmission, attempts have been made to avoid using homologous blood transfusions for trauma and reconstructive orthopedic procedures. The effect of postoperative collection and reinfusion of unwashed, filtered, salvaged blood alone and combined with preoperative predeposited blood on the transfusion requirements of patients undergoing a total hip or total knee replacement was investigated.

Methods.—Three hundred seventy-five patients were included in the prospective study. Two hundred eight patients were treated with postoperative blood salvage using the CBC ConstaVac autotransfusion system and closed suction drainage. Another 50 patients predeposited 1 to 4 units of autologous blood, which they received in addition to blood salvaged postoperatively. The remaining 117 patients served as control subjects, receiving transfusions with homologous blood from the blood bank.

Findings.—Postoperative reinfusion of salvaged blood reduced the need for homologous transfusion after hip and knee arthroplasty, compared with the need of the control subjects. These 2 groups needed a mean of 2.7 and 4.2 units, respectively. The combination of postoperative reinfusion of salvaged blood and predeposited autologous blood was associated with the lowest requirement for homologous blood transfusions: a mean of 1.7 units.

Conclusion.—The use of preoperatively deposited autologous blood and postoperatively salvaged unwashed, filtered blood minimizes the need for transfusion of homologous blood in patients undergoing total hip or total knee arthroplasty. Patients scheduled for orthopedic surgeries associated with significant blood loss should deposit at least 3 units of autologous blood before the procedure.

▶ This report offers information that is intuitively obvious. A re-infusion of salvage blood will lessen the need for transfusions, whether it be homologous or autologous. Although there is relatively little question of effectiveness of either re-infusion, or autologous collection and re-infusion, there is a growing debate with regard to the cost-effectiveness of either option. The small, but real, reaction that occurs even with the autologous collection and the high discard rate have prompted some practices to question the validity of the routine use of this clinical practice.

B.F. Morrey, M.D.

Mortality and Rehabilitation Following Hip Fracture: A Study of 202 Elderly Patients

Stavrou ZP, Erginousakis DA, Loizides AA, et al (Evangelismos Hosp, Athens, Greece)
Acta Orthop Scand 68:89S–91S, 1997   3–9

Introduction.—With the growing elderly population, it is important to determine the optimal management, prevention, and economic impact of hip fractures. It is estimated that by the year 2050, the incidence of hip fracture will triple in elderly people. Risk factors that contribute to mortality and compromise rehabilitation were assessed in 202 elderly patients with hip fracture.

Findings.—The mean age of 149 female and 53 male patients was 76 years. A compression screw and plate was used for pertrochanteric fractures in 149 patients, and Thompson's hemiarthroplasty with acrylic cement was used in 46 patients. Thirty-seven patients (18%) died during the first year after the fracture. Mortality was associated with increasing age (Fig 1). Patients with surgical delay of more than 3 days had a higher rate of mortality, compared with patients who underwent surgery within 3 days of fracture (68% vs. 32%). The incidence of mortality was significantly increased (30%) after hip fracture in patients with cardiovascular disease. Patients who underwent hemiarthroplasty had a higher mortality

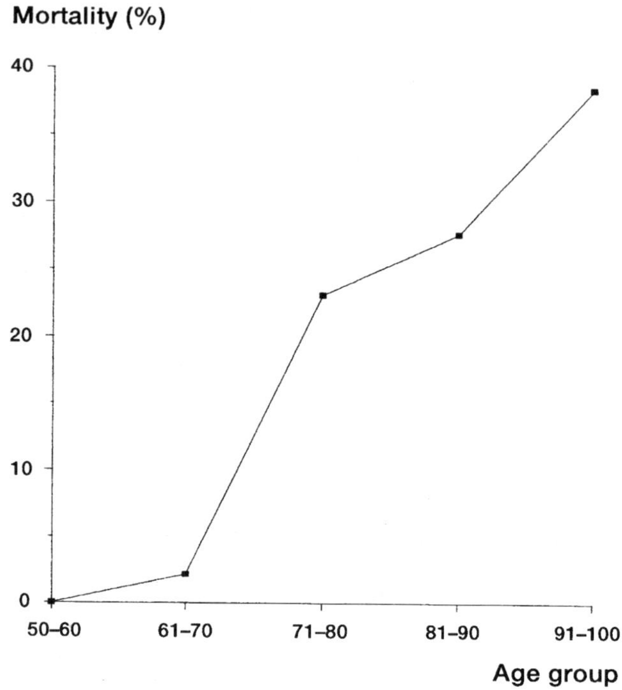

FIGURE 1.—Percentage of mortality according to the patient's age, with dramatic increase after the age of 60 years. (Courtesy of Stavrou ZP, Erginousakis DA, Loizides AA: Mortality and rehabilitation following hip fracture: A study of 202 elderly patients. *Acta Orthop Scand* 68:89S–91S, 1997.)

rate, compared with patients who underwent screw and plate fixation (33% vs. 25%). Half of the patients with preoperative walking problems remained bedridden after surgery.

Conclusions.—The general health of elderly patients with hip fracture, along with age, type of surgical procedure, and timing of surgery (on or within 3 days of fracture) are important determinants of survival and rehabilitation outcome.

▶ The major value of this report is the relatively large number of elderly patients in which the demographics allow the calculation of mortality rates shown in Figure 1. The exponential rise in mortality as a function of age strongly correlates with the increase of cardiovascular diseases, which follows a similar curve.

B.F. Morrey, M.D.

Hip Fracture in Elderly Men: Prognostic Factors and Outcomes
Diamond TH, Thornley SW, Sekel R, et al (St George Hosp, Sydney, Australia)
Med J Aust 167:412–415, 1997   3–10

Introduction.—Hip fracture is associated with increased morbidity and mortality in elderly females, but published data on hip fracture in elderly males are limited. Mortality and functional outcome were assessed in all elderly males aged 60 years and older admitted for hip fracture at a 650-bed tertiary care center during a 1-year period.

Methods.—All males admitted for hip fracture during 1995 were recruited retrospectively from medical records and evaluated prospectively at 6 and 12 months after the fracture occurred. Data were gathered for 51 males aged 60 years and older and 51 age-matched females regarding age; prognostic factors, such as pre-existing illness and osteoporotic risk factors; and outcome data, such as fracture-related complications, mortality, and level of function as determined by the Barthel index of activities of daily living at 6 and 12 months after occurrence of the fracture. Patients with local bone disease or high-impact injuries were excluded.

Results.—The median age of 51 males was 80. Forty-one of the 51 males (80%) were available for 6- and 12-month assessments. The proportions of males and females who came from institutions (32% vs. 28%, respectively) or required institutionalization after discharge (18% vs. 14%, respectively) were similar. The mean length of stay was similar for both sexes. Significantly more males died during hospitalization, compared with females (14% vs. 6%). Males had significantly more risk factors for osteoporosis, compared with females. Physical functioning deteriorated significantly in males from 14.9 at baseline to 13.4 at 6 months and 12.4 at 12 months after fracture. Males had a significantly higher prevalence of excessive alcohol consumption and current smoking, compared with females.

Conclusions.—Elderly males with hip fracture had significantly higher mortality and more risk factors for osteoporosis, compared with females. Males with hip fracture were similar to females in that they were usually fragile and had pre-existing medical illness and fracture-related complications contributing to their overall poor outcomes. Males had significantly higher rates of excessive alcohol consumption and current smoking, compared with their female counterparts.

▶ The significance of this paper is that it emphasizes issues referable to the male gender regarding hip fractures. The fact that males only represent approximately one third of the population sustaining hip fractures indicates that those who do sustain this injury may have factors that put them at increased risk. In fact, this study shows that this is the case, with the observation that this group of males with an average age of 80 years had higher-than-average osteoporosis risk factors than other males of comparable age. The significant observation that there is a higher prevalence of alcohol ingestion and smoking compared with that seen in females is particularly relevant. The analysis itself is less than ideal in that the females were matched with the males only as a function of age and possibly fracture type, and the control group of 51 females comes from a sample of 132, calling into question the validity of this particular sample as a control group. Nonetheless, the salient observation that males sustaining hip fractures are at increased risk with a higher short-term mortality rate is important information of which the orthopedic surgeon should be aware.

B.F. Morrey, M.D.

Development and Validation of a Clinical Prediction Rule for Prolonged Nursing Home Residence After Hip Fracture

Steiner JF, Kramer AM, Eilertsen TB, et al (Univ of Colorado, Denver)
J Am Geriatr Soc 45:1510–1514, 1997   3–11

Introduction.—The long-term consequences after hip fracture are substantial in most older adults. Clinical prediction rules are helpful in assessing prognosis and informing prognostic discussions with patients and caregivers. Clinical prediction rules based on risk factors for hip fracture have not been developed. The development and validation of a clinical prediction rule for prolonged nursing home residence 6 months after hip fracture is described.

Methods.—The prediction rule was created and validated from 2 prospective cohort investigations of patients age 65 and older with hip fracture. One investigation was a development study (DS) and the other a validation study (VS). Patients (344) with hip fracture admitted to 92 rehabilitation units or skilled nursing facilities were included in the DS. The VS included 239 patients with hip fracture from 11 integrated health care systems. Hospital records, nursing evaluations, and patient questionnaires were used to gather information about demographics, comorbidity, and physical and neuropsychological function. Predictors for a risk score to assess the likelihood of nursing home residence were identified.

Results.—In the DS group, 18.7% of patients resided in nursing homes 6 months after hip fracture. There were 4 independent risk factors for institutionalization: incontinence, being unmarried, dependence in ambulation, and cognitive impairment. At 6 months after institutionalization, 73.2% of patients with all 4 risk factors were hospitalized, compared with 0% of patients with none of the risk factors. In the VS group, 6.1% of patients resided in nursing homes 6 months after hip fracture. At this time, 50% of patients with all 4 risk factors resided in nursing homes, compared with 0% of patients with no risk factors.

Conclusion.—A clinical prediction rule was developed and validated; it accurately differentiated older patients with hip fracture who were at high risk for institutionalization at 6 months from patients who were able to return to community living.

▶ With increasing needs to optimally manage all of our patients, the disposition of individuals sustaining hip fractures is becoming even more challenging. This study provides 4 indicators that suggest long-term nursing home residence is required after hip fracture. They include being unmarried, incontinence, dependence in ambulation, and cognitive alteration. This paper provides statistical validity to these clinical impressions and is worthy of emphasis. The logical implication is that social services or other support groups will be consulted immediately when a patient with a fractured hip is brought into the emergency room.

B.F. Morrey, M.D.

Does Indomethacin Reduce Heterotopic Bone Formation After Operations for Acetabular Fractures?: A Prospective Randomised Study

Matta JM, Sienbenrock KA (Univ of Berne, Switzerland)
J Bone Joint Surg Br 79-B:959–963, 1997   3–12

Objective.—The incidence of heterotopic ossification (HO) after repair of fractures of the acetabulum ranges from 18% to 90%. Nonrandomized, retrospective studies have shown that indomethacin reduces the incidence of significant ectopic bone after surgery by 30% to 45%. The effect of indomethacin was assessed in a prospective, randomized trial of patients having operative treatment for acute fracture of the acetabulum.

Methods.—After surgery to repair a fracture of the acetabulum, 107 patients received either 25 mg indomethacin 3 times daily for 6 weeks ($n = 61$) or no prophylactic treatment ($n = 46$). Heterotopic ossification was evaluated at an average of 7.9 months using CT and an anteroposterior radiograph of the pelvis. Loss of more than 20% of movement and presence of grade 2 HO were defined as significant ossification.

Results.—There were 104 patients available for follow-up. Thirty indomethacin patients (52.6%) had no radiographically detectable ossification, compared with 19 control patients (43.2%). Four indomethacin patients (7%) and 1 control patient (2.3%) had grade 2 ossification. Three-dimensional CT showed that indomethacin patients had a median volume for HO of 1.5 cm³ and control patients had a median volume of 4.0 cm³. For patients having the Kocher-Langenbeck or extended iliofemoral approach only, 3-dimensional CT showed that the median volume of HO was 1.7 cm³ for the indomethacin patients and 3.6 cm³ for control patients. Three indomethacin patients and 1 control patient had grade 2 ossification. None of these differences was significant. Only male sex was significantly associated with median volume of HO. Measurement of HO by CT and plain radiographs were significantly correlated.

Conclusion.—Prophylactic indomethacin treatment after surgery for fracture of the acetabulum was not effective in preventing ectopic bone formation.

▶ Concern about the development of ectopic bone after acetabular fractures continues to be a major issue for the traumatologist, particularly when dealing with a male patient in whom the delay in treatment is required. The particular value of this investigation is that it represents a careful analysis of a cohort of patients studied in a prospective manner. As designed, the study shows no statistical difference between those receiving indomethacin and those in the control group.

Although the authors are to be commended on the careful design of their study, the percentage differences in the 2 groups is noted to represent approximately twice the frequency of extensive bone in those not given indomethacin treatment, compared with the treated group. The reason this has not reached statistical significance in all probability is because of the relatively small sample size. The real issue, of course, is whether indomethacin changes the clinical course by decreasing the incidence of clinically relevant ectopic bone. This study suggests that this probably is not the case and that treatment with this medication does not protect the patient in a measurable manner. This finding, therefore, should be of value to those dealing with ectopic fracture.

B.F. Morrey, M.D.

Detrimental Effect of Aging on the Endurance of Bone Cement: An In Vivo and In Vitro Study in Rabbits

Ioannidis TT, Kavadias C, Sdrenias C, et al (Athens Univ, Greece)
Acta Orthop Scand 68:115S–118S, 1997   3–13

Introduction.—Better and stronger bone cements are continually being sought for fixating prosthetic devices. Only a few trials have addressed the effect of degradation or aging on bone cement. The effect of aging on the compressive endurance of cement was compared during in vivo and in vitro conditions.

Methods.—Cement molds were implanted in the dorsum of rabbits. Other molds were maintained in stable conditions and darkness. Four in vivo and 4 in vitro molds were compared at 15 days and 1, 3, 6, 12, and 24 months. When rabbits were sacrificed, the molds were removed with surrounding soft tissues, which were histologically examined. Molds were tested in compression until failure, using an Instron machine (1 ton at a speed of 25 mm/min).

Results.—At all time points, the in vitro molds had significantly greater endurance than in vivo molds, with the exception of the 6-month period, when differences were not significant. Both the in vivo and in vitro molds had an increase in compression endurance up to 3 months. The in vivo molds were encased in a well-defined layer of fibrous tissue that increased in cellularity up to the third month, then almost disappeared by 1 year. There was a reappearance of macrophages and foreign body cells at 2 years, suggesting a "chemical aging" effect in the in vivo environment.

Conclusions.—Bone cement ages with a significant decrease in compressive endurance in the in vivo environment. The reappearance of inflammatory and foreign body cells at a later stage raises questions about the use of bone cement in joint replacement.

▶ This is an interesting and important clinical question, and the methodology provokes some question as to validity given the very brief duration of the in vivo and in vitro study samples. The obvious limitations of a prolonged in vivo experiment provide an understandable explanation of the in vivo testing in less than 2 years. It is particularly surprising to find that even with this very brief period, some in vivo mechanism seems to accelerate the degradation of the mechanical properties of the cement. The mechanism of such a process of course is not explained. The ultimate conclusion of the article, however, must be questioned—that these findings provide a basis for questioning the validity of the use of cement in joint replacement arthroplasty. Three decades of a high success rate would seem to effectively neutralize this position.

B.F. Morrey, M.D.

Coexistence of Dissimilar Metals After Conversion of Intertrochanteric Osteotomy to Total Hip Arthroplasty: 18 Patients Followed for 5–20 Years After Conversion

Papapolychroniou T, Vafiadis J, Zacharopoiulos K, et al (NIMTS, Hosp, Athens, Greece)

Acta Orthop Scand 68:38S-41S, 1997   3–14

Introduction.—The extraction of old internal fixation devices, especially those used up until the late 1970s, may cause excessive trauma to the femoral shaft in patients with conversion of failed intertrochanteric osteotomy to total hip arthroplasty (THA). The outcome of leaving part or all of the old osteosynthetic material during conversion of failed intertrochanteric osteotomy to THA to decrease the risk of excessive trauma was studied.

Methods.—Between 1975 and 1991, conversion of failed intertrochanteric osteotomies to THA were performed in 48 patients who had previously undergone internal fixation. During surgery, it was not possible to remove the osteosynthetic material without a high risk of severe complications in 10 of 48 patients. Screw fragments were left in the canal in an additional 8 patients. Insertion of the cement and prosthetic stem was completed with unexpected ease in the 18 patients in whom osteosynthetic material was left. The internal fixation device was successfully removed from 29 hips. In 1 patient, removal was so tedious that the shaft of the femur was extensively damaged and surgery needed to be terminated. The patient underwent revision 3 weeks later.

Results.—There were no clinical problems in the 37 patients available at a mean follow-up of 10 years. There were no signs of loosening and only occasional osteoporosis of the greater trochanter on radiographic follow-up. Clinical and radiographic findings were similar for 20 patients in whom osteosynthetic material was completely removed and 11 patients in whom at least part of the material was still in place.

Conclusions.—Theoretically, the coexistence of different materials in the femoral shaft should be avoided, but none of the patients in this cohort seemed to have difficulty with some or all of the osteosynthetic device remaining and the addition of new material. There seems to be no disadvantage to performing THA and leaving the old internal fixation material in place.

▶ This paper offers an interesting observation, with significant long-term follow-up of 10 years of a reasonably large cohort of 48 patients. The central issue is one that commonly occurs in the course of performing difficult reoperations in which all or a part of the previous fixation device is, of necessity, left in situ and a dissimilar metal is inserted juxtaposed or in close proximity. Although the interaction of dissimilar metals is known to theoretically pose potential problems, relatively little clinical information validates this concern. This study further supports the practice of avoiding the difficult removal of some metal fixation devices brought about by concern of the reaction of the dissimilar metals.

B.F. Morrey, M.D.

Chronic Exertional Compartment Syndrome: MR Imaging at 0.1 T Compared With Tissue Pressure Measurement
Eskelin MKK, Lötjönen JMP, Mäntysaari MJ (Central Military Hosp, Helsinki; Helsinki Univ)
Radiology 206:333–337, 1998   3–15

Background.—In patients with chronic exertional compartment syndrome, repetitive muscle loading causes increased intracompartmental pressure, probably as a result of tissue edema. This leads to reductions in arteriovenous pressure gradient and muscle perfusion. The ability of MRI to detect changes in water distribution has led to its use to visualize muscles involved in compartment syndromes. Compartment syndromes are usually diagnosed by invasive intracompartmental pressure measurement. Low–field-strength MRI was studied as an alternative approach to diagnosis of chronic exertional compartment syndrome.

Methods.—The study included 13 soldiers in training who developed clinical evidence of chronic exertional compartment syndrome in the anterior tibial compartment. Before and immediately after a standardized treadmill exercise protocol, the subjects were examined with MRI using a 0.1-T scanner and wih intracompartmental pressure measurements. Four controls without lower leg pain were also examined with MRI. The MRI signal intensity in the suspected involved compartment was compared with that in unaffected lower leg tissues, such as the subcutaneous fat, tibial bone marrow, or the superficial posterior compartment.

Results.—The results of intracompartmental pressure measurements were positive for compartment syndrome in 6 of the 13 patients, borderline in 2, and negative in 5. For patients with suspected compartment syndrome, the exercise-related change in normalized MR signal intensity was significantly correlated with the change in measured intracompartmental pressure and the absolute measured pressure after exercise. For patients in whom invasive measurements showed increased compartment pressures after exercise, the increase in normalized signal intensity from rest to exercise was significantly greater than in the control group or in patients with a normal or borderline increase in intracompartmental pressure. The control group and the "normal or borderline" group had a similar MR signal response to exercise.

Conclusions.—Low–field-strength MRI, performed at rest and immediately after exercise, may be a useful approach to diagnosis of chronic exertional compartment syndrome. The study shows a high correlation between the increases in intracompartmental pressure and in MR signal intensity after exercise, suggesting that MRI is also useful in assessing the severity of compartment syndrome. The combination of MRI findings and physiologic measurements may be of value in the pathophysiology of compartment syndrome.

▶ Fortunately, chronic exertional compartment syndrome is not too common except in a certain patient population type. Because this can be such a disabling disease, and since the diagnosis is often difficult and requires an invasive technique, this is an important contribution as a reliable, noninvasive method of making the diagnosis.

The experimental design is well thought out and has been carefully executed. The sample size is sufficiently large to allow the question to be adequately addressed. Finally, the results as statistically analyzed do show a conclusion that is supported by the authors' intrepretation of the data. Thus, this is a strong contribution to the literature and provides a significant enhancement of our ability to diagnose chronic exertional compartment syndrome in a noninvasive manner. While the calculation of the diagnosis was significantly different from controls, it would be helpful to have had a sensitivity, specificity, and accuracy calculation as well.

B.F. Morrey, M.D.

4 Trauma and Amputation Surgery

Introduction

In this year's crop of 35 peer-review articles, an unusually strong group pertaining to amputation surgery should advance our knowledge and the care of patients. Enhanced techniques in the management of postoperative and phantom pain are apparent, as are fresh visits to the issue of techniques to determine amputation level and the high morbidity of foot wounds in the diabetic. An excellent article points out that this surgery is not to be left to inexperienced surgeons for optimum patient outcome.

In the Trauma section of this chapter, we have an excellent randomized controlled trial on hip fracture management (Abstract 4–22) and a well-done outcome study of pelvic fractures in women (Abstract 4–20). This year, we have not increased the numbers of articles cited in the YEAR BOOK OF ORTHOPEDICS Trauma section that have as their foundation excellent research design. We need to continue to work to improve the knowledge foundation on which we practice the subspeciality of orthopedic traumatology and pay careful attention to the highest quality research designs.

There are several good basic science projects that add to the knowledge on which we base our practice. These concepts need to be tested by using the above-noted improved experimental designs in the clinical setting at this point. This year's selected articles also bring us increased knowledge of adult respiratory distress syndrome as it relates to femur trauma, as well as new techniques and approaches for managing complex femur and tibia fractures. There is so much more work to be done. . . .

Marc F. Swiontkowski, M.D.

Amputation Surgery

Lower Limb Amputation and Grade of Surgeon

White SA, Thompson MM, Zickerman AM, et al (Leicester Gen Hosp, England)

Br J Surg 84:509–511, 1997   4–1

Introduction.—A goal of lower limb amputation is to balance the patient's ability to remain mobile with a prosthetic limb against an acceptable level of morbidity and mortality. None of the tests used to predict successful wound healing and limb fitment, such as Doppler indices and skin perfusion pressure, have gained widespread acceptance. Patients who underwent major lower limb amputations during a 5-year period were reviewed for clinical and operative factors predictive of independent ambulation.

Methods.—Patients were treated at 2 major teaching hospitals between 1989 and 1993. The 172 patients had 193 lower limb amputations for peripheral vascular disease. Amputations were below-knee in 98 cases, above-knee in 86, and through-knee in 9. The patients were classified according to mobility levels and divided into those who could walk with a prosthetic limb and those who were unable to walk independently.

Results.—After amputation, 110 patients were considered unsuitable for prosthetic limb fitting and walking rehabilitation. The remaining 62 patients were referred for prosthetic limbs and walking training. Significantly more of the former group had undergone above-knee amputations. In the latter group, 72% could walk independently, either with or without walking aids, after rehabilitation. Among patients who could walk, the median duration of rehabilitation from surgery to discharge was 125 days. Walkers and non-walkers did not differ significantly in most risk factors (Table 1), but there was a trend toward independent ambulation in those having a below-knee amputation. Final outcome did appear to be influ-

TABLE 1.—Risk Factor Analysis for Nonwalkers vs. Walkers

Risk	Non-walkers n = 18)	Walkers (n = 44)
Median age (years)	71	72
Sex (male)	11 (61)	26 (59)
Rest pain	6 (33)	15 (34)
Gangrene	12 (66)	26 (59)
Diabetes	8 (44)	20 (45)
Ischaemic heart disease	4 (22)	10 (23)
Smoking	6 (33)	18 (41)
Vascular reconstruction	12 (66)	31 (70)
Grade of surgeon (junior)*	12 (66)	18 (41)
Amputation level (below-knee)	9 (50)	32 (73)

Note: Values in parentheses are percentages.

*P < 0.05.

(Courtesy of White SA, Thompson MM, Zickerman AM, et al: Lower limb amputation and grade of surgeon. *Br J Surg* 84:509–511. Copyright 1997, Blackwell Science Ltd.)

TABLE 2.—Risk Factor Differences Between Junior and Senior Surgeons

Risk	Junior surgeons operating (*n* = 30)	Senior surgeons and consultants operating (*n* = 32)
Median age (years)	72	72
Gangrene	19 (63)	16 (50)
Diabetes	16 (53)	11 (34)
Ischaemic heart disease	10 (33)	6 (19)
Smoking	11 (37)	12 (38)
Vascular reconstruction	24 (80)	20 (63)
Amputation level (below-knee)	13 (43)	17 (53)
Stump complications*	15 (50)	8 (25)
Independent ambulation*	18 (60)	27 (84)

Note: Values in parentheses are percentages.
*P < 0.05.
(Courtesy of White SA, Thompson MM, Zickerman AM, et al: Lower limb amputation and grade of surgeon. *Br J Surg* 84:509–511. Copyright 1997, Blackwell Science Ltd.)

enced, however, by grade of the surgeon. Those operated on by a junior surgeon were more likely to have stump-related complications than those operated on by a senior surgeon or consultant (50% vs. 25%), and these complications were associated with nonwalking (Table 2).

Conclusion.—Independent ambulation after lower limb amputation is influenced by the presence of stump-related complications, and the rate of such complications is related to the experience of the operating surgeon. Senior trainees or consultants should perform surgery in patients likely to be referred for ambulatory training.

▶ This retrospective review points out the critical element of a surgeon's experience as it relates to patient outcome. The same phenomenon has been identified as a critical factor for the management of hip fractures. In order to give our patients the best functional results, great care must be taken with the technical aspects of adjusting the length of the bone and the management of the flap closure. These skills require experience and judgment.

M.F. Swiontkowski, M.D.

Phantom Pain and Sensation Among British Veteran Amputees

Wartan SW, Hamann W, Wedley JR, et al (Guy's Hosp, London)
Br J Anaesth 78:652–659, 1997
4–2

Background.—Virtually all patients undergoing amputation have various types of persisting phantom sensations. The relationship between such sensations and phantom pain remains unclear. The reported frequency of chronic phantom limb pain has a vast range—from 1% to 98%. The incidence and time course of phantom limb and stump pain in long-standing amputees, the possible relationship between phantom sensation and phantom pain, and the choice and efficacy of treatment were investigated in the current study.

Methods and Findings.—Five hundred ninety veterans with amputations were surveyed by mail. The response rate was 89%. Fifty-five percent of the subjects reported phantom limb pain, and 56% stump pain. Phantom pain and phantom sensation were highly correlated. The intensity of phantom sensation significantly predicted the time course of phantom pain. The condition worsened in only 3% of subjects with phantom pain. One hundred forty-nine subjects with phantom pain had discussed the pain with their family physicians. Forty-nine of these subjects were told there was no available treatment. Satisfactory methods for controlling phantom limb pain included transcutaneous nerve stimulation (TENS), analgesics, and nonsteroidal anti-inflammatory drugs (NSAIDs).

Conclusions.—Phantom pain is a major problem among long-standing amputees, with 47% reporting continuing pain. Equally common was stump pain, which is more treatable. Treatment with TENS, analgesics, and NSAIDs appears to be beneficial.

Randomised Trial of Epidural Bupivacaine and Morphine in Prevention of Stump and Phantom Pain in Lower-limb Amputation
Nikolajsen L, Ilkjaer S, Christensen JH, et al (Univ of Aarhus, Denmark)
Lancet 350:1353–1357, 1997   4–3

Introduction.—The development of phantom pain has been associated with severe preamputation pain. Previous studies have shown that the rate of phantom pain was lower among patients receiving epidural treatment for pain before the amputation; however, these studies have had small sample sizes, insufficient randomization, and nonblinded assessment of treatment and pain. Extra hospital costs are associated with the administration of an epidural treatment before rather than at the time of amputation. Whether postoperative stump and phantom pain is reduced by preoperative pain treatment with epidural bupivacaine and morphine was investigated in a randomized, double-blind trial.

Methods.—There were 60 patients scheduled for lower-limb amputation who were randomly assigned to morphine (0.16–0.28 mg/hr) and epidural bupivacaine (0.25%, 4–7 ml/hr) for 18 hours before and during the operation. There were 29 patients in the blockade group and 31 in the control group of epidural saline and oral or IM morphine. General anesthesia was administered to all patients for the amputation. After 1 week, and then after 3, 6, and 12 months, all patients were asked about stump and phantom pain. Consumption of opioids, intensity of stump and phantom pain, and rate of stump and phantom pain were measured.

Results.—In the blockade group, the median duration of preoperative epidural blockade was 18 hours, and in the saline group, it was 18.5 hours. In both groups, the combined median duration of postoperative epidural pain treatment was 166 hours. Phantom pain was seen in 14 patients

(52%) in the blockade group and in 15 (56%) in the control group after 1 week. At 3 months, phantom pain was seen in 14 patients in the blockade group (82%) vs. 10 patients in the control group (50%). At 6 months, phantom pain was seen in 13 patients in the blockade group (81%) vs. 11 in the control group (55%). At 12 months, phantom pain was seen in 9 patients in the blockade group (51%) and in 11 patients in the control group (69%). In both groups at all 4 postoperative interviews, intensity of stump and phantom pain and consumption of opioids were similar.

Conclusion.—Phantom or stump pain is not prevented by preoperative epidural blockade started a median of 18 hours before the amputation and continued into the postoperative period. Preoperative ischemic pain and postoperative stump pain, however, are reduced with epidural pain treatment.

▶ In the first study (Abstract 4–2), the prevalence of self-reported phantom limb pain following amputation is documented at 56%. This was a mail survey with a high response rate (89%). This is the first large study to document, in a community sample, the efficacy of transcutaneous electrical nerve stimulation units as well as nonsteroidal anti-inflammatory drugs in the management of this condition.

In the second article (Abstract 4–3), the efficacy of epidural bupivacaine vs. morphine is documented in a well-designed, randomized, controlled trail of 60 lower limb amputees. Although phantom and stump pain is not improved with bupivacaine epidural, postoperative stump pain is clearly affected. These techniques deserve further investigation in a larger sample. The use of perineural catheters for postoperative pain management also needs further investigation in clinical trial format.

M.F. Swiontkowski, M.D.

Surgical Morbidity and the Risk of Amputation Due to Infected Puncture Wounds in Diabetic Versus Nondiabetic Adults

Armstrong DG, Lavery LA, Quebedeaux TL, et al (Univ of Texas, San Antonio; Brooke Army Med Ctr; Mexican American Med Treatment Effectiveness Research Ctr, San Antonio, Tex)
South Med J 90:384–389, 1997   4–4

Background.—The majority of lower extremity amputations performed each year are related to diabetes mellitus. Outcomes between diabetic and nondiabetic patients admitted to the hospital for foot infections resulting from puncture wounds were compared in a retrospective survey.

Methods.—The study group consisted of patients admitted to a university hospital from 1985 to 1992 for foot infections resulting from a puncture wound. There were 77 diabetic patients and 69 nondiabetic patients. All patients had plain radiographs, incision, drainage, and exploration of the puncture site and collection of tissue samples for analysis and culture. All patients received parenteral antibiotics.

Results.—There were 32 lower extremity amputations in this study group. Diabetic patients were about 46 times more likely to have an amputation than nondiabetic patients. Diabetic patients were 5 times more likely to require multiple operations than nondiabetic patients. The average length of stay was twice as long for diabetic patients. The diabetic patients were older and more likely to have retinopathy, nephropathy, neuropathy, peripheral arterial occlusive disease, and osteomyelitis than the nondiabetic patients. The interval from injury to surgery was significantly longer in diabetic patients. There was a significant difference in hemoglobin, hematocrit, albumin values, and total lymphocyte counts between these 2 groups.

Conclusions.—As expected, morbidity from an infected puncture wound of the foot was much higher in diabetic than in nondiabetic patients. The diabetic patient is at a significantly higher risk for amputation and multiple operations after a puncture wound to the lower extremity.

Seasonal Variations in Lower Extremity Amputation

Armstrong DG, van Houtum WH, Lavery LA, et al (Univ of Tex, San Antonio)
J Foot Ankle Surg 36:146–150, 1997   4–5

Background.—A major etiologic factor for amputation among diabetic persons is infected neuropathic ulceration caused or exacerbated by increased activity. Because ambulation and activity are reduced in the winter, it may be expected that the prevalence of amputation among diabetic persons would be lower in that season. Seasonal variations in nontraumatic amputations among diabetic and nondiabetic adults were investigated.

Methods.—Data on 14,555 amputations performed in 1990 and 1991 were obtained from a New York state database. Amputations were classified by level (foot, leg, or thigh).

Findings.—Lower-extremity amputations in diabetic patients were most commonly done in spring. Among nondiabetic persons, such an amputation usually occurred in winter. Fewer amputations at the foot level were done in winter among diabetic patients compared with nondiabetic persons. The least common season for amputation at any level in either group was fall. More diabetic patients had an admission diagnosis of vascular disease at that time.

Conclusions.—These data appear to support the notion that cold weather, by limiting activity, protects against amputation in diabetic patients. Prospective studies that control for potential confounding variables are needed to further explore the relationship between season and nontraumatic amputation.

▶ It is a well-established fact that diabetics are at higher risk for limb loss following foot puncture wounds. In the first study (Abstract 4–4), this is nicely documented in a retrospective study. In the second study (Abstract 4–5), we note that summer is the most common season for this type of clinical phenomenon. It is apparent that foot protective mechanisms are not widely employed in the summer time, though in the winter they are clearly mandatory. Efforts should be directed toward educating diabetic patients about protective footwear, and frequent examinations for wounds should be performed. Puncture wounds, when they occur, are deserving of prompt aggressive treatment.

M.F. Swiontkowski, M.D.

Determination of Amputation Level in Ischemic Limbs: Reappraisal of the Measurement of TcPo$_2$

Wütschert R, Bounameaux H (Univ Hosp of Geneva)
Diabetes Care 20:1315–1318, 1997   4–6

Introduction.—Selection of the optimal amputation level in ischemic limbs requires a balance between the need to obtain primary wound healing and the desire to maintain maximum limb length to achieve successful rehabilitation. One method of predicting stump healing, the measurement of transcutaneous partial pressue of oxygen (TcPO$_2$), has been promoted as an aid in defining jeopardized extremities in patients with diabetes. A MEDLINE search was conducted to determine a critical TcPO$_2$ level at which the rates of stump failure and too-proximal amputation would be clinically acceptable.

Methods.—The computerized search for the period from January 1985 to November 1996 identified all studies with the keywords of transcutaneous oxygen tension and amputation. Selected studies had to be prospective, to have information about the outcome of the stump for levels of TcPO$_2$ ranging from 0 to 50 mm Hg, and to have the level of amputation determined by a surgeon mainly on clinical assessment and without knowledge of TcPO$_2$. Data from eligible studies were analyzed by means of receiver operating characteristic (ROC) curve.

Results.—Ten studies with 615 patients (51% diabetic) fulfilled selection criteria. The stump failed to heal in 101 cases (16.4%). Patients had a median TcPO$_2$ value of 35 mm Hg at the level of amputation. It was not possible to identify a threshold value below which the stump definitely failed to heal. The optimal TcPO$_2$ value appeared to lie between 10 and 20 mm Hg (Fig 1), and the difference of accuracy within this range did not reach statistical significance. Healing was predicted with an 80% accuracy with this cutoff.

Discussion.—When combined with clinical factors, preoperative measurement of TcPO$_2$ may help to predict stump outcome and level of ampu-

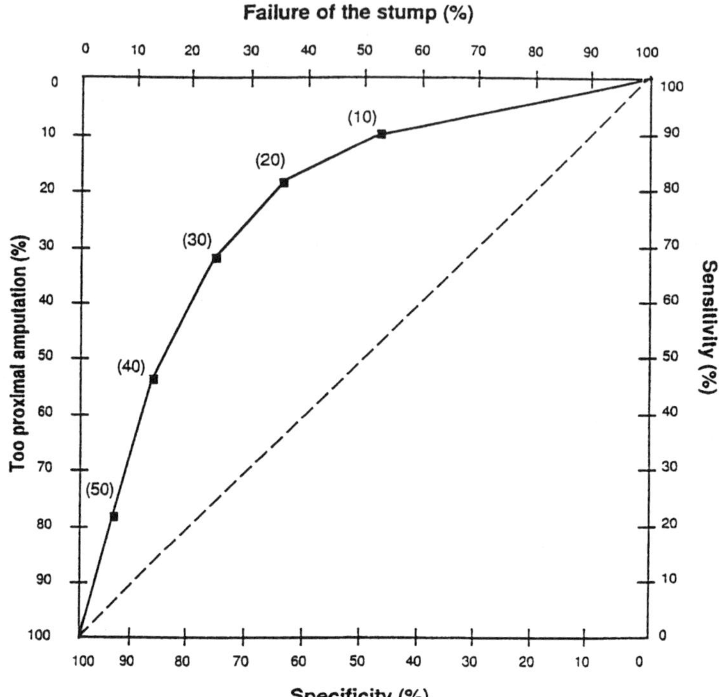

FIGURE 1.—Receiver operating characteristic curve analysis of accuracy of transcutaneous partial pressure of oxygen (TcPo$_2$) levels to predict optimal amputation level in 615 lower-limb amputations. The figures between *brackets* along the curve represent the respective TcPo$_2$ cutoff values. (Courtesy of Wütschert R, Bounameaux H: Determination of amputation level in ischemic limbs: Reappraisal of the measurement of TcPo$_2$. *Diabetes Care* 20:1315–1318, 1997.)

tation. Analysis indicates that 20 mm Hg is the optimal cutoff in the average situation, and that the cutoff should not be set above 30 mm Hg because of the rapid decrease in negative predictive value and accuracy beyond this threshold.

► We revisit the utility of TcPo$_2$ measurement in this structured literature review. This is not a formal meta-analysis because there are inadequate numbers of randomized control trials on which to base that research technique. In this literature review, TcPo$_2$ could be used as a predictor of amputation level with 80% accuracy. The compilation of information would suggest that 20 mm of mercury is a reasonable number to use in preoperative planning.

M.F. Swiontkowski, M.D.

The Performance of the ICEROSS Prostheses Amongst Transtibial Amputees With a Special Reference to the Workplace: A Preliminary Study
Dasgupta AK, McCluskie PJA, Patel VS, et al (St Mary's Hosp, Portsmouth, England)
Occup Med 47:228–236, 1997

4–7

Background.—The Icelandic Roll on Silicone Socket (ICEROSS) prosthesis, made from a silicone rubber sheet, is used primarily for suspension for transtibial prostheses. The ICEROSS is rolled over the stump, providing good skin contact, securing a good fit, and improving weight-bearing ability. The performance of the ICEROSS prosthesis among transtibial amputees in the workplace was investigated.

Methods.—Twenty-seven men with transtibial amputations were included. Sixteen were employed (group 1), and 11 were not (group 2). Data were collected by questionnaire interview, clinical assessment, and objective testing.

Findings.—Men in group 1 were younger than those in group 2. The main cause of amputation was trauma. Group 1 men with ICEROSS suspension performed better and had improved mobility. The men performed fewer dynamic activities than static activities in the workplace. Overall, the comfort and performance of men with ICEROSS were improved.

Conclusions.—The overall performance of the ICEROSS in cosmosis, suspension, and mobility appears to be better than that of the old prostheses. The ICEROSS can be worn successfully in the workplace.

▶ In this, the only study selected in the amputation section this year regarding prosthetic techniques, the silicone socket with the patellar tendon–bearing prosthesis yielded improved functional performance in a relatively young group of post-traumatic amputees. There is much to be gained from a structured, continued engineering approach to redesigning socket material and suspension systems for below-knee amputees.

M.F. Swiontkowski, M.D.

Musculoskeletal Trauma

A Critical Assessment of Factors Influencing Reliability in the Classification of Fractures, Using Fractures of the Tibial Plafond as a Model
Dirschl DR, Adams GL (Univ of North Carolina, Chapel Hill; Eastern Carolina Univ, Greenville, NC)
J Orthop Trauma 11:471–476, 1997

4–8

Objective.—Interobserver and intraobserver reliability for systems of fracture classification are disappointing. In a study of the Rüedi-Allgöwer classification of fractures, the tibial plafond was used as a model for factors that may influence reliability of the classification system: quality of

TABLE 1.—Interobserver Reliability of the Classification of Fractures of the Tibial Plafond and Effects of Level of Training

	Rüedi-Allgöwer classification of radiographs	Mean Kappa ± SEM Binary decision tree classification of radiographs	p value
All observers	0.43 ± 0.048	0.35 ± 0.038	> 0.25
PGY-3 eliminated	0.52 ± 0.072	0.39 ± 0.035	> 0.25

(Courtesy of Dirschl DR, Adams GL: A critical assessment of factors influencing reliability in the classification of fractures, using fractures of the tibial plafond as a model. *J Orthop Trauma* 11:471–476, 1997.)

the radiographs, ability of the observer to identify the fracture fragments, and the use of binary decision making.

Methods.—To test interobserver reliability, 2 orthopedists, 2 PGY-5 orthopedic residents, and 2 PGY-3 orthopedic residents (none of whom had knowledge of the classification of the fractures) reviewed pretreatment radiographs of 25 patients with fractures of the tibial plafond and classified fractures according to the Rüedi-Allgöwer system. Three months later, the observers classified the same fractures by marking the fragment of the tibial articular surface on the radiograph and classifying the fracture according to the binary classification system. Interobserver reliability was evaluated using a weighted kappa statistic.

Results.—The kappa coefficient averaged 0.43 for the Rüedi-Allgöwer system and 0.35 for the binary system. The difference was not significant. Level of training affected interobserver reliability (Table 1). Radiographs were evaluated as of adequate quality for classification purposes in 44% and 52% of fractures, respectively. The kappa statistic for agreement of adequacy of radiographs for classification purposes was 0.38 for the Rüedi-Allgöwer system and 0.25 for the binary system. Marking fragments on radiographs did not improve interobserver reliability. When the segments were premarked by the senior investigator, interobserver reliability improved significantly (kappa = 0.54).

Conclusion.—Interobserver reliability of fracture classification is low because of difficulty in identifying fracture fragments.

Assessment of the AO/ASIF Fracture Classification for the Distal Tibia
Martin JS, Marsh JL, Bonar SK, et al (Univ of Iowa, Iowa City; Rockhill Med Plaza, Kansas City, Mo; Univ of New Mexico, Albuquerque)
J Orthop Trauma 11:477–483, 1997   4–9

Purpose.—The classification is widely used in the assessment of diaphyseal and articular fractures. However, there have been no extensive assessments of its reliability and reproducibility, nor any comparisons with other common classification systems. The Association for the Study of the Problems of Internal Fixation Classification System (AO/ASIF) was compared with the Rüedi and Allgöwer system for fractures of the distal tibia.

The study also evaluated the benefit of CT scanning and the effect of observer reliability on fracture classification and other characteristics.

Methods.—The study included radiographs of 43 fractures of the distal tibia, including 14 cases in which CT scans were available. The images were evaluated by readers with greater and lesser degrees of experience, who classified them using the AO/ASIF and Rüedi and Allgöwer systems. The kappa coefficient of agreement was calculated. This information was used to compare the 2 classification systems for interobserver reliability and intraobserver reproducibility, and to examine the value of observer experience and CT scanning.

Results.—The AO/ASIF system showed good interobserver and intraobserver agreement in classification of fractures into types, significantly better than the Rüedi and Allgöwer system. However, classification of fractures into AO/ASIF groups was associated with poor agreement. Experienced readers generally showed better interobserver agreement, but there was no significant difference in intraobserver agreement. The CT scans led to better agreement on the percentage of articular surface involved. However, in both classification systems, the CT scans had no impact on interobserver reliability or intraobserver reproducibility.

Conclusions.—This study documents good observer agreement at the type level when the AO/ASIF classification is used to assess fractures of the distal tibia. However, agreement at the group level is poor. Although interobserver agreement improves with experience, the same is not true for intraobserver agreement. Although CT scans lead to better agreement on articular surface involvement, they do not improve agreement on classification. More study is needed to define those characteristics which can be reliably and reproducibly assessed on plain films and/or CT scans.

▶ In these 2 assessments (Abstracts 4–8 and 4–9) of AO/OTA and Rüedi–Allgöwer fracture classifications for the distal tibia, we identify problems regarding inter-observer reliability. These difficulties have been identified in hip fracture classification systems and distal radius fracture classifications systems, as well as soft tissue injury classification systems. The problem is not that of a poor classification system, but rather the necessity of forcing a continuous clinical/radiographic variable into a dichotomous variable (the classification system). We do not need new and different fracture classification systems. Instead, we should use them, when applying them to retrospective reviews of radiographs to document injury severity, in more thoughtful fashion. Separate radiographic grading should be performed by individuals blinded to treatment and outcome; 2 or more observers should be used. When there is a lack of agreement, consensus methodology should be used to reach agreement. The most senior and experienced surgeons should be used to classify radiographs whenever they are available.

M.F. Swiontkowski, M.D.

Open Fractures

Benzalkonium Chloride: A Potential Disinfecting Irrigation Solution
Gainor BJ, Hockman DE, Anglen JO, et al (Univ of Missouri, Columbia)
J Orthop Trauma 11:121–125, 1997   4–10

Introduction.—Débridement and copious irrigation of surgical wounds has reduced the incidence of infection, a serious complication that results in increased morbidity. When previous studies showed Castile soap to be more effective than some commonly used antibiotic solutions in reducing bacteria, other detergents/surfactants were investigated as potential irrigating agents. The disinfecting properties of benzalkonium chloride, a cationic disinfectant were examined.

Methods.—In this in vitro study, pieces of bovine muscle (2.5 cm $\times$ 0.5 cm $\times$ 0.5 cm) were aseptically cut from the center of freshly harvested beef muscle, then incubated with 1.0×10^7 colony-forming units of bacteria for 15 minutes. The muscle strips were irrigated with 100 mL, 1 L, or 10 L of benzalkonium chloride at a 1:2000 concentration in normal saline; control strips were irrigated with normal saline only. Adherent bacteria was removed from the muscle strips by sonication, and the sonicate was cultured to determine the number of living organisms.

Results.—Strips of bovine muscle were contaminated with *Staphylococcus aureus*, slime producing *Staphylococcus epidermidis*, and *Pseudomonas aeruginosa*. In all experiments, benzalkonium chloride was superior to normal saline in decreasing bacteria in bovine muscle. No living bacteria could be recovered from the muscle strips when 10 L of benzalkonium chloride was used for irrigation. Increases in volume of benzalkonium chloride, but not normal saline, led to greater decreases in the amount of remaining bacteria.

Discussion.—Although the use of broad-spectrum antibiotic solutions for irrigation of orthopedic wounds is widely accepted, little experimental evidence supports this practice. Copious irrigation with normal saline has also been popular, but the findings of this in vitro study suggest that benzalkonium chloride solution may be superior. Previous problems with this disinfectant were traced to a contaminated shelf supply.

▶ In this in vitro study assessing the efficacy of benzalkonium chloride, the compound was identified to be superior to saline in terms of its bacterial side effects. Follow-up studies will be required to assess the impact of this compound on viable muscle, bone, and cartilage. One clear message from this study is that adequate solution volumes must be used to flood the surface area of the muscle tissue.

M.F. Swiontkowski, M.D.

Biomechanical, Scanning Electron Microscopy, and Microhardness Analyses of the Bone–Pin Interface in Hydroxyapatite Coated Versus Uncoated Pins

Moroni A, Caja VL, Maltarello MC, et al (Bologna Univ, Italy)
J Orthop Trauma 11:154–161, 1997   4–11

Introduction.—Pin tract infection, a major disadvantage of external fixation, appears in the areas in which pin is in contact with bone. Many methods have been used to avoid pin loosening and arrest pin tract infection. The bone–pin interface in hydroxyapatite-coated vs. uncoated pins was evaluated. This coating is now applied to several implant devices, including hip prostheses and dental implants.

Methods.—A test group of 14 sheep had 84 bicylindrical stainless steel external fixation pins implanted. Half of the pins were coated with hydroxyapatite and half were left uncoated. Seven sheep had 6 coated pins implanted in the left tibia, and the other 7 had 6 uncoated pins implanted in the left tibia; all right tibias were left intact. A linear external fixator was mounted on the pins, the medial tibial middiaphysis was exposed, and a 5-mm resection osteotomy was performed.

The animals were killed 6 weeks after the implant surgery. Four pins removed from each animal had extraction torque measured, and all pins were examined radiographically for pin tract rarefaction (defined as 0.5 mm or greater of radiolucency around a pin at the entry or exit cortex, or both). Two pins from each sheep were used for histologic, scanning electron microscopy (SEM), and microhardness analysis.

Results.—The pins coated with hydroxyapatite showed significantly lower radiographic pin tract rarefaction than did the uncoated pins. Group average insertion torque was greater in coated than in the uncoated pins

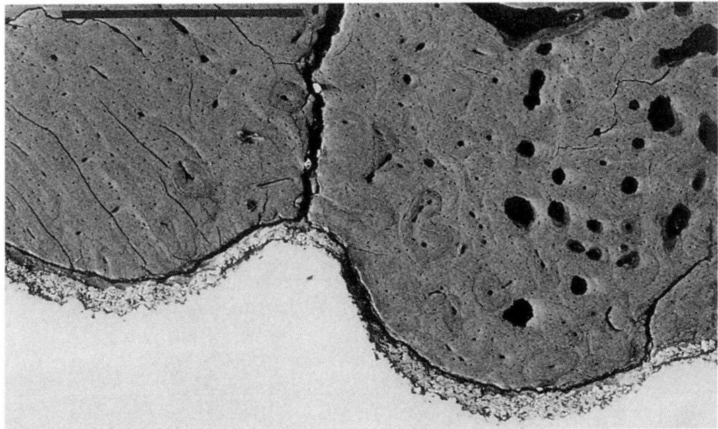

FIGURE 4.—Scanning electron microscopy showing extensive bony coverage of a hydroxyapatite coated pin. No coating delamination or resorption is visible. (Courtesy of Moroni A, Caja VL, Maltarello MC, et al: Biomechanical, scanning electron microscopy, and microhardness analyses of the bone-pin interface in hydroxyapatite coated versus uncoated pins. *J Orthop Trauma* 11:154–161, 1997.)

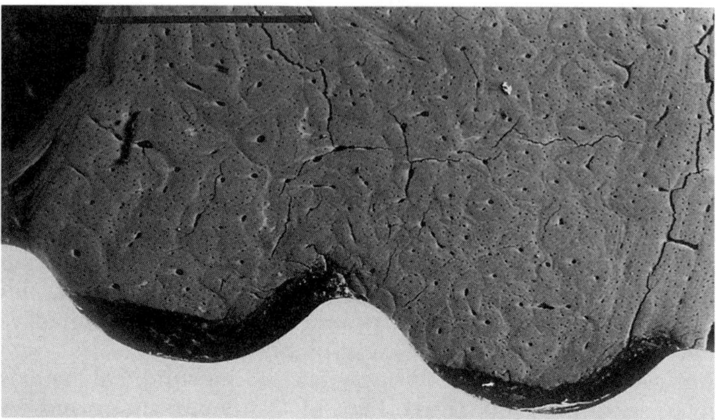

FIGURE 3.—Scanning electron microscopy showing a severe gap around an uncoated pin. (*Bar* = 1 mm.) (Courtesy of Moroni A, Caja VL, Maltarello MC, et al: Biomechanical, scanning electron microscopy, and microhardiness analyses of the bone-pin interface in hydroxyapatite coated versus uncoated pins. *J Orthop Trauma* 11:154–161, 1997.)

(960 N/mm vs. 709 N/mm), but the difference was not significant. Differences in group average extraction torque were significant: 1,485 N/mm in the coated group vs. 298 N/mm in the uncoated group. Histologic and SEM analysis revealed extensive bony coverage of the hydroxyapatite-coated pins (Fig 4). In contrast, uncoated pins (Fig 3) had many bone resorption areas, fibrous tissue proliferation, and encapsulation. Bone tissue close to the pins was softer than bone tissue far from the pins.

Conclusions.—Hydroxyapatite-coated pins significantly improved the bone-pin interface, compared with uncoated pins. Use of this bioceramic material may substantially enhance the stability of external fixation.

▶ External fixation is a critical piece of the armamentarium for the orthopedic surgeon in the management of open fractures. Hydroxyapatite coating for external fixation pins has be hypothesized to improve fixation and duration of pin-bone interface. In this animal model, the advantages of the coating are apparent. Utility for the trauma patient must now be documented in a controlled clinical trial setting, optimally with blinding of the observers determining loosening, pin track infection, and radiographic lucency.

M.F. Swiontkowski, M.D.

Intraarticular Findings After Gunshot Wounds Through the Knee

Tornetta P III, Hui RC (Kings County Hosp Ctr, Brooklyn, NY)
J Orthop Trauma 11:422–424, 1997   4–12

Objective.—Because gunshot wounds are becoming more common, appropriate treatment of gunshot wounds through the knee should be defined. The arthroscopic and radiographic findings in patients who had low-velocity missiles penetrating their knee joints were compared and arthroscopic management of these injuries was evaluated.

Methods.—Records of 33 patients (5 female), aged 13–62 years, with low-velocity gunshot wounds through the knee without significant soft-tissue or fracture injury were reviewed retrospectively. Radiographs were obtained of all knees, and arthroscopy was performed in 32 patients.

Results.—Radiographs showed bony fragments in 16 patients, bullets in 19, and debris in 10. No bullets, fragments, or debris were found in 7 patients. At surgery, 5 chondral injuries and 14 miniscal injuries were found. Debris was found in 17 knees. Of 7 patients without abnormal radiographic findings, 5 had a meniscal tear and 5 had floating debris on arthroscopy. Miniarthrotomies were performed to remove 7 bullets and to débride wound edges in 5 knees. The average hospital stay was 3 days, and no patient was readmitted for an infection.

Conclusion.—Because most soft-tissue injuries were not visible on radiographs, operative treatment is recommended for patients with low-velocity gunshot wounds through the knee. Wounds can be managed arthroscopically with bullet removal and débridement.

The Impact of Gunshot Wounds on an Orthopaedic Surgical Service in an Urban Trauma Center
Brown TD, Michas P, Williams RE, et al (Tulane Univ, New Orleans, La)
J Orthop Trauma 11:149–153, 1997   4–13

Background.—Little information exists on the impact of gunshot injuries on orthopedic practice in urban trauma centers. The prevalence of gunshot wound-related orthopedic injuries in 1 such center was determined.

Methods.—This retrospective study included 284 patients admitted in 1994 through the emergency department with a gunshot wound for which the orthopedic surgery service was consulted. Patients who died before or during attempts at resuscitation in the emergency department and those treated as outpatients were excluded.

Findings.—The 284 patients studied comprised 24% of all orthopedic admissions, 33% of the mean daily orthopedic census, and 14% of all patients undergoing orthopedic surgery. Eighty-seven percent of the patients were male. Ninety-four percent were African American (mean age, 27 years). About half were tested for alcohol or drug use or both; 45% were positive for alcohol, and 65% for drugs. Only 4% had private insurance.

Conclusions.—During this period of study, more orthopedic trauma resources were devoted to gunshot wound injuries than to any other single diagnosis. Discussions of the high percentage of U.S. resources devoted to health care compared with that in other nations should include considerations of the immense resources devoted to problems almost unique to the United States, such as the care of victims of violent crime.

▶ In the second article of this pairing (Abstract 4–13), the reality of the impact of gunshot wounds on an inter-city orthopedic trauma service is documented. The inter-relationship between assault with firearms and drug and alcohol abuse is apparent in this population. Continued efforts must be directed toward teaching youths in the urban setting conflict resolution and the elimination of routine carrying of hand weapons. Orthopedic surgeons can play an important role as educators, both in the community and in the school systems.

In the first article (Abstract 4–12), the authors delineate the impact of trans-articular knee wounds. Because of the high incidence of associated intraarticular pathology, operative management for transarticular knee wounds is recommended.

M.F. Swiontkowski, M.D.

Efficacy of Cultures in the Management of Open Fractures
Lee J (Univ of California, Sacramento)
Clin Orthop 339:71–75, 1997 4–14

Background.—The need for sequential or multiple cultures of open fracture wounds and the interpretation of such cultures are debated. The roles of pre-débridement and post-débridement bacterial cultures of open fracture wounds were further defined.

Methods and Findings.—Two hundred forty-five open fractures were analyzed retrospectively. Only 8% of the organisms grown before débridement eventually caused infection. Seven percent of the fractures with negative pre-débridement cultures became infected. Among the fractures that became infected, pre-débridement cultures grew the organisms responsible only 22% of the time. Infection was predicted more accurately by post-débridement cultures. However, of the fractures that became infected, the infecting organism was found in only 42% of the post-débridement cultures.

Conclusion.—Pre-débridement and post-débridement bacterial cultures from open fracture wounds appear to be of no value. The authors recommend that such cultures not be done.

▶ For years, individuals have been recommending pre-débridement and post-débridement intraoperative cultures as excellent predictors of deep infection. This retrospective review documents that this is a waste of resources. I am in agreement and have not used intraoperative cultures for the past 13 years. When there is concern regarding wound fluctuants or drainage, then it is the appropriate time to obtain a culture.

M.F. Swiontkowski, M.D.

Compartmental Syndrome

The Effect of Early Versus Late Fasciotomy in the Management of Extremity Trauma

Williams AB, Luchette FA, Papaconstantinou HT, et al (Univ of Cincinnati, Ohio)

Surgery 122:861–866, 1997   4–15

Introduction.—Fasciotomy for compartment syndrome is most effective when performed soon after the injury to the extremity. Recent studies report that the risk of infectious complications is increased when fasciotomy is undertaken more than 12 hours after the injury, and that nonoperative management is preferable in such cases. Rates of infection, neurologic sequelae, and limb salvage were retrospectively compared in 88 patients who underwent fasciotomy either early (less than 12 hours after injury) or late (more than 12 hours after injury), before and after 12 hours of injury.

Methods.—Patients were treated at the study institution during a 6-year period (1990–1995). Records were reviewed for demographics, injury severity score, associated vascular and orthopedic injuries, compartment pressures, details of fasciotomy, complications, and outcome. Follow-up data for more than 1 month were obtained for 76 patients.

Results.—Fasciotomy was performed early in 61 (69%) patients and late in 27 (31%). The involved compartments were in the leg in 59 cases, the forearm or hand in 15, the thigh in 12, and the foot in 2. Although the early group had a significantly lower rate of infection than the late group (7.3% vs. 28%), the 2 groups did not differ significantly in rates of limb salvage and neurologic sequelae (Table 1). Except for missile injuries, which occurred only in the early fasciotomy group, early and late groups did not differ in mechanisms of injury. The 3 patients who died had

TABLE 1.—Outcome of Compartment Syndrome After Fasciotomy

	Early (≤12 hr)	*Late (>12 hr)*	*>36 hr**
N	61	27	8
Male/Female	55/8	27/3	8/0
Age (yr)	35 ± 2.02†	33 ± 2.7	33 ± 3.7
ISS	16.1 ± 1.3	14.0 ± 1.7	14.5 ± 2.5
Compartment pressure (mm Hg)	66 ± 3.6	60 ± 4.9	58 ± 16
Infection	4 (7.3)	7 (28)‡	4 (50)‡
Neurologic injury	17 (29)	6 (22.2)	4 (50)
Amputation	2 (3.3)	2 (7.4)	2 (25)
Death (%)	1 (1.6)	2 (7.4)	0

Note: Numbers in parentheses indicate percentage of cohort.
*The >36 hour group is a subset of the late fasciotomy group.
†Mean ± SEM.
‡*P* ≤ 0.05 chi-squared analysis vs. early group.
Abbreviation: ISS, injury severity score.
(Courtesy of Williams AB, Luchette FA, Papaconstantinou HT, et al: The effect of early versus late fasciotomy in the management of extremity trauma. *Surgery* 122:861–866, 1997.)

significant associated injuries. No relationship was found between outcome and age, gender, presence of hypotension, mechanism of injury, vascular or orthopedic injury, or length of time to fasciotomy.

Discussion.—Fasciotomy for compartment syndrome should be performed as soon as possible after the injury, but many patients have subacute compartment syndrome after a delay of 24–48 hours. Although infection developed more often in patients who underwent fasciotomy after a delay of 12 or more hours, these patients had similar rates of limb salvage as those who were treated early. Thus, fasciotomy should be used aggressively, even when diagnosis of compartment syndrome is delayed.

▶ This retrospective review studies the outcomes of patients with compartmental syndrome released within 12 hours of and 12 hours after examination. The authors have identify similar rates of limb salvage and neurologic sequella. The rate of deep infection for those released after 12 hours is more than 4 times that of the patients released early. Since the authors judge only the outcome of limb salvage, which is a treatment decision, their recommendation of aggressive fasciotomy even 24 hours after the onset of the compartmental syndrome is called to question. Functional evaluations on patients released late with a subgroup treated without fasciotomy should be performed.

M.F. Swiontkowski, M.D.

Adult Respiratory Distress Syndrome

Experimental Fat Embolism Induces Urine 2,3-Dinor-6-Ketoprostaglandin $F_{1\alpha}$ and 11-Dehydrothromboxane B_2 Excretion in Pigs
Rautanen M, Gullichsen E, Riutta A, et al (Univ of Turku, Finland; Univ of Tampere, Finland; Inst of Isotopes of the Hungarian Academy of Sciences, Budapest, Hungary)
Crit Care Med 25:1215–1221, 1997   4–16

Introduction.—Patients with multiple fractures are at risk for the fat embolism syndrome, a condition whose pathophysiologic mechanisms are poorly understood. The hypothesis that altered prostanoid metabolism may be related to the development of pulmonary dysfunction in fat embolism was tested.

Methods.—The study was carried out on 27 male and female Finnish Landrace pigs with a mean weight of 26.7 kg. Anesthetized and mechanically ventilated animals were subjected to an intracaval infusion of 10% allogeneic bone marrow suspension (100 mg/kg over 5 minutes; 18 pigs) or to control saline infusion (9 pigs). Nine pigs in the bone marrow suspension group received an IV bolus of aspirin (300 mg) 1 hour before the infusion, then a dose of 150 mg/hr for 2 hours (aspirin-treated group); the remaining 9 received only the bone marrow suspension (fat embolism group). Hemodynamic and oxygen transport data were obtained for a period of 5 hours after the infusions.

Results.—The animals with fat embolism had unchanged mean arterial pressure and relatively stable central venous pressure and pulmonary artery occlusion pressure over time, but cardiac index decreased within 30 minutes. There was an immediate increase in mean pulmonary arterial pressure and pulmonary vascular resistance after infusion of the bone marrow suspension (from 23 to 34 mm Hg and from 305 to 585 dyne·sec/cm^5, respectively, and these variables remained elevated during the monitoring period. The fat embolism group also exhibited persistent increases in pulmonary shunt, together with instant and gradual decreases in PaO_2, hemoglobin oxygen saturation, and oxygen delivery. Aspirin treatment ameliorated the changes in pulmonary arterial pressure and partial pressure of arterial oxygen (PaO_2), abolished changes in pulmonary shunt and oxygen saturation in arterial blood (SaO_2), and significantly reduced urinary excretion of measured prostanoid metabolites relative to the fat embolism group. And, starting at 1 hour, excretion of the metabolites was also reduced when compared with the control group.

Conclusions.—This fat embolism model was characterized by pulmonary hypertension, increased pulmonary vascular tone, and increased pulmonary shunt. Hemodynamic effects of fat embolism may be associated with the changed relation of thromboxane A_2/prostacyclin, key agents in the pathogenesis of various forms of acute pulmonary insufficiency.

Pulmonary Effects of Fixation of a Fracture With a Plate Compared With Intramedullary Nailing: A Canine Model of Fat Embolism and Fracture Fixation
Schemitsch EH, Jain R, Turchin DC, et al (St Michael's Hosp, Toronto; Mount Sinai Hosp, Toronto; Univ of Toronto)
J Bone Joint Surg Am 79–A:984–996, 1997   4–17

Introduction.—Patients with a fracture of a long bone and multiple injuries are at risk for the development of fat embolism syndrome and adult respiratory distress syndrome (ARDS), and the mortality rate in such patients is reported to be 10%. Early fixation of the fracture is advised, but intramedullary nailing may cause additional embolization of marrow fat and exacerbate pulmonary dysfunction. The pulmonary effects of the timing and method of fracture fixation were examined by using a canine embolism model.

Methods.—Fat embolism was created in a group of skeletally mature mixed breed dogs. Reaming of the ipsilateral femur and tibia was followed by pressurization of the intramedullary canal. Eight control dogs had induction of fat embolism alone; 33 dogs had induction of fat embolism and internal fixation of a transverse fracture of the middle of the contralateral femoral shaft. Four control dogs were killed 4 hours after induction of fat embolism and 4 after 24 hours. Experimental animals had a femoral fracture created and fixation performed either 4 hours (15 dogs) or 24 hours (18 dogs) after embolic showering. Fixation was performed with

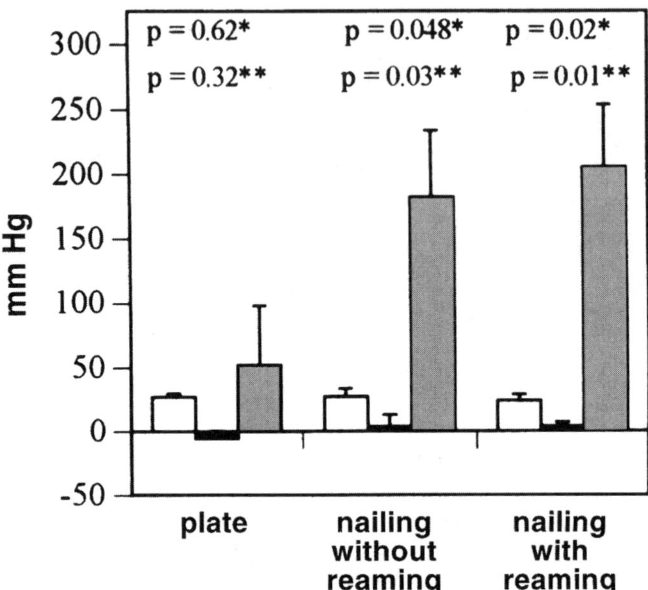

FIGURE 5.—Bar graph showing the alveolar-arterial P_{O_2} gradients over time in the group in which the fracture was fixed at 4 hours. The time intervals are baseline (*white bar*), 4 hours after induction of embolism (*black bar*), and 1 hour after fixation (*gray bar*). *Asterisk*, P values derived from comparison of the measurements made after fixation with baseline measurements; *double asterisk*, P values derived from comparison of the measurements made after fixation with those made 4 hours after embolization. (To convert millimeters of mercury to kilopascals, multiply by 0.1333.) (Courtesy of Schemitsch EH, Jain R, Turchin DC, et al: Pulmonary effects of fixation of a fracture with a plate compared with intramedullary nailing: A canine model of fat embolism and fracture fixation. *J Bone Joint Surg Am* 79-A:984–996, 1997.)

application of a plate, nailing with reaming, or nailing without reaming. Measurements of pulmonary arterial pressure and the alveolar-arterial gradient were obtained preoperatively, during induction of fat embolism, and up to 1 hour after fixation. The lungs, brain, and kidneys were examined for evidence of intravascular fat.

Results.—Control and experimental animals did not differ significantly in pulmonary artery pressure at baseline or at 4 and 24 hours after induction of fat embolism. Neither creation nor fixation of the fracture affected pulmonary arterial pressure. Fixation with a plate had no significant effect on the alveolar-arterial gradient, but this value was raised above baseline in animals that had fixation of a fracture 4 hours after embolization (Fig 5). Compared with animals that had fixation with a plate, alveolar-arterial gradients were 4 and 3.5, respectively, times higher in those that had nailing with reaming and nailing without reaming 4 hours after embolization. When fixation was performed 24 hours after embolization, the alveolar-arterial gradient was not affected by fixation method (Fig 6). The amount of embolic fat in lungs, brain, and kidneys was not affected by fixation at either 4 or 24 hours. Fixation increased pulmonary edema scores, but no differences among scores were associated with the 3 methods of fixation.

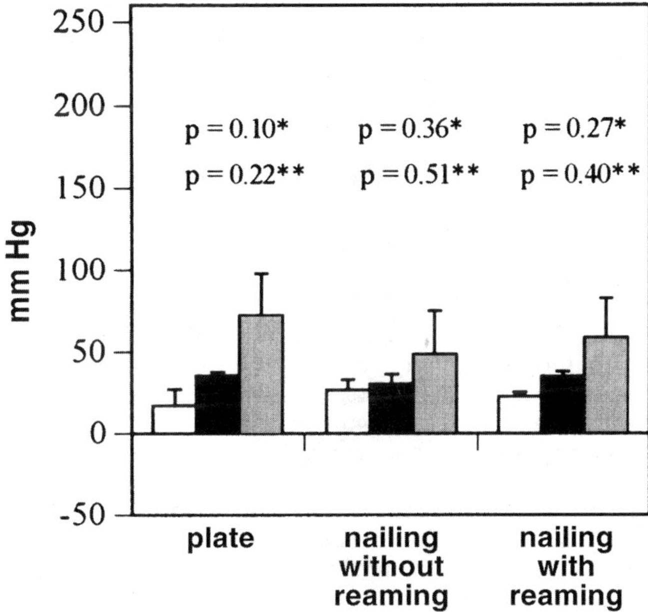

FIGURE 6.—Bar graph showing the alveolar-arterial P_{O_2} gradients over time in the group in which the fracture was fixed at 24 hours. The time intervals are baseline (*white bar*), 24 hours after induction of embolism (*black bar*), and 1 hour after fixation (*gray bar*). *Asterisk,* P values derived from comparison of the measurements made after fixation with baseline measurements; *double asterisk,* P values derived from comparison of the measurements made after fixation with those made 24 hours after embolization. (To convert millimeters of mercury to kilopascals, multiply by 0.1333. (Courtesy of Schemitsch EH, Jain R, Turchin DC, et al: Pulmonary effects of fixation of a fracture with a plate compared with intramedullary nailing: A canine model of fat embolism and fracture fixation. *J Bone Joint Surg Am* 79-A:984–996, 1997.)

Conclusions.—Method of fixation of a fracture appears to play only a minor role in the development of pulmonary dysfunction. Fixation produced no substantial evidence of acute inflammation of the end organ or effects on pulmonary artery pressure.

▶ In these 2 well-designed animal studies (Abstracts 4–16 and 4–17), we learn that pulmonary hypertension and increased pulmonary vascular tone with shunting are the major hemodynamic effects of fat embolism. The first study identifies thromboxane A_2 as the key compound. This information can be used to design future pharmacologic intervention for the pathophysiologic process.

In the second article, referencing techniques for internal fixation of associated femur fracture with adult respiratory distress syndrome, the authors identify in a dog model that the technique for fixation plays only a minor role. Similarly, they identify atrioventricular shunting and pulmonary hypertension as the major elements of pathophysiology. This basic research dovetails nicely with the clinical studies we've reviewed in the last 2 years. There does not seem to be solid evidence linking reamed femoral nailing in the multiple injured patient with a higher incidence of adult respiratory distress syndrome.

M.F. Swiontkowski, M.D.

Reamed Femoral Nailing in Patients With Multiple Injuries: Adverse Effects of Tourniquet Use
Pollak AN, Battistella F, Pettey J, et al (Univ of California, Davis)
Clin Orthop 339:41–46, 1997   4–18

Background.—Pulmonary microvascular injury can result from limb perfusion after tourniquet ischemia and from microembolization (such as that associated with reamed femoral nailing). Both processes lead to increases in pulmonary capillary membrane permeability and edema. However, the relationship between femoral nailing followed by tourniquet ischemia and clinical lung injury has not been reported.

Methods.—Seventy-two patients with femoral shaft fractures and tibial or ankle fractures treated by internal fixation between 1987 and 1993 were studied. Reamed intramedullary nails were used to treat the femoral shaft fractures. Tibial and ankle injuries were treated surgically with a tourniquet in 34 patients (group T) and without a tourniquet in 38 patients (group NT). Group T patients were further divided according to length of tourniquet time: T1 patients had the tourniquet applied for 90 minutes or less and T2 patients for more than 90 minutes. The groups were matched for injury severity.

Findings.—The NT group were dependent on the ventilator for fewer days and spent less time in intensive care than did the T group. The number of days spent dependent on the ventilator and in intensive care increased as tourniquet time increased.

Conclusions.—Combining reamed femoral nailing with fracture fixation under tourniquet control appears to increase pulmonary morbidity in patients with multitrauma. Further research is needed to measure pulmonary injury associated with ischemia reperfusion and intramedullary nailing in such patients.

▶ According to this retrospective case review, the use of tourniquets with reamed femoral nailing appears to be associated with increased pulmonary morbidity in multiply injured patients. It is likely that the products of tourniquet ischemia, in terms of platelet adherence and subsequent mobilization of thrombi, play a role in this phenomenon.

M.F. Swiontkowski, M.D.

Pelvic Fractures

Iliosacral Screw Fixation: Early Complications of the Percutaneous Technique

Routt MLC Jr, Simonian PT, Mills WJ (Harborview Med Ctr, Seattle)
J Orthop Trauma 11:584–589, 1997   4–19

Introduction.—There is ongoing debate over the operative treatment of displaced posterior pelvic ring disruption. Wound problems can result from open reductions performed through a posterior surgical exposure. An increasingly popular option for posterior pelvic internal fixation is iliosacral screws inserted from the lateral ilium across the sacroiliac joint and into the upper sacral vertebral body. Early complications associated with percutaneous placement of iliosacral screws are reported.

Methods.—The prospective study included 177 consecutive patients undergoing treatment for unstable pelvic ring fractures. There were 102 males and 75 females, mean age 32 years. In each case, closed manipulative reduction of the posterior pelvic ring was attempted. If fluoroscopy showed unacceptable reduction—more than 1 cm in any field of fluoroscopic imaging—open reduction was performed. A total of 244 percutaneous iliosacral screws were placed. Follow-up imaging studies included plain inlet and outlet radiographs at 6 weeks, 3 months, and 12 months; postoperative pelvic CT scanning; and yearly pelvic radiographs.

Results.—Postoperative assessment was available in 159 patients. None had posterior pelvic infections, and there were minimal problems with blood loss. Sources of complications included inadequate imaging, surgeon error, and failed fixation. In 18 patients, obesity or abdominal contrast led to inadequate fluoroscopic imaging. Surgeon error led to screw misplacement in 5 cases, 1 associated with a transient L5 neuropraxia. Seven patients had failed fixation; the causes were craniocerebral trauma, delayed union, noncompliance, or a deep anterior pelvic infection related to a urethral tear. Two patients had sacral nonunion, necessitating débridement, bone grafting, and repeat fixation. The best imaging study for assessment of reduction quality and implant safety was the postoperative CT scan, which revealed 19 malreductions.

Conclusions.—This experience underscores the difficulty of iliosacral screw fixation of displaced posterior pelvic ring disruptions. Although the sacral anatomy is variable, iliosacral screw insertion is safe if good triplanar fluoroscopic images of the accurately-reduced posterior pelvic ring are obtained. Supplementary techniques of posterior pelvic fixation may be needed for patients with anticipated compliance problems or those with craniocerebral trauma. There are few problems with infection, blood loss, or fracture nonunion.

▶ Late migration of posterior pelvic ring fractures with malunion and functional disability is a major problem. Over the past 5 years, percutaneous screw fixation has evolved as the optimal management for maintenance of reduction of these injuries. It should be done within the first 3–4 days after the injury to allow manipulative reductions without wide surgical exposures. The senior author of this publication has documented patient issues associated with imaging difficulties, as well as the difficulty in achieving anatomic reductions. The incidence of infection and non-union appears to be acceptably low. It is a technique which demands a high degree of conscientiousness in terms of preoperative planning, patient positioning, and screw placement.

M.F. Swiontkowski, M.D.

Effect of Trauma and Pelvic Fracture on Female Genitourinary, Sexual, and Reproductive Function

Copeland CE, Bosse MJ, McCarthy ML, et al (Univ of Maryland, Baltimore; Johns Hopkins Univ, Baltimore, Md)
J Orthop Trauma 11:73–81, 1997   4–20

Introduction.—Pelvic trauma in women can result in adverse effects on genitourinary and reproductive function. The impact of pelvic fracture on women's physical, sexual, and reproductive functioning were evaluated retrospectively, and findings were correlated to the mechanism, severity, and displacement of the pelvic injury.

Methods.—Eligible multitrauma patients were aged 16–44 years at the time of injury; excluded were those with spinal cord injury, severe head injury, psychiatric problems, or limb amputation. The final study group consisted of 241 women, 123 subjects with pelvic fracture and 118 controls with at least 1 extremity fracture but no pelvic fracture. Most women sustained multiple injuries in addition to the study injury. Those with and without pelvic fracture were matched for age, year of discharge, and severity of orthopedic injury. Patients were interviewed at an average of 4.1 years after the injury. The questionnaire stressed comparison of preinjury and postinjury status.

Results.—Urinary complaints were more common in women with pelvic fractures (Fig 1) than in controls (21% vs. 7%). Specific complaints reported significantly more frequently in the pelvic fracture vs. the control group were stress incontinence, frequency, and nocturia. Findings that correlated with the likelihood of urinary tract complaints included severity of the pelvic injury, initial fracture displacement of 5 mm or more, residual fracture displacement of 5 mm or more, and displacement of the hemipelvis in a lateral or vertical direction. Bowel complaints were also more common in subjects than in controls. Among those who were pregnant at the time of injury, the rate of fetal death was 80% in subjects and 25% in controls. The 2 groups did not differ in miscarriage or infertility rates, but subjects had an increased rate of cesarean section after the pelvic fracture. Pain during sex was reported by 43% of women with pelvic fractures displaced 5 mm or greater. Physiologic problems with arousal or orgasm were uncommon in both groups.

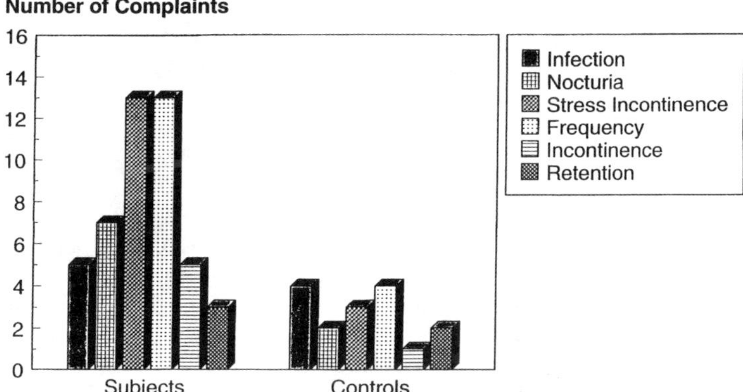

FIGURE 1.—Graphic analysis of urinary tract complaints as reported by 26 subjects (21%) and 9 controls (7%) ($P = 0.003$). Individuals could report 1 or more complaints. Considering each complaint individually, the following complaints were reported significantly more frequently in subjects than in controls: nocturia ($P = 0.04$), stress incontinence ($P = 0.007$), and frequent urination ($P = 0.02$). (Courtesy of Copeland CE, Bosse MJ, McCarthy ML, et al: Effect of trauma and pelvic fracture on female genitourinary, sexual, and reproductive function. *J Orthop Trauma* 11:73–81, 1997.)

Conclusions.—Despite a very low incidence of frank genitourinary injuries and no significant gastrointestinal injuries in these patients, a history of pelvic fracture was associated with the development of urinary complaints, gynecologic pain, and an increased rate of cesarean section. Orthopedic surgeons need to discuss these potential problems with their female patients and refer them for rehabilitation if needed.

▶ In this well-designed outcome study on women with pelvic trauma, the high frequency of urinary complaints, gynecologic pain, and dyspareunia are identified. Although the questionnaire used in this study was not validated psychometrically, it did address all of the important concerns expressed by female patients with pelvic fracture. The higher incidents of these complications is well documented and is deserving of further investigation using optimum clinical research design.

M.F. Swiontkowski, M.D.

Hip Fractures

Hip Screw Augmentation With an In Situ–setting Calcium Phosphate Cement: An In Vitro Biomechanical Analysis
Moore DC, Frankenburg EP, Goulet JA, et al (Univ of Michigan, Ann Arbor)
J Orthop Trauma 11:577–583, 1997   4–21

Objective.—In patients undergoing sliding hip screw fixation for intertrochanteric hip fractures, screw cut-out is the most frequent device-related complication. In certain situations, injecting polymethylmethacrylate (PMMA) into the screw track or packing it into the femoral head is thought to reduce stresses at the screw-bone interface by increasing the implant of the surface area. However, this use of PMMA also carries the risk of intraoperative and long-term complications. Newer in situ-setting calcium phosphate cements may be a useful alternative. Cut-out resistance was compared in screws augmented with calcium phosphate cement versus PMMA.

Methods.—The study used compression hip screws placed in paired cadaver proximal femurs. Mean participant age was 75 years. Cut-out testing was performed before and after the screws were augmented with PMMA or calcium phosphate cement. The bilateral study design permitted pairwise comparisons of the augmentation materials, with repeated tests to provide an internal control for bone quality. Two-way repeated measures analysis of variance was performed to compare the initial fixation strength of screws augmented with the 2 materials.

Results.—The 2 groups of augmented screws were not significantly different in their cut-out behavior. Yield strength was increased by 16% with calcium phosphate cement and 28% with PMMA; the difference was significant only with PMMA. In both groups, energy to yield increased significantly by 41%. Stiffness increased by only 6% with PMMA augmentation, and decreased by 10% with calcium phosphate cement augmentation.

Conclusions.—The cut-out resistance of compression hip screws in senile trabecular bone was augmented to a similar extent with in situ–setting calcium phosphate cement and with PMMA. The newer calcium phosphate cements may be useful substitutes for PMMA in the salvage of compression hip screw fixation in elderly osteopenic patients with complex intertrochanteric fractures. The authors call for more study of calcium phosphate cements for this purpose.

▶ In this proximal femur cadaveric study, the utility of calcium phosphate cement to increase yield strength is well documented. Improvement in this yield strength and stiffness is not quite as high as with PMMA. The calcium phosphate cement, however, can be completely remodelled, and patients can bear weight in the early postoperative phase. The concept that cement can be used to provide a more anatomical proximal femoral anatomy with healing is deserving of further investigation, and clinical trials looking at both functional outcomes as well as objective measures of gait and abductor strength are required.

M.F. Swiontkowski, M.D.

Intraoperative Intravascular Volume Optimisation and Length of Hospital Stay After Repair of Proximal Femoral Fracture: Randomised Controlled Trial

Sinclair S, James S, Singer M (Univ College London)
BMJ 315:909–912, 1997

4–22

Background.—Many patients with a femoral neck fracture are in poor general health, and surgical repair is a further stressor that contributes to long hospitalizations and poor recovery. Some researchers have reported that the optimization of cardiac output and tissue oxygen delivery improves outcomes in high-risk patients. These authors used Doppler esophageal US to monitor and optimize circulatory parameters in a high-risk group of patients undergoing femoral neck repair.

Methods.—Elderly (older than 55 years) patients with a first-time femoral neck fracture, who did not have fracture caused by neoplasm or hospital falls and who did not undergo regional anesthesia, were eligible. All patients underwent routine perioperative monitoring, including the placement of a Doppler US probe into the esophagus. All patients received conventional treatment with crystalloid, hydroxyethyl starch colloid, or blood to replace fluid losses and maintain blood pressure and heart rate. In the control group ($n = 20$), this conventional treatment was all that was used; but in the protocol group ($n = 20$), hydroxyethyl starch colloid was given to correct stroke volume and flow time, based on results of the esophageal Doppler monitor.

Findings.—Compared with the control group, patients in the protocol group received significantly more colloids (0 vs. 750 mL) and had higher stroke volumes (-6 vs. 13 mL), cardiac output (-0.25 vs. 1.0), and corrected flow times (24 vs. 38.5 msec). Blood pressure and heart rate did not differ between the groups. All but 1 of the patients in the protocol group survived (1 death occurred 36 days after surgery as the result of pre-existing amyloid cardiac failure), and all but 2 patients in the control group survived (1 death was caused by a cerebrovascular accident shortly after surgery and one 65 days after surgery was caused by congestive cardiac failure). Of the survivors, postoperative hospitalization rates were

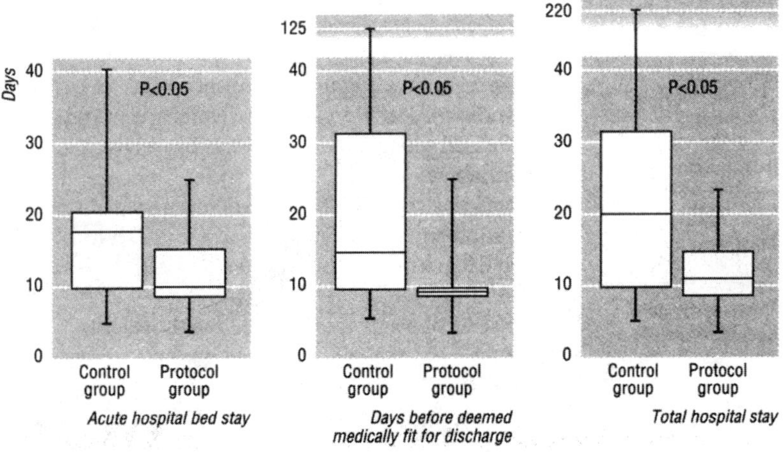

FIGURE 2.—Acute bed stay, days before deemed medically fit for discharge, and total duration of hospital stay for survivors. Median, quartiles, and extremes are shown for 18 control patients and 19 protocol patients. (This figure was first published in the *BMJ*, Sinclair S, James S, Singer M: Intraoperative intravascular volume optimisation and length of hospital stay after repair of proximal femoral fracture: Randomised controlled trial. *BMJ* 315:909-912, 1997, and is reproduced by permission of the BMJ.)

significantly better in patients in the protocol group (Fig 2). No complications related to the Doppler probe developed.

Conclusion.—Doppler US monitoring to optimize stroke volume and hypovolemia resulted in significantly improved hemodynamics and a shorter hospital stay. In fact, with Doppler monitoring, the stroke volume and cardiac output actually increased, whereas in the control group, both of these values fell during surgery. This method of intravascular volume optimization was safe and effective and should be considered in high-risk patients undergoing femoral neck fracture repair.

▶ In this optimally designed, randomized controlled trial, the utility of Doppler US in monitoring cardiac volumes is documented. Although the numbers were small and the confidence intervals for the statistics were not reported, it seems wise for the anesthesiologist to optimize hemodynamic status in the highest risk hip fracture patients.

M.F. Swiontkowski, M.D.

Femur

Proximal Thigh Pain After Femoral Nailing: Causes and Treatment

Dodenhoff RM, Dainton JN, Hutchins PM (Royal Cornwall Hosp, Truro, England)

J Bone Joint Surg Br 79-B:738–741, 1997

4–23

Background.—Intramedullary nailing is often used to treat fractures of the femur, and it is often associated with persistent pain in the proximal thigh after union. This article assesses the incidence of pain after femoral nailing and attempts to determine causal factors.

Methods.—Ninety-eight femoral fractures were fixed with a Grosse-Kempf nail. Patients ranged in age from teenagers to nonagenarians, with most fractures due to a traffic accident or a severe fall. Radiographic films were evaluated to exclude tumor metastasis and to identify areas of nail protrusion, heterotopic bone formation, and implant failure or fracture.

Findings.—Over a mean follow-up of 21 months, 80 patients were evaluated. Of these 80, 33 patients (41%) had femoral pain that was significant enough to interfere with their mobility or lifestyle (Table 3).

TABLE 3.—Associated Findings in 33 Patients with Delayed Pain

Finding	Number	Percentage
Heterotopic ossification grades 2 to 4	21	64
Prominent locking screw	3	9
Implant fracture	2	6
Nonunion	2	6
Paget's disease of the femur	1	3
No abnormality detected	4	12

(Courtesy of Dodenhoff RM, Dainton JN, Hutchins PM. Proximal thigh pain after femoral nailing: Causes and treatment. *J Bone Joint Surg [Br]* 79B:738–741, 1997.)

Heterotopic ossification was closely associated with pain: 21 of 24 patients (88%) with heterotopic ossification had pain, and patients reporting pain were significantly more likely to have new bone formation. Nails were removed after 18 months in 27 of these 80 patients (34%); pain was the most common reason (17 of 27 patients). However, in 6 patients, removal of the nail did not cause the pain to resolve. Nail prominence had no significant association with pain. In the 3 patients with locking screw prominence who complained of pain, removal of the implant resolved the pain.

Conclusions.—Heterotopic bone formation and pain were significantly associated with each other, although heterotopic bone formation may not be the cause of the pain. Injury to the soft tissues when the nail was inserted may be cause of pain in such instances of new bone growth. In any case, removal of the nail does not always resolve the pain.

▶ This is a retrospective study of patients managed with a Grosse-Kempf nail for femoral shaft fractures. This nail has a rather large locking bolt head and has been known to have a higher incidence of proximal trochanter as well as distal femoral irritation caused by the large bolt head size. We are encouraged that the majority of patients who had proximal thigh pain were improved with nail removal. It is likely that injury to the gluteus medius tendon with nail insertion is at the root cause of the pain, which explains why nail removal is not always successful.

M.F. Swiontkowski, M.D.

Bridge Plating Osteosynthesis of 20 Comminuted Fractures of the Femur
Chrisovitsinos JP, Xenakis T, Papakostides KG, et al (Hatzikostas Gen Hosp, Ioannina, Greece; Univ of Ioannina, Greece)
Acta Orthop Scand 68:72–76, 1997   4–24

Background.—The importance of preserving the viability and integrity of the soft-tissue envelope of metaphyseal and diaphyseal fractures has been emphasized in recent research. A 2- to 3-week delay has been found to help the soft-tissue envelope recover in patients with comminuted fractures of the metaphysis and diaphysis. This type of indirect fixation, called *bridge plating,* is part of the new concept of biological internal fixation. The outcomes of treatment of comminuted subtrochanteric, diaphyseal, and supracondylar fractures of the femur using indirect reduction and bridge plating were analyzed retrospectively.

Methods.—Data were obtained on 20 comminuted fractures of the femur in 20 patients. Mean follow-up was 1.5 years, with a range of 1–4.5 years. Eleven fractures were subtrochanteric; 6, complex diaphyseal; and 3, supracondylar. Three fractures were open. Subtrochanteric fractures were treated with a 95-degree dynamic condylar screw or a 135-degree hip screw. For 4 patients, autocompression plate implants were used for diaphyseal fractures. In 2, limited contact dynamic compression plate implants were used. A 95-degree dynamic condylar screw implant and the Condylar Buttress Plate were used to treat the 3 supracondylar fractures. Bone grafting was used for 11 fractures.

Findings.—No complications occurred in the immediate postoperative period. All fractures were united at a mean of 5 months, regardless of bone grafting use. Late complications included mild knee stiffness in 4 patients and shortening of 1–2 cm in 4 patients.

Summary.—In this series, bridge plating with indirect fracture reduction resulted in a rapid union of all comminuted fractures of the femur. No major complications occurred.

▶ A surgeon must have in his or her armamentarium the use of plating for infrequent indications in the management of femoral shaft fractures. In this series of 20 patients, fractures of either end of the femur were the main indication. The authors of this retrospective review show that limited soft tissue striping, the use of longer implants, and indirection reduction of fragments produce an excellent union rate with minimal complications.

M.F. Swiontkowski, M.D.

Technical Notes on a Radiolucent Distractor for Indirect Reduction and Intramedullary Nailing
Dahners LE (Univ of North Carolina, Chapel Hill)
J Orthop Trauma 11:374–377, 1997   4–25

Introduction.—The fracture table has been the standard for the application of distraction forces required to allow coaxial alignment of long-bone fractures during internal fixation procedures. There are various drawbacks to the fracture table, however, including its cumbersome size, high cost, and the need for an assistant outside the sterile field to adjust the table. A version of a "low-tech" distraction device that the author has used since 1985 was described. A similar device is now on the market.

Methods.—The device consists of a perineal post, a longitudinal distraction beam, and a second post for application of distraction to a standard Kirschner wire bow. In the commercially available version (Kairos Orthopaedics, Sacramento, Calif), the distraction beam has a screw-driven carriage with a mounting site for the wire tensioner. The carriage allows distraction forces to be applied by turning the knob at the end of the distraction bar. Distraction of the femur is able to be applied in the lateral position (Fig 2), the "floppy lateral" position, or the supine position. The device can be sterilized and used in the surgical field. A patient with multiple trauma who is placed on a radiolucent table for thoracoabdominal procedures can undergo intramedullary nailing without being transferred to a fracture table.

Discussion.—For institutions with a radiolucent table, a radiolucent distractor offers a cost-effective means for achieving fracture reduction. In

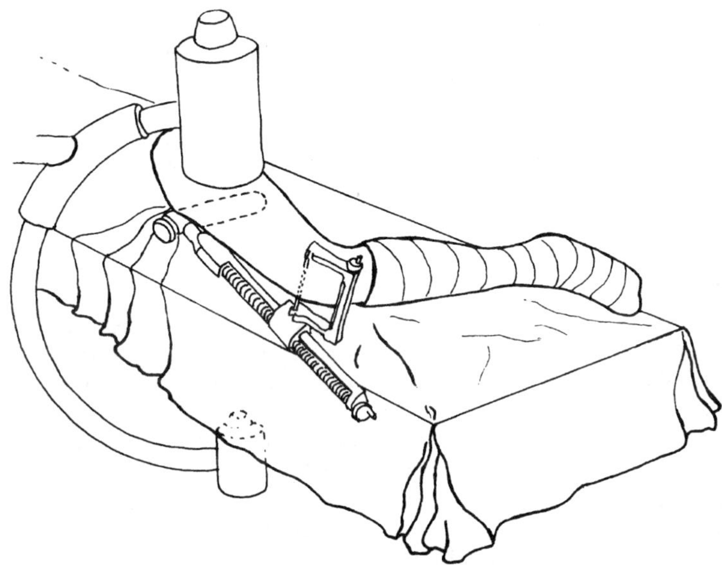

FIGURE 2.—Distractor in position for femoral nailing in the lateral position. Note than the C-arm is brought in anteriorly with the image intensifier on top. (Courtesy of Dahners LE: Technical notes on a radiolucent distractor for indirect reduction and intramedullary nailing. *J Orthop Trauma* 11:374–377, 1997.)

addition to its application in femur and tibia nailing, the device can be used as a distractor of knee and ankle fractures and for hip or ankle arthroscopy. When the device has a perineal post, surgeons should be cautious of the position of the male genitalia, especially in the floppy lateral or supine positions.

▶ This new device may have some real advantages in terms of managing the multiple injured patient. Based on the work of Johnson et al.,[1] we have learned how to manage these patients on radiolucent tables in the semi-supine position. This manipulative reduction device may make that treatment even easier.

M.F. Swiontkowski, M.D.

Reference

1. McFarran M, Johnson KD: Intramedullary nailing of acute femoral shaft fractures with the use of the femoral distractor. *J Orthop Trauma* 6:479, 1992.

Tibia

Closed Fractures of the Tibial Shaft: A Meta-analysis of Three Methods of Treatment
Littenberg B, Weinstein LP, McCarren M, et al (Dartmouth-Hitchcock Med Ctr, Lebanon, NH; Amercian Academy of Orthopaedic Surgeons, Rosemont, Ill)
J Bone Joint Surg Am 80-A:174–183, 1998   4–26

Background.—The best method for treating closed fractures of the tibial shaft is not clear. Immobilization in a cast, open reduction and internal fixation, and fixation with an intramedullary rod are used most often. The literature was reviewed to determine the clinical outcomes of these treatments.

Methods.—Of 2,372 reports published between 1966 and 1993, 19 met the inclusion citeria for the current analysis. Six controlled studies and 27 patient groups were included. Outcomes of controlled studies were summarized using odds ratios and risk differences. Outcomes from case series were summarized by the medians of the reported results.

Findings.—Comparative studies demonstrated that treatment with a cast was associated with a lower rate of superficial infection than open reduction and internal fixation. Open reduction and internal fixation were associated with a greater rate of union by 20 weeks than treatment with a cast. No other significant correlations were identified. Data were not sufficient for assessment of any aspect of functional status, level of pain, or other patient-reported outcomes.

Conclusions.—The published literature to date provides inadequate information for determining the best treatment for closed fractures of the tibia. In general, the studies reviewed included few patients and were poorly designed.

▶ In this structured literature review, the lack of knowledge regarding comparative outcomes with operative vs. cast/functional brace treatment for closed fractures of the tibia is apparent. With the data available, most of which is based on an uncontrolled case series with passive follow-up, we are left with little hard information. Not surprisingly, cast treatment is associated with a low rate of superficial infection and a higher rate of delayed union by 20 weeks. We desperately need better information on which to base treatment recommendations for our patients with closed fractures of the tibial shaft.

M.F. Swiontkowski, M.D.

Acceleration of Tibia and Distal Radius Fracture Healing in Patients Who Smoke

Cook SD, Ryaby JP, McCabe J, et al (Tulane Univ, New Orleans, La; Exogen, Piscataway, NJ; Health Products Development, Lancaster, Pa; et al)
Clin Orthop 337:197–207, 1997   4–27

Background.—Cigarette smoking can profoundly affect bone and bone healing. Previous studies have shown that pulsed US accelerates the normal fracture repair process in animals and human beings. The efficacy of a low-intensity US device as an accelerator of cortical and cancellous bone fracture healing was assessed in smokers and nonsmokers.

Methods and Findings.—Sixty-seven patients with tibial and 61 with distal radius fractures were studied. Half the patients in each fracture group were treated with active US, and half were treated with a placebo device. The use of the active US device reduced healing time 41% in smokers and 26% in nonsmokers with tibial fractures. Among patients with distal radius fractures, active treatment decreased healing time by 51% in smokers and 34% in nonsmokers. Active treatment also markedly decreased the incidence of tibial delayed unions in both smokers and nonsmokers.

Conclusions.—Active US treatment accelerates cortical and cancellous bone fractures. It substantially mitigates the delay in healing noted in cigarette smokers. It also accelerates return to normal activity and decreases the long-term complications of delayed union.

▶ This data is part of 2 double-blind, randomized, controlled trials of patients with tibia fractures and distal radius fractures subjected to US devices. In a comparison between smokers and the non-smokers, it seems the advantage of US to accelerate fracture healing is even greater for the former. These data are derived from well-designed clinical trails. Therefore, our confidence in the quality of the information should be relatively high.

M.F. Swiontkowski, M.D.

Intramedullary Nailing of Unstable Diaphyseal Fractures of the Tibia With Distal Intraarticular Involvement

Konrath G, Moed BR, Watson JT, et al (Henry Ford Hosp, Detroit)
J Orthop Trauma 11:200–205, 1997   4–28

Introduction.—Recent studies of diaphyseal tibia fractures with ipsilateral ankle fractures recommend operative stabilization of both fractures. The authors of this study, however, have been treating the diaphyseal fracture component with an intramedullary nail. Supplemental open reduction and internal fixation or percutaneous screw fixation are used to stabilize contiguous ipsilateral distal intra-articular fracture extensions and noncontiguous ipsilateral ankle fractures.

Methods.—Twenty-eight patients who sustained an unstable tibial diaphyseal fracture with distal intra-articular involvement were treated with intramedullary nailing from 1990 to 1994; 20 were available for follow-up. Fractures were open in 5 cases and closed in 15. All were stabilized with lag screw fixation of the intra-articular fracture extension or ankle fracture and intramedullary nailing of the diaphyseal fracture. Lag screw fixation was performed with or without supplemental plates. Patients were followed for an average period of 22 months for time to bony union, malunion, knee and ankle range of motion, early arthrosis, and complications.

Results.—Nineteen diaphyseal fractures achieved union at an average of 17 weeks and had excellent alignment. Union did not occur in a type IIIB open diaphyseal fracture and a compartment syndrome, but the fracture healed after exchange reamed nailing and fibular osteotomy. Three of the healed diaphyseal fractures had required additional procedures. All distal fracture extensions and ipsilateral noncontiguous ankle fractures healed without complications. One patient with an ipsilateral anterior cruciate ligament tear had a decrease in knee motion, but all others had normal knee motion. Ankle pain was reported by 3 patients; none complained of knee pain. Implant removal was required in 6 patients because of irritation from locking screws or the intramedullary nail.

Conclusions.—These combined ipsilateral tibial shaft and ankle injuries were treated successfully with intramedullary nailing and stabilization with lag screw fixation. Outcome was comparable to that reported for isolated tibial shaft fractures and ankle injuries.

Decision Making Errors in the Use of Interlocking Tibial Nails
Templeman D, Larson C, Varecka T, et al (Hennepin County Med Ctr, Minneapolis, Minn)
Clin Orthop 339:65–70, 1997   4–29

Background.—Three types of modes are used for the insertion of interlocking nails for the stabilization of tibial fractures, but guidelines for the optimal mode of interlocking for each fracture type do not exist. Whether there are fracture types that are prone to postoperative alignment changes when the dynamic or nonlocked mode of interlocking nails is employed was determined in a retrospective study.

Methods.—Loss of alignment was defined as 1 cm or more of shortening or angulation greater than 5 degrees in the frontal plane or 10 degrees in the sagittal plane. From 1989 to 1993, 71 tibial fractures treated with unlocked or dynamically locked intramedullary nails were available for study. The study group consisted of 54 men and 17 women, with an average age of 34 years. Fracture geometry was classified according to the Association for the Study of the Problems of Internal Fixation Classification System (AO/ASIF).

TABLE 2.—Changes in Alignment That Occurred Respective to Fracture Pattern

AO Classification	Number	Tibial Diaphysis Change in Alignment
A1 spiral	18	
A2 obligue	4	A = 7
A3 transverse	27	
B1 spiral wedge	4	
B2 bending wedge	9	B = 1
B3 fragmented wedge	2	
C1 complex spiral	1	C = 0
C2 complex segmental	6	

(Courtesy of Templeman D, Larson C, Varecka T, et al: Decision making errors in the use of interlocking tibial nails. *Clin Orthop* 339:65–70, 1997.)

Findings.—Changes in postoperative alignment occurred in 11% of the 71 tibial fractures in this series. Changes in alignment developed in 4 of 18 spiral fractures, 3 of 4 oblique fractures, and 1 of 13 wedge fractures. Nine complex fractures were treated without a change in alignment (Table 2). Changes in alignment were also more common in the fractures of the proximal and distal third of the tibia (Table 5).

Conclusions.—A review of tibial fractures treated with intramedullary nails demonstrated that spiral and oblique fractures were not sufficiently stabilized by nonlocked and dynamically locked modes of interlocking nails. These fractures should be treated with statically locked interlocking tibial nails to prevent postoperative changes in alignment. Fractures outside of the middle third of the tibia should also be treated with static interlocking tibial nails. When unlocked or dynamically locked tibial nails are employed, frequent postoperative radiographs should be used to monitor alignment changes.

TABLE 5.—Patient Data

Case	Age (years)	Mechanism of Injury	Site	AO	Locking	Complication
1	65	Motor vehicle accident	M3	A2:2		Shortening 1.0 cm
2	20	Bicycle accident	P3	B2:3	2 proximal	Shortening 1.0 cm; procurvatum 12°
3	48	Pedestrian versus motor vehicle	P3	A2:1	2 proximal	Shortening 1.0 cm; varus 5°
4	32	Motor vehicle accident	D3	A1:2	0	Shortening 1.5 cm
5	23	Motor vehicle accident	D3	A2:3	1 distal	Shortening 1.0 cm
6	61	Assault	D3	A1:2	2 distal	Shortening 2.5 cm
7	32	Logging	D3	A1:2	1 proximal	Shortening 1.0 cm
8	63	Fall	D3	A1:2	0	Shortening 1.6 cm

Abbreviations: P3, proximal ⅓; *M3*, middle ⅓; *D3*, distal ⅓.

(Courtesy of Templeman D, Larson C, Varecka T, et al: Decision making errors in the use of interlocking tibial nails. *Clin Orthop* 339:65–70, 1997.)

A Technique for Intramedullary Nailing of Proximal Third Tibia Fractures

Buehler KC, Green J, Woll TS, et al (Oregon Health Sciences Univ, Portland)
J Orthop Trauma 11:218–223, 1997   4–30

Introduction.—Intramedullary nailing, the standard treatment for most tibia shaft fractures, can fail to obtain an acceptable reduction of proximal third tibia fractures. Because of the inherent advantages of intramedullary fixation over other methods, a technique was developed that would allow intramedullary nailing to be used successfully in treating proximal third tibia fractures. This technique was used in 14 cases.

Methods.—Tibial shaft fractures of the proximal third were within 10 cm of the joint line in all 14 cases. Ten patients had been struck by an automobile, and 4 were injured in motor vehicle accidents. Open fractures were present in 5 cases. The intramedullary nailing procedure was performed after initial resuscitation and stabilization of the patient. Fractures were reduced and an AO femoral distractor was placed on the medial aspect of the tibia in 12 cases. The technique involves correct overlapping

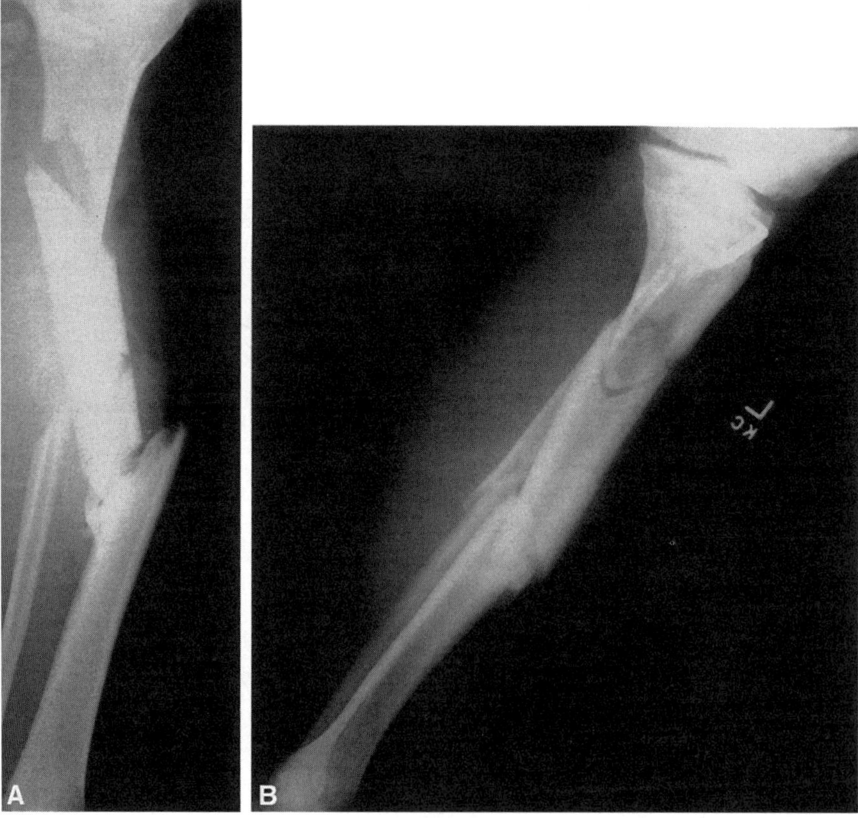

(*Continued*)

FIGURE 4 (cont.)

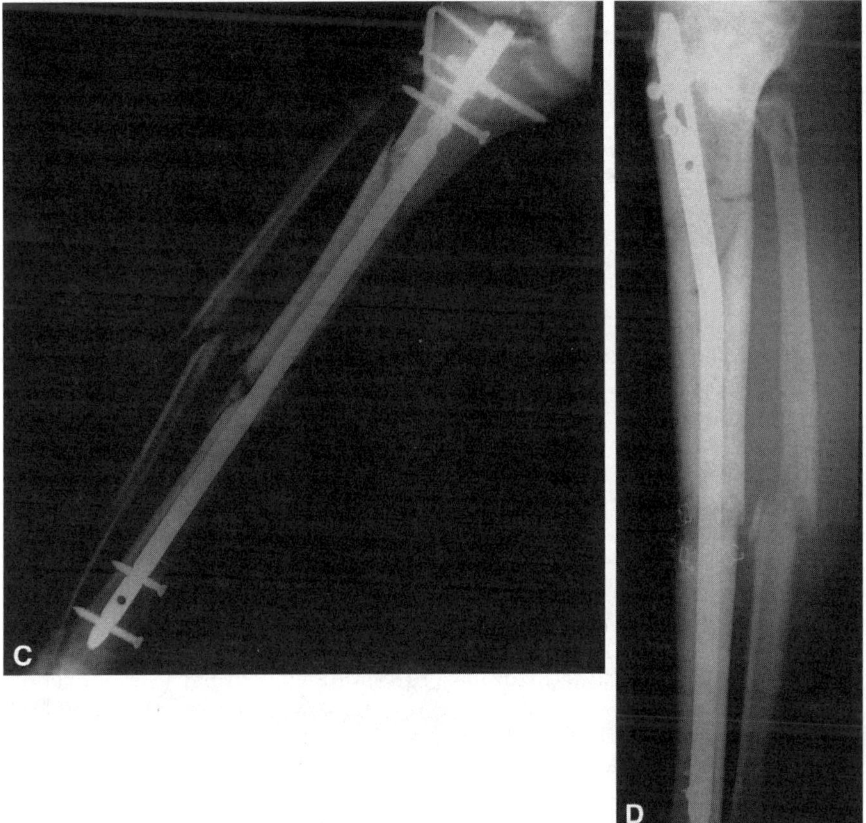

FIGURE 4.—**A and B,** preoperative anteroposterior (AP)/lateral radiograph of segmental proximal tibia fracture. Patient had a previous high tibial osteotomy. **C and D,** Postoperative AP/lateral radiograph of successfully reduced segmental tibia fracture with intramedullary fixation. (Courtesy of Buehler KC, Green J, Woll TS, et al: A technique for intramedullary nailing of proximal third tibia fractures. *J Orthop Trauma* 11:218–223, 1997.)

of posterior walls with distraction and Schanz screw if needed, a proximal and lateral starting point in line with the lateral intercondylar eminence, hyperflexion of the knee for nail insertion, a sagittal plane entry point parallel to the anterior cortex of the proximal fragment under radiographic control, and proximal interlocking with the knee in full extension.

Results.—All patients were followed up for more than 6 months. None had intraoperative or postoperative complications associated with use of the technique. Immediately postoperatively, fracture alignment was 2.0 mm average anterior displacement of the proximal fragment; average coronal plane alignment was 2.0 degrees of valgus (Fig 4). One patient died a week after the injury. Two patients required revision postoperatively, with nail removal, open reduction, and plate fixation. Outcome was satisfactory in the remaining cases.

Discussion.—Proximal third tibia fractures treated with intramedullary nailing have a high incidence of malalignment. The success of the technique described depends upon neutralizing factors contributing to malreduction: wide effective diameters of tibial nails, narrow diameter of the medial tibial metaphysis, and a posteriorly directed sagittal plane entrance angle.

The Role of Fibular Fixation in Combined Fractures of the Tibia and Fibula: A Biomechanical Investigation

Weber TG, Harrington RM, Henley MB, et al (Univ of Washington, Seattle)
J Orthop Trauma 11:206–211, 1997   4–31

Introduction.—A subset of fractures of the tibia and fibula requires internal fixation to maintain alignment and length during healing. Fixation of the fibula has been recommended for treating fractures of the tibia and fibula, but little is known about the mechanical effect of the intact tibia on internally fixed tibia fractures. Whether adjunctive plating of the fibula with tibial fixation enhanced stability under combined compressive and bending loads was examined using a cadaveric model of fractures of both the tibia and fibula.

Methods.—Ten matched pairs of fresh lower extremities, intact from mid-thigh to foot, were studied. Six pairs considered suitable were frozen until the experiments were conducted. Each specimen was mounted on the table of a materials testing machine. With an intramedullary rod locked in the distal femur, it was possible for compression and flexion, valgus bending, or varus bending loads to be transmitted from the actuator of the testing machine to the knee. Intact tibial deformations under load were measured by means of 3 transducers mounted on the tibia at anterior, posterolateral, and posteromedial positions. A 2-cm osteotomy was created near the tibial midshaft in 1 specimen of each pair. Tibial gap displacements were measured under 4 conditions: intact fibula, osteotomized fibula, fibula fixed with a plate, and fibula fixed with an Enders intramedullary nail. Tibial fixation was performed with an interlocked unreamed intramedullary nail in the other specimens of the pair.

Results.—Although tibial osteotomy site motions were significantly greater in all directions of loading after osteotomy of the tibia, no significant increases in motion were found across the tibial defect after fibular osteotomy when an interlocked intramedullary rod was used to fix the tibia. When the tibial defect was fixed using an external fixator, plating the fibula led to decreased motion in flexion, which was significant in valgus loading. With intramedullary rod fixation of the tibia, osteotomizing the fibula did not affect defect site motion or its subsequent stabilization with a plate or intramedullary rod.

Conclusions.—Plating of the fibula can decrease motion across a tibial defect only when less rigid fixation is used. In cases of severely unstable tibia/fibula fractures treated with an external fixator, plating the fibula may decrease the load on pins and pin/bone interfaces, thus increasing the life span of the fixation.

Knee Pain After Intramedullary Tibial Nailing: Its Incidence, Etiology, and Outcome

Court-Brown CM, Gustilo T, Shaw AD (Royal Infirmary of Edinburgh, Scotland)

J Orthop Trauma 11:103–105, 1997 4–32

Background.—Tibial fractures are often treated with intramedullary nailing of the tibia. Unfortunately, this procedure has been reported to cause anterior knee pain that sometimes necessitates nail removal. These authors examined the incidence of nail-related knee pain and its effects on nail removal.

Methods.—A Grosse Kempf intramedullary nail was used for stabilization in 169 patients with diaphyseal fractures of the tibia. The fracture classification, the extent of patellar tendon damage, the type of skin incision, any proximal locking screws, and any hematomas or superficial sepsis were recorded. Anterior knee pain related to the nail entry site was rated on a 10-point analogue scale (0 = no pain; higher than 6 = severe pain). Pain was assessed during activities of daily life such as kneeling, running, and climbing stairs. Pain after removal of the nail was also assessed.

Findings.—Of the 169 patients who underwent tibial nailing, 95 (56%) reported pain of the anterior knee that was related to the nail site; these

TABLE 1.—Comparison of the Descriptive Indices Between the Pain and No Pain Groups

	Pain	No Pain	P
Male (%)	84.2	73.4	NS
Age (yr)	31.5	44.2	<0.001
AO			
Type A (%)	61.1	54.7	NS
Type B (%)	20.0	31.2	NS
Type C (%)	18.9	14.1	NS
Open fracture (%)	18.9	29.7	NS
Type III open fracture (%)	61.1	57.9	NS
Tscherne C1 and C2 fracture (%)	62.5	81.1	NS
Transverse skin incision (%)	98.9	96.5	NS
Proximal screws (%)	75	83.6	NS
Wound complications (%)	9.5	9.3	NS
Patellar tendon			
Split (%)	45.2	29.8	NS
Medial (%)	54.8	70.2	NS
Nail removal (%)	65.2	37.5	<0.001

Note: The only significant differences are in patient age and the incidence of nail removal.
Abbreviation: NS, not significant.
(Courtesy of Court-Brown CM, Gustilo T, Shaw AD. Knee pain after intramedullary tibial nailing: Its incidence, etiology, and outcome. *J Orthop Trauma* 11:103–105, 1997.)

TABLE 2.—Overall Incidence of Knee Pain

	Number	%
No pain	74	43.8
Mild pain (analogue <4)	65	38.5
Moderate pain (analogue 4–6)	21	12.4
Severe pain (analogue >6)	9	5.4

Note: For the purposes of defining the incidence of nail-related anterior knee pain, the no-pain group includes the 10 patients with diffuse knee pain unrelated to nailing.
(Courtesy of Court-Brown CM, Gustilo T, Shaw AD. Knee pain after intramedullary tibial nailing: Its incidence, etiology, and outcome. *J Orthop Trauma* 11:103–105, 1997.)

were called the pain group. Of the remaining 74 patients, 10 experienced mild, episodic pain that was not considered to be related to the tibial nailing; these patients were excluded from further analysis. The 64 patients who reported no pain were referred to as the no-pain group. Comparisons between the pain and no-pain groups revealed significant differences only in patient age (younger patients were more likely to have pain) and nail removal (those with pain were more likely to undergo nail removal (Table 1). In 27% of patients, nail removal completely resolved the pain; another 69% had marked improvement, and only 3.2% had worse pain after nail removal. Of the patients who experienced pain, less than 20% reported moderate or worse pain (Table 2). Pain differed for various activities; only 33% of patients in the pain group reported pain with rest, whereas 92% reported pain with kneeling and 61% had pain with squatting.

Conclusion.—Anterior knee pain after intramedullary tibial nailing could be caused by the presence of the nail or to tissue damage during insertion of the nail. However, given that nail removal caused at least marked improvement in all but 2 of 95 patients with anterior knee pain, the cause of the pain is likely the nail itself. In this series, more than half of the patients (56%) experienced pain related to the nail entry site. Thus, patients undergoing intramedullary tibial nailing should be counseled that postoperative pain may occur, but that if it does, it can be treated with nail removal.

▶ Intramedullary interlocking nailing is the treatment of choice in most centers for dealing with unstable diaphyseal fractures of the tibia. In the first study in this group (Abstract 4–28), the situation of associated distal intra-articular involvement is investigated in a retrospective study design. Lag screw fixation, which can be done percutaneously followed by intramedullary interlocking nailing, provides excellent clinical outcomes comparable with those obtained when there is no intraarticular extension. It is the authors' experience that these articular extensions are usually nondisplaced. Therefore, one would expect similar results in 2 contrasting groups.

When the fractures occur in the upper portion of the tibia, special techniques need to be used to prevent displacement with nailing (Abstracts 4–29 and 4–30). These authors have worked for several years to develop surgical techniques to prevent anterior displacement of the proximal fragment relative to the distal fragment. They describe a proximal and lateral starting point relative to the patellar tendon, hyperflexion of the knee for nail insertion, and then extension before placement of the interlocking bolts. Specialized instruments are required with attention to detail.

The question has arisen frequently whether augmentation with fibular fixation is helpful with the management of ipsilateral tibia and fibula fractures. In this biomechanical study of a cadaveric model (Abstract 4–31), fixation of fibular fractures with plate and Enders nailing is investigated. It seems beneficial only with the most flexible tibial fixation. It is, therefore, not necessary with the routine use of intramedullary interlocking nails unless the tibular fracture involves the ankle joint.

Anterior knee pain associated with tibial nailing is a common occurrence. This article (Abstract 4–32) gives us a strong indication that the anterior knee pain can be resolved with nail removal in the vast majority of cases. Removing the implant seems to be necessary only about 50% of the time.

M.F. Swiontkowski, M.D.

Miscellaneous

Implementation of the Ottawa Knee Rule for the Use of Radiography in Acute Knee Injuries

Stiell IG, Wells GA, Hoag RH, et al (Univ of Ottawa, Ont; Queensway-Carleton Hosp, Nepean, Ont; Univ of Toronto; et al)
JAMA 278:2075–2079, 1997   4–33

Objective.—More than 1 million adults annually in the United States and Canada have an acute knee injury. Because the accumulated cost of routine radiographs is high, the Ottawa Knee Rule was developed and validated as a clinical decision rule for radiography. The impact of implementing the Ottawa Knee Rule on actual use of radiography, waiting times, and direct medical charges was assessed.

Methods.—This non-randomized, controlled clinical trial involved a before and after comparison of 3,907 nonpregnant adult patients with an acute knee injury seen at 1 teaching and 1 community intervention hospital (using the Ottawa Knee Rule) and at 1 teaching and 1 community control hospital from July 1, 1994 to June 30, 1995 and from September 1, 1995 to August 31, 1996. The outcomes were the proportion of patients referred for knee radiographs, patient satisfaction with treatment, and charges.

Results.—In before and after periods, there was a 26.4% reduction in referrals for knee radiography in the intervention group (77.6% vs. 57.1%) compared to a 1.3% reduction in the control group (76.9%vs. 75.9%). At intervention hospitals, physicians interpreted the rule accurately for 97.7% of patients with excellent interobserver agreement ($\kappa = 0.91$). In the after-intervention period, patients who did not have knee radiography spent significantly less time in the emergency department than patients undergoing radiography (85.7 vs. 118.8 minutes). When surveyed, 95.7% and 98.7% of these respective patients were satisfied with the care. Mean charges were significantly lower in the nonradiography group than in the radiography group ($80 vs. $183). All clinically important fractures were identified by the Ottawa Knee Rule for a sensitivity of 1.0 and a negative predictive value of 1.0.

Conclusion.—The Ottawa Knee Rule identified all important knee fractures while reducing radiographic utilization and medical costs significantly. The Rule is extremely sensitive and accurate.

▶ This manuscript is of value for emergency room physicians and orthopedic surgeons alike. The authors have successfully documented that the widespread overuse of knee radiographs on presentation can be decreased by the use of simple rules. These rules must be taught to assessing clinicians, and this is where orthopedic surgeons can play a major role. Patient satisfaction, lower costs, and low rate of missed injury are the reward for these efforts.

M.F. Swiontkowski, M.D.

Reliability of Fat-pad Sign in Radial Head/Neck Fractures of the Elbow

Irshad F, Shaw NJ, Gregory RJH (Dryburn Hosp, Durham, England)
Injury 28:433–435, 1997 4–34

Background.—Fat-pad signs on radiographs indicate an effusion in the elbow joint. These signs appear as translucent areas on the lateral radiograph of the elbow flexed to a right angle. They can be on the anterior or posterior aspect of the distal humerus. The reliability of fat-pad signs in radial head and neck fractures of the elbow was tested.

Methods.—One hundred ninety-three patients with elbow injuries were included in the prospective study. Standard radiographs were obtained. The presence and absence of fractures and fat-pad signs were reported for 181 films.

Findings.—The fat-pad sign had a sensitivity and specificity of 85.4% and 50%, respectively, for radial head and neck fracture of the elbow. Negative and positive predictive values were 87% and 47%, respectively.

Conclusions.—The interpretation of the fat-pad sign as an indicator of radial head and neck fractures of the elbow requires caution. Its absence is a more reliable predictor of no such fracture than its presence is an indication of such fracture.

▶ In the prospective uncontrolled study, the sensitivity of the fat-pad sign is examined. The specificity appears to be only 50%. A careful examination of the patient with placement of pressure over the proximal radius and passive pronation and supination of the wrist is advised. With the careful examination by palpation and passive range of motion, plus the evaluation for signs of effusion, 90% of radial head/neck fractures can be identified. It is always appropriate to rely more on physical exam than on radiographs in determining initial diagnosis and treatment plans.

M.F. Swiontkowski, M.D.

Open Reduction Internal Fixation of Displaced Transverse Patella Fractures With Figure-Eight Wiring Through Parallel Cannulated Compression Screws
Berg EE (New Hampshire Bone and Joint Inst, Bedford)
J Orthop Trauma 11:573–576, 1997   4–35

Background.—In displaced transverse patellar fractures, operative fixation is performed to provide rigid restoration of the quadriceps mechanism and articular surface congruity, thus permitting early motion. In the traditional method, a tension band is applied anteriorly over parallel Kirschner wires. However, there are problems with this technique, including loss of reduction and implant migration resulting from soft tissue atrophy and lack of fixation rigidity. A new technique of transverse patella fracture fixation—using a tensioned anterior figure-eight wire placed through parallel cannulated screws—was prospectively evaluated.

Technique.—The technique is performed through a longitudinal midline incision, as used for total knee arthroplasty. The fracture is reduced and articular surface congruity is confirmed. Two 1.25 or 2.0 mm guide pins are placed into the patella in parallel fashion in a cephalocaudal direction, with the fragments drilled to permit lagged interfragmentary compression. Large or small cannulated screws are selected according to bone quality and fragment size. To prevent anterior fracture angulation on knee flexion, an 18-gauge wire that fits both large and small AO cannulated screw systems is placed in figure-8 fashion through the 2 screws. The wire is tensioned with a Kirschner traction bow and secured with a square knot. The knee is put through a range of motion to confirm fixation stability.

Outcomes.—This technique was used in 10 patients with displaced transverse patella fractures. All patients went through a standardized rehabilitation protocol, including early continuous passive knee motion. Average clinical union time was 8 weeks and radiographic union time 13 weeks. Most of the patients were elderly, with osteopenic bone. However, continuous passive motion had no ill effect on the quality of fracture reduction. The results, assessed using Hospital for Special Surgery Knee scores, were good or excellent in 70% of patients.

Conclusions.—A new fixation technique, using a tensioned anterior figure-8 wire placed through parallel cannulated screws, was evaluated for use in transverse patella fractures. The results were comparable to those of modified tension band wiring. The new technique offers a low-profile construct with reduced irritation of local soft tissues. The ability to use early restricted motion is an important advantage. The technique provided good salvage in 3 patients with osteoporotic bone in whom traditional tension band wiring did not maintain anatomic reduction.

▶ This is an important technique of which the reader should be aware. It is particularly useful in osteopenic individuals and is a technique for failed tension band wire fixation. Although it need not be used universally, it is a handy technique. One important technical aspect is that the threads of the screw in the proximal pole of the patella must not penetrate the bone cortex, lest the wires which go through the cannulation fatigue and break.

M.F. Swiontkowski, M.D.

5 Forearm, Wrist, and Hand

Introduction

The publications of 1997 written on disorders of the forearm, wrist, and hand can largely be characterized as the reworking and refinement of old problems rather than as innovation. As in 1996, the treatment and complications of complex fractures of the distal radius continued to compel numerous investigators to present variations on accepted forms of treatment. Just as important, many articles presented longer term follow-up and, thus, clearer scrutiny of recent breakthroughs in the treatment of these difficult fractures. From these it would appear that the ice has finally been broken, and now open reduction, bone grafting, and internal fixation of acute unstable distal radius fractures may finally be accepted by the mainstream of orthopedics. I consider this to be a welcome trend, because the treatment of malunions is by far more difficult to do well than operatively addressing the acute fractures in the first place.

Another message can be inferred by the sheer number of publications on problem distal radius fractures presented in recent years: we are seeing greater numbers of complex fractures owing to recent changes in our leisure activities. Specifically, the baby boomers and the X generation continue to invent ways to smash this vulnerable part of their anatomy in the pursuit of happiness, what with the rising popularity of in-line skating, rock climbing, mountain biking, and snowboarding. Not to be outdone by the younger generations, our current crop of retirees is perhaps the first generation in the history of the world not to go away quietly after retirement. This latter group is perhaps the most demanding of all, who, unlike their own parents and grandparents, will not accept a "silver fork deformity" malunion of a distal fracture as an acceptable heirloom. Indeed, the 65-and-older generation is not only informed but savvy regarding what functional limitations they are willing to accept (and guard jealously) and what capacities they wish to retain; this presses us to provide them with the very best of treatment outcomes. Therefore, like my predecessor, I too have chosen a number of articles for your review which I hope will provide insight and technical help to assist in the treatment of these injuries.

In keeping with the "refinement rather than innovation" theme of 1997, several excellent articles offer insight and important restatement of two important, yet dreaded, complications of surgery: neuromas and reflex sympathetic dystrophy. The treatment of these conditions can be so difficult, unnerving, and unpleasant (what with the added burden of workman's compensation, litigation, and the complexities of health care maintenance organizations) that we may all understandably contemplate a change in careers should we encounter another one of these problems. The key to successful treatment of these disorders depends on the knowledge and adherence to a well thought out and defined treatment protocol. Two excellent ones are offered here for your review.

Finally, I am certain that, in the past year, we have all begun to experience the vagaries of "allowable" options as deemed appropriate by the clinical decision makers of many health maintenance organizations with respect to the evaluation and diagnosis of disorders of the wrist. It would seem that we finally had a superior diagnostic tool with a proven record of efficacy—the wrist arthroscope—with which to proceed in the evaluation and treatment of soft tissue injuries of the wrist. Recently, however, wrist arthroscopy has been denied by these decision makers, who, instead, grant equally expensive radiographic imaging studies (remember, financial reimbursement deals can be made with hospital-based radiologists and their equipment). Fortunately, important innovations in imaging techniques have been offered in this year's literature—particularly in the area of refined MRI technology for the diagnosis of subtle disruptions of both the intercarpal ligaments and the triangular fibrocartilage complex which approaches, but does not equal, the specificity, sensitivity, and reliability of wrist arthroscopy. We may yet win this battle in the end, but for now I have selected several articles that reveal the current possibilities of the latest imaging techniques.

Stephen D. Trigg, M.D.

Evaluation and Diagnosis

The Scapholunate Interosseous Ligament in MR Arthrography of the Wrist: Correlation With Non-enhanced MRI and Wrist Arthroscopy

Scheck RJ, Kubitzek C, Hierner R, et al (Ludwig-Maximilian-Univ, Munich)
Skeletal Radiol 26:263–271, 1997   5–1

Background.—The scapholunate interosseous ligament (SLIL) contributes to the functioning and stability of the entire wrist. Three-compartment MR arthrography is an imaging method that can obtain multidirectional images of pathologic changes in the wrist. Three-compartment MR wrist arthrography was compared with nonenhanced MRI and wrist arthroscopy, to examine the potential of MR arthrography to visualize and diagnose all SLIL defects.

Methods.—The study group consisted of 41 patients, with an average age of 34 years, who were seen between 1994 and 1996 with chronic wrist pain, but without radiographic evidence of instability. All patients were examined by nonenhanced MRI and 3-compartment MR wrist arthrography. These results were compared with those of wrist arthroscopy.

Findings.—All 3 segments of the SLIL were identified in 88% of wrists by nonenhanced MRI and in all patients by MR arthrography. The SLIL could be examined with a high confidence level in 42% of segments with nonenhanced MRI arthrography and in 90% of segments with MR arthrography. No assessment could be made in 18% of SLIL segments with nonenhanced MRI, but all segments could be assessed in all patients with MR arthrography (Fig 3). Compared to wrist arthroscopy, nonenhanced MRI classified SLIL defects as positive in 2 of 4 cases for dorsal, 9 of 14 for central, and 4 of 11 for palmar defects. This represents a 52% overall true positive rate for detecting and localizing defects. Magnetic resonance arthrography had a 90% overall true positive rate. The overall true negative rate was 34% for nonenhanced MRI and 87% for MR arthrography.

Conclusions.—Magnetic resonance arthrography had 90% sensitivity and 87% specificity for the detection and localization of scapholunate interosseous ligament defects; it can detect defects in all regions of the SLIL and correlates well with the findings at arthroscopy. Magnetic resonance arthrography has the potential to replace arthroscopy, which is expensive and invasive, in the identification and diagnosis of SLIL defects.

▶ Atraumatic attritional and traumatic partial ruptures of the SLIL, which result in nondissociative carpal instability, are one of the causes of chronic wrist pain. When suspected clinically, and when radiographs including stress views fail to show evidence for scapholunate dissociation, the most accurate diagnostic method for determining disruptions of this ligament has been proved to be wrist arthroscopy. However, in the current practice environment, often HMOs do not approve this diagnostic surgical procedure and require other diagnostic tools. Traditional arthrograms and nonenhanced MRI for the diagnosis of intercarpal ligament tears are often inconclusive. The authors of this study conclude that MR arthrography produces images that consistently result in a higher degree of interpretation with confidence of partial ligament tears over arthrography and nonenhanced MRI, and can further better delineate the dorsal and palmar structural elements of the SLIL from the nonstructural central membranous portion of the ligament. Central portion leakage is most often from attritional age-related perforations that can be misinterpreted as significant ruptures. Although MR arthrography is a more labor-intensive radiographic technique and requires specialized wrist coils to produce the anatomical detail noted in this study, this technique may be considered as a reasonable second best diagnostic tool to wrist arthroscopy.

S.D. Trigg, M.D.

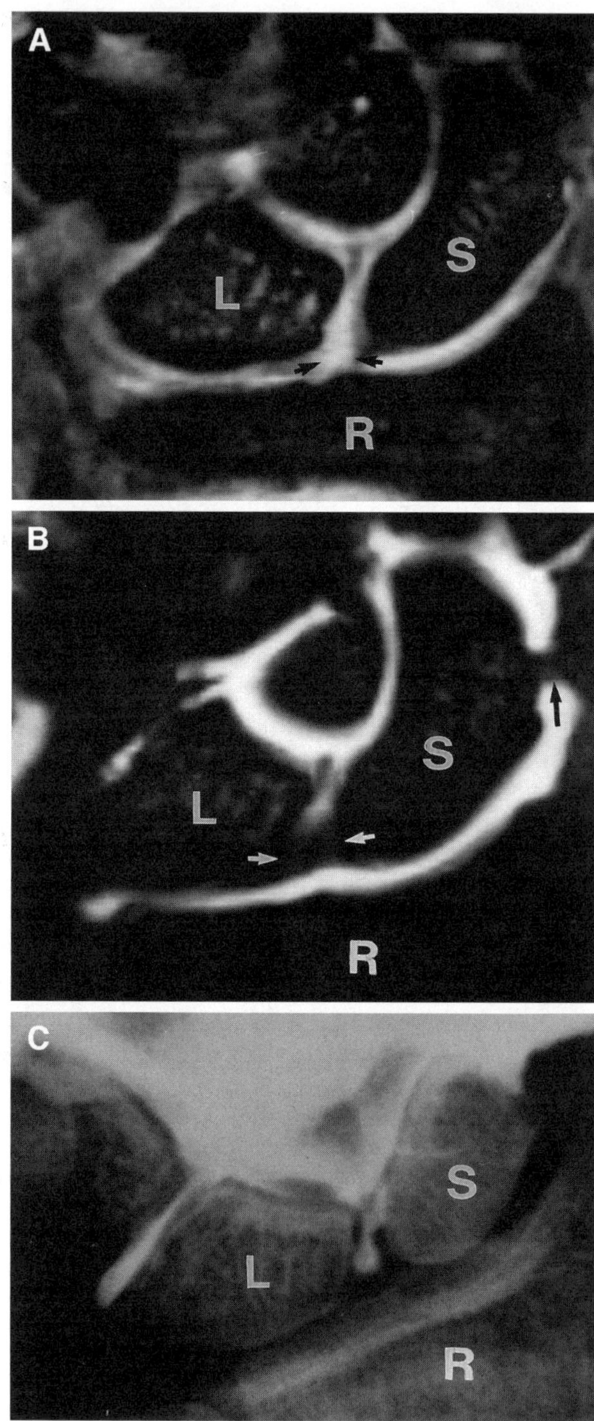

(Continued)

The Utility of High-Resolution Magnetic Resonance Imaging in the Evaluation of the Triangular Fibrocartilage Complex of the Wrist
Potter HG, Asnis-Ernberg L, Weiland AJ, et al (Hosp for Special Surgery, New York)
J Bone Joint Surg Am 79-A:1675–1684, 1997   5–2

Introduction.—Tears of the triangular fibrocartilage complex of the wrist may not be readily apparent on physical examination because many other lesions may produce pain on the ulnar side. Arthrograms of the wrist have been used to detect these tears, but their ability to localize the tear and provide information regarding adjacent soft-tissue structures may be limited. A prospective study assessed the value of high-resolution MRI in the detection and localization of tears of the triangular fibrocartilage complex.

Methods.—Seventy-seven patients—all with pain, ligamentous instability, and/or occult ganglia—were evaluated from January 1993 to April 1996. The MRI studies used a dedicated surface coil and 3-dimensional gradient-recalled techniques. Images were assessed for radial or ulnar avulsion, central defects, degenerative intrasubstance changes, joint fluids, and complex tears of the triangular fibrocartilage complex. Findings of MRI were compared with those of arthroscopy.

Results.—Fifty-nine of 77 patients appeared to have a tear of the triangular fibrocartilage complex at MRI; 57 cases were confirmed at arthroscopy. Fourteen of 21 partial tears identified at MRI were confirmed on arthroscopic examination. Twenty-nine tears were ulnar, 8 were radial (Fig 5), 9 were central, and 11 were complex. When arthroscopy was used as the standard, MRI had a sensitivity of 100%, a specificity of 90%, and an accuracy of 97% for detection of a tear of the triangular fibrocartilage complex of the wrist. In 53 of 57 tears, MRI provided accurate localization; sensitivity was 100%, specificity 75%, and accuracy 92%.

Discussion.—Subtle morphologic changes in the triangular fibrocartilage complex can be detected if proper MRI technique is used. All imaging in these patients used a 1.5-tesla superconducting magnet and either a 5-inch curved receive-only surface coil or quadrature design phased-array wrist coil. The coronal volumetric acquisition was centered over the proximal aspect of the lunate, and the slice thickness was 1 mm. No contrast medium was used.

FIGURE 3 (cont.)
    FIGURE 3.—In a woman 24 years of age with posttraumatic radial wrist pain for 1 month, **A,** non-enhanced coronal gradient-echo image shows areas of intermediate to high signal intensity between the scaphoid and lunate bones (palmar SLIL segment, *arrows*). This was interpreted as SLIL perforation. **B,** MR arthrography demonstrates the intact and taut palmar SLIL (*white arrows*), which was proved arthroscopically. Note the ligament carrying the main vascular supply to the scaphoid (*black arrow*). **C,** arthrogram, obtained after a midcarpal injection, shows no evidence of SLIL perforation. *Abbreviations:* *SLIL,* scapholunate interosseous ligament; *R,* radius; *S,* scaphoid bone; *L,* lunate bone. (Courtesy of Scheck RJ, Kubitzek C, Hierner R, et al: The scapholunate interosseous ligament in MR arthrography of the wrist: Correlation with non-enhanced MRI and wrist arthroscopy. *Skeletal Radiol* 26:263–271. Copyright 1997, Springer-Verlag.)

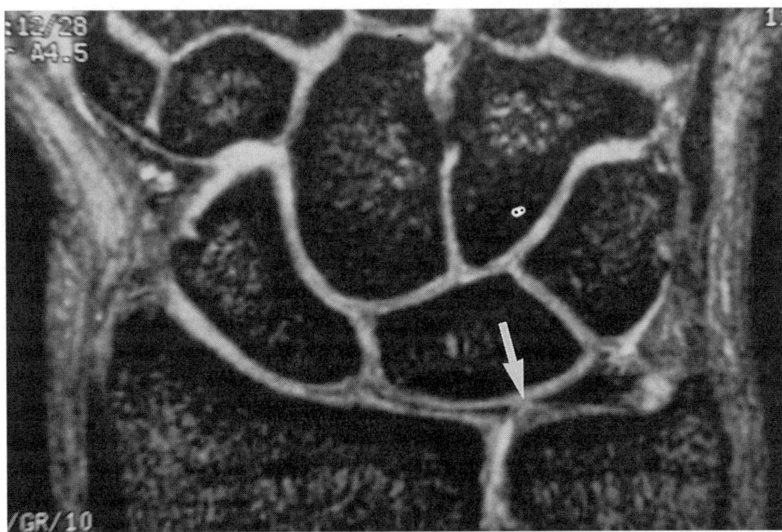

FIGURE 5.—Coronal gradient-echo image of a 46-year-old man who had had a previous twisting injury, demonstrating a radial detachment of the articular disk *(arrow)*. The detachment was confirmed at the time of arthroscopy. (Courtesy of Potter HG, Asnis-Ernberg L, Weiland AJ, et al: The utility of high-resolution magnetic resonance imaging in the evaluation of the triangular fibrocartilage complex of the wrist. *J Bone Joint Surg Am* 79-A:1675–1684, 1997.)

▶ Many of the early literature studies reporting the usefulness of MRI for the diagnosis of tears of the triangular fibrocartilage complex of the wrist used low-contrast, thick-section image acquisition, often with relatively large fields of view and conventional spin-echo pulse-sequencing techniques. Not surprisingly, many of these studies reported less than acceptable degrees of sensitivity and specificity when compared with subsequent arthroscopic operative findings. The authors of this study have shown that with refinement of the MRI technique and the use of smaller fields of view, the level of agreement between MRI and arthroscopy is significantly improved with respect to localization of complete tears and only slightly less accurate for detection of partial tears.

Arthroscopy remains the most accurate, sensitive, and specific diagnostic tool for the detection of abnormalities of the triangular fibrocartilage complex of the wrist when used by experienced surgeons. However, arthroscopy cannot detect many other sources of ulnar-sided wrist pain and, therefore, when the clinical examination is uncertain or there is a suspicion of multiple problems, high-resolution MRI may provide significant of information with a relatively high degree of accuracy.

S.D. Trigg, M.D.

Arthroscopic Diagnosis of Intra-articular Soft Tissue Injuries Associated With Distal Radial Fractures
Richards RS, Bennett JD, Roth JH, et al (Univ of Western Ontario, London, Ont; St Joseph's Health Centre, London, Ont)
J Hand Surg [Am] 22A:772–776, 1997   5–3

Introduction.—About 10% of all bony injuries and up to 75% of all fractures of the forearm are fractures of the radius. Arthrography and stress radiographs do not provide the anatomical detail of arthroscopy. Soft-tissue injuries present in intra-articular and extra-articular fractures of the radius were examined. The value of preoperative radiographs in predicting associated soft-tissue injury was evaluated.

Methods.—One hundred eighteen patients with distal radial fractures that required surgical reduction and fixation because of failure to obtain or maintain reduction underwent arthroscopy. Intra-articular bleeding and the amount of irrigation fluid required were minimized by performing arthroscopic reduction of fractures 48 hours after injury. Radial-sided triangular fibrocartilage complex (TFCC) injuries and scapholunate (SL) and lunotriquetrol (LT) ligament injuries were treated arthroscopically.

Results.—Of 118 patients, 46 had TFCC tears. The TFCC tears were present in 35% of intra-articular fractures and in 53% of extra-articular fractures. There was a higher incidence of Palmer 1D radial tears in patients who had a 3-part fracture, compared with other fracture types. In 88 patients with intra-articular fractures; SL ligament injuries with SL instability were observed in 19 patients (21.6%); 6 patients (6.8%) had LT ligament injuries; and 6 patients had combined SL and LT ligament injuries. Preoperative radiographs were not predictive of SL injury; 60% of all SL tears had a normal SL interval of 2 mm or less. There was no association between ulnar styloid fractures and TFCC injuries. Initial displacement was associated with the presence of a TFCC injury. Patients with an intact TFCC had an average ulnar variance of 2.5 mm positive, compared with an average variance of 4.6 mm positive in patients with a torn TFCC. The average dorsal angulation was 12 degrees and 24 degrees, respectively, in patients with an intact and torn TFCC. Patients with 4-part fractures with a coronal fracture of the lunate facet had a lower incidence of radial TFCC tears than those with extra-articular fractures or 3-part fractures. Differences for ulnar variance, dorsal angulation, and fracture types were significant.

Conclusion.—The association between arthroscopically detected intra-articular distal radial fractures and ligament injuries was reported earlier; the large number of associated soft-tissue injuries with extra-articular distal radial fractures have not been reported before. Tears of the radial aspect of the TFCC were observed for both types of fractures. The preoperative degree of displacement was associated with the presence of a TFCC injury. Preoperative radiographs were not useful in predicting the presence of SL or LT ligament injuries. The SL and LT ligament injuries were observed in severely comminuted intra-articular fractures and minimally displaced extra-articular fractures.

▶ As if the technical difficulties inherent in the successful reduction, stabilization, and eventual anatomical healing of fractures of the distal radius are not enough to contend with, the information learned from this study regarding the prevalence of associated soft-tissue injuries about the carpus presents additional treatment considerations in some cases. Fortunately, from experience, it would appear that the majority of these soft-tissue disruptions heal by the time of fracture union. However, important predictive information is given by the authors, particularly with respect to the association of TFCC injuries and degree of initial displacement of the fracture fragments. If signficant displacement is noted, additional investigation in the acute setting should be done to assess distal radioulnar joint and ulnar-carpal stability. Furthermore, any persistence of pain or symptoms of instability or both after fracture healing may be a sequela of incomplete healing of these soft-tissue elements and thus warrants a more focused clinical examination to determine insufficiency of the TFCC and the SL and LT interosseous ligaments.

S.D. Trigg, M.D.

Wrist

Treatment of Unstable Distal Radius Fractures: Methods and Comparison of External Distraction and ORIF Versus External Distraction-ORIF Neutralization
Putnam MD, Fischer MD (Univ of Minnesota, Minneapolis)
J Hand Surg (Am) 22A:238–251, 1997   5–4

Objective.—Unstable distal fractures are characterized by the presence of fragments, intra-articular extension, and soft tissue injury. Because of the deleterious effects of prolonged mobilization, external fixation to facilitate reduction and protect against shortening, and internal fixation to restore anatomy and permit early mobility are recommended. Results of a defined protocol of external distraction, internal fixation, early removal of external fixation, and mobilization are assessed.

Methods.—For 3 years 26 patients, part of a larger group treated according to the protocol, were followed-up for an average of 14 months (Fig 1). Reduction was unacceptable if there was radial shortening > 2 mm, angulation > 5 degrees dorsal or > 15 degrees volar, or an intra-articular stepoff > 1 mm. Radiographs were taken before and after reduction. Fractures were classified according to the AO/ASIF method as 1 (A-2), 6 (A-3), 1 (B-3), 2 (C-1), 13 (C-2), and 3 (C-3) and, according to the Frykman method, as 17 grade VIII, 5 grade VII, 3 grade VI, and 1 grade V.

Technique.—The fracture is exposed radially and traction is applied. The radius is exposed through the fourth compartment using either a dorsal or volar approach depending on the direction of displacement of the distal fragment. Reduction is performed

Management Algorithm

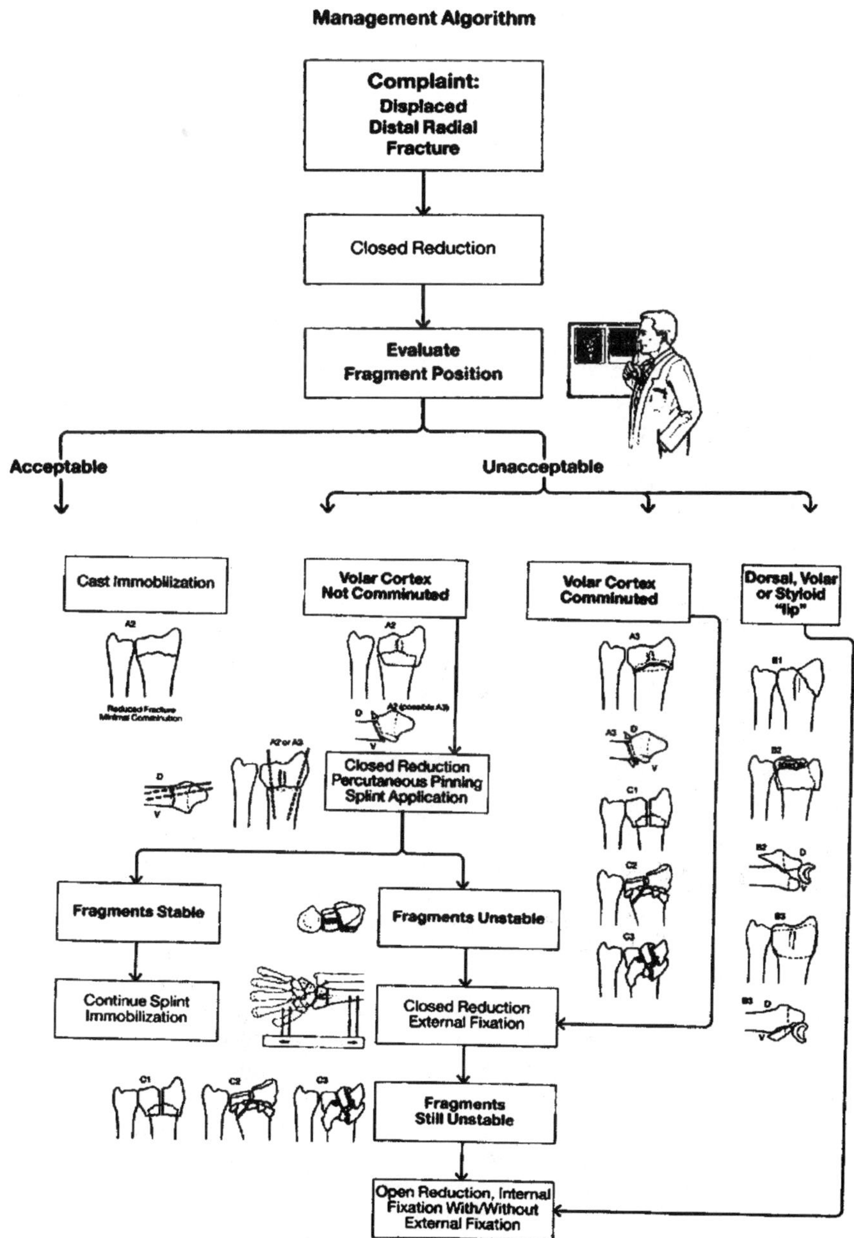

FIGURE 1.—The management algorithm currently used by the authors for all distal radius fractures. (Courtesy of Putnam MD, Fischer MD: Treatment of unstable distal radius fractures: Methods and comparison of external distraction-ORIF neutralization. *J Hand Surg [Am]* 22A:238–251, 1997).

with the aid of distraction provided by the external fixator. Fixation is accomplished with Kirschner wires and a 3.5-mm oblique T-plate. A bone graft may be necessary. The external fixator is removed, and the stability of the radius is assessed by direct visual fluoroscopy. If the repair is unstable, the fixator is left in place for as long as 4 weeks.

Results.—Bone grafts were required in 25 of 26 patients. External fixation was applied for a mean of 24 days. Intra-articular stepoff was graded 0 in 21 patients and graded 1 in 15 patients. Active range of motion was 82% of unaffected side, flexion was 77% of unaffected side, and grip strength was 73% of unaffected side. Five patients had pain on heavy activity, 10 had occasional aches, and 11 were pain free. All 18 employed patients returned to work, with 1 requiring employment modification. When the group requiring postoperative external fixation was compared with the group requiring intraoperative external fixation, no differences were observed in any measurements. Two complications in the latter group included a collapse of volar support and volar migration and a failure of fixation, leading to deformity. Complications reported in other studies include failure to achieve intra-articular reduction, loss of reduction after removal of the fixator, or high rates of pin track problems.

Conclusion.—The need for external fixation of unstable distal radius fractures was determined by the stability of internal fixation. Use of bone grafts, plates, and screws or external fixation lessened the risk of loss of reduction.

▶ The authors of this study have presented yet another approach to the management of complex, unstable distal radius fractures using a defined protocol. Their use of an external fixation device in all cases where open reduction, bone grafting, and internal fixation was done served two important purposes. First, the external fixation device, like other methods of intraoperative traction, greatly facilitates the reduction and provisional stabilization of these unstable fractures. Second, once bone grafting and internal fixation was carried out, the fixator was removed and fracture stability was assessed; when the construct was judged to be possibly unstable, the fixator was then reassembled to act as a neutralization device with early removal of the device (mean 24 days). These results appear to have excluded many of the problems of long-term fixator placement, including pin tract infection and arthrofibrosis. The treatment protocol allows use of the best features of both stabilization techniques: internal fixation for early mobilization when ridged internal fixation is achieved and the use of external fixation as a temporary neutralization device to allow initial healing of more unstable ORIF constructs. This approach should be strongly considered when the treatment of more complex distal radius fractures is undertaken by operative means.

S.D. Trigg, M.D.

Prospective Multicenter Trial of a Plate for Dorsal Fixation of Distal Radius Fractures

Ring D, Jupiter JB, Brennwald J, et al (Harvard Med School, Boston; Univ of Basel, Switzerland; Inselspital, Bern, Switzerland; et al)

J Hand Surg (Am) 22A:777–784, 1997   5–5

Introduction.—Stable internal fixation of fractures of the distal end of the radius has been problematic because of inadequate plate design, including poor adaptation to the pathologic anatomy of the distal radius, difficult contouring or trimming of the plate, difficulty securely fixing small articular fracture fragments, and irritation of the overlying extensor tendons from the bulk of the hardware. Outcome of a plate design intended to facilitate management of complex wrist pathology was evaluated in 22 patients with complex fractures who underwent internal fixation.

Methods.—The plate was used only in patients for whom open reduction and internal fixation was appropriate, including 16 patients with

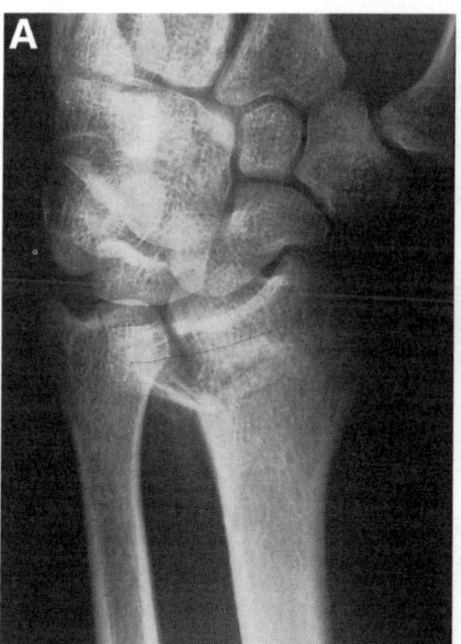
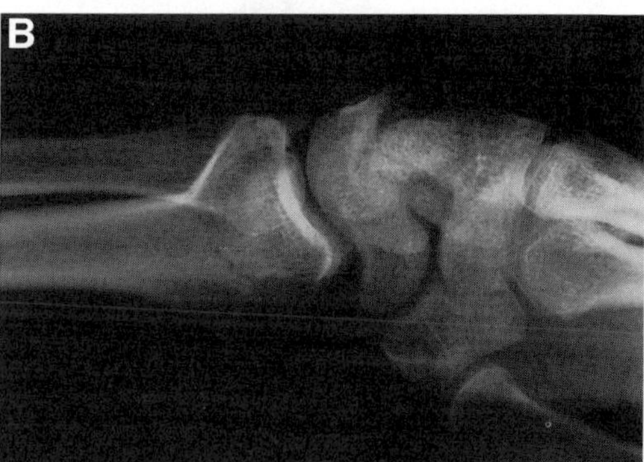
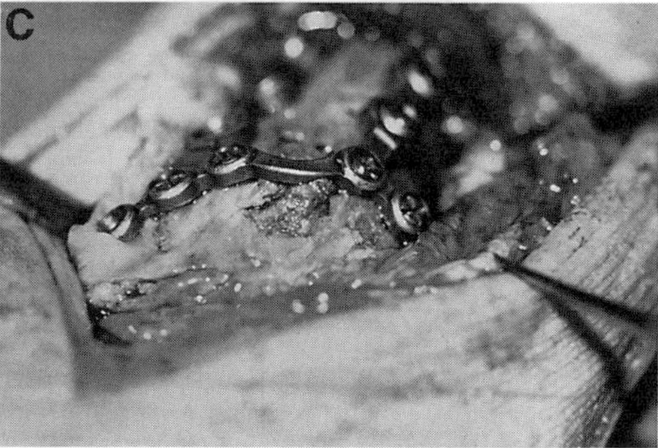

(*Continued*)

FIGURE 2 (cont.)

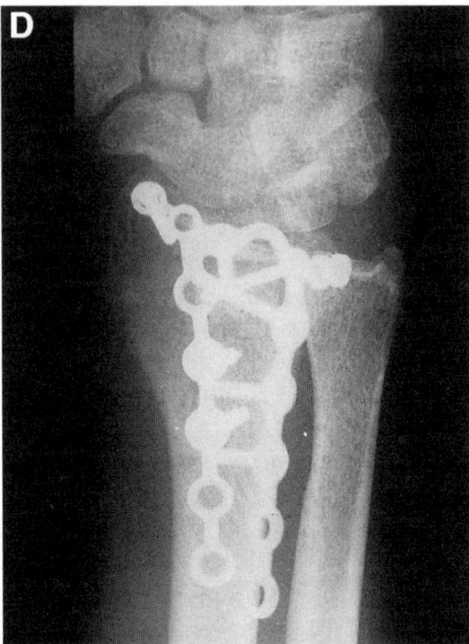

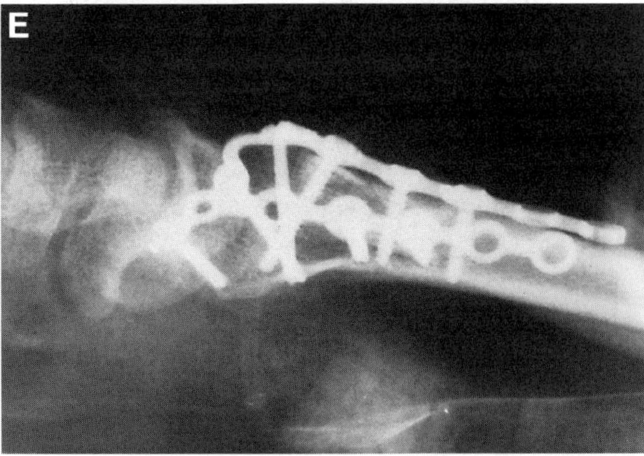

FIGURE 2.—A 51-year-old executive fell, sustaining this dorsal bending fracture of the distal radius. He was seen 3.5 weeks after closed reduction and splint immobilization. Two oblique radiographs (**A, B**) demonstrate marked dorsal angulation (**C**). The fourth extensor compartment with the enclosed extensor tendons is elevated subperiosteally. A dorsal capsulotomy is made to inspect the scapholunate interosseous ligament and articular surface of the distal radius. Osteotomy through the fracture site and callus was required to improve the reduction. Anteroposterior (**D**) and lateral (**E**) radiographs obtained 1 year later demonstrate a healed fracture in good alignment. The hardware is intact. (Courtesy of Ring D, Jupiter JB, Brennwald J: Prospective multicenter trial of a plate for dorsal fixation of distal radius fractures. *J Hand Surg [Am]* 22A:777–784, 1997.)

complex intra-articular fracture (C2 or C3 fractures) and 2 patients with dorsal articular shearing-type fractures. Six patients also underwent supplemental fixation (4 with an external fixator, 1 with a volar T-shaped plate, and 1 with a 3.5-mm interfragmentary compression screw). All except 3 patients had autograft cancellous bone (harvested from the iliac crest) placed into metaphyseal defects.

Surgical Technique.—Finger trap traction or temporary external fixation was used to produce continuous distraction of the distal fracture in most patients. Articular reconstruction was supported with the 1.0-mm buttress pins to provide fixed anchor points not dependent upon screw thread-bone in patients with severe comminution or poor bone quality. Full active digit motion and forearm rotation were recommended immediately after surgery. Wrist motion was usually possible after a short period of splint immobilization.

Results.—Final follow-up was an average of 14 months after surgery. At an average of 6 weeks after surgery, radiographic evidence of union was documented. Average parameters were: palmer tilt 5 degrees, radial inclination 18.5 degrees, radial shortening 0 mm, and maximum articular incongruity 0.5 mm. There was no loss of reduction from immediate postoperative radiographs to those taken at final follow-up evaluation. Residual deformity occurred in arms with incomplete reduction of complex and challenging fractures. No evidence of carpal instability was detected on follow-up radiographs. On final follow-up, average range of motion and grip strength were 76% and 56% of the contralateral side, respectively. There were no infections, nonunions, wound problems, or plate failures. Four of 5 patients who had extensor tendon irritation had their plates removed. Tendonitis in all patients occurred in the second dorsal compartment, rather than the fourth, which is typical for patients who have undergone dorsal plate fixation. There were 6, 7, and 9 excellent, good, and fair results, respectively, according to the rating scale of Gartland and Werley.

Conclusion.—One of the goals of this plate design was to minimize extensor tendon irritation, thus making dorsal plate fixation a more attractive option. Five of 22 patients (23%) had extensor tendonitis within the follow-up period. The surgical technique has been altered to reduce the rate of tendonitis. A retinacular flap is now used to protect the second-compartment extensor tendons. The plate provided fixation secure enough to allow immediate postoperative immobilization in patients with relatively simple fracture patterns (Fig 2).

▶ The successful management of complex unstable fractures of the distal radius remains as yet an unsolved problem. The more recent trend toward management of these fractures by open reduction, bone grafting, and internal fixation was borne out of the frustrations of unpredictable outcomes when external fixation alone was used. External fixation often yielded unacceptable restoration of anatomy and was frequently associated with multiple postoperative complications. The message of this present study is not about this particular plate design, itself, as other recently introduced dorsal plate designs can claim similar results. Rather, this and other preliminary studies appear to show a more favorable clinical outcome with internal fixation when compared with studies using external fixation for comparable complex fractures. The progress in plate design, and as importantly, the operative techniques learned by their investigators should be carefully followed by all orthopedists because of the growing functional expectations of our patients after treatment of these common skeletal injuries.

S.D. Trigg, M.D.

The Risks of Kirschner Wire Placement in the Distal Radius: A Comparison of Techniques

Hochwald NL, Levine R, Tornetta P III (Univ Hosp of Brooklyn, NY; Univ of Medicine and Dentistry of New Jersey, Newark)
J Hand Surg (Am) 22A:580–584, 1997   5–6

Introduction.—Kirschner wires (K-wires) are frequently used in the fixation of distal radius fractures. Optimal placement is controversial, as there is concern about injury to the extensor tendons and branches of the superficial radial nerve. The incidence of potential nerve or tendon injury associated with 2 K-wire placement techniques was compared using fresh cadaver wrists.

Methods.—Eighty-eight K-wires were inserted into 44 cadaver wrists. Kirschner wires were placed percutaneously at the radial styloid and Lister's tubercle in 22 wrists. In the remaining 22 wrists, K-wires were

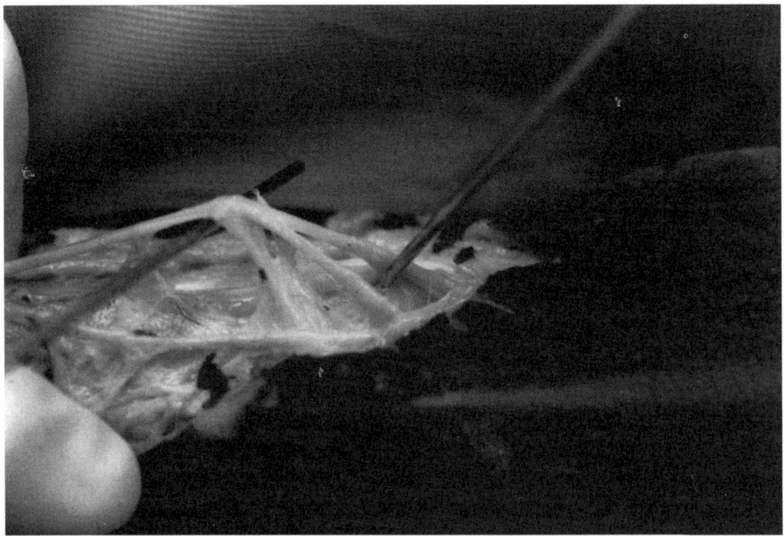

FIGURE 1.—A percutaneously placed Kirschner wire (K-wire) at the radial styloid is shown displacing a superficial radial nerve branch. Note the close proximity of the nerve arborization to the K-wire position. (Courtesy of Hochwald NL, Levine R, Tornetta P III: The risks of Kirschner wire placement in the distal radius: A comparison of techniques. *J Hand Surg [Am]* 22A:580–584, 1997.)

inserted at the same site through a limited open incision. After K-wire placement, wrists were dissected under a 3.5× loupe magnification. The sensory branch of the radial nerve was located and traced distally through its arborization. The first 3 extensor compartments were dissected for visualization. Measurements were taken from the K-wires to the branches of the radial sensory nerve and to the closest aspect of individual extensor compartments. Structures were considered potentially injured if they were displaced, notched, pierced, or touched the K-wires.

Results.—In the percutaneous group, pins touched or pierced an extensor tendon in 2 of 22 (9%) wrists at the radial styloid and 9 (41%) at Lister's tubercle; and the superficial radial nerve in 7 (32%) at the radial styloid and 1 (5%) at Lister's tubercle. None of the nerve branches were pierced. In the limited open technique group, pins did not touch extensor tendons at the radial styloid. One pin in 1 wrist (5%) entered the first extensor compartment between tendon slips, 1 (5%) extensor tendon was punctured at Lister's tubercle, and the superficial radial nerve was touching or displaced by the K-wire in 1 (5%) wrist at the radial styloid and at Lister's tubercle (Fig 1).

Conclusion.—Percutaneous insertion of K-wires yielded a significantly higher rate of potentially injured nerves and tendons than the limited open technique. Blunt dissection down to bone and the use of a soft-tissue protector for K-wire insertion into the distal radius is recommended to decrease the risk of potential injuries.

▶ Kirschner wires (K-wires) are among the most commonly utilized devices for provisional intra-operative fracture stabilization as well as for more permanent fixation in the operative treatment of distal radius fractures. The radial styloid fragment often remains largely intact in such fractures, and for this reason, K-wires are frequently placed through this fragment as a first step in the reduction and reassembly of the bone fragments. The authors of this study clearly point out the dangers of percutaneous placement resulting from the proximity and variability of branches of the superficial branch of the radial nerve as they course over the radial styloid. The secondary danger of impaling adjacent tendons is also noted. With appropriate caution, the authors strongly suggest using a limited open incision and blunt dissection to bone with K-wire placement performed under direct visualization, thus reducing potential injury to these structures.

S.D. Trigg, M.D.

Corrective Osteotomy for Malunited, Volarly Displaced Fractures of the Distal End of the Radius

Shea K, Fernandez DL, Jupiter JB, et al (Massachusetts Gen Hosp, Boston; Kantonspital, Aarav, Switzerland)
J Bone Joint Surg Am 79-A:1816–1826, 1997

5–7

Background.—Malunion after a volarly displaced fracture of the distal metaphysis of the radius causes a decrease in grip strength, cosmetic deformity, and incongruence and instability of the joint. The results of

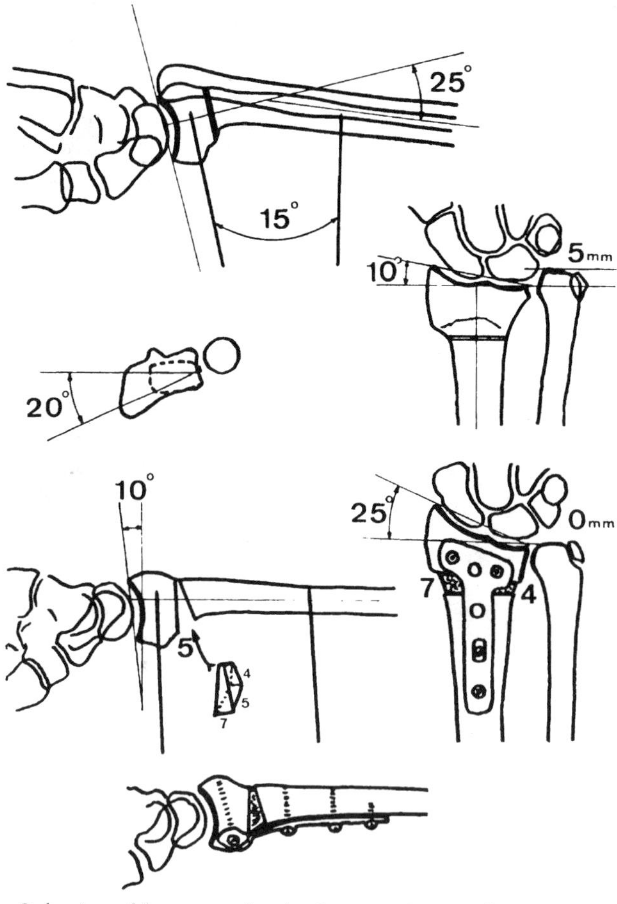

FIGURE 1.—C, drawings of the preoperative plan for a man, 57 years of age, who had had a malunited Smith fracture associated with dorsal subluxation of the distal radioulanr joint for 6 months. The involved wrist had volar inclination of 25 degrees compared with 10 degrees on the normal side, 10 degrees of ulnar inclination compared with 25 degrees on the normal side, −5 mm of ulnar variance compared with −1 degree on the normal side, and a pronation deformity of 20 degrees. Use of a corticocancellous wedge graft measuring 7 × 5 × 4 mm was planned to support the correction. (Courtesy of Shea K, Fernandez DL, Jupiter JB, et al: Corrective osteotomy for malunited, volarly displaced fractures of the distal end of the radius. *J Bone Joint Surg Am* 79-A:1816–1826, 1997.)

corrective osteotomy for a volarly angulated, posttraumatic deformity of the distal end of the radius were retrospectively analyzed in a series of 25 patients.

Methods.—The study group consisted of 25 patients aged 21–84 years who had corrective osteotomy for malunited volarly angulated fractures of the distal end of the radius from 1986 to 1995. The indications for osteotomy were pain or functional limitations. The initial treatment had been closed reduction and immobilization for 22 and operative intervention for 3 patients. The patients were referred an average of 8 months after fracture. All patients reported wrist pain. All had limited wrist motion and decreased grip strength. Posttraumatic osteoarthritic changes were detected in the majority of patients. The goals of the opening-wedge osteotomy included anatomical restoration and improvement of joint range of motion (Fig 1, C). Postoperatively, the wrist was supported with a splint for 2 weeks, unless more than 10 mm of lengthening was required. In that case, a cast was worn for 6 weeks. After removal of the external support, exercises and activities of daily living were resumed, but resistance and manual labor were not permitted until radiographically confirmed union, at about 8 weeks.

Findings.—The 25 patients in the study group were followed up for an average of 61 months after the osteotomy. Of the 25 patients, 11 had an additional operative procedure. The procedures included removal of the plate and screws in 7 patients, removal of the hardware plus a Bowers procedure and ulnar shortening, a Darrach resection, and a carpal tunnel release in 1 patient each. In 1 patient, the osteotomy did not heal, requiring an additional bone graft with new plate and screws. Union of the fracture was documented in the other 24 patients by 8 weeks. At the last follow-up, 13 patients were free of pain, 10 had mild pain, and 2 had severe pain. Ability to work was normal in 20 and reduced in 5 patients. After surgery, average supination of the forearm increased from 41 to 69 degrees, average pronation of the forearm increased from 64 to 75 degrees, average wrist extension increased from 25 to 55 degrees, average wrist flexion increased from 53 to 55 degrees, and average grip strength increased from 17 kg to 30 kg. Sensory examination demonstrated sensitivity comparable with the contralateral hand in all patients. Recent radiographs demonstrated union at the osteotomy site in all 25 patients. Average ulnar inclination improved from 14 to 22 degrees, average volar inclination improved from 24 to 5 degrees, and average ulnar variance improved from 5 to 0 mm. The overall functional results were rated very good in 10, good in 8, fair in 3, and poor in 4 patients in the study group.

Conclusions.—In retrospective series of 25 patients who had corrective osteotomy for malunited volarly displaced fracture of the distal end of the radius, the functional result was very good in 10, good in 8, fair in 3, and poor in 4. Every effort should be expended to create and maintain anatomical reduction in the treatment of volarly displaced fractures of the distal end of the radius.

▶ Malunion of the volarly displaced fractures of the distal radius result in adverse alterations in the function on the hand, wrist, and forearm and are associated with arthrofibrosis and posttraumatic arthrosis similar to the more common dorsally displaced distal radius fracture malunions. This study shows, not surprisingly, that after successful corrective osteotomy, there is an improvement of function equivalent to that noted after similar procedures done for the dorsally displaced malunions. However, as for the dorsally displaced fracture malunions, pain and instability about the distal radioulnar joint (DRUJ) remains the most perplexing and as yet unresolved postoperative problem. Whether or not an additional procedure should be done about the DRUJ (e.g., hemiresection arthroplasty or ulnar shortening) at the time of the osteotomy should be based on preoperative radiographic assessment and intraoperative findings of residual instability, articular congruency, and arthrosis. Nonetheless, as the authors learned, even such well-done additional procedures about the DRUJ are unfortunately associated with a higher percentage of unfavorable outcomes. Our inability, therefore, to reliably predict whether or not these secondary procedures about the distal end of the radius will be successful should compel us to counsel patients in the acute situation, that open reduction and internal fixation of displaced distal radius fractures should be strongly considered as the best initial treatment.

S.D. Trigg, M.D.

Repeat Screw Stabilization With Bone Grafting After a Failed Herbert Screw Fixation for Acute Scaphoid Fractures and Nonunions
Inoue G, Kuwahata Y (Nagoya Univ, Japan; Kuwahata Orthopaedic Clinic, Shizuoka, Japan)
J Hand Surg (Am) 22A:413–418, 1997   5–8

Introduction.—The reported success rate for Herbert screw internal fixation for acute scaphoid fractures and nonunions is 80% to 90%. Failures do occur, and there is little in the literature that addresses the optimal treatment for patients with a persistent nonunion after a failed Herbert screw procedure. Outcomes of a series of 8 patients who underwent repeat Herbert screw internal fixation and bone grafting for both acute scaphoid fractures and nonunions were evaluated.

Methods.—All patients were males with an average age of 26 years. Three patients underwent their original procedure for an acute scaphoid fracture and 6 for nonunion. The average interval from initial to second surgery was 13 months. All patients had a fracture that passed through the middle third of the scaphoid.

Surgical Technique.—The loosened screw was removed and bone fragments were cleared. The flexion deformity was rectified and an iliac crest–wedge-shaped bone graft was introduced. Cancellous bone chips were packed into the cavity and the region of the previous screw hole. The appropriate screw length was determined, and the scaphoid was drilled along the same course as the pilot hole, then tapped. The screw was inserted freehandedly. Wrists were immobilized for about 7 weeks.

Results.—Average follow-up was 19 months after the last operation. Six patients achieved union after the second Herbert screw fixation by an average of 12 weeks. They were pain free and were able to return to their previous occupations. Compared with the uninvolved wrist, the average range of motion (ROM) of the treated wrist was 87% and average grip strength was 93%. Two patients, 1 who was treated by a lag screw fixation, did not achieve union. One patient achieved union 3 months after a third procedure involving an inlay bone graft and K-wire fixation (wrist ROM 57%; grip 69%). Another patient with a 20-year nonunion history and mild osteoarthritic changes underwent a third procedure. The posterior interosseous nerve was denervated at the wrist and this provided pain relief (wrist ROM 54%; grip 73%). Both patients needed a change of employment to lighter work.

Conclusion.—Repeat bone grafting using supplemental K-wire internal fixation might be the treatment of choice for patients with failure of the Herbert screw. Four to 5 months of immobilization of the wrist may be required for subsequent procedures. The most frequent cause of failure of the Herbert screw is improper screw placement.

▶ Herbert screw fixation of scaphoid fractures has revolutionized the treatment of both acute scaphoid fractures and scaphoid fracture nonunion. The reported union rates utilizing this device remain very favorable (80% to 90%). Most surgical procedures for nonunions after Herbert screw fixation failures have resorted to Russe-type grafting, a technique that requires long periods of postoperative casting, often with resultant complications common after prolonged immobilization. The authors of this study present their experience with repeat Herbert screw fixation and bone grafting of scaphoid wrist fracture nonunions. Although apparently technically difficult as a second procedure, their reported success rate gives creditablity to this as a viable secondary procedure alternative to the more common Russe-graft techniques. One may also consider the use of this approach alone or with a vascularized bone graft, which theoretically may improve the union rate of the second procedure.

S.D. Trigg, M.D.

Radial Recession Osteotomy for Kienböck's Disease

Quenzer DE, Dobyns JH, Linscheid RL, et al (Mayo Clinic and Found, Rochester, Minn)
J Hand Surg [Am] 22A:386–395, 1997
5–9

Background.—Radial recession decreases joint compressive forces in patients with negative ulnar variance resulting from Kienböck's lunatomalacia. The clinical and radiographic outcomes of 68 radial recession osteotomies for Kienböck's disease were examined to determine risks and benefits of this procedure. In 25 of these patients, concomitant procedures were also performed.

Study Group.—Clinical records, plain radiographs, and trispiral tomographs were reviewed for the 68 consecutive patients who underwent radial recession osteotomy for unilateral Kienböck's disease. One half of the patients reported injuries, and symptoms had been present at least 6 months before diagnosis. None of the patients had a medical disease associated with avascular necrosis or had diabetes. Of the 68 patients in this series, 26 performed heavy labor and 12 performed moderate labor. Five patients were receiving disability payments. All patients reported wrist pain. Range of motion and grip strength were decreased in all patients.

Methods.—The radial recession osteotomies were performed between 1978 and 1992. A supplemental surgical procedure was performed for 25 of the 68 patients in the study group. No patient had intercarpal arthrodesis. During the osteotomy, an attempt was made to correct ulnar variance to neutral or slightly positive, by removing an average of 3.0 mm of radius. The postoperative follow-up ranged from 12 to 133 months.

Results.—Healing of the radius was radiographically confirmed by 16 weeks in 64 patients and by 6 months in the remaining 4 patients. Complications occurred in 6 patients, including the delayed healing, and injuries to the extensor pollicus longus. The plate and screw were removed in 11 patients. Three patients had lunate cheilectomy to relieve pain and improve motion. A successful tendon transfer was performed in 1 patient. At the 6-month follow-up, 97% of patients reported improvement and 13% were free of pain. At the 12-month follow-up, 93% reported improvement and 43% were free of pain. Range of motion was improved in 52% and worsened in 19%. Grip strength was improved in 74%. In this series, 74% returned to their original jobs, including 81% of heavy laborers. There were no differences in outcome for the workers' compensation patients and the group as a whole. Ulnocarpal impingement developed in 2 patients.

Clinical outcome was not significantly different for those patients who underwent supplemental procedures. Three of the patients who had supplemental procedures had complications related to those procedures. Surgical change in ulnar variance averaged 2.8 mm. Five patients had formation of new lunate fossa bone formation. Radial inclination was reduced an average of 41 degrees. Of 35 patients studied for at least 12 months, 12 had improvement in lunate density, fracture healing, and joint space preservation. Radiographic findings were not changed in 16 patients and 7 had further lunate collapse. Lunate density improved in 40%, was unchanged in 46%, and worsened in 14%. Lunate bone collapse was improved in 31%, unchanged in 66%, and worsened in 1 patient. Lunate fragmentation improved in 5, was unchanged in 28, and worsened in 2 patients. Radiographic evidence of arthritis was observed in 23%. Carpal height increased in 29%, was unchanged in 43%, and decreased in 29%. Among the 25 patients with supplemental procedures, 50% had radiographic improvement with a minimum of 18 months of follow-up. Of the 12 patients who had lunate revascularization or vascularized bone grafting, 55% had improvement in appearance. Of the 8 patients who had nonvascularized bone grafts, 1 was improved. Of 9 patients who had open reduction and internal fixation, only 1 had radiographic evidence of success.

Conclusions.—Radial recession osteotomy is an effective procedure that provides pain relief for more than 90% of patients with Kienböck's disease. Radial recession does not always correct avascular necrosis of the lunate bone, and fractures and collapse may occur. Radial recession may be combined with other procedures, such as lunate revascularization.

▶ Ever since Hulten associated negative ulnar variance with Kienböck's disease in 1928, a majority of operative procedures have focused upon either lunate decompression, joint leveling, or both. Radial recession osteotomy has been shown in several biomechanical studies to decrease the joint compressive forces at the radiolunate joint. The authors of this study, similar to other reported studies on this procedure, have shown that the vast majority of patients had reduction of their preoperative pain postoperatively, and improved strength and motion. The authors mention, and I concur, that radial recession osteotomy is technically easier than ulnar lengthening, the latter requiring bone grafting. Nonetheless, as in other studies on the results of radial recession osteotomy, the appearance of the lunate often does not change over the long term despite the clinical improvements. Knowing this preoperatively, the authors have added numerous other adjuvant procedures, including bone grafting without revascularization, attempted osteosynthesis, and revascularization procedures to many of the osteotomies. Important to note is their conclusion that attempted osteosynthesis of an associated lunate fracture is not recommended based upon their failures of fixation. Additionally, bone grafting without revascularization was not successful in apparent revascularization of the lunate, except in 1 patient, whereupon 55% of patients undergoing vascularized lunate bone grafting showed evidence of revasculazation. It remains a matter of future study as to whether or not these vascularized grafting procedures done alone can compare with the clinical improvements noted with radial recession osteotomies.

S.D. Trigg, M.D.

Arthroscopic Synovectomy of the Rheumatoid Wrist: A 3.8 Year Follow-up

Adolfsson L, Frisén M (Univ Hosp, Linköping, Sweden)
J Hand Surg (Br) 22B:711–713, 1997

5–10

Objective.—Whether there is a long-term benefit of surgical synovectomy for joints affected by rheumatoid arthritis is controversial. Furthermore, there are no studies comparing arthroscopic synovectomy with open synovectomy. Results of a prospective study evaluating the long-term outcome after arthroscopic synovectomy are presented.

Methods.—Arthroscopic wrist synovectomy using the Whipple technique, including a traction device, a 2.4-mm arthroscope, continuous irrigation, and a motorized shaver system, was performed on 24 wrists in 19 patients (3 men), average age 46 years. Four dorsal incisions and 1 radial portal were used to visualize the radiocarpal and midcarpal space; another portal for the distal radioulnar joint was used in patients with intact triangular fibrocartilage. The average duration of surgery was 50 minutes. Range of motion (flexion-extension and pronation-supination) was measured preoperatively and repeated at an average of 3.8 years. Patients' subjective assessments of symptoms and function were obtained and compared with the normal wrist.

Results.—Seventeen (70.8%) of the 24 wrists showed improved ROM (Table 1). Although no long-term results of arthroscopic synovectomy have been published for comparison, this study indicates improvements of arthritic symptoms and function lasting an average of 3.8 years after arthroscopic synovectomy. This minimally invasive procedure allows immediate mobilization, probably because the technique reduces postoperative pain. Because radiography shows an increased risk of further degeneration if significant arthritic damage is present at surgery, early synovectomy may decrease joint destruction. Other studies have found no link between early synovectomy and long-term radiographic appearance.

Conclusion.—Radiographic findings and clinical results are not correlated and suggest that wrist arthroscopic synovectomy should be performed on patients with LDE grades 0 to III arthritis. Arthroscopic synovectomy does not affect the long-term outcome of the rheumatoid wrist.

TABLE 1.—Pre- and Postoperative (Mean 3.8 Years) Range of
Motion Values

	Preoperative	Postoperative
Average ROM flexion-extension	74°	87°
Average ROM pronation-supination	138°	152°
Average score	43	55

(Courtesy of Adolfsson L, Frisén M: Arthroscopic synovectomy of the rheumatoid wrist: A 3.8-year follow-up. *J Hand Surg [Br]* 22B:711–713, 1997.)

▶ Joint synovectomy for patients with inflammatory arthritis has proved to be an important procedure in the early stages of the disease when pharmacologic management has failed to resolve residual synovitis. The benefits of the procedure are usually improvement of pain, motion, and function. Arthroscopic synovectomy of the knee, shoulder, and elbow have proved to be as effective as an open synovectomy and is associated with less postoperative morbidity. Wrist synovectomy for inflammatory arthritic diseases has been infrequently reported, and then only with a short-term follow-up. The authors of this present study have shown that, at an average of 3.8 years after surgery, the majority of patients continued to have improved outcomes when compared with their preoperative status. However, as reported elsewhere in the literature, synovectomy may not alter the radiographic progression of the degenerative changes despite reported clinical improvements. Nonetheless, synovectomy should still be considered in patients with refractory synovitis, and, on the basis of this longer term study, arthroscopic synovectomy in the hands of experienced surgeons apparently offers distinct advantages over an open procedure.

S.D. Trigg, M.D.

Forearm

Reconstruction of the Interosseous Membrane of the Forearm in Cadavers

Skahen JR III, Palmer AK, Werner FW, et al (State Univ of New York, Syracuse)
J Hand Surg (Am) 22A:986–994, 1997   5–11

Introduction.—Proximal migration of the radius after resection of the radial head in the treatment of the Essex-Lopresti lesion can cause pain and disability of the distal radioulnar joint. Resection of the radial head by itself can aggravate this problem and should not be pursued, if possible. Present surgical approaches include: resection of the radial head and pinning of the distal radioulnar joint until soft tissues heal, silicone arthroplasty of the proximal radius, and construction of a single-bone forearm. Outcomes are inconsistent and do not solve the entire problem. When the radial head is lost, the central band (CB) of the interosseous membrane (IOM) resists proximal migration of the radius by shifting load to the ulna. It may be possible that reconstruction of a damaged IOM of the forearm with a load-sharing graft may prevent proximal migration of the radius. The biomechanical function of the IOM of the forearm was analyzed in 12 fresh cadaver forearms to determine the axial stabilization roles of the forearm, specifically the IOM and the triangular fibrocartilage complex (TFCC).

Findings.—Specimens were transected at the junction of the middle and distal thirds of the humerus. Dissection of the IOM of the forearm revealed that the CB was the most dominant and consistent structure. The palmaris longus and one half of the flexor carpi radialis were not adequate as graft material; thus, the full flexor carpi radialis tendon was used for grafting

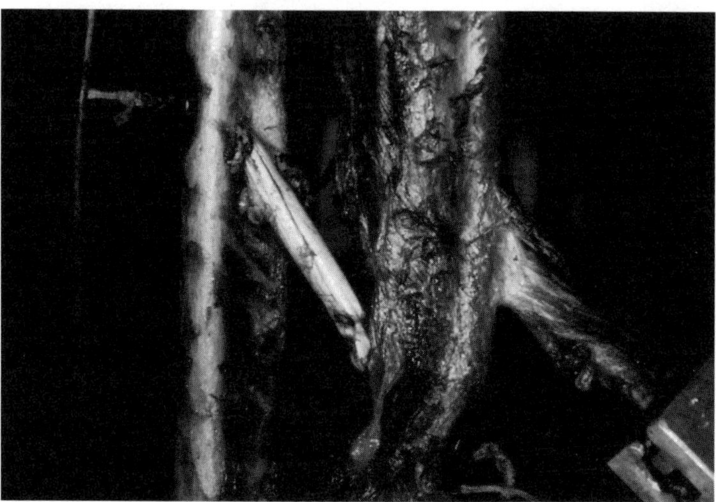

FIGURE 1.—A reconstruction graft for the central band of the interosseous membrane. Flexor carpi radialis autograft is secured in the position and orientation of the original central band. Each end of the flexor carpi radialis is held with a #5 nonabsorbable braided polyester suture using a whipstitch, passed through oblique holes in the radius and ulna, maximally tensioned, and tied to a nylon button. The ulna is on the left, the radius is on the right, and distal is at the top. (Courtesy of Skahen JR III, Palmer AK, Werner FW, et al: Reconstruction of the interosseous membrane of the forearm in cadavers. *J Hand Surg [Am]* 22A:986–994, 1997.)

(Fig 1). Strain in the CB of IOM was the least in full supination and progressively increased to a maximum in full pronation in intact specimens. This relationship was not dependent on direction of rotation, because data obtained during full supination to full pronation showed the same trend. Excision of the radial head did not alter this relationship. The strain in the CB was greater throughout forearm rotation. The rise in strain after radial head excision was significant from full pronation to 36 degrees of supination. Complete proximal migration of the radius to the point where the stump abutted the capitellum happened only after complete release of the IOM and TFCC.

Conclusion.—The Essex-Lopresti injury includes fracture of the radial head, disruption of the IOM, and disruption of the TFCC. This injury causes global instability of the forearm. Optimal treatment cannot be realized without addressing each component of the injury. The CB was a primary stabilizer of the forearm. Strain response to physiologic loading was found to be predictable, consistent, and dependent on position of forearm rotation. Excision of the radial head markedly increased the strain experienced by the CB. When the IOM and TFCC are competent, they can resist proximal migration of the radius.

▶ The proximal migration of the radius after resection of the radial head for treatment of the Essex-Lopresti injury often results in functional disability, pain, and eventual arthrosis of the distal radioulnar joint. This migration is often gradual and is hypothesized to be a result of attenuation of the IOM with repetitive force load. The authors of this cadaveric study have furthered our knowledge of the importance of the radial head as the primary stabilizer to proximal radius migration and, secondly, the role of the CB of the IOM and TFCC as the most important secondary stabilizers. The authors present from their laboratory studies a viable reconstructive procedure of the CB using a flexor carpi radialis graft that may have future clinical application in correcting radius migration.

S.D. Trigg, M.D.

Anatomy of the Posterior Interosseous Nerve in Relation to Fixation of the Radial Head

Tornetta P III, Hochwald NL, Bono C, et al (Kings County Hosp, Brooklyn, NY)
Clin Orthop 345:215–218, 1997   5–12

Background.—Although nonoperative management of radial head and neck fractures is accepted, operative management appears to give better results for displaced fractures. If internal fixation is employed, the head must be fixed to the shaft, but extension of the approach distal to the annular ligament may put the posterior interosseous nerve at risk. The risk of blind subperiosteal dissection distal to the annular ligament for the placement of a plate across the radial neck was examined in cadaverous specimens.

Methods.—The investigations were performed with 50 fresh cadaverous arms. A standard posterolateral approach to the radial head was used in each arm. The forearm was pronated to identify the most anterior aspect of the safe zone and then supinated to identify the most posterior aspect of the safe zone for plate placement. No specific attempts were made to locate the posterior interosseous nerve. A small key elevator stripped an area large enough for placement of a 4-cm minifragment plate on the radius. The forearm was supinated and a longitudinal anterolateral incision was made from above the elbow to the midforearm. The radial nerve was dissected under loupe magnification and all branches were followed distal to the plate. The distance from the radiocapitellar joint to the branch point of the nerve, to the extensor carpi radialis longus, to the posterior inter-osseous nerve, and from the posterior interosseous nerve to the closing point of the plate with the arm in neutral were measured. Structural damage to the posterior interosseous nerve was assessed.

Results.—The take-off of the muscular branch to the extensor carpi radialis longus was approximately 7.1 mm proximal to the radiocapitellar joint. The posterior interosseous nerve originated approximately 1.2 mm from the radiocapitellar joint. In 31 arms, the take-off was proximal, and in 19, it was distal to the joint. The posterior interosseous nerve was intramuscular in 49 of 50 arms and lay on the radius in 1 arm. There was no damage to the posterior interosseous nerve or branches. The plate did not trap any nerve branches. The distance from the posterior interosseous nerve to the plate was about 5 mm. In 2 cases, the nerve passed over the distal end of the plate within the supinator, approximately 3.5 cm and 4 cm distal to the radial neck.

Conclusions.—This investigation of 50 cadaverous arms indicates that the posterior interosseous nerve is not at risk for structural injury during distal subperiosteal dissection along the radius. Plating the radial neck by distal extension of the posterolateral approach with subperiosteal dissection is safe. Tension should always be avoided on the nerve, as it could lead to physiologic injury.

▶ Several recent studies have shown improved results after operative management of displaced radial head and neck fractures as an alternative to excision, particularly involving those fractures associated with injuries to the distal radioulnar joint or the interosseous membrane or both. There have been recent improvements in smaller osteosynthesis plates and interfragmentary screw systems that facilitate the assembly and stabilization of these often difficult fractures, and the so-called safe zones for placement of internal fixation hardware have been established.[1] Often, with the more complex fractures, particularly those involving extension into the neck and proximal diaphyseal portions, the posterolateral operative exposure can be limited by a surgeon's tolerance of potential injury to the posterior interosseous nerve with distal dissection. This cadaveric study shows that with subperiosteal dissection, and with the forearm in pronation, exposure distal to the annular ligament, the nerve appears safe following subsequent anatomical dissection after blind application of the plate. The posterior interosseous nerve was shown to lie largely in an intramuscular location in all but 1 specimen and no direct injury to the nerve could be detected. An alternative to the posterolateral approach is the anterior approach, which has its own inherent dangers and often requires a greater degree of dissection. Knowing the location of the posterior interosseous nerve from this study, then, may give the surgeon an added measure of confidence when addressing operative treatment of these fractures.

S.D. Trigg, M.D.

Reference

1. Smith G, Hotchkiss R: Radial head and neck fractures: Anatomic guidelines for proper placement of internal fixation. *J Shoulder Elbow Surg* 5:113–117, 1996.

Hand

Ligament Reconstruction Basal Joint Arthroplasty Without Tendon Interposition

Gerwin M, Griffith A, Weiland AJ, et al (Hosp for Special Surgery, New York)
Clin Orthop 342:42–45, 1997   5–13

Introduction.—Tendon interposition is often used to maintain joint space in patients undergoing basal joint resection arthroplasty with ligament reconstruction. A prospective, randomized study was conducted to examine the necessity of tendon interposition during this procedure.

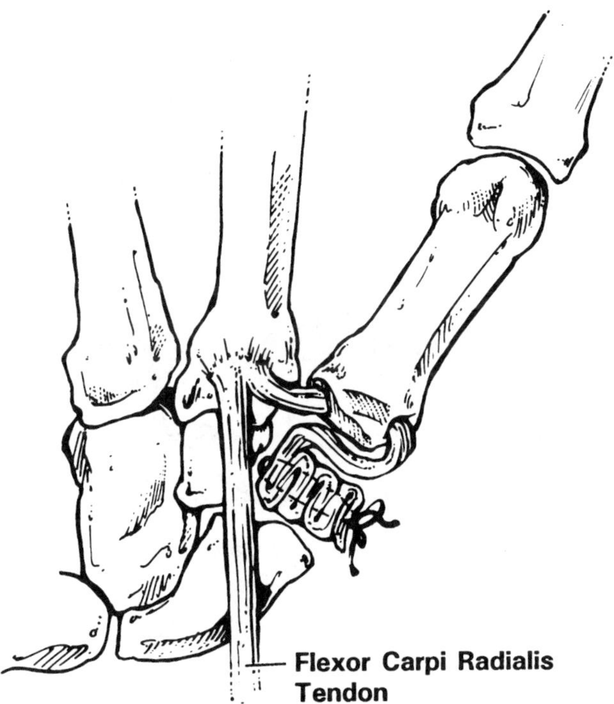

FIGURE 1.—Group I: ligament reconstruction basal joint arthroplasty with tendon interposition. Half the flexor carpi radialis tendon is rolled and placed in the void created by resection of the trapezium. (Courtesy of Gerwin M, Griffith A, Weiland AJ, et al: Ligament reconstruction basal joint arthroplasty without tendon interposition. *Clin Orthop* 342:42–45, 1997.)

Methods.—Twenty patients scheduled for basal joint arthroplasty and ligament reconstruction were enrolled in the study from September 1, 1992 through March 1, 1994. Nine were randomized to have the procedure with tendon interposition (group I) and 11 without tendon interposition (group II). In group I, half of the flexor carpi radialis tendon was harvested for placement in the void created by resection of the trapezium (Fig 1). In group II patients, no rolled tendon spacer was placed within the void of the resected trapezium (Fig 2). Patients were followed for an average of 23 months and assessed for radiographic outcome, hand function, and their overall satisfaction with the procedure.

Results.—The 2 groups had no significant difference in range of motion of the thumb interphalangeal joint, metacarpophalangeal joint, or palmar abduction, or the ability of the thumb to touch the volar aspect of the fifth metacarpophalangeal joint. Two-point pinch strength and 3-point grip strength were both slightly greater in group II, a difference that was statistically significant. Grip strength and lateral strength were similar in the 2 groups, and all patients were able to perform the 6 activities of daily living that were evaluated. Radiographic findings were also similar with and without tendon interposition. Subjective satisfaction was 72% in group I and 76% in group II.

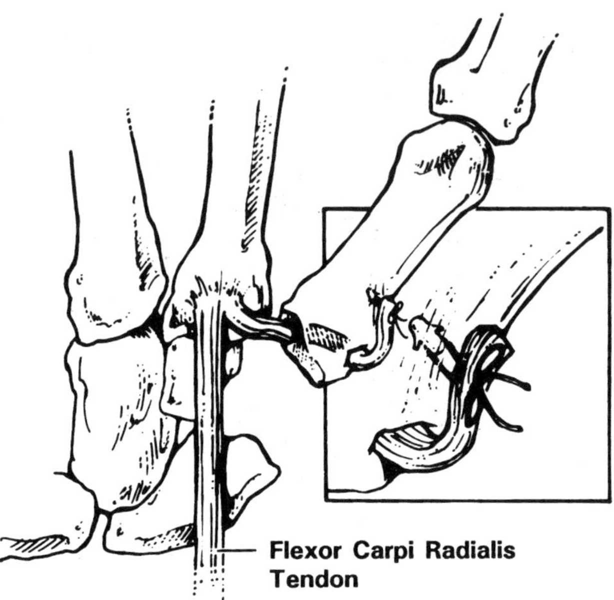

FIGURE 2.—Group II: ligament reconstruction basal joint arthroplasty without tendon interposition. No rolled tendon interposition is placed in the void of the resected trapezium. (Courtesy of Gerwin M, Griffith A, Weiland AJ, et al: Ligament reconstruction basal joint arthroplasty without tendon interposition. *Clin Orthop* 342:42–45, 1997.)

Conclusion.—Tendon interposition did not improve functional outcome or subjective satisfaction for patients undergoing basal joint arthroplasty, and all surgeons thought that the surgery was easier to perform when this element of the procedure was omitted.

▶ Every year or so, there appears yet another well-designed study advocating a variation on some form of trapezium resection, with or without tendon interposition, for the treatment of painful basal thumb joint arthritis. Taken as a whole, most of these various techniques report postoperative improvement in pain and thumb ray mobility. Recently, the majority of procedures report some form of ligament reconstruction and suspension of the thumb metacarpal, begging the question as to whether the addition of interposition material is structurally and, thus, clinically irrelevant. The authors of this study appear to make this conclusion rather convincingly, albeit from a study of a small group of patients. Certainly, the basal thumb joint ligament reconstruction advocated by the authors is technically simpler than most other ligament reconstruction techniques, which require additional length of tendon graft for the interposition and apparently producing similar favorable results.

S.D. Trigg, M.D.

Early Active Mobilization for Extensor Tendon Injuries: The Norwich Regime

Sylaidis P, Youatt M, Logan A (West Norwich Hosp, England)
J Hand Surg [Br] 22B:594–596, 1997   5–14

Background.—After extensor tendon repair, dynamic splinting has been found to provide better results than static splinting, but involves clumsy splints and complicated protocols. A controlled, active mobilization protocol without dynamic splinting, the Norwich regime, has been created and results of a series of 27 consecutive patients were assessed.

Study Group.—All patients who had primary finger extensor tendon repair for complete division between the proximal half of the proximal phalanx and the wrist were eligible for the study. The 27 patients in this series were all male, aged 19–81. Of these 27 patients, 17 had simple tendon injuries and 10 had complex injuries.

Methods.—After extensor tendon repair, tension was controlled by wrist extension and avoidance of composite metacarpophalangeal and interphalangeal flexion. The hand was rested on a palmar splint with the wrist at 45 degrees extension, metacarpophalangeal joints flexed to at least 50 degrees, and interphalangeal joints extended (Fig 1). Controlled active mobilization was initiated on the first day after surgery. The patient performed 2 exercises: combined interphalangeal and metacarpal phalangeal extension and metacarpal phalangeal joint extension with interphalangeal joint flexion. These exercises were performed no more than 4 times per session for 4 sessions daily for 4 weeks. Then the splint was worn only at night and the exercises were replaced with gentle flexion of the metacarpophalangeal and interphalangeal joints, increasing over time to full flexion and power grip. Progress was evaluated at 4 and 6 postoperative weeks with the Dargan criteria. Time to return to work was also noted.

Results.—Among those patients with simple tendon injuries, 2 were lost to follow-up between the fourth and sixth postoperative week. Of the remaining patients, there were 14 excellent, 8 good, and 2 fair results at 6-week follow-up. Of the patients with complex fractures, 2 were lost to follow-up between the fourth and sixth postoperative week. Of the remaining patients, there were 9 excellent, 2 good, and 2 fair results. The average time to return to work was 6.5 weeks for simple tendon injuries and 8.5 weeks for complex injuries in this study group.

Conclusions.—The results of this prospective study of early active mobilization of extensor tendon injuries using the Norwich regime are comparable with those after dynamic splinting. The Norwich regime does not require complicated splintage and exercise protocols to achieve these results.

▶ The development of the now well-accepted protocols for early mobilization of postlaceration flexor tendon repairs, and, more recently, encouraging results with some active early mobilization techniques with improved suturing methods, were curiously slow to be similarly applied to extensor tendon injuries. This trend, despite several well-done studies, nonetheless shows

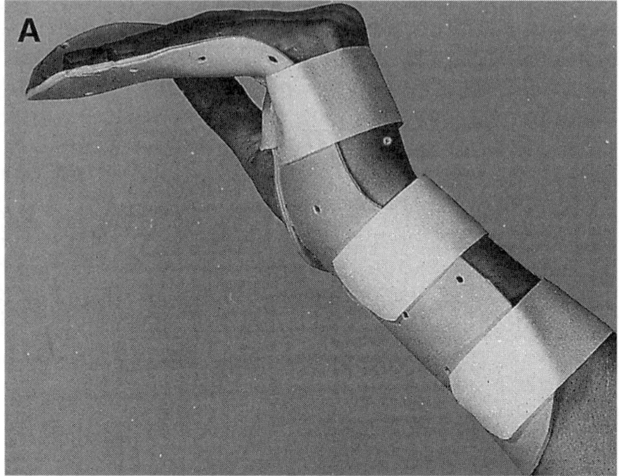

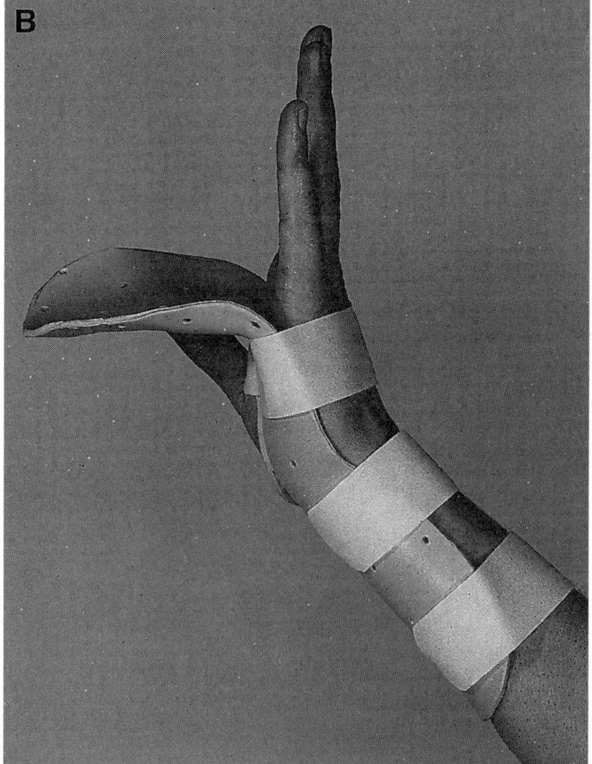

(Continued)

FIGURE 1 (cont.)

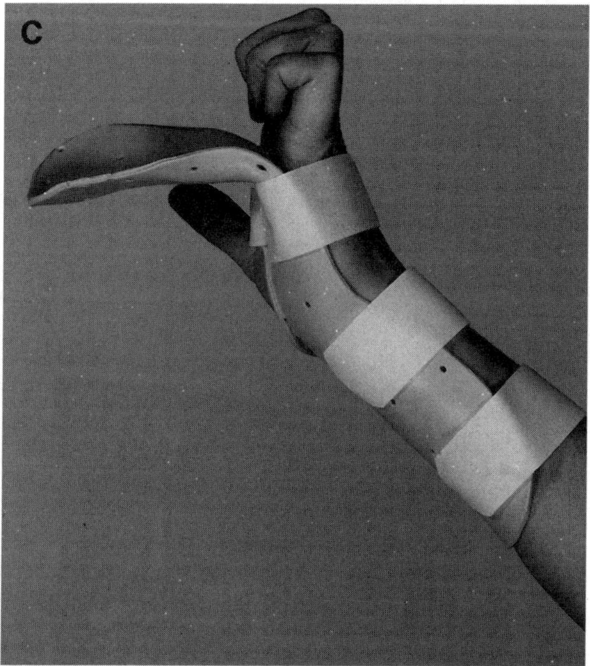

FIGURE 1.—**A,** resting splint; **B,** combined extension exercise; **C,** interphalangeal flexion exercise. (Courtesy of Sylaidis P, Youatt M, Logan A: Early active mobilization for extensor tendon injuries: The Norwich Regime. *J Hand Surg [Br]* 22B:594–596, 1997.)

the efficacy of early extensor tendon mobilization using dynamic extension splints and adapted mobilization methods. Often, however, I have found that the dynamic mobilization splints require frequent adjustments, and therefore, more therapy visits, even in compliant patients. The authors of this study report on a simple active mobilization technique for extensor tendon injuries that initially requires only 2 exercises in the first 4 weeks, and only another additional exercise thereafter, until the program is discontinued at an average of 6 weeks. Their reported results appear comparable with other studies that utilized dynamic splints. One may be encouraged by their results to consider this simpler, and likely more cost-effective, method of treatment for these injuries.

S.D. Trigg, M.D.

Suggested Reading

Blair, WF, Steyers, CM: Extensor tendon injuries. *Orthop Clin North America* 23:141–147, 1992.

Evans, RB: Clinical application of controlled stress to the healing extensor tendon: A review of 112 cases. *Phys Ther* 69:1041–1049, 1989.

Sagittal Band Reconstruction

Watson HK, Weinzweig J, Guidera PM (Univ of Connecticut, Hartford; Yale Univ, New Haven, Conn; Univ of Massachusetts, Worcester; et al)
J Hand Surg (Am) 22A:452–456, 1997

5–15

Background.—The occurrence of extensor tendon subluxation at the metacarpophalangeal joint in patients without rheumatoid arthritis is rare. In almost all such patients reported, disruption of the radial sagittal band with ulnar subluxation of the extensor tendon was noted. A technique for sagittal band reconstruction was described that effectively recentralizes and stabilizes the extensor tendon by using the deep transverse metacarpal ligament, the normal volar attachment of the sagittal band, thus avoiding the need to distort normal collateral ligament or lumbrical anatomy.

Methods and Outcomes.—Twenty-one sagittal band reconstructions were done in 16 patients. There were 18 cases of ulnar subluxation caused by radial sagittal band disruption and 3 cases of radial subluxation caused by ulnar sagittal band disruption. The technique involved weaving a retrograde segment of extensor tendon on itself after passing it through the deep transverse metacarpal ligament. The procedure eliminated pain in all patients. There were no recurrences of extensor tendon subluxation.

Conclusion.—The technique effectively produces a stable mechanism for maintaining the centralized position of the extensor tendon without disrupting normal anatomy or limiting the range of motion of the metacarpophalangeal joint. It involves weaving a retrograde segment of extensor tendon on itself after passing it through the deep transverse metacarpal ligament, which serves as a pulley.

▶ Sagittal band disruption or attenuation in nonrheumatoid patients, resulting in ulnar translation of the extensor tendon at the metacarpophalangeal joint, is a disconcerting and often disabling condition. The authors present their reconstructive technique, which restores the anatomical and structural function of the sagittal band, producing excellent postoperative stability and range of motion.

S.D. Trigg, M.D.

Distal Interphalangeal Joint Silicone Interpositional Arthroplasty of the Hand

Shaw Wilgis EF (Union Mem Hosp, Lutherville, Md)
Clin Orthop 342:38–41, 1997

5–16

Background.—The pain of degenerative arthritis can be relieved by arthrodesis, but loss of motion of the distal joint and of fine control of the fingertip accompanies this procedure. This may be restrictive for patients with multiple digit involvement or those requiring flexion for fine motor activities. Silicone interpositional arthroplasty can provide pain relief, while retaining limited stable flexion of the distal joint. The results of this procedure performed in 38 digits were reviewed.

Study Group.—The study group consisted of 18 female patients, aged 47–70 years, who had 31 silicone interpositional arthroplasties of the distal interphalangeal joint. Of the 31 implants, 28 remained in place after an average follow-up of 10 years, for a survival rate of 90%.

> *Surgical Procedure.*—A dorsal T-shaped incision proximal to the germinal nail matrix is used to approach the joint. The extensor tendon is divided proximal to the distal interphalangeal joint. The distal interphalangeal joint is exposed by hyperflexion of the distal phalanx. The head of the middle phalanx is removed transversely. The intramedullary canals of the middle and distal phalanges are prepared for implants. The prosthesis is inserted with a no-touch technique. The joint is reduced by extending the distal phalanx. The extensor tendon is repaired with nonabsorbable sutures. A Kirschner wire is inserted retrograde through the distal phalanx to engage the volar portion of the flexor sheath. After surgery, the distal joint is externally splinted in full extension for 4 weeks. The pin is removed and the joint is maintained in full extension for 4 more weeks. Graduated active motion of the distal joint is encouraged after 8 weeks. Night splinting is used for the third and fourth postoperative months.

Findings.—All patients had reduced pain postoperatively. Cosmetic appearance was improved in 27 of 31 digits. Power was improved in 22 and dexterity improved in 25. Overall satisfaction was improved in 27 of the 31 digits. An extension lag was detected in 18 of 23 digits examined, with an average of 12.7 degrees. The active range of motion was 10–50 degrees in these digits. Of the 23 joints examined, 10 were stable to lateral stress, and 1 was grossly unstable. Three silicone implants were removed because of complications.

Conclusions.—Distal interphalangeal joint silicone arthroplasty is effective for relief of pain from degenerative arthritis, while providing for retention of some movement with stability of the distal joint. This procedure is an alternative to arthrodesis of the distal interphalangeal joint.

▶ Despite the commonality of painful degenerative osteoarthritis of the distal interphalangeal joints of the fingers, silicone implant arthroplasty has been infrequently reported as a treatment alternative when compared with arthrodesis, the more commonly done procedure. Certainly, arthrodesis is the more accepted technique for the majority of patients; however, in certain patients, preservation of motion is desirable, which may include some wind and string musicians, artists, and hobbyists for whom some motion of the distal interphalangeal (DIP) joints is desirable. Furthermore, patients having undergone multiple arthrodesis procedures often complain of diminished composite hand function. The author reports overall favorable results with a high degree of patient satisfaction at long-term follow-up in the majority of the patients who underwent silicone DIP joint arthroplasty. The author did not mention any evidence of silicone synovitis. On the basis of the outcomes of this study and other series reports, we should perhaps not have a knee-jerk reaction to perform an arthrodesis in all patients having a painful degenerative DIP joint.

S.D. Trigg, M.D.

Neurovascular

Evaluation and Treatment of the Painful Neuroma
Mackinnon SE (Washington Univ, St Louis)
Tech Hand Upper Extrem Surg 1:195–212, 1997   5–17

Introduction.—Nearly 150 different techniques have been reported for controlling painful neuroma, indicating that there is no general consensus for surgical management. Traditional treatment involves excision of the neuroma and capping of the nerve with various materials. Transposition of a sensory nerve into innervated muscle or into bone has been used to decrease sensory regeneration and to treat painful neuroma formation. These approaches produce acceptable long-term results in about 65% of patients. A surgical algorithm for management of painful neuroma was presented (Fig 1), and evaluation and treatment were reviewed.

Diagnosis.—It is generally agreed that a diagnosis of neuroma may be made if there is pain in the region of a scar associated with altered sensibility in the distribution of a peripheral nerve. A painful Tinel-like response in the distribution of the nerve when the scar is palpated is commonly associated with hyperalgesia in the distribution of the injured nerve. The diagnosis of painful neuroma is straightforward, but patient selection is not. Selection of appropriate patients for surgical intervention is as crucial as nuances in surgical technique.

Indications/Contraindications.—Patients who are comfortable with massage and palpation of the affected area are not good surgical candidates. Presence of a Tinel sign proximal to the area of actual neuroma formation along the course of the involved nerve is helpful in discerning sensations. A 3-part Pain Rating Scale modified from the Hendler's Back Pain Scale and the McGill Pain Questionnaire that includes a visual analogue scale and questions regarding pain and functional limitations is helpful in choosing appropriate candidates for surgical intervention. Patients who score positive on all 3 scales are not appropriate surgical candidates; those who score positive on 2 of 3 scales should undergo psychological evaluation before being considered for surgery. Patients who describe increased pain after anesthetic nerve blocks are not good surgical candidates. Patients chosen for surgical intervention should undergo a short preoperative course of desensitization. If they do not respond to these techniques in the course of 1 month, they are not likely to respond to desensitization. Neuropathic drugs (Neurontin, Elavil, and Tegretol) may be helpful as initial alternatives to surgical intervention and are

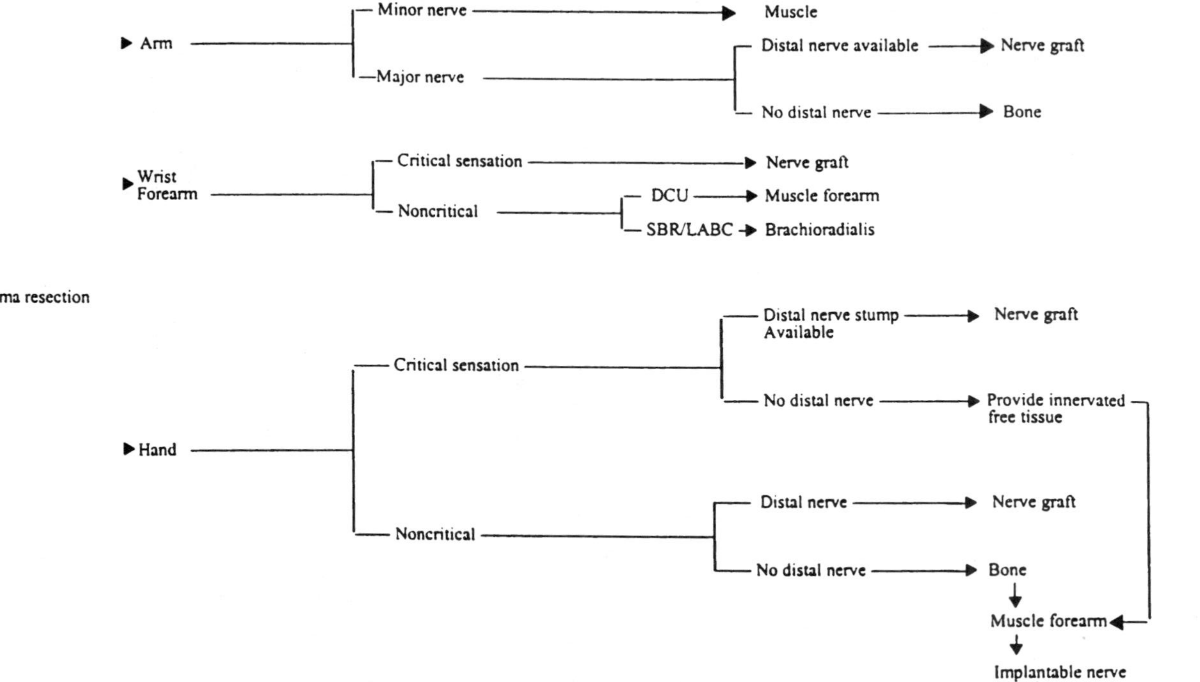

FIGURE 1.—Surgical algorithm for management of painful neuroma. *Abbreviations*: *LABC*, lateral antebrachial cutaneous; *DCU*, dorsal cutaneous ulnar; *SBR*, superficial radial. (Modified with permission from Mackinnon SE, Dellon AL: Algorithm for management of painful neuroma. *Contemp Orthop* 13:15–27, 1986. Courtesy of Mackinnon SE: Evaluation and treatment of the painful neuroma. *Tech Hand Upper Extrem Surg* 1:195–212, 1997.)

commonly used for postoperative pain management. The surgeon may also consider an excellent pain management group to make sure medical intervention cannot control the patient's pain. For difficult patients, the Minnesota Multiphasic Personality Inventory evaluation may be useful. The surgeon must be prepared to help with postoperative pain control in the event of surgical failure. The most important complication of surgical intervention is failure to relieve pain. The failure can represent inappropriate patient selection as much as failure of the surgical procedure itself. Surgeons should admit defeat and avoid the temptation to offer further surgery if an initial procedure does not provide pain relief. Referral should be made to a pain management group. Postoperative management of patients undergoing surgery for neuroma is crucial to outcome. Surgical result can be identified within a few days of operation. Patients should be encouraged to return to some type of limited employment soon after surgery.

Conclusion.—Patients undergoing surgery for painful neuroma should be carefully selected and followed up to maximize optimal outcome.

▶ The persistence of a painful neuroma after injury often overshadows the morbidity of the original injury, no matter how severe, and can leave the patient with significant functional impairment as well as the possibility of long-term employment problems and psychological disturbances. The author of this study, one of the most noted investigators in this field, presents a modification of her treatment algorithm based upon experimental data and a wealth of clinical experience. The initial diagnosis, and localization, of a painful neuroma is well within the capacities of all orthopedists, whether or not the actual surgical treatment (often requiring microsurgical experience) is undertaken. Perhaps most importantly, this article presents many of the pitfalls of treatment based, no doubt, upon the author's own failures of treatment, which can give us all wise counsel when tackling these difficult neural lesions.

S.D. Trigg, M.D.

Reflex Sympathetic Dystrophy in the Upper Extremity
Gellman H, Nichols D (Univ of Arkansas, Little Rock)
J Am Acad Orthop Surg 5:313–322, 1997   5–18

Introduction.—Reflex sympathetic dystrophy (RSD) may be the most challenging and frustrating pain syndrome to manage. The primary signs of this disorder are pain, swelling, and autonomic dysfunction. Early diagnosis and treatment are crucial. Reflex sympathetic dystrophy of the upper extremity was reviewed.

Pathophysiology.—The etiology of RSD has not been elucidated. Several factors seem to be involved. An injury normally activates the sympathetic nervous system, causing vasoconstriction in the limb and a decrease in sympathetic tone. If the decrease in sympathetic tone continues inappro-

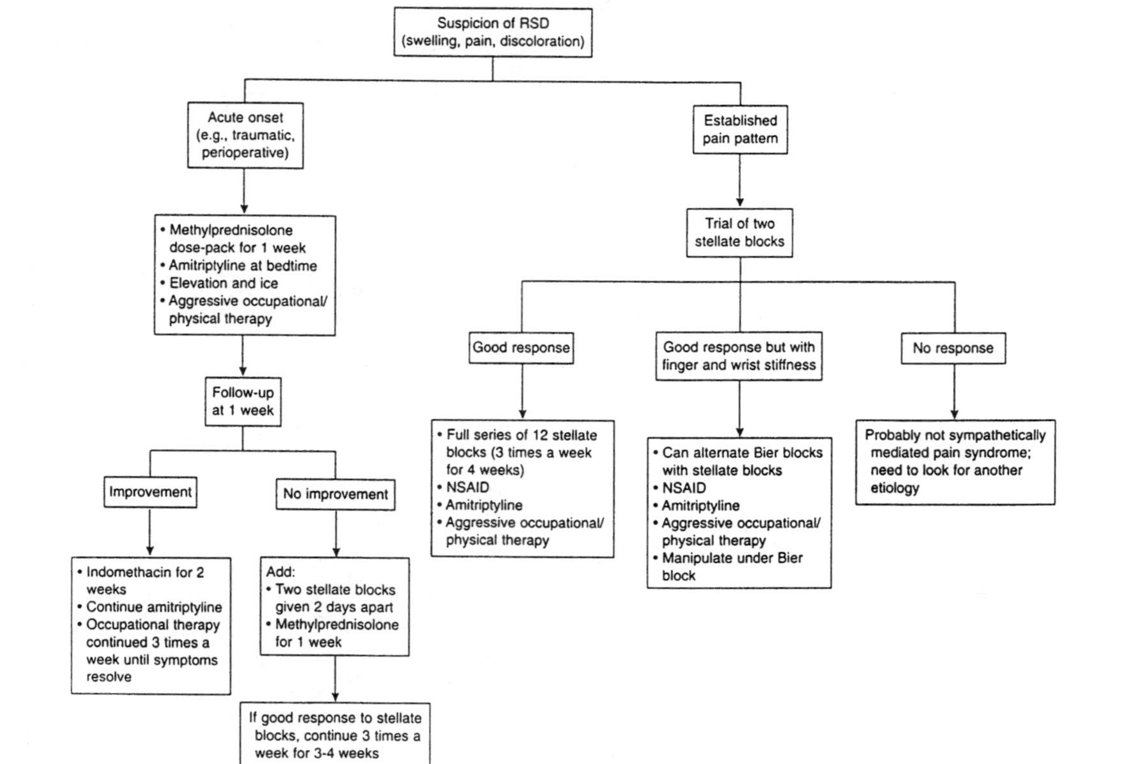

FIGURE 2.—Algorithm for recommended evaluation and treatment of upper-extremity reflex sympathetic dystrophy *Abbreviations*: *NSAID*, nonsteroidal anti-inflammatory drug; *RSD*, reflex sympathetic dystrophy. (Reprinted with permission, from Gellman H, Nichols D: Reflex sympathetic dystrophy in the upper extremity. *J Am Acad Orthop Surg* 5:313–322. Copyright 1997, American Academy of Orthropaedic Surgeons.)

priately, an abnormal feedback mechanism may develop and cause an atypical sympathetic reflex. This can result in tissue edema and capillary collapse and ischemia that can cause pain. The pain signal may then re-excite the sympathetic nerves, thus creating a positive feedback circuit. Sympathetic stimulation usually suppresses C-fiber nociceptor activity. After injury, ectopically firing C fibers are stimulated by sympathetic activity; successful treatment of RSD may be dependent upon interrupting this abnormal continuous-feedback loop. Other theories include a possible genetic diathesis in RSD or even suggest RSD is a neuroimmune disorder.

Diagnosis.—Because RSD is sympathetically mediated, the diagnosis may be substantiated on the basis of response of the pain to sympathetic blockade. When signs and symptoms of RSD are subtle or a detailed medical history is not possible, 3-phase bone scan, cold-stress testing, thermography, and resting blood flow and muscle temperature may be used to help determine diagnosis.

Treatment.—Treatment delay can prolong rehabilitation and may allow pain and physical alterations to become established and refractory to treatment. Patients with diagnostic and treatment delays over 6 months after onset have poorer prognosis than patients treated within 3 weeks of onset. Treatment is multifaceted (Fig 2) and includes: appropriate exercise programs and static splinting; treatment with α-adrenergic blocking agents, mood-elevating drugs, calcium channel blockers; and IV regional blocks and stellate ganglion blocks. New treatment approaches include electroacupuncture, transcutaneous electric nerve stimulation, and bio-feedback.

Conclusion.—There is no definitive approach to the diagnosis and treatment of RSD. A high index of suspicion is important. Prognosis is guarded at best. Patients with early diagnosis and multifaceted treatment have a better chance for good response than those with delayed diagnosis and treatment.

▶ Reflex sympathetic dystrophy and other complex regional pain disorders remain among the most perplexing and difficult postinjury and postsurgical complications to treat. Moreover, successful treatment of these disorders is extremely time-consuming and is often associated with significant psycho-social, workers' compensation, and legal variables that only add to the complexity of the clinical treatment. We, as orthopedists, are almost always the first to recognize the problem, and our patients rightfully have an expectation that we will be the principal physician to initiate treatment, but then may call upon other physicians and therapists to assist in resolving the disorder. This article presents an algorithmic approach to the problem based upon known successful treatment practices and includes new research information as to the etiology of RSD. Thus, it sheds new light on possible future pharmacologic intervention strategies.

S.D. Trigg, M.D.

The Role of Epineurotomy in the Operative Treatment of Carpal Tunnel Syndrome

Leinberry CF, Hammond NL III, Siegfried JW (Saint Joseph Hosp, Reading, Pa; Lankenau Hosp, Wynnewood, Pa)
J Bone Joint Surg Am 79-A:555–557, 1997   5–19

Background.—It has been suggested that in addition to operative release of the transverse carpal ligament for treatment of carpal tunnel syndrome, adjuvant manipulation of the median nerve is beneficial. The effect of epineurotomy of the median nerve on the outcome of operative treatment of chronic median nerve compression in the carpal canal was investigated.

Study Group.—A prospective, randomized clinical study was performed with 50 hands of 44 patients with carpal tunnel syndrome who were treated operatively from 1986 through 1989. Criteria for inclusion were symptoms of dysfunction of the median nerve, as a result of compression in the carpal canal that were not responsive to conservative treatment and electromyographic studies that suggested advanced nerve compression. The patients ranged from ages 38 to 100. Average symptom duration was more than 2 years.

Methods.—Hands were randomly chosen to receive operative decompression of the median nerve by longitudinal incision of the transverse carpal ligament alone (group 1) or operative decompression plus longitudinal opening of the epineurium in the carpal canal region (group 2). Patients were examined and had an electrophysiologic study performed in a blinded fashion 12 months postoperatively.

Results.—No significant differences in outcome were detected between these 2 treatment groups.

Conclusions.—The addition of adjuvant epineurotomy to ligament release provided no additional benefit to patients with carpal tunnel syndrome.

▶ Adjuvant surgical procedures about the median nerve done, in addition to transection of the transverse carpal ligament for the surgical treatment of carpal tunnel syndrome, have long been held by a significant number of hand surgeons to be important in the resolvement of this condition. Previously, Gelberman et al.[1] showed that one of the most common adjuvant procedures, internal neurolysis, was of no benefit to the resolvement of the condition when compared with simple transection of the transverse carpal ligament. Epineurotomy without internal manipulation of the fascicles, likewise, remains a commonly performed adjuvant procedure. The authors have shown in this well-done, prospective study that epineurotomy, while appearing to cause no harm, nonetheless shows no clinical or electrophysiologic benefit at 1 year. The etiology of carpal tunnel syndrome appears to be a multifactorial process in susceptible individuals, and when conservative measures fail, the surgical treatment seems to require only simple decompression of the nerve without adjuvant procedures, even in clinically severe cases.

S.D. Trigg, M.D.

Reference

1. Gelberman RH, Pfeffer GB, Galbraith RT, et al: Results of treatment of severe carpal tunnel syndrome without internal neurolysis of the median nerve. *J Bone Joint Surg Am* 69A:896–903, 1987.

6   Elbow

Introduction

Over the last year, several articles have reflected an increased interest in the treatment of tennis elbow, including the management of the failed surgical procedure. Additionally, the effectiveness of a time-honored synovectomy is evaluated both as an open and as an arthroscopic procedure. Several topics relating to trauma include joint replacement, which has not been previously addressed in the literature. Overall, these articles provide a spectrum of emerging surgical options that (hopefully) will allow improved management of patients with these problems.

Bernard F. Morrey, M.D.

Tennis Elbow

The Efficacy of an Injection of Steroids for Medial Epicondylitis: A Prospective Study of Sixty Elbows

Stahl S, Kaufman T (Rambam Med Ctr, Haifa, Israel)
J Bone Joint Surg Am 79-A:1648–1652, 1997   6–1

Objective.—Although a variety of nonoperative measures have been used to treat medial epicondylitis, the long-term benefits of local injection of steroids are disputable, and complications have been reported. Results of a randomized, prospective, double-blind study analyzing the short-term and long-term effects of local injection of steroids to treat medial epicondylitis were presented.

Methods.—A modification of the Nirschl and Pettrone pain assessment grading system (0 to 4) and a visual-analogue scale for pain intensity were administered to 58 patients (60 elbows) before and at 6 weeks, 3 months, and 1 year after 1 injection of 40 mg (1 mL) methylprednisolone with 1 mL 1% lidocaine ($n = 30$ elbows) or 1 injection of 1 mL 1% lidocaine with 1 mL saline solution ($n = 30$ elbows). Patients with elbow injury, carpal tunnel syndrome, lateral epicondylitis, or ulnar neuropathy were excluded. Local complications were assessed by interviews and physical examinations. Pain scores were analyzed statistically.

Results.—No patients were lost to follow-up. Pain scores before injection were similar (2.4 for the test group and 2.3 for the control group). After 6 weeks, the test group had significantly lower pain scores than the control group (1.2 vs. 1.9). The group scores did not differ significantly at 3 months or 1 year (1.2 vs. 1.3 and 0.5 vs. 0.6, respectively). Whereas the test group had a significant decrease in mean pain-phase score at 6 weeks, there was no significant difference in intensity of pain between groups at 6 weeks. There were no local complications.

Conclusion.—Local injection of steroids for medial epicondylitis provides short-term benefits only.

▶ Epicondylitis is probably the most common elbow condition for which medical attention is sought. Although there appears to be a tendency to lessen the frequency with which cortisone is injected, there remains little well-developed clinical information regarding the effectiveness of cortisone injections. This paper, therefore, is particularly valuable in that it offers a prospective study of a large number of elbows with the less common medial epicondylitis treated with cortisone injection.

The findings could be predicted by those who deal with this condition on a regular basis and may be extrapolated to the management of lateral epicondylitis. Specifically, cortisone is of value in altering short-term pain and should be used when the condition is "hot." However, this study confirms the fact that a cortisone injection does not alter the natural history of the process. Although the subject is not specifically addressed, there is also no evidence to indicate that cortisone provides any detrimental effects in the long-term analysis.

B.F. Morrey, M.D.

Bilaterally Decreased Motor Performance of Arms in Patients With Chronic Tennis Elbow
Pienimäki TT, Kauranen K, Vanharanta H (Oulu Univ, Finland)
Arch Phys Med Rehabil 78:1092–1095, 1997   6–2

Background.—Repeated movement is one possible cause of lateral epicondylitis. The motor performance of arms in patients with chronic unilateral tennis elbow was measured in a current study.

Methods.—Thirty-two patients with chronic unilateral tennis elbow syndrome and 32 healthy controls matched for age and sex were studied. Arm motor performance was measured with the Human Performance Measurement/Basic Elements of Performance system using the module for hands and the device protocol. Reaction times, speed of movement, and coordination as a combination of speed of movement and accuracy were determined.

Findings.—Simple 1- and 2-choice reaction times were 19% to 36% slower in patients than in control subjects. The speed of movement was 31% to 32% slower in patients than in controls. These differences were significant. The coordination results were 9.6 and 9.7 bits/sec in the patients and controls, a nonsignificant difference. Reaction times and speed of movement between affected and unaffected arms of the patients did not differ. Patients' healthy arms had significantly slower reaction times and speed of movement than the corresponding arms of control subjects.

Conclusions.—Patients with unilateral chronic tennis elbow have a bilateral reduction in reaction times and speed of movement of arms compared to control subjects. The reduced motor performance may be primary, with an increased susceptibility to development of tennis elbow syndrome, or it may result from chronicity.

► The value of this presentation is to call attention to the medical community of an effort to measure objective performance changes in patients with lateral epicondylitis. As would be expected, there are major problems with any effort to offer such information. The report is of a small sample size. There is an inherent difference between the dominant and nondominant sides. The spectrum of severity in the study group is reflected by the fact that the chronic nature varied from 15 to 102 months. There is additional question as to the validity of the instrument and even the methodology. This last observation is supported by the conflicting and illogical finding that patients with the tennis elbow condition had better coordination of hands with their involved arms than on the uninvolved side. Over and above these concerns is the fact that females have been shown to have a slower reaction time than males, which further underscores the complexity of measuring small differences.

In spite of all this, I do think it is worthwhile to at least be aware of the effort to demonstrate objective changes in performance. Once again, in spite of these shortcomings, the fact that statistically significant differences were found is probably a sufficiently valid observation to at least adopt the position that some impairment in speed and performance is expected in those with chronic lateral epicondylitis.

B.F. Morrey, M.D.

Salvage Surgery for Lateral Tennis Elbow
Organ SW, Nirschl RP, Kraushaar BS, et al (Nirschl Orthopaedic Sportsmedicine Clinic, Arlington, Va)
Am J Sports Med 25:746–750, 1997   6–3

Objective.—A large number of patients fail surgical intervention for repair of lateral tennis elbow possibly because surgeons fail to identify and resect pathologic tissue. Records of patients who had failed surgical intervention for lateral tennis elbow were analyzed retrospectively before salvage surgery.

Methods.—Salvage surgery was performed between 1979 and 1994 in 35 elbows in 34 patients (16 men), aged 28–70 years. Sixteen patients (17 elbows) were workers' compensation patients, 12 were athletes, and 6 were non–workers' compensation patients with occupational injuries. Previous surgeries included 19 slide and release procedures, 6 slide and release procedures with partial resection of the annular ligament (Bosworth), 7 unknown procedures, 2 primary radial nerve decompressions, and 1 Nirschl procedure.

Results.—At surgery, 34 elbows showed residual tendinosis in the extensor carpi radialis brevis tendon origin; in 27 elbows, pathologic changes in that tendon had not been addressed, and intervention was incomplete in 7 elbows. In these 7 elbows, extensor carpi radialis brevis tendon origin surgical trauma was apparent. Scarred or altered areas over the extensor aponeurosis were debrided or repaired in 34 elbows. Results of salvage surgery were excellent in 20 elbows, good in 9, fair in 5, and poor in 1, at an average of 64 months after surgery. Patients with good or excellent results were able to return to their preinjury work or activity levels.

Conclusion.—For lateral tennis elbow, identification and resection of pathologic tissue, usually seen in the extensor carpi radialis brevis tendon, improves outcome after salvage surgery. Release operations, which weaken the extensor aponeurosis, should be avoided.

▶ There is very little information regarding this subject. The points worth emphasizing are the fact that, at least in the authors' experience, failure to address the pathology in the extensor carpi radialis brevis, either in whole or in part, was the most common cause of surgical failure. The second salient point is the fact that, although reoperation in this patient population is obviously very difficult and potentially problematic, the authors were able to produce good to excellent results in 83% of patients with the revision surgery. From our experience, we would concur that the inadequate addressing of the extensor carpi radialis brevis is 1 of the most common problems. We have found other possible explanations for the lack of surgical success and believe that this differential diagnosis should continue to be considered: entrapment of posterior interosseous nerve and ligament injury.

B.F. Morrey, M.D.

Synovectomy

Synovectomy of the Elbow and Radial Head Excision in Rheumatoid Arthritis: Predictive Factors and Long-term Outcome
Gendi NST, Axon JMC, Carr AJ, et al (Basildon Hosp, England; Queen Elizabeth II Hosp, Welwyn Garden City, England; Queen Elizabeth Hosp, Adelaide, Australia, et al)
J Bone Joint Surg Br 79-B:918–923, 1997
6–4

Objective.—The elbow is affected in more than 70% of patients with rheumatoid arthritis (RA), resulting in pain, weakness, stiffness, and instability that interfere with a variety of daily activities. Elbow RA is often managed with elbow synovectomy (ES), usually combined with radial head excision (RHE). Although studies have shown very high rates of pain relief with ES, there are questions about the final results, including the possibility of deterioration over time. The 20-year results in a large group of rheumatoid elbows undergoing ES are reported.

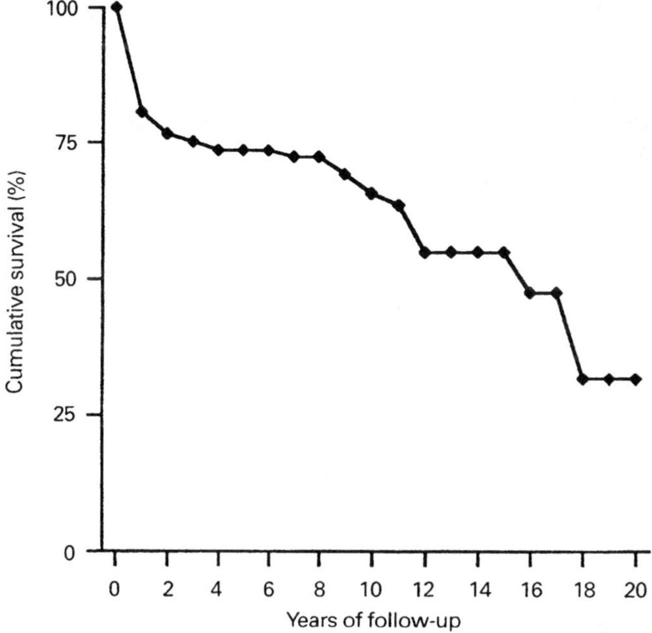

FIGURE 1.—Survival analysis of elbow synovectomy and radial head excision in rheumatoid arthritis. (Courtesy of Gendi NST, Axon JMC, Carr AJ, et al: Synovectomy of the elbow and radial head excision in rheumatoid arthritis: Predictive factors and long-term outcome. *J Bone Joint Surg Br* 79B:918–923, 1997.)

Methods.—Survival analysis was performed in 171 elbows undergoing ES, usually with RHE. For this analysis, treatment failure was defined as the wish for or performance of revision surgery or the presence of significant to severe pain. Follow-up data were available for 115 elbows of 95 patients.

Findings.—One-year cumulative survival was 81%. After the first year, survival decreased on average by 2.6% per year (Fig 1). A low preoperative range of supination-pronation was the factor most strongly related to success with ES. Surgical failure was also predicted by a low range of flexion-extension. When these 2 factors were combined, their predictive value was even better. However, the failure rate was high for patients with a long duration of elbow symptoms. Surgery produced a mean 50-degree gain in supination-pronation and an 11-degree gain in flexion-extension. Both of these variables were related to successful surgery. Surgical failure was related to recurrent synovitis, elbow instability, ulnar neuropathy, poor general mobility, and poor upper extremity function. Upper extremity function was related to the severity of RA in that shoulder.

Conclusions.—For patients with RA involving the elbow, ES plus RHE provides good short-term results. However, the results deteriorate over time, except in patients with more than 50% limitation of forearm rotation with no severe limitation of flexion-extension. Synovectomy with

RHE can be recommended for such patients, with a high probability of success.

▶ This presentation is one that represents the largest experience to date with RA of the elbow. Although it was a retrospective analysis, the large numbers are of particular value since over 30 patients had a potential for >5-year surveillance. The major value is clearly in the calculation of the anticipated Kaplan-Meier survival curve, but the particular value showed a linear downward trend after the 10-year mark, with a recognized relatively flat survival curve from the second to the tenth years. Although over this period of time one may legitimately question the variation in surgical techniques and selection criteria, the careful analysis of a large sample with long-term follow-up provides the most comprehensive such review to date in the literature. The authors make a credible effort to provide predictive factors that might predict the outcome. However, it is difficult to understand why limitation in supination and forearm rotation is one of the strongest positive predictive values. The duration of symptoms before surgery is a recognized factor that portends a poorer outcome. The finding that the extent of involvement did not play a predictive role is in contrast with what is generally accepted in the literature and what is felt to be clinically true by most surgeons. The limited flexion arc of <60 degrees, which also predicted a failure rate of 60%, is an important finding in the selection factors.

The predictive factors are of the initial success and not necessarily the long-term result. Thus, the loss of supination before surgery predicts a high likelihood of success afterward since it is likely that improved supination will be obtained with the procedure. One deficiency of this paper is the surgical technique. The authors do not explain to any extent the precise procedure performed. It was implied that the radial head was excised in all patients, but this is not discussed to any extent, nor is whether any selection factors were used in making this determination rather than a routine procedure, which was considered an essential portion of the synovectomy.

B.F. Morrey, M.D.

Arthroscopic Synovectomy of the Elbow for Rheumatoid Arthritis: A Prospective Study
Lee BPH, Morrey BF (Singapore General Hosp; Mayo Clinic and Found, Rochester, Minn)
J Bone Joint Surg Br 79-B:770–772, 1997   6–5

Background.—Elbow involvement is common in rheumatoid arthritis (RA). Synovectomy has been the conventional treatment for RA of the elbow after failure of conventional treatment. Previous reports have described the use of arthroscopic synovectomy, which carries a risk for nerve injury. This study examined the long-term risks and benefits of arthroscopic elbow synovectomy.

Methods.—The authors' experience included 11 consecutive patients undergoing a total of 14 arthroscopic synovectomies of the elbow over a 4-year period. The patients were 8 women and 3 men, and they had been receiving medical treatment on average for 8 years. None had had previous elbow surgery. Arthroscopic debridement was performed using a 4-mm reciprocating device with vacuum control. Extreme caution was used to prevent injury to vessels and nerves around the joint. The results were assessed using the Mayo Elbow Performance Score (MEPS). The patients were followed up on average for 42 months.

Results.—Pain improved in all patients, improving by 2 grades in 10 elbows. Mean arc of flexion improved from 91 to 98 degrees, and mean arc of rotation from 111 to 120 degrees. According to the MEPS, a short-term rating of good to excellent was achieved in 93% of cases. However, at last follow-up only 57% of patients had continued good or excellent results. Total joint replacement had been performed in 4 elbows. There was 1 case each of transient neurapraxia of the ulnar and radial nerves.

Conclusions.—Arthroscopic synovectomy shortens rehabilitation time in patients with RA involvement of the elbow. However, the results are not as long-lasting as with open synovectomy. The short-term gain and risk for serious nerve injury must be borne in mind when arthroscopic synovectomy is considered. The authors currently offer this procedure to patients younger than 50 who have more than 90 degrees of movement, grade III or lower radiologic changes, and inadequate response to 6 months of treatment with anti-inflammatory agents.

▶ With the obvious success of total joint replacement, synovectomy for RA has received much less attention in recent years. Arthroscopic synovectomy of the elbow is being performed in a number of centers, and Lee and Morrey have reported their early experience with this procedure. The promising message from this paper is that 93% of their 14 patients received a good or excellent result in the short term. They did not experience any serious complications. They expressed concern regarding the fact that after an average of 3½ years following surgery, the good and excellent results had fallen to 57%. Let us not be discouraged but encouraged by this article. Although not fully discussed in the paper, the synovectomies that were performed in those patients were not complete synovectomies, which can now be performed in a much more technically reproducible manner. Also, capsulectomies and removal of osteophytes were not performed in this series. It is well recognized that patients with RA have pain at the end points of motion and avoid those extremes of motion even when the total arc of motion is already diminished. Capsulectomy and removal of osteophytes can restore that motion, and experience in patients subsequent to those reported in this series would strongly suggest that a total synovectomy with restoration of motion to the joint can offer very promising results. Further follow-up in such a group of patients will be necessary to determine the role of synovectomy of the elbow for RA and to clarify the relationship between preoperative motion, extent of involvement of the joint, and final outcome.

S.W. O'Driscoll, M.D., Ph.D.

Trauma

Transolecranon Fracture–Dislocation of the Elbow

Ring D, Jupiter JB, Sanders RW, et al (Massachusetts Gen Hosp, Boston; Tampa Gen Hosp, Fla; Wayne State Univ, Detroit)
J Orthop Trauma 11:545–550, 1997   6–6

Purpose.—Anterior elbow dislocation without fracture of the proximal ulna is an uncommon occurrence. It has been shown that "transolecranon fracture-dislocation of the elbow" can produce a complex and comminuted proximal ulnar fracture. A series of 17 patients with transolecranon fracture-dislocation of the elbow is reported.

Patients.—Thirteen patients were identified from a 10-year review of Monteggia fractures in adults seen at Massachusetts General Hospital; the other 4 came from the practice of 1 of the authors. The patients were 14 men and 3 women, average age 38 years. Most were injured in high-energy traumatic incidents, most often a motor vehicle accident. Complex, comminuted fractures of the proximal ulna were present in 14 patients, 7 having fragmentation of the olecranon, 8 having large coronoid fragments, and 6 having segmental fractures of the ulna (Fig 1, B). The remaining 3

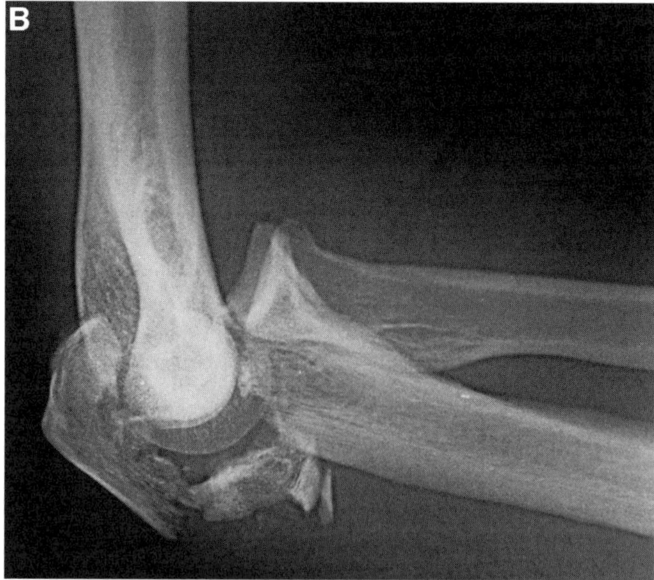

FIGURE 1.—Translocation fracture of the elbow is defined as complex by the extent of comminution of the greater sigmoid notch and proximal ulnar metaphysis. (Courtesy of Ring D, Jupiter JB, Sanders RW, et al: Transolecranon fracture–dislocation of the elbow. *J Orthop Trauma* 11:545–550, 1997.)

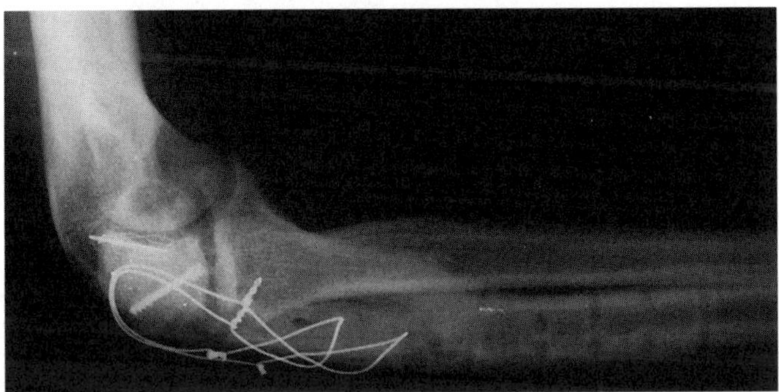

FIGURE 2.—A 19-year-old student sustained a transolecranon fracture-dislocation of the right elbow in a motor vehicle accident. F, lateral radiograph of the healed ulna following plate removal of 18 months after the initial injury. (Courtesy of Ring D, Jupiter JB, Sanders RW, et al: Transolecranon fracture-dislocation of the elbow. *J Orthop Trauma* 11:545–550, 1997.)

patients had simple, oblique, olecranon fractures. Surgical management was with open reduction and internal fixation, in most cases with a plate and screws. The results were evaluated using the elbow performance rating of Broberg and Morrey. The average follow-up was 25 months.

Outcomes.—Within 6 weeks after their initial operation, 2 patients needed one-third tubular plates switched to 3.5 mm dynamic compression plates. There were no other early complications, and all fractures healed. At follow-up, the results were considered excellent in 7 patients, good in 8, and fair in 2. There were 2 cases of mild posttraumatic arthritis. All 10 patients who were employed before injury were able to return to their previous jobs without modifications. Good results were achieved, even in elbows with large coronoid fragments and extensive comminution of the trochlear notch, as long as the fracture was stably fixed in anatomic position (Fig 2, F).

Conclusions.—An experience with management of transolecranon fracture-dislocation of the elbow is presented. Most anterior elbow dislocations are fracture-dislocations, occurring when the distal humerus is driven through the olecranon. This results in a complex, comminuted proximal ulnar fracture. Radiocapitellar dislocation is clearly observed, sometimes causing confusion with anterior Monteggia lesions. The injury must be managed as a complex disruption of the ulnohumeral articulation. In most such injuries, good results can be achieved with stable restoration of the contour and dimensions of the trochlear notch of the ulna.

▶ The value of this article is that it emphasizes the previous observation of the relatively uncommon, but extremely difficult, management of fracture-dislocations of the elbow at the ulnohumeral joint. This type of injury, which has been termed a type III olecranon fracture in Mayo's classification system, may be successfully treated if the ulnohumeral relationship is restored and stability is realized by virtue of the fixation employed. In most instances this includes at least a single plate, and typically tension band wires, as a single screw and wires are usually inadequate. In our practice we have used the dynamic joint distractor, and the authors have also demonstrated the effectiveness of supplemental stabilization with a rigid external fixation device. The most important principle in management is that stabilizing the ulnohumeral joint, achieved by rigidly stabilizing the fracture, provides an opportunity for a successful outcome.

B.F. Morrey, M.D.

Total Elbow Arthroplasty as Primary Treatment for Distal Humeral Fractures in Elderly Patients
Cobb TK, Morrey BF (Mayo Clinic, Rochester, Minn)
J Bone Joint Surg Am 79-A:826–832, 1997   6–7

Introduction.—In well-selected elderly patients, total elbow arthroplasty can be a useful treatment for posttraumatic elbow deformities. Joint replacement is indicated only if there is no other appropriate alternative. An experience with total elbow arthroplasty in 20 older adults with severely comminuted elbow fractures is reported.

Patients.—Total elbow arthroplasty was performed in 21 of 129 acute fractures of the distal aspect of the humerus over an 11-year period. The patients were 15 women and 5 men, mean age 72 at the time of injury. Most of the injuries occurred as a result of minor falls. Rheumatoid arthritis was present in 10 elbows of 9 patients, in whom it affected the choice of treatment. Because of the degree of comminution and poor bone stock, open reduction and internal fixation was not a usable option. Joint replacement was performed a mean of 7 days after the injury. The patients remained in the hospital a mean of 7 days after the operation, and were followed up for a mean of 3 years. All patients were followed up for at least 2 years, and none was lost to follow-up.

Outcomes.—At last follow-up, 20 of the 21 implants were intact. In the remaining elbow, another fall led to fracture of the ulnar component of the artificial joint, leading to revision total elbow arthroplasty. According to the Mayo Elbow Performance Score, the results were excellent in 15 elbows and good in 5. The patients were satisfied with the results in every case. The joints had a mean arc of flexion of 25 to 130 degrees, with no radiographic evidence of loosening. There were 2 cases of postoperative ulnar neurapraxia, and 1 of reflex sympathetic dystrophy. There was 1 case each of intraoperative myocardial infarction and stroke.

Conclusions.—For older adults with severely comminuted fractures of the distal humerus, total elbow arthroplasty can be a useful treatment option. Joint replacement can be performed even in elbows with rheumatoid arthritis. Strict selection criteria must be observed; total elbow arthroplasty is not a valid alternative to osteosynthesis in younger patients.

▶ This clinical report represents an important transition in our thinking regarding the management of elderly patients with comminuted fractures of the distal humerus, which are notoriously difficult to fix. As with hemiarthroplasty for displaced femoral neck fractures, prosthetic replacement offers some advantages over internal fixation for comminuted distal humeral fractures in this patient population. In the absence of complications, the results are uniformly satisfactory, and rehabilitation is impressively quicker and easier. Several points merit emphasis: (1) This is a relatively uncommon treatment; the authors report fewer than 1 case per year of nonrheumatoid patients treated in this manner; (2) the triceps should be left attached, because it is not necessary to remove it and the rehabilitation is vastly different if it is retained; and (3) not addressed in the article but being recognized, these patients do not have the normal stabilizing mechanisms around the elbow, and, therefore, the forces are more directly transmitted through the prosthesis to the coupling mechanism.

S.W. O'Driscoll, M.D., Ph.D.

Ligamentomuscular Protective Reflex in the Elbow

Phillips D, Petrie S, Solomonow M, et al (Louisiana State Univ, New Orleans)
J Hand Surg (Am) 22A:473–478, 1997   6–8

Introduction.—The ligamentomuscular protective reflex has been demonstrated in the knee, shoulder, and ankle. It is uncertain, however, whether this reflex exists in all other major joints and which specific nerves, muscles, and ligaments are associated with the reflex in a given joint. Whether a ligamentomuscular protective reflex arc exists from the elbow ligaments to the associated muscles was determined using a feline model.

Methods.—Six anesthetized adult cats underwent dissection of each hindlimb. A bipolar stimulating stainless-steel electrode probe applied 100 µsec supramaximal pulses at a rate of 10 pulses/sec to the animals' articular nerve branches. Fine-wire electrodes were inserted into the muscle bellies to assess reflex activation of any muscles around the elbow joint. The M-wave discharge of each muscle was recorded, and the conduction time from application of the stimulus to the nerve to the appearance of the reflexive M-wave was calculated. The M-wave, or electromyographic response to each pulse, is the synchronous discharge of all active motor units in the muscle.

Results.—The feline model confirmed the existence of a reflex arc from the medial elbow ligaments to the forearm pronator muscles. Stimulation of the articular nerve elicited myoelectric activity in a number of monitored muscles: the flexor digitorum superficialis, flexor digitorum profundus, flexor carpi radialis, flexor carpi ulnaris, and pronator teres. The afferent nature of the articular nerve was confirmed by the disappearance of myoelectric activity in the muscles when this nerve was severed between the electrodes and the median nerve.

Discussion.—Findings in this feline model document the existence of a fast-acting reflex arc from sensory elements in the medial ligaments of the elbow to the flexor-pronator muscles of the forearm. This reflex is mediated by the median nerve and its articular branch. Elbow repair procedures should preserve the neural supply of the ligaments and elbow capsule.

▶ This animal study does demonstrate a potentially protective fast-acting reflex arc that has been shown to exist in other joints. This may have some potential implications for rehabilitation. Clinically, it would be expected that a tear of this ligament would in all likelihood disrupt the nerve responsible for the reflex arc. Finally, it is not practical to consider this nerve identifiable or salvageable in most ligamentous surgery, and there is no clinical information that arthrotomies or exposures to the elbow that may disrupt the nerve place the patient in a vulnerable position for ligamentous injury caused by loss of the reflex arc.

B.F. Morrey, M.D.

Miscellaneous

Snapping of the Medial Head of the Triceps and Recurrent Dislocation of the Ulnar Nerve: Anatomical and Dynamic Factors

Spinner RJ, Goldner RD (Duke Univ, Durham, NC)
J Bone Joint Surg Am 80-A:239–247, 1998   6–9

Objective.—Snapping in the elbow is usually ascribed to recurrent dislocation of the ulnar nerve. However, snapping can also result from dislocation of the medial head of the triceps muscle or tenson over the medial epicondyle. If this occurs along with dislocation of the ulnar nerve, at least 2 snaps will be heard, regardless of whether medial elbow discomfort or ulnar neuropathy is present (Fig 1). Seventeen patients with recurrent dislocation of the ulnar nerve and snapping of the medial head of the triceps were described.

Patients.—The experience included 22 elbows of 17 patients with snapping of both the ulnar nerve and the medial head of the triceps over the medial epicondyle. The snapping was painless in 2 cases, associated with medial elbow pain in 5, associated with ulnar nerve symptoms only in 5, and associated with ulnar nerve snapping and symptoms in 7. In 5 cases, snapping was an incidental finding in asymptomatic patients; 1 of these patients had snapping and ulnar nerve symptoms in the other elbow. The diagnosis was confirmed at surgery in the first 3 patients, and by CT and/or MRI in the rest.

Outcomes.—Symptoms were enough of a problem to require surgery in 7 cases. In 6 of these cases, ulnar nerve symptoms were associated with lateral transposition or excision of the dislocating medial head of the triceps, in addition to decompression and transposition of the ulnar nerve. Two patients required surgery to correct snapping occurring immediately after a previous ulnar nerve transfer; these cases resulted from unrecognized dislocation of the medial head of the triceps and from an accessory triceps tendon, respectively. Valgus osteotomy of the distal humerus was performed to correct the line of pull of the triceps in 1 patient with medial

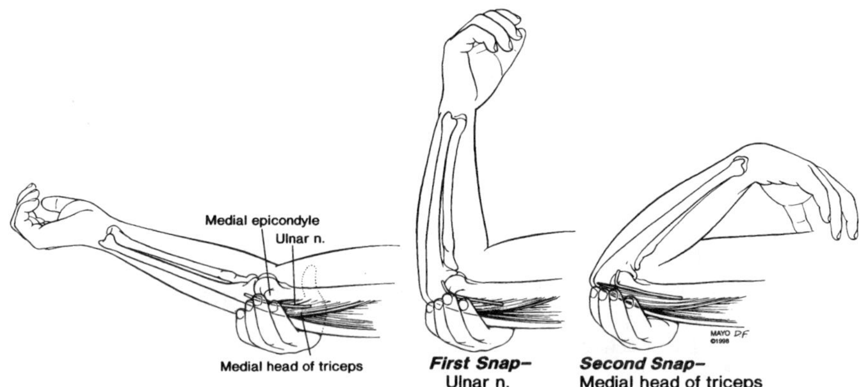

FIGURE 1.—Illustrations showing how the position of the ulnar nerve and the medial head of the triceps can be determined relative to the medial epicondyle as the elbow is flexed and extended actively or passively. In a patient who has snapping of the medial head of the triceps and dislocation of the ulnar nerve, the ulnar nerve dislocates at 90 degrees and the medial head of the triceps dislocates at approximately 110 degrees. (Printed by permission of the Mayo Foundation from Spinner RJ, Goldner RD: Snapping of the medial head of the triceps and recurrent dislocation of the ulnar nerve: Anatomical and dynamic factors. *J Bone Joint Surg [Am]* 80-A:239–247, 1998. Printed by permission of the Mayo Foundation.)

elbow pain, snapping, and cubitus varus. At 4.5 years postoperatively, all surgically treated patients had excellent results, with no snapping, no ulnar nerve symptoms, and full range of motion. The remaining patients received nonoperative treatment, which controlled ulnar nerve symptoms in 4 cases and snapping-related pain in 4.

Conclusions.—Dislocation of the ulnar nerve is not the only cause of snapping on the medial side of the elbow. This is so even when ulnar nerve symptoms are present. When ulnar nerve transposition is present, particularly if there is dislocation of the ulnar nerve, the elbow should be examined in flexion and extension during surgery to be sure the medial head of the triceps is not snapping over the medial epicondyle. If snapping of the medial head of the triceps accompanying ulnar nerve dislocation is not recognized, the patient may have persistent, symptomatic snapping after an otherwise successful ulnar nerve transposition.

▶ The authors highlight this relatively uncommon etiology for ulnar nerve symptomatology in those with spontaneous subluxation of the ulnar nerve. As emphasized, these patients often have a snapping sensation along the medial aspect of the elbow. The clinician must be very careful in the assessment to determine whether this is caused by a spontaneous subluxation of the ulnar nerve or by, at least in part, a hypermobile medial head of the triceps. As the authors emphasize, the distinction is important because symptoms can persist even after ulnar nerve translocation if the existence of a hypermobile muscle is not identified and addressed.

B.F. Morrey, M.D.

Validity of Observer-based Aggregate Scoring Systems as Descriptors of Elbow Pain, Function, and Disability

Turchin DC, Beaton DE, Richards RR (Scarborough, Ont; Inst for Work and Health, Toronto; St Michael's Hosp, Toronto)

J Bone Joint Surg Am 80-A:154–162, 1998   6–10

Purpose.—Currently used elbow scoring systems rely on observer assessments of clinical and functional criteria. After these criteria are scored separately and aggregated, the aggregate score is ranked as poor to excellent. The various systems use different outcome criteria, weight the criteria differently, and assign different values to each category ranking (Table 1). The validity of differing elbow scoring systems was evaluated by using 5 systems to assess the same group of patients.

Methods.—The study sample comprised 69 patients with elbow problems seeking care at referral clinics. The 5 systems assessed were the Mayo elbow-performance index and the scoring systems described by Broberg and Morrey, Ewald et al., The Hospital for Special Surgery, and Pritchard. Various instruments were used to evaluate the validity of the scoring systems, including visual analogue scales for pain and function, physician and patient ratings of the severity of elbow impairments, and 2 patient-completed functional questionnaires. The raw aggregate scores of the various systems were compared, and the level of agreement among categorical rankings was assessed.

Results.—Comparison of raw scores showed good correlation among the various systems. However, comparison of categorical rankings revealed only slight-to-moderate correlation. The most discriminating systems on validity testing were that of Ewald et al. and the Mayo elbow-performance index, followed by the systems of The Hospital for Special Surgery and of Broberg and Morrey, and, lastly, the system of Pritchard. Correlation with the functional score on the visual analogue scale was only moderate for the 5 scoring systems, but moderate to good for the patient-completed functional questionnaires.

Conclusions.—The 5 elbow scoring systems evaluated disagree substantially when used to evaluate the same group of patients. The results of these systems should be expressed as raw scores rather than categorical rankings, the findings suggest. Patient-completed functional question-

TABLE 1.—Distribution and Weighting of Domains in the Elbow-scoring Systems

| | | | Score *(Points)* | | | | |
Instrument	Pain	Motion	Strength	Stability	Function	Deformity	Total
The Hospital for Special Surgery	30	28	10	0	20	12	100
Ewald et al.	50	10	0	0	30	10	100
Pritchard	50	25	25	0	0	0	100
Broberg and Morrey	40	25	10	10	15	0	100
Mayo elbow-performance index	45	20	0	10	25	0	100

(Courtesy of Turchin DC, Beaton DE, Richards RR: Validity of observer-based aggregate scoring systems as descriptors of elbow pain, function, and disability. *J Bone Joint Surg [Am]* 80-A:154–162, 1998.)

naires give a better picture of perceived functional loss than the elbow scoring systems do. The findings show that it is not valid to compare the results of studies using different scoring systems. The best approach to evaluating the outcomes of treatment for elbow problems is a patient-derived functional assessment, a clinical examination, and a pain assessment.

▶ There has been a marked increase in methods of assessing radiographs, and clinical and functional outcomes in orthopedics. This study points out the lack of rigorous validation of these various systems. One question, of course, is what is the standard against which these various systems are compared. The intracorrelation among the various systems was surprisingly good, which is not surprising because most of the functional assessment systems inquire about the same issues but only place a different importance factor to each of the categories. Finally, it should be emphasized that just as with the knee, there is no one functional score that is an accurate reflection of the improvement of treatment for all disease entities. Thus, one score may be particularly effective in revealing an accurate improvement after joint replacement arthroplasty and may not in any way discriminate improvement after tennis elbow or medial collateral ligament surgery. More studies such as this are needed to better understand and appreciate the strengths and limitations of these scoring systems.

B.F. Morrey, M.D.

7　Shoulder

Introduction

The number of contributions to the literature regarding the definition and management of shoulder pathology has increased regularly over the last several years. A variety of articles have been selected to discuss various aspects of rotator cuff repair. The impact of suture anchors, arthroscopic procedures, and the management of massive tears are all considered. A number of contributions have been added regarding the management of shoulder instability and stiffness. The emerging role of arthroscopy is discussed, as are long-term results from open procedures. The final section of this chapter deals with an array of topics ranging from the value of arthrodesis in today's era of arthroplasty to thoughtful reviews of the psychological and occupational factors relating to overuse syndromes and the effectiveness of classification for shoulder fractures. Overall, this year's literature has proved to be of significant value with regard to the full spectrum of shoulder pathology. I hope you will find it useful in your orthopedic practice.

Bernard F. Morrey, M.D.

Cuff

Non-operative Treatment of Subacromial Impingement Syndrome

Morrison DS, Frogameni AD, Woodworth P (Southern California Ctr for Sports Medicine, Long Beach; Med College of Ohio, Toledo)
J Bone Joint Surg Am 79-A:732–737, 1997　　　　　　　　　　　　7–1

Objective.—Patients with subacromial impingement have encroachment of the coracoacromial arch on the underlying rotator cuff. Nonoperative treatment may be recommended to reduce inflammation, permit rotator cuff healing, and restore shoulder function. The results of nonoperative treatment for subacromial impingement syndrome are reviewed.

Methods.—The analysis included 636 shoulders of 616 patients with subacromial impingement syndrome. There were 386 males and 230 females, average age 42 years. The symptoms had been present for an average of 16 months. All patients had a positive impingement sign with no other shoulder abnormalities, such as full-thickness rotator cuff tears, acromioclavicular joint osteoarthrosis, glenohumeral joint instability, or adhesive capsulitis. Treatment included anti-inflammatory medication and supervised physical therapy, with isotonic exercises to strengthen the rotator cuff. The patients were followed for an average of 27 months. The results of treatment were analyzed, including the effects of potentially confounding variables.

Results.—Conservative treatment gave satisfactory results in 67% of patients. Twenty-eight percent of patients showed no improvement, and eventually underwent arthroscopic subacromial decompression. Another 5% of patients had unsatisfactory results, but refused surgery. Of the patients with successful conservative treatment, 18% had recurrent symptoms during follow-up. In each case, the symptoms were successfully managed with rest or resumption of physical therapy. On analysis of confounding variables, the results were better for patients aged 20 years or younger and those aged 41–60 years than for those aged 21–40 years. However, the worst results were seen in patients over age 60. The rate of satisfactory results was 78% for patients who had had symptoms for less than 4 weeks, compared with 63% for those who had had symptoms for 1–6 months and 67% for those whose symptoms had been present longer than 6 months. The success rate was 91% for patients with a type I acromion, compared with 68% for those with a type II acromion and 64% for those with a type III acromion. The results were unaffected by sex, dominant side, or concomitant acromioclavicular joint tenderness.

Conclusions.—This retrospective study suggests that two thirds of patients with subacromial impingement syndrome do well with nonoperative treatment. The authors' treatment program stresses isotonic exercise to strengthen the rotator cuff, thus addressing the extrinsic theory of this condition. The results are influenced by age, symptom duration, and acromial shape.

▶ As the diagnosis of impingement syndrome has become familiar to virtually all orthopedic surgeons, the literature is filled with discussions of surgical procedures to treat this condition. What is distinctly absent from the literature is information that allows the surgeon to arrive at some estimation as to the frequency with which patients fail nonoperative treatment. In fact, it is the common belief that many patients have relatively little nonoperative experience before they undergo the procedure. The large number of surgical procedures of various types suggests this liberal surgical indication philosophy. Thus, this article outlining the manner in which over 600 patients were evaluated and treated prior to undergoing surgical intervention is particularly relevant. The article clearly demonstrates that a reasonable percentage of patients rapidly responded to nonoperative treatment and did not even keep their return appointment. Approximately 25% of the patients' failure to respond otherwise to nonoperative treatment and, thus, their need for surgical ontervention provides some information with regard to what might be expected, at least based on these surgeons' nonoperative treatment protocol and therapy program. Finally, the morphology of the acromion has been debated with regard to the origin and persistence of impingement symptoms. This variable was specifically assessed, but the small percentage

(6%) of type I acromion makes interpretation of the findings somewhat difficult. Nonetheless, as might be expected, those with the flat (type I) acromion had a high percentage of success with nonoperative treatment, while those with the type II or III were associated with a more frequent need for surgery. Overall, this is a very informative article which deserves to be read in its entirety by those interested in the subject.

B.F. Morrey, M.D.

Traumatic Tears of the Subscapularis Tendon: Clinical Diagnosis, Magnetic Resonance Imaging Findings, and Operative Treatment
Deutsch A, Altchek DW, Veltri DM, et al (Case Western Reserve Univ, Cleveland, Ohio; Hosp for Special Surgery, New York)
Am J Sports Med 25:13–22, 1997   7–2

Objective.—Rotator cuff tears rarely involve the subscapularis tendon. The symptoms, diagnoses, MRI evaluations, and operative treatment of 13 patients with 14 rotator cuff tears involving the scapularis tendon are reported.

Methods.—Charts of 13 male patients, aged 18–64, seen between 1991 and 1993, were retrospectively reviewed. All patients had had traumatic injury an average of 3 weeks before the initial visit. Two shoulders were diagnosed with a rotator cuff tear isolated to the subscapularis tendon. The remaining 12 shoulders were treated nonoperatively and did not improve in strength and function. Correct diagnoses were delayed for 4–24 months. Ultimately, arthroscopic surgery was performed on 1 shoulder and arthrotomies on the remaining 13. All shoulders were evaluated with MRI.

Results.—Seven shoulders were injured during sports, and 11 injuries were the result of traumatic hyperextension or external rotation of the abducted arms. All patients reported pain and weakness. Plain radiographs revealed bony abnormalities in 6 shoulders. MR images revealed 13 full-thickness tears and 1 partial-thickness tear. MRI and arthroscopic findings showed 6 shoulders with a medial subluxation of the biceps tendon and 1 shoulder with a biceps rupture. Surgery revealed subscapularis injury in 7 of 13 shoulders only after scar tissue was removed. After surgical repair of the subscapularis tendon, 6 shoulders still had biceps tendon instability and required tenodesis of the biceps tendon to the intertubercular groove for stabilization. Shoulders were placed in slings for 5–6 weeks, and range-of-motion exercises were begun at 1 week, elevation and passive rotation exercises at 4 weeks, deltoid and rotator cuff muscle isometric exercises at 8 weeks, and resistance exercises at 3 months. Return to sports was not allowed for at least 6 months. At an average follow-up of 2 years, pain and weakness was completely relieved in 10 shoulders, strength was normal in all shoulders, and external motion was somewhat decreased in 5 shoulders. All patients have returned to work, and 12 have returned to their sports activities.

TABLE 2.—Clinical Findings in 14 Shoulders With Traumatic Tears of the Subscapularis Tendon

Finding	Number
Range of active forward flexion	
Normal (equal to uninjured side)	10
Reduced (10° to 60° less than uninjured side)	4
Range of passive external rotation*	
Normal	4
Reduced (5° to 15°)	3
Increased (5° to 25°)	7
Range of passive internal rotation*	
Normal	12
Reduced (2 vertebral levels)	2
Strength of internal rotation†	
Normal	1
Grade 4	13
Strength of external rotation†	
Normal	8
Grade 4	6
Strength of supraspinatus muscle‡	
Normal	9
Grade 4	5
Lift-off test	
Pathologic conditions	2
Inconclusive (secondary to tenderness)	12
Impingement sign§	
Painless	4
Slightly painful	10
Instability testing	
Negative	13
Positive	1
Yergason's test	
Negative	7
Tenderness at intertubercular groove	7
Speed's test	
Negative	7
Tenderness at intertubercular groove	7

Note: All measurements are based on comparisons with the contralateral uninjured arm.
*Tested with the arm at the side.
†MRC grades 0 to 5, manually tested with the arm at the side in neutral rotation.
‡Jobe and Jobe.
§Hawkins and Kennedy. Neer and Welsh.
(Courtesy of Deutsch A, Altchek DW, Veltri DM, et al: Traumatic tears of the subscapularis tendon: Clinical diagnosis, magnetic resonance imaging findings, and operative treatment. *Am J Sports Med* 25:13–22, 1997.)

Conclusion.—Proper diagnosis and early surgical repair of tears of the subscapularis tendon result in less pain and improved shoulder function.

▶ Acceptance of the diagnosis of subscapularis muscle tear independent of shoulder dislocation is difficult. Early literature regarding recurring instability of the shoulder clearly implicated a deficient subscapularis muscle, presumably due to tearing and stretching with the initial injury. In this particular series, however, there is little question, based on the careful history and analysis of symptoms, that shoulder instability was not a concurrent finding in this patient population. This paper does, therefore, in our judgment, adequately document the "isolated" tear of the subscapularis tendon. Having said this, the association with tears of the biceps should be noted. Another salient feature is the rather protean nature of the clinical presentation (Table 2). Lacking any specific or discreet pathognomonic findings, a high level of suspicion, and awareness of the condition are essential to make the proper diagnosis. In fact, the subtlety of the diagnosis escaped the arthroscopic assessment of half the initial surgical explorations. Nonetheless, when the diagnosis is established, repair of the torn muscle tendon complex is associated with virtually 100% improvement of patient's symptoms. The value of the report is identifying an uncommon injury that may masquerade as several other pathologic events occurring around the shoulder, offering further value of emphasizing that even delayed surgical repair is of value in restoring or improving function.

B.F. Morrey, M.D.

Arthroscopic Rotator Cuff Repair: Analysis of Technique and Results at 2- and 3-Year Follow-up

Tauro JC (New Jersey Med School, Toms River)
Arthroscopy 14:45–51, 1998   7–3

Background.—Arthroscopic techniques of rotator cuff repair have been developed to reduce the morbidity of open repair while improving the functional results of cuff débridement alone. Preliminary reports have suggested promising results. An experience with completely arthroscopic rotator cuff repair, including 2- to 3-year follow-up data, is reported.

Methods.—The experience included 53 patients who were followed for at least 2 years after arthroscopic rotator cuff repair. Some were patients in whom nonoperative treatment for chronic, full-thickness rotator cuff tears had failed; others were high-demand patients undergoing early treatment for acute tears. Most patients had avulsions of the supraspinatus from the greater tuberosity, sometimes with associated longitudinal tears. The avulsions were repaired with nonretrievable suture anchors, while the longitudinal tears were repaired with a side-to-side suturing technique. As indicated, the surgeons arthroscopically performed such open-mobilization techniques as elevation of the cuff off the glenoid neck and scapular fossa and cutting of the coracohumeral ligament. The suture repairs were done using 0-polydioxarone (PDS) or 1-PDS suture, a 7-mm suture punch, and simple and mattress suture configurations. The clinical evaluations were done using a modified 45-point UCLA rating system, which included additional points for abduction range of motion and strength.

Results.—The patients' average rating scale scores improved from 17 points preoperatively to 41 points postoperatively. The results were considered excellent in 36 patients, good in 13, fair in 1, and poor in 3. Anchor pullout sometimes occurred during the operation, but never postoperatively. The patients with fair and good results were all operated on early in the experience, when 0-PDS suture was used; 1-PDS was used later on. Compared with patients having open repair, patients treated arthroscopically had less scarring, a shorter hospital stay, less postoperative pain, and easier rehabilitation.

Conclusions.—In properly selected cases performed by an experienced shoulder arthroscopist, arthroscopic rotator cuff repair is technically feasible and clinically preferred. The arthroscopist must be able to see the tear well, and to mobilize it back to the tuberosity under only moderate tension. The authors recommend the use of an anterolateral operative portal, which improves both the angle of entry for instruments with anchors and visualization in the subacromial space. The repair is not technically difficult when 1-PDS suture is used in simple configurations. Simple techniques of arthroscopic cuff mobilization permit the repair of large tears.

▶ Arthroscopic repair of the rotator cuff continues to emerge as a technically feasible procedure. This study includes avulsion as well as the more readily addressed longitudinal tears, with a modest minimum 2-year surveillance. Results in 49 of 53 patients were reported as satisfactory, with the vast majority being rated as excellent. This is certainly impressive. Although the authors do describe the inclusion criteria as relating primarily to the ability to mobilize the tendon, we are now providing information about what percentage of patients in the overall population so evaluated were actually amenable to this procedure. Furthermore, as noted in the discussion, there was not a control group to determine whether débridement alone may have been sufficient in some of the small tears, although, clearly, débridement as a salvage for a massive tear would apply to a patient population entirely different from that studied in this article. It is difficult to understand and, therefore, bothersome that the size of the tear did not directly correlate with the overall outcome of the procedure. Larger series with additional studies and surveillance of longer duration are necessary to appreciate the value and utility of this approach fully.

B.F. Morrey, M.D.

Massive, Irreparable Tears of the Rotator Cuff: Results of Operative Débridement and Subacromial Decompression

Gartsman GM (Methodist Hosp, Houston)
J Bone Joint Surg Am 79-A:715–721, 1997   7–4

Background.—There are various treatment options for surgeons who encounter a massive, irreparable defect of the tendons of the rotator cuff during an operation. A common treatment includes débridement of the edges of the necrotic tendon, decompression of the subacromial space with an anterior and inferior acromioplasty, resection of the coracoacromial ligament, removal of the subacromial bursa, and meticulous repair of the deltoid. Rehabilitation is then started immediately.

Methods.—The effectiveness of operative débridement and subacromial decompression of the shoulder was evaluated preoperatively and postoperatively in 33 patients with irreparable tear of the rotator cuff. Pain, ability to perform activities of daily living (ADL), range of motion, strength, and patient satisfaction were evaluated. The Shoulder Score Index of the American Shoulder and Elbow Surgeons and the scoring systems of the University of California at Los Angeles and Constant and Murley were used.

Results.—Follow-up was a minimum of 2 years in all 33 patients. At follow-up, 26 patients believed that their shoulder had improved, 3 believed it was unchanged, and 4 believed that it was worse. Patients reported significant decreases in pain, significant increases in range of motion and ability to perform ADL, and decreases in strength with elevation.

Conclusion.—The improvements in pain, range of motion, and functioning in ADL in this study were inferior to improvements reported in other studies of repaired torn rotator cuffs. According to the scoring systems used in this study, the results of operative débridement and subacromial decompression are inferior to the results of operative decompression and repair of a torn rotator cuff.

▶ Controversy over the management of the massive rotator cuff continues. Some have stated that there is no tear so massive that it cannot be reconstructed or repaired. There is no question that the best function comes about when the supraspinatus and remaining cuff tissue can be reattached. If, however, the lesion is extensive, Gartsman and others have demonstrated that débridement is effective in decreasing pain and, thus, to some extent, improving motion. Strength is not improved.

There is also some evidence that the benefit observed after the initial procedure does not persist over long periods and symptoms recur. Although there is no perfect solution to this difficult clinical problem, it would seem that débridement does offer some benefit, particularly for those patients in whom the technical ability to obtain a functional reconstruction is not possible.

B.F. Morrey, M.D.

A Biomechanical Evaluation of Suture Anchors in Repair of the Rotator Cuff

Rossouw DJ, McElroy BJ, Amis AA, et al (Royal Berkshire Hosp, Reading, England; St Mary's Hosp, London; Imperial College of Science, Technology and Medicine, London)
J Bone Joint Surg Br 79-B:458–461, 1997   7–5

Background.—In the repair of rotator cuff tears, there is a need for secure reattachment and early mobilization. Suture anchors may be used during arthroscopic rotator cuff repair, but have yet to be fully evaluated. Because of concerns about disuse osteoporosis, the greater tuberosity may be an inappropriate site for fixation of a suture anchor. The adjacent

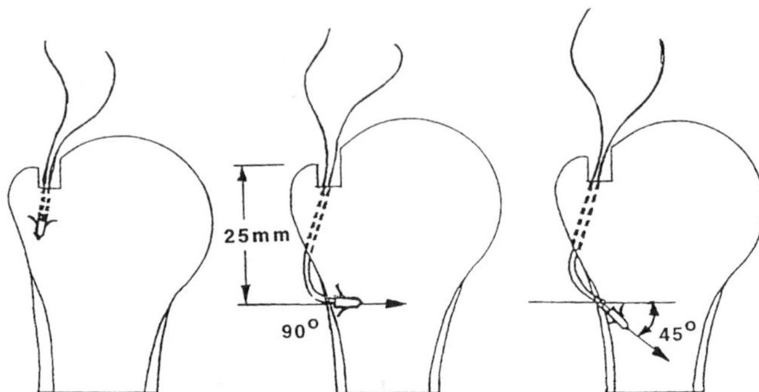

FIGURE 1.—The 3 sites of insertion of the suture anchor. (Courtesy of Roussouw DJ, McElroy BJ, Amis AA, et al: A biomechanical evaluation of suture anchors in repair of the rotator cuff. *J Bone Joint Surg Br* 79B:458–461, 1997.)

lateral humeral cortex may provide stronger anchorage. This biomechanical study evaluated the strength of suture anchors in rotator cuff repair.

Methods.—Suture anchors were placed in 3 locations in cadaver shoulders, either in the base of the trough or in the lateral cortex of the humerus (Fig 1). Static tensile tests of suture-anchor attachment and of rotator cuff repair were performed. Cyclic load tests were also performed as a more realistic method of evaluating the repair.

Findings.—Suture anchors placed in the lateral cortex of the humerus produced a significantly stronger repair than those placed in the greater tuberosity. On cyclic loading, repair failure occurred at low loads. The mechanism of failure was tearing into the bones and tendons. Suture anchor repairs were not significantly stronger than conventional transosseous attachments.

Conclusions.—Rotator cuff repairs with suture anchors placed in the lateral cortex of the humerus appear strong enough for early rehabilitation with assisted passive movement. However, these experimental results question the integrity of such repairs for postoperative early motion. Suture anchor repairs are no stronger than conventional repairs. More research— including cyclic and static loading—is needed to assess the strength of various attachment techniques and to reduce the high repair failure rate.

▶ The attractiveness of suture anchors continues to prompt expansion of surgical indications. Because of the well-recognized technical problems of secure reattachment of the torn rotator cuff, the use of these devices for this clinical entity is logical and is expanding clinically. Articles such as this, therefore, are important to provide some objective basis or insight as to what might be expected with the use of suture anchors in osteoporotic bone commonly encountered in the greater tuberosity. The variation in technical application is significant because the line of pull is a crucial variable in the stability of these devices. The conclusion should be noted carefully: the in vitro strength of the suture anchors is not superior to the conventional transosseous tunnel technique to the extent that early motion for rotator cuff repair is a goal. This and other articles provide some doubt as to the utility of suture anchors for rotator cuff repair, particularly when the site of attachment is osteoporotic.

B.F. Morrey, M.D.

Instability

Bankart Repair for Anterior Instability of the Shoulder: Long-term Outcome

Gill TJ, Micheli LJ, Gebhard F, et al (Children's Hosp, Boston; Univ of Mannheim, Germany)

J Bone Joint Surg Am 79-A:850–857, 1997   7–6

Background.—Anterior instability of the shoulder is frequently encountered in orthopedic practice, and is most often treated surgically with the Bankart procedure. It is the only surgical procedure that corrects the primary pathologic defect, the so-called Bankart lesion, present in as many as 85% of dislocations. There is no information on the long-term outcome or functional results of this procedure.

Methods.—In 60 shoulders in 56 patients, range of motion, stability, and strength were evaluated a minimum of 8 years after the Bankart procedure. There were 39 male patients, and the mean patient age at operation was 21.4. Patients completed a questionnaire about the history of the instability, participation in sports, pain, and functional ability at home and work.

Results.—At a mean of 11.9 years postoperatively, the mean loss of external rotation was 12 degrees. Differences in forward elevation, abduction, and internal rotation between the involved and normal shoulder were not significant. Crepitus on glenohumeral motion was noted in 1 patient. Of the 56 patients, 55 returned to their previous work. Mild pain with strenuous activity was reported by 28 patients, and pain at rest was reported by 1 patient. Three patients had a new dislocation of the involved shoulder more than 3 years after surgery. Results were rated excellent or good by 52 patients, fair by 3 patients, and poor by 1 patient. Fifty-four patients stated they would undergo the Bankart procedure again.

Discussion.—A modified shoulder rating system was used that emphasized pain-free function, stability, and motion. In the patients who rated their results as fair or poor, the most common problems were decreased range of motion and intermittent pain, not instability.

Clinical Significance.—The Bankart procedure for anterior instability of the shoulder offers excellent long-term results and high patient satisfaction. At least 6 weeks of formal physical therapy is recommended after the procedure.

▶ The authors provide us with a significant contribution to the literature inasmuch as long-term functional assessment of a standardized surgical procedure is documented. The proposed methodology, while appearing to provide increased insight as to the effectiveness of this procedure, remains to be validated by other investigators. Nonetheless, the effort at assessing not just stability as the end point, but the presence or absence of pain and functional activity is important information, particularly given that the mean follow-up exceeds 10 years. The recurrence rate, which has been carefully documented, also serves as a standard against which newer arthroscopic techniques should be compared. This contribution, therefore, is of merit from several perspectives and deserves to be read in its entirety.

B.F. Morrey, M.D.

Anterior Dislocation of the Shoulder in Elderly Patients

Gumina S, Postacchini F (Univ 'La Sapienza', Rome)
J Bone Joint Surg Br 79-B:540–543, 1997   7–7

Introduction.—Relatively little is known about the problem of shoulder dislocation in the elderly, including its prevalence, associated lesions, and the frequency of redislocation. The findings in elderly patients with shoulder dislocation were reviewed, including 7-year follow-up data.

Patients.—Over a 2-year period, 108 of 545 patients treated for anterior shoulder dislocation were aged 60 years or older, for a prevalence of 20%. In 94% of patients, general anesthesia was needed for relocation of the humeral head. Nine percent of patients had injuries to the axillary nerve, but all of these injuries resolved completely within 3–12 months. At a mean follow-up of 7 years, 95 patients were interviewed and examined: 77 women and 18 men, mean age 72 years.

Findings.—At follow-up, 22% of patients had at least 1 recurrent dislocation, and 10 had 2 or more. Patient age did not affect the tendency to redislocate. Sixty-one percent of patients had rotator cuff tears diagnosed on clinical grounds or from imaging studies. All of the patients with recurrent dislocations had rotator cuff tears. Surgery was performed in 16 patients, consisting of rotator cuff repair only in 8 patients with a single dislocation and a cuff tear. Five of the 8 surgical patients with recurrent dislocations also had a torn rotator cuff; they were managed with cuff repair, with or without a stabilizing procedure. Satisfactory results were achieved in most surgical patients. The exceptions were 2 patients with multiple redislocations and rotator cuff tears who were managed with cuff repair only.

Conclusions.—Anterior shoulder dislocation appears to be a common problem in patients over age 60. The redislocation rate is 20%, and the rate of rotator cuff tear is 60%. Some of these patients will need surgery to repair the rotator cuff or to stabilize the shoulder. For patients who experience multiple redislocations, both procedures should probably be performed.

▶ With the multiplicity of reports regarding anterior shoulder dislocation, the implication of this problem for the elderly patient is readily emphasized. This article, therefore, is of value in reporting a surprisingly high (20%)

incidence of dislocations occurring in patients over 60 years of age. As has been well documented in the literature, the tendency for recurrence is not as high as in younger patients, but still, in this series of over 100 patients, it remains surprisingly high, with a recurrence in approximately 20%. Nonetheless, the shoulder generally stabilizes and does not require surgical intervention. The need for rotator cuff repair if surgery is required is noted in this article, as it has been documented in the past. It is encouraging, likewise, to note that patients with the appropriate intervention, either for recurrence or for rotator cuff tear, may be expected to have a satisfactory outcome if the primary pathology is addressed.

B.F. Morrey, M.D.

Two- to Five-Year Followup of Arthroscopic Bankart Reconstruction Using a Suture Anchor Technique

Koss S, Richmond JC, Woodward JS Jr (Tufts Univ, Boston)
Am J Sports Med 25:809–812, 1997   7–8

Background.—A Bankart lesion, separation of the inferior glenohumeral ligament-anterior labral complex from the glenoid rim, is found in the majority of traumatic anterior shoulder dislocations. The most common repair technique is the open Bankart procedure, although shoulder arthroscopic techniques are now being employed. This report describes results of an arthroscopic procedure used to repair anterior shoulder instability.

Methods.—From 1990 to 1993, arthroscopic Bankart reconstruction was performed on 27 patients with recurrent anterior shoulder instability. The average number of shoulder dislocations prior to surgery in this study group was 5. The surgical technique consisted of arthroscopic placement of suture anchors along the anteroinferior glenoid, which were used to repair the capsulolabral detachment. Of the 27 patients in this series, 20 returned for a follow-up visit, 26–64 months after surgery, consisting of a physical examination, pain and function questionnaires, and radiographs. Two patients were interviewed by telephone. Five patients in whom the procedure was unsuccessful had undergone open surgical stabilization.

Results.—The average Bankart rating score in this study group was 88, with 70% good-to-excellent results and 30% fair-to-poor results. The average University of California, Los Angeles shoulder function score was 32. The average loss of external rotation in abduction was 1 degree. The procedure failed in 8 patients who had recurrence of shoulder instability. In 7 of the failures, there were repeat traumatic events. Multivariate analysis indicated that success was correlated with fewer shoulder dislocations prior to repair.

Conclusions.—This study describes the results of arthroscopic Bankart reconstruction using a Mitek suture anchor technique. After a follow-up period of 2–5 years, there was a 30% failure rate with recurrent shoulder instability. In 7 of these 8 failures, there was repeat trauma. Because of this high failure rate, this arthroscopic stabilization technique is not recommended for patients who plan to return to contact sports. It should be considered for patients who value maintenance of external rotation or improved cosmetic results.

▶ Although the numbers are not large, the relatively long-term follow-up does allow interpretation and some legitimacy to the outcome and the reasons for failure. The 30% failure rate is worthy of note. The risk factors for recurrence support other reports and, thus, merits emphasis. The technique is best reserved for those desirous of a cosmetic result, near normal function but not requiring the degree of stability that would be expected in those engaged in contact sports or sports with the force being imparted to the shoulder joint. It is, of course, arguable that a better or different surgical technique could extend the indications and provide more favorable results than reported here. More data are necessary to draw such a conclusion—a conclusion that cannot be derived from this paper.

B.F. Morrey, M.D.

Assessment of Failed Arthroscopic Anterior Labral Repairs: Findings at Open Surgery

Mologne TS, McBride MT, Lapoint JM (Naval Med Ctr, San Diego, Calif)
Am J Sports Med 25:813–817, 1997   7–9

Background.—Arthroscopic techniques have recently been used to repair traumatic anterior glenohumeral instability. Twenty patients with postoperative instability after arthroscopic Bankart repair were examined at open Bankart stabilization to determine the cause of persistent instability.

Study Design.—A retrospective review of patients who underwent open shoulder stabilization procedures between 1990 and 1995 detected 19 male and 1 female patient who had previously had an arthroscopic stabilization procedure. At the time of the arthroscopic stabilization procedure 15 patients had recurrent dislocations and 5 had recurrent subluxations. The arthroscopic procedure was performed with transglenoid sutures in 10, 8 mm Suretac devices in 7, G-II Mitek Suture Anchors in 2, and an arthroscopic Dyonics screw in 1 patient. Five patients recalled an injury prior to recurrence of instability. The average time from the arthroscopic procedure to the open procedure was 17.9 months.

Findings.—Of the 20 patients in the study group, 12 had healed Bankart lesions and 8 had persistent lesions. Fifteen had attenuated and redundant anterior capsules. Seven of 9 patients with postarthroscopic dislocation had persistent Bankart lesions, while only 1 of 11 with subluxation had a persistent Bankart lesion. The presence of a persistent Bankart lesion was correlated with postarthroscopic dislocation. All 11 patients with postarthroscopic recurrent subluxation had redundant anterior capsules.

Conclusions.—Twenty patients who had undergone open shoulder stabilization for recurrent instability following arthroscopic shoulder stabilization were studied to evaluate their capsulolabral lesions. The presence of a persistent Bankart lesion was significantly correlated with postarthroscopic dislocation, and the presence of persistent capsular laxity was significantly correlated with postarthroscopic subluxation. Failure to successfully treat either the Bankart lesion or capsular laxity arthroscopically may lead to persistent postoperative instability.

▶ This detailed analysis is of value in emphasizing that failure to successfully reattach the Bankart labral lesion is a major cause of arthroscopic shoulder stabilization failure. However, the persistence of a lax capsule is also a common cause for failure of this technique. The authors appropriately emphasize the difficulty of estimating capsular laxity as well as the difficulty of accurately estimating the tension of the reconstruction. This particular contribution compliments other data emerging in the literature that will allow the surgeon to properly select the patient population as well as correctly execute the essential steps of the arthroscopic repair.

B.F. Morrey, M.D.

Arthroscopic Capsular Release for the Stiff Shoulder: Description of Technique and Anatomic Considerations

Zanotti RM, Kuhn JE (Univ of Michigan, Ann Arbor)
Am J Sports Med 25:294–298, 1997   7–10

Purpose.—Arthroscopic capsular release has become an option for the treatment of primary or secondary stiff shoulder. However, there is concern about the possible risk to certain neurovascular structures. Studies in cadavers were performed to evaluate the anatomic proximity of these neurovascular structures to the arthroscopically released joint capsule.

Methods.—Complete arthroscopic capsular release was performed in 7 cadaver shoulders with the use of electrocautery (Fig 1). All shoulders underwent circumferential release, performed about 1 cm lateral to the glenoid rim. The shoulders were then frozen in the lateral arthroscopic position (i.e., 45 degrees of abduction and 20 degrees of flexion). Dissections were then carried out to define the anatomic relationships among the released capsule and the axillary nerve, posterior circumflex humeral artery, and brachial artery.

Results.—The axillary nerve was located an average of 7.04 mm from the capsular release, with a 95% confidence interval of 5.62–8.47 mm. Average distance to the posterior circumflex humeral artery was 8.2 mm (95% confidence interval, 6.41–9.99 mm), and average distance to the brachial artery was 15.97 mm (95% confidence interval, 9.85–22.09 mm). Dissection following the axillary nerve medially from the released capsule revealed interposition of the inferior border of the subscapularis muscle between the capsule and nerve.

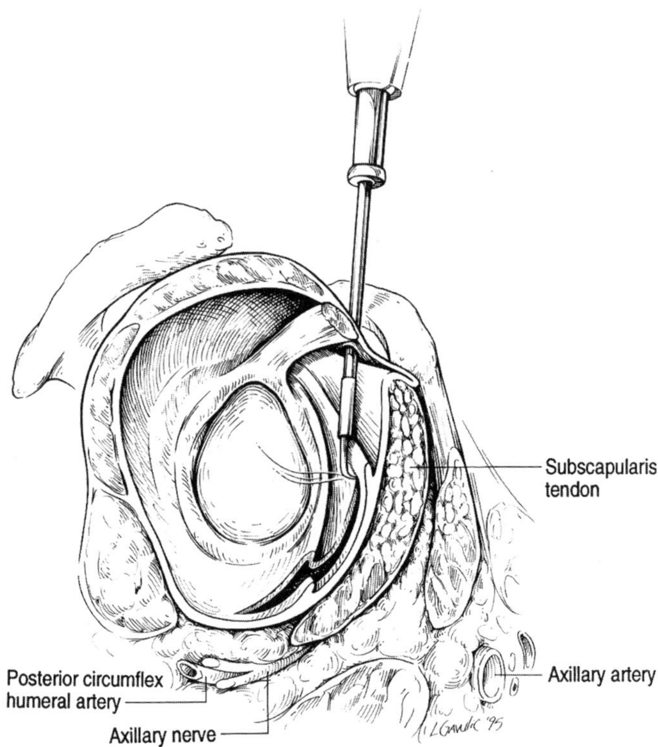

FIGURE 1.—Schematic drawing of the capsular release with the aid of the electrocautery device inserted through the anterior portal. The electrocautery unit has released the anterior band of the inferior glenohumeral ligament and is approaching the middle glenohumeral ligament. Neighboring anatomic structures are labeled. (Courtesy of Zanotti RM, Kuhn JE: Arthroscopic capsular release for the stiff shoulder: Description of technique and anatomic considerations. *Am J Sports Med* 25:294–298, 1997.)

Conclusions.—This study helps to define the anatomic proximity of various neurovascular structures in shoulders undergoing arthroscopic capsular release. Performing the capsular release within 1 cm of the glenoid rim will provide a relatively safe margin of protection for these structures. The capsule should be penetrated no deeper than 4.5 mm, the distance from the bend to the tip of the electrocautery device. The results apply to normal shoulders studied in lateral arthroscopic position.

▶ As arthroscopic intervention for the spectrum of shoulder pathology increases, greater awareness of the regional anatomy becomes more important. These authors emphasize the relationship and proximity of the axillary nerve as well as the posterior circumflex artery to the various regions of the shoulder capsule. Both these structures' location less than 1 cm from the capsule is of specific importance, and the article also has the more general value of emphasizing the intra-specimen variation of the findings. As would be expected, the axillary nerve is particularly vulnerable. One practical value of this article is the definition of the safe margin between the capsule and the neurovascular structures, with the recommendation that capsule release should occur approximately 1 cm from the glenoid rim (Fig 1).

B.F. Morrey, M.D.

Arthroscopic Release of Postoperative Capsular Contracture of the Shoulder
Warner JJP, Allen AA, Marks PH, et al (Univ of Pittsburgh, Pa; Hosp for Special Surgery, New York, Northwest Private Hosp, Burnie, Australia)
J Bone Joint Surg Am 79-A:1151–1158, 1997   7–11

Objective.—Some patients with loss of motion after a shoulder operation need surgical release. Open shoulder release techniques can improve motion, but require extensive dissection. The results of an arthroscopic capsular release technique are presented.

Methods.—The experience included 18 patients with postoperative shoulder stiffness. In each case, physical therapy and closed manipulation had failed to restore joint motion. None of the patients had known extra-articular contractures. Thirteen patients underwent arthroscopic anterior capsular release. Eleven patients had posterior capsular releases, including 6 patients with persistent limitations of flexion and internal rotation after anterior release (Fig 1). Concomitant procedures included arthroscopic acromioplasty for concomitant impingement disease in 8 patients and débridement of cartilaginous injuries in 2.

Results.—In 5 of 13 patients, anterior capsular release was sufficient to restore shoulder motion. Six required posterior release as well. In the remaining 2 patients, extra-articular scarring involving the subscapularis made it impossible to complete the arthroscopic release. Both patients underwent successful open release. The 5 patients managed with posterior release had loss of only internal rotation and flexion. The 11 patients undergoing anterior or combined anterior/posterior release had a mean 43-point improvement in the Constant and Murley score. All improvements in motion were significant, including a mean 51-degree improvement in flexion, a 31-degree improvement in external rotation in adduction, a 40-degree improvement in external rotation in abduction, a 6 spinous-process improvement in internal rotation in adduction, and a 41-degree improvement in internal rotation in abduction. For the 5 patients undergoing posterior release only, Constant and Murley score improved by a mean of 20 points, and improvements in motion were significant. This group had a mean 4 spinous-process improvement in internal rotation in adduction and a 42-degree improvement in internal rotation in abduction. Persistent pain related to previous articular cartilage injury was noted in 1 patient who had combined release and 1 who had posterior release.

Conclusions.—In selected patients with postoperative shoulder stiffness, arthroscopic capsular release can reliably restore shoulder motion. The arthroscopic approach minimizes morbidity. This technique is not suitable

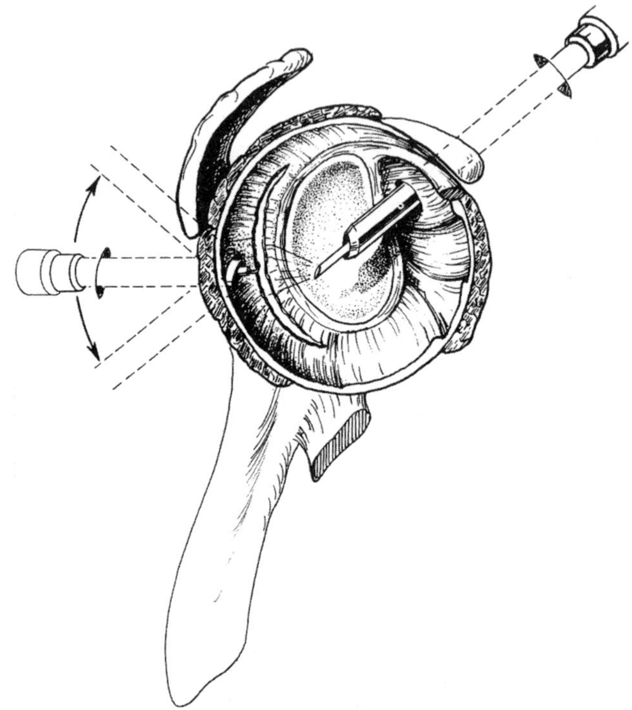

FIGURE 1.—Drawing showing division of the posterior aspect of the capsule along the glenoid rim with use of a hooked electrocautery device placed through the posterior portal. The arthroscope is in the anterior-superior portal. (Courtesy of Warner JJP, Allen AA, Marks PH, et al: Arthroscopic release of postoperative capsular contracture of the shoulder. *J Bone Joint Surg [Am]* 79A:1151–1158, 1997.)

for use in patients with known extra-articular contractures. Conversion to open release is possible if the arthroscopic procedure cannot be completed.

▶ The title of this article belies its true significance. The authors very carefully discuss the concise surgical indications and the clinical evaluation used to determine the need for not just posterior capsular but also anterior and inferior capsular release. It should be noted that the arthroscopic procedure was not successful in all instances and the surgeon must be prepared to perform an open procedure; thus, the appropriate discussion must be carried out with the patient.

B.F. Morrey, M.D.

Miscellaneous

The Role of Shoulder Fusion in the Era of Arthroplasty

González-Díaz R, Rodríguez-Merchán EC, Gilbert MS (La Paz Univ, Madrid; Mount Sinai School of Medicine, New York)
Int Orthop 21:204–209, 1997   7–12

Objective.—Shoulder fusion is an uncommon operation, but it can provide relief of pain and improved function when arthroplasty is contraindicated. The indications for and surgical techniques, complications, and results of shoulder fusion were presented.

Indications.—There are 12 indications for shoulder fusion (Table 1). Best results are obtained when the trapezius muscle has a fair degree of function and there is some flexion in the serratus anterior and the rhomboid. The acromioclavicular and sternoclavicular joints must be able to take additional stress after fusion. Immobilization is contraindicated if rheumatoid arthritis is present in the elbow and wrist. Bilateral fusion should not be performed in 1 stage.

Techniques.—The arthrodesis can be either extra-articular, intra-articular, or combined, with the combined procedure recommended for children. A compression plate and screws without a cast is recommended, although the pelvic reconstruction plate is an alternative and does not usually need to be removed. Necessary tendon transfers and nerve grafts should be performed with the upper limb maintained in a good position to assure a useful hand and elbow. External fixation using iliac crest bone grafts has failed to achieve fusion for a long period.

Results.—Complications include functional limitation, pseudoarthrosis, malposition, deterioration of function in the distal joints, fracture of the

---

TABLE 1.—Indications for Shoulder Fusion

1. Bacterial infection
2. Paralytic disorders of infancy
3. Combined deltoid muscle and rotator cuff paralysis
4. Post-traumatic paralysis of the brachial plexus in adults
5. Inflammatory arthritis with severe rotator cuff involvement
6. Failed arthroplasty
7. Recurrent dislocation
8. Tumour resection
9. Irreparable rotator cuff tear
10. Painful arthritis in a patient with activities that require power and not unrestricted motion
11. The immunocompromised patient
12. Tuberculosis

(Courtesy of González-Díaz R, Rodríquez-Merchán EC, Gilbert MS: The role of shoulder fusion in the era of arthroplasty. *Int Orthop* 21:204–209. Copyright 1997, Springer-Verlag.)

same limb, acromioclavicular dislocation, traction neuritis of the supra-scapular nerve, infection, failure or migration of the internal fixation device, epiphyseal problems, and the requirement for large allografts. The position of the shoulder must be correct to assure satisfactory function, with the degree of internal rotation being the most important factor. Arthrodesis in shoulders of children must take into account the fact that the proximal humeral epiphysis does not fuse until age 17 to 21 years. Epiphyseal damage can result in a very short upper limb. Progressive loss of abduction after fusion should be avoided. The optimal position for children is abduction, 45 degrees; flexion, 25 degrees; and internal rotation, 25 degrees. For adults, the best position is abduction, 20 degrees; flexion, 30 degrees; and internal rotation, 40 degrees. Rotation is more important in children than in adults.

Conclusion.—Shoulder fusion is an acceptable alternative for patients with contraindications for arthroplasty or failed arthroplasty.

▶ It is worthwhile revisiting nonreplacement reconstructive options. The authors provide a litany of potential indications for surgical fusion (Table 1). The justification for fusion will vary depending upon the experience of the surgeon performing the joint reconstruction, such that the absolute indication for fusion probably remains limited to the chronic refractory infection case. The optimum position of fusion remains controversial but is easiest to remember as 30 degrees abduction (± 10), 30 degrees forward flexion (−10), and 30 degrees internal rotation (±10). The ability to accurately replicate these 3 angular positions justifies some range in the accepted or anticipated position.

The surgical techniques for obtaining shoulder fusion have de-emphasized the large plates that can be bothersome to the point of requiring removal, and most now favor the compression screw technique. Nonetheless, the complication rate remains high—emphasizing, once again, the well-recognized tenet that shoulder arthrodesis remains a salvage procedure.

B.F. Morrey, M.D.

Psychosocial Factors and the Rehabilitation of Patients With Chronic Work-related Upper Extremity Disorders
Burton K, Polatin PB, Gatchel RJ (Univ of Texas, Dallas)
J Occup Rehabil 7:139–153, 1997   7–13

Introduction.—The incidence of upper extremity injuries, and particularly of repetitive strain injuries, is rapidly increasing in the workplace. Patients with repetitive strain injuries experience pain, weakness, and numbness or paresthesia. If symptoms of repetitive strain injury persist despite treatment, chronic pain can lead to anxiety, depression, and substance abuse. A prospective study investigated the effects of psychosocial factors on long-term employment outcome in a cohort of patients with chronic, work-related, upper extremity pain disorder.

Methods.—Seventy patients participated in the study. In all cases, acute conservative care failed or was judged unnecessary, surgery was unsuccessful or not an option, and severe functional limitations remained more than 4 months after the injury. All patients completed an interdisciplinary functional restoration program that included occupational therapy, cognitive-behavioral therapy, ergonomic consultation, and biofeedback. The study group had a mean age of 39 years; 47 patients were women and 37 were white. Patients were evaluated for Diagnostic and Statistical Manual of Mental Disorders, Third Edition, axis I and axis II diagnoses, history of childhood abuse, pain intensity, perceived level of disability, and level of depression.

Results.—In univariate analysis, return-to-work status 1 year after rehabilitation was predicted by the number of axis I disorders, a past diagnosis of substance abuse, a past and/or current diagnosis of an anxiety disorder, a diagnosis of borderline personality disorder, childhood abuse, self-reported depressed mood, and a moderate-to-high level of perceived disability. Age, race, length of disability, and past surgical treatment also predicted return to work. In multiple logistic regression analysis, patients significantly less likely to return to work at 1-year follow-up were older and were white, had a current diagnosis of anxiety disorder, and had a worse perception of their disability after the rehabilitation program.

Conclusion.—Among patients with upper extremity disability, psychosocial variables were found to influence return to work 1 year after completion of a rehabilitation program. A majority of patients in this study met criteria for 1 or more axis I disorders before their injuries, suggesting a predisposition to a chronic upper-extremity pain disorder post injury. Rehabilitation programs need to address these psychosocial issues.

▶ This carefully performed study provides objective support for the clinical impression of many orthopedic surgeons that the so-called axis I disorders—major depression, substance abuse, and anxiety disorders—are significantly associated with pain and impairment after injury. However, it should be emphasized that the cause and effect is not clearly defined, as most of the participants in this study also met criteria for classification of their injuries as axis I disorders before the injury! The associated finding that over 80% of patients had a personality pathology is also not particularly surprising, but, once again, it adds some objective evidence to our clinical impression.

The observation that length of disability is a major determinant of a patient's ability to return to work has also been documented in the literature and is, once again, confirmed by this study. A worthwhile benchmark in treating these patients is the fact that patients have a higher return-to-work rate less than 8 months after injury, compared with those whose injury occurred more than 15 months previously. The fact that those with borderline personality disorder have major problems returning to work has been shown by other investigations and is confirmed by this study.

Finally, it is particularly important for the surgeon to recognize that patients who had had at least 1 surgical procedure returned to work at a statistically significantly lower rate than those who had had no surgery. This puts a considerable burden on the surgeon to accurately identify these patients and avoid offering ill-advised procedures. This is a difficult task when we feel sympathy for patients and their circumstances and believe we can assist them with surgical intervention. A study such as this, however, provides some insight into the need for avoiding such a mistake.

B.F. Morrey, M.D.

Occupational Factors Related to Shoulder Pain and Disability

Pope DP, Croft PR, Pritchard CM, et al (Univ of Manchester, England; Univ of Keele, Stoke-on-Trent, England)
Occup Environ Med 54:316–321, 1997   7–14

Background.—Studies have found a higher incidence of shoulder symptoms in occupational groups than in the general population. Shoulder symptoms in occupational settings may be related to the physical and psychosocial aspects of the work and to the work environment. Occupational factors related to shoulder pain and disability were examined using population-based data.

Methods.—The study was based on a random sample of 50 patients from an English general practice. In a mail questionnaire, the patients were asked about shoulder-related symptoms and resultant disability. The questionnaire also asked about lifetime occupational history, including information on physical exposures, working conditions, and psychosocial factors for each workplace. For subjects with shoulder pain and disability, occupational factors at the time of symptom onset were compared with those of patients without symptoms.

Results.—Of 217 employed respondents, 39 met the study criteria for shoulder pain. Compared with symptom-free patients, those with shoulder pain were older, more likely to have long-term illness or instability, to have seen a physician for back pain, to have a recent history of neck pain, and to have other joint problems. Analysis of occupational factors found more than a 5-fold increase in shoulder pain and disability among men who carried weights on one shoulder. The risk of shoulder problems was approximately doubled for those who worked with their hands above shoulder levels, performed repetitive wrist or arm movements, or stretched down to reach below knee level. Risk of shoulder pain and disability was increased 4-fold for men who worked in very cold conditions and 6-fold for those who worked in damp conditions. Risk was nearly doubled for subjects of both sexes who reported a lot of work-related stress and tripled for those whose work was very monotonous. The work-related factors—including physical exposures, working conditions, and psychosocial factors—were independently associated with shoulder symptoms.

Conclusions.—Many work-related factors influence the risk of shoulder pain and disability, this population-based study suggests. The findings underscore the multifactorial etiology of shoulder pain, similar to the situation with back pain. Measures to prevent occupational musculoskeletal disorders should address not only heavy physical work but also working conditions and the workplace environment.

▶ This is one of an increasing number of reports attempting to correlate clinical presentations with the workplace environment. The authors provide a rather rigorous statistical analysis based on a prospective protocol of the independent correlations of the workplace environment, psychological aspects of the patient, and the specific activity, all relating to the occurrence of shoulder symptoms. The importance of this communiqué is the recognition by the clinician of the multifactorial nature of the condition of overuse pain in the shoulder girdle. This would logically lead away from surgical intervention and to a reliance on nonsurgical treatment modalities.

B.F. Morrey, M.D.

Poor Reproducibility of Classification of Proximal Humeral Fractures: Additional CT of Minor Value

Sjödén GOJ, Movin T, Güntner P, et al (Huddinge Univ, Sweden)
Acta Orthop Scand 68:239–242, 1997   7–15

Objective.—Although fractures of the proximal humerus should be classified carefully for planning treatment and evaluating outcome, shoulder surgeons sometimes find it difficult to categorize fractures from plain radiographs. Whether CT improves reproducibility of classification of proximal humeral fractures was evaluated.

Methods.—One 45-degree anteroposterior view, and 1 scapular conventional radiograph, and CT examinations were performed on 26 proximal humeral fractures. Five orthopedic specialists and 5 radiology specialists reviewed each and classified the fractures, using the Neer and AO classifications. Classifications were repeated 2 months later. Interobserver reliability (kappa statistic) and intraobserver reproducibility were assessed.

Results.—The mean kappa coefficient was 0.42 in the first viewing and 0.43 in the second viewing with the Neer system. With the AO system, the respective kappa coefficients were 0.31 and 0.26, respectively. Intraobserver reproducibility ranged from 0.20 to 0.85 with the Neer system and from 0.16 to 0.60 with the AO system.

Conclusion.—Neither the Neer nor the AO fracture classification system provide sufficiently consistent and reproducible results, even with the addition of CT to plain radiographs.

▶ This relatively brief report adds some fuel to the ongoing controversy regarding the value of radiographic fracture classification, particularly that involving the proximal humerus. This was a well-done study, and the conclusions confirming the observation that current classification systems of proximal humeral fractures have a low consistency of interpretation would appear to be valid. As the authors point out, this compromises the ability to compare fracture management among different studies. As noted by Neer, the concept of the classification, however, remains useful for developing a surgical plan. This fact would appear to be true even if the final classification—and, therefore, the final surgical strategy—is defined only at the time of surgery.

B.F. Morrey, M.D.

Shoulder Strength and Range of Motion in Symptomatic and Pain-free Elite Swimmers

Bak K, Magnusson SP (Univ of Copenhagen; Team Denmark Test Ctr, Copenhagen)
Am J Sports Med 25:454–459, 1997   7–16

Purpose.—Swimmers are prone to coracoacromial impingement in the shoulder, often associated with glenohumeral instability or excessive shoulder laxity. To prevent these problems, exercises to improve external rotational strength have been prescribed. However, the relationship between shoulder pain and shoulder strength and movement is unclear. This study compared shoulder strength and range of motion in swimmers with and without shoulder pain.

Methods.—The study included 15 swimmers, 7 with unilateral swimming-related shoulder pain and 8 with no current or past shoulder pain (Table 1). The 2 groups underwent internal and external isokinetic shoulder-strength testing and measurements of shoulder flexion and abduction strength. The relationship between these measurements and shoulder strength was assessed.

Results.—The swimmers with shoulder pain showed reduced concentric and eccentric internal rotational torque in both intergroup and side-to-side comparisons. Internal rotational torque was reduced, leading to significantly increased concentric and eccentric external-to-internal rotational strength ratios in the painful shoulders. In addition, the painful shoulders

TABLE 1.—Personal Data and Training History for Both Test Groups*

Variable	Group 1	Group 2
No.	7	8
Sex (F/M)	3/4	3/5
Age (years)	18 (16–19)	19 (15–25)
Competive swimming experience (years)	7.1 [2.2]	8.3 [3.4]
Training amount (km/year)	1675 [218.6]	1750 [492.8]
Strength training (No.)†	5	2

*Age is shown as median with ranges in parentheses. Other values are shown as mean values with standard deviations in brackets.

†Number of swimmers practicing strength training regularly for a minimum of 2 years before the investigation.

(Courtesy of Bak K, Magnusson SP: Shoulder strength and range of motion in symptomatic and pain-free elite swimmers. *Am J Sports Med* 25:454–459, 1997.)

showed a significantly increased functional ratio, defined as the ratio of eccentric external rotation to concentric internal rotation. Both symptomatic and nonsymptomatic swimmers had above-normal external range of motion and below-normal internal range of motion, with no differences between groups or on side-to-side comparison.

Conclusions.—Just strengthening external rotation of the shoulder may not be sufficient to prevent or correct shoulder-pain problems in swimmers. In addition, it may be effective to address the potential deficit in internal rotational strength; swimmers with painful shoulders need balanced strength training of the shoulder girdle. Shoulder range of motion appears unrelated to shoulder pain in swimmers. The motion changes observed in these athletes may reflect an adaptation to repetitive stress.

▶ This carefully performed study offers the provocative conclusion that in addition to the obvious need to enhance flexibility and strength of external rotators of the shoulder joint in swimmers, the need to provide complementary strength and stretching exercises to the internal rotators may also be important. This finding is consistent with other studies demonstrating that the antagonist as well as the agonist may require attention during the rehabilitation effort, particularly in high-performance and elite athletes. With increasing pressure to manage patients' postoperative pain, a number of modalities are being investigated, primarily relating to local blocks and intra-articular injections. The authors accurately describe the deficiency of the most popular modalities currently employed, specifically including inter-scalene blocks, primarily due to relatively high incidence of potential side effects and the less than optimally effective intra-articular injection. This carefully controlled study does offer a strong case for the utility of a supra-scapular nerve block in controlling post-arthroscopic shoulder pain. The authors reviewed a number of variables, including functional ones as well as complications and side-effects. It is not clear whether this particular modality is more effective for some procedures than for others, but the authors do show that it is superior to the saline control.

B.F. Morrey, M.D.

Comparison of the Accuracy of Steroid Placement With Clinical Outcome in Patients With Shoulder Symptoms
Eustace JA, Brophy DP, Gibney RP, et al (St Vincent's Hosp, Dublin)
Ann Rheum Dis 56:59–63, 1997   7–17

Background.—Steroid injection has long been performed for the relief of localized rheumatic symptoms. However, studies of the effectiveness of this treatment have yielded widely varying results. This may reflect variations in how often the steroid is actually injected into the desired target. The accuracy of steroid injection was assessed, along with its impact on the effectiveness of local steroid injection.

Methods.—The study included 37 patients with a total of 38 localized steroid injections into the glenohumeral joint (24 injections) or subacromial bursa (14 injections). The steroid was mixed with contrast material to show the accuracy of the injection. All injections were given in the radiology department, followed immediately by radiography. The patients were evaluated 2 weeks after the injection, without knowledge of the radiographic findings. The patients were asked to rate the maximum and current effectiveness of steroid injection on a 5-point scale, and whether they would have it repeated if necessary. The ratings of benefit were compared for shoulders with accurate and inaccurate injection.

Technique.—The injections were made by a standard technique, as described by Dixon and Graber. An anterior approach to the glenohumeral joint was used, with a 21G × 1.5-inch needle placed 2.5 cm below the tip of the coracoid process and 2.5 cm medial to the head of the humerus. A lateral approach was taken to the subacromial bursa, with the needle placed through the deltoid muscle and directed medial and slightly anterior under the lateral end of the acromion process. Glenohumeral injection was performed in patients with adhesive capsulitis or acute synovitis. Subacromial injection was performed in patients with rotator cuff syndrome, unless the point of maximal tenderness was over the anterior glenohumeral joint line.

Results.—The steroid was accurately placed in 37% of joints, including 29% of attempted subacromial injections and 42% of attempted glenohumeral joint injections. The shoulders with accurate and inaccurate injection were significantly different in terms of stiffness, functional loss, and change in flexion and abduction. Patients with accurate injection had a significant improvement in perceived maximum benefit of the injection. At follow-up, there was a nonsignificant difference in current benefit.

Conclusions.—Though generally well tolerated, local steroid injections into the shoulder joint are often inaccurate. In this study, only 42% of glenohumeral joint injections made by a standardized anterior approach reached their desired target. Patients with accurate injections show significantly greater benefit than those with inaccurate injections. The findings confirm previous studies suggesting that fewer than half of attempted shoulder injections are accurately placed.

▶ This study is of particular interest because it assesses one of the most obvious questions in medicine: To what extent is the success of a steroid injection influenced by the accuracy of needle placement? While it would seem as though the answer is axiomatic, this particular question has been rarely addressed in the literature. This carefully done study suffers somewhat from relatively small sample size and is limited only to the shoulder. However, given that, it is of interest to note that only a third of the injections were accurately placed. Particularly notable is the inaccuracy of the subacromial injection (29%). The fact that a standardized system was used as described in a textbook may limit the accuracy in that most orthopedic surgeons carefully palpate the location that dictates the site of needle entry. Although it may be self-serving, there is also some question as to the accuracy of an injection when performed by various specialties, apparently in this instance by those trained in rheumatology rather than orthopedic surgery. Nonetheless, the topic is of particular value in emphasizing the need for accurate placement of the injection and in providing objective evidence that the variation in response is, in all probability, at least to some extent related to the accuracy of the placement.

B.F. Morrey, M.D.

Results of Nerve Grafting for Injuries of the Axillary and Suprascapular Nerves

Mikami Y, Nagano A, Ochial N, et al (Univ of Tokyo; Univ of Tsukuba, Japan; Tokyo Metropolitan Geriatric Hosp)
J Bone Joint Surg Br 79-B:527–531, 1997   7–18

Objective.—Injuries to the axillary and suprascapular nerves make it impossible to elevate and externally rotate the shoulder. Results of nerve grafting of 1 or both of these nerves were evaluated.

Methods.—Between 1984 and 1995, 33 patients (1 female), aged 13–38 years, with combined injuries of the axillary and suprascapular nerves had nerve grafting. Thirty injuries resulted from motorcycle accidents, 1 from a bicycle accident, 1 from skiing, and 1 from a car accident. The average length of time between injury and repair was 3 months. The average follow-up was 27 months.

Technique.—The anterior and posterior axillary nerve is exposed through a deltopectoral approach and explored. After detachment of the trapezius and the posterior deltoid, the suprascapular nerve is explored from the upper trunk of the brachial plexus to the motor branch of the infraspinatus. The sural nerve from the same side leg is used if a graft is required.

Results.—Both nerves were repaired by grafting in 22 patients, the axillary nerve was treated by grafting in 8, and the suprascapular nerve was repaired by grafting in 3. The mean lengths of axillary and suprascapular nerve graft were 70 and 90 mm, respectively. The deltoid recovered to M3 or better in 16 (73%) patients and the infraspinatus to M3 or better in 15 (68%). Fifteen (68%) patients had excellent shoulder function. Results were most satisfactory when nerve grafting was performed within 4 months of injury.

Conclusion.—Nerve grafting for injuries of the axillary and suprascapular nerves resulted in satisfactory recovery of muscle and shoulder function when surgery was performed within 4 months of injury.

▶ The authors present a large series of patients with combined axillary and suprascapular nerve injuries and make several important points. Visualization is important and a combined anterior and posterior approach should be used. These are typically high-energy injuries and the nerves should be explored along their entire length, although most common sites of rupture in the authors' series were the scapular notch (suprascapular nerve) or between the posterior cord and quadrangular space (axillary nerve). Most important, the authors had superior results (M4–M5) if the procedure was performed within 4 months of injury. As we have become more aggressive in treating nerve injuries, results have continued to improve.

J.A. Katarincic, M.D.

8   Hip Reconstruction

Introduction

This year's focus on the hip has continued to be joint replacement arthroplasty. This chapter includes several high quality, long-term studies investigating the implications of a specific diagnosis and patient age; they will be of particular benefit to those doing these procedures. There has been increased interest and information regarding acetabular revision, particularly dealing with the implications of bone graft. These data are of particular benefit given the recognized relatively high incidence of acetabular failure, particularly in the younger patient, and the increasing number of revisions for osteolysis. Discussions of management of several complications of the joint replacement arthroplasty as well as avascular necrosis round out this section of interesting and clinically relevant articles.

Bernard F. Morrey, M.D.

Primary Total Hip Arthroplasty

The Long-term Results of Charnley Low-Friction Arthroplasty in Young Patients Who Have Congenital Dislocation, Degenerative Osteoarthrosis, or Rheumatoid Arthritis

Sochart DH, Porter ML (Wrightington Hosp, Wigan, England)
J Bone Joint Surg Am 79-A:1599–1617, 1997   8–1

Introduction.—This study reviews the long-term results of 226 Charnley hip replacements in a young population group, average age 31.7 years. This represents a small select of the almost 10,500 procedures done between 1966 and 1978 at the same institution.

Methods.—The operative diagnosis was developmental dysplasia of the hip in 60, degenerative osteoarthritis in 66, and rheumatoid arthritis in 100. Overall females outnumbered males by a 2:1 ratio. The mean surveillance was 19.7 years (range, 2–35 years). The outcome according to loosening, wear, and revision was carefully documented.

Results.—Radiographic loosening of the cup was greatest in those with dissociated double hypertropia (DDH) (37%) and least with rheumatoid arthritis (15%). Radiographic loosening on the femoral side was greatest in those with osteoarthritis (26%) and was only 10% in those with DDH and rheumatoid arthritis. Assessing the status at 25 years revealed an 81%

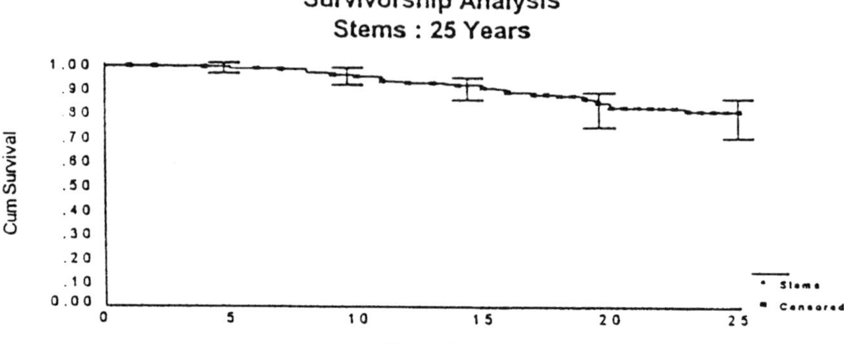

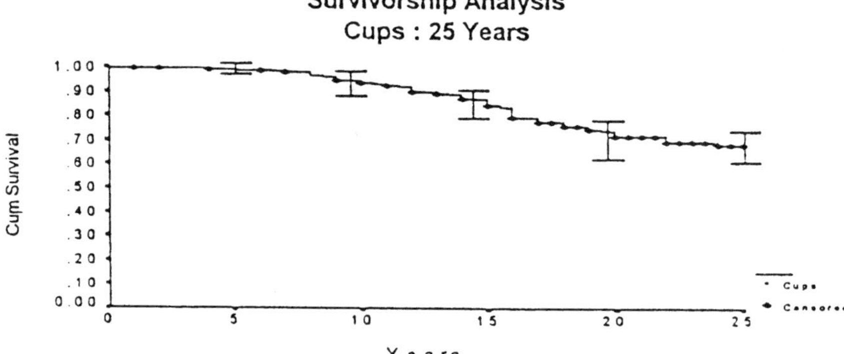

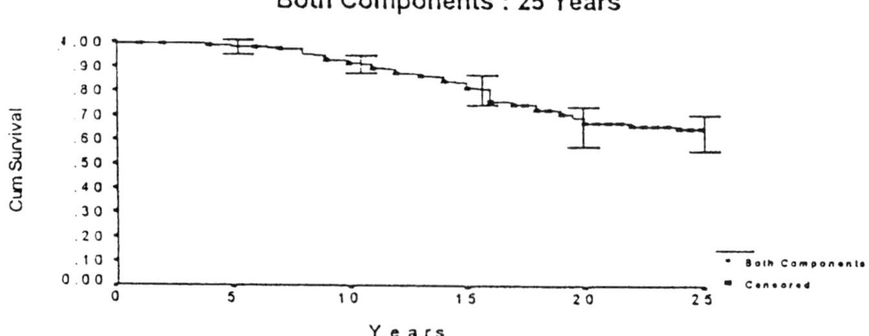

FIGURE 7.—Individual 25-year survivorship curves for the entire series, showing the acetabular and femoral components separately and in combination, with 95% confidence intervals. (Courtesy of Sochart DH, Porter ML: The long-term results of Charnley low-friction arthroplasty in young patients who have congenital dislocation, degenerative osteoarthrosis, or rheumatoid arthritis. *J Bone Joint Surg Am* 79-A:1599–1617, 1997.)

femoral survival rate for the overall series (Fig 7). The 25-year survival for the acetabular implant free of revision was 68%. Survival free of revision was analyzed further by diagnosis. In those with developmental dysplasia survival of the femoral component was 89%, in those with rheumatoid arthritis it was 85%, and in patients with degenerative osteoarthritis it was 74%. Survival of the acetabulum was less than favorable with a mean of 58% in those with developmental dysplasia, 79% in the group with rheumatoid arthritis, and 59% in patients who had degenerative arthrosis.

Conclusion.—Major factors that influence the long-term result in this particular study were wear in those with osteoarthritis and cup loosening in those with DDH.

▶ This is an excellent study from the cradle of low-friction arthroplasty. The authors provide an extremely detailed and rigorous analysis of the 3 diagnoses commonly associated with the younger patient population. The meticulous records kept at Wrightington and the careful scrutiny of these radiographs allows the message to be clearly and definitively made. The overall survival for the younger patient population with these 3 diagnoses is approximately 80%, the limiting factor being the acetabular component. The acetabular component is particularly vulnerable in DDH largely because of fixation and in patients with osteoarthritis primarily because of activity level. Moreover, as with other replacements, individuals with rheumatoid arthritis have a lower incidence of implant failure from loosening or wear for either the femoral or acetabular implant.

B.F. Morrey, M.D.

Factors Affecting Aseptic Failure of Fixation After Primary Charnley Total Hip Arthroplasty: Multivariate Survival Analysis

Kobayashi S, Takaoka K, Saito N, et al (Shinshu Univ, Matsumoto, Japan)
J Bone Joint Surg Am 79-A:1618–1627, 1997   8–2

Introduction.—The authors perform a rigorous analysis of their data with an interpretation using the multi-variant Cox proportional hazards model to determine factors which influence aseptic failure of fixation for hip joint replacement.

Methods.—In a consecutive series of 293 procedures, the average age of the patients was 59 years. All received the Charnley type implant with a mean surveillance of 13 years (range, 1 month to 23 years). The authors delineate the criteria for defining radiographic failure in both the femoral and acetabular components. Zonal analysis and grading of the interface resulted in 24 specific measurements on the acetabular side and 30 data points for the femoral analysis. The authors use radiographic evidence of failure as the end point of the study. In this instance, the failure is defined as progression of at least 1 of 5 postoperative signs: subsidence, fracture of the cement, endosteal cavitation, demarcation of the cement, and separation of the component from the cement.

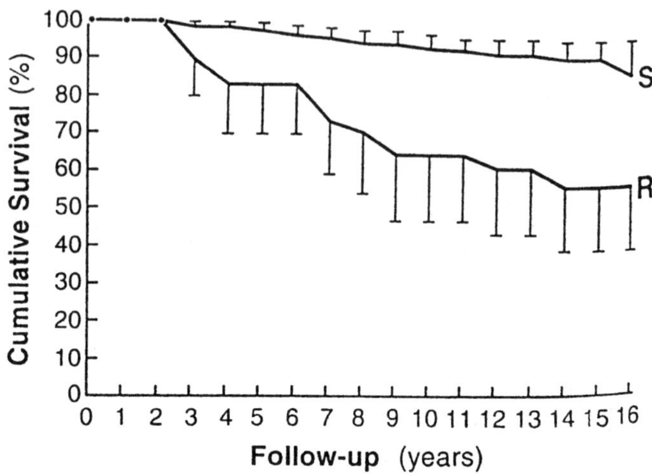

FIGURE 7.—Graph comparing the radiographic survival between the 31 sockets that had rapid wear of the polyethylene (R) and the 262 that did not have rapid wear (S). The 95% confidence intervals are shown on only 1 side of each curve. At 16 years, the cohorts consisted of 12 hips (R) and 76 hips (S); the cumulative rates of survival (average and 95% confidence interval) were 56.8% ± 17.0% and 87.0% ± 8.8%, respectively. (Courtesy of Kobayashi S, Takaoka K, Saito N, et al: Factors affecting aseptic failure of fixation after primary Charnley total hip arthroplasty: Multivariate survival analysis. *J Bone Joint Surg Am* 79-A:1618–1627, 1997.)

Results.—Based on this definition of failure, the 16-year survival rate was 83.6% for the acetabular component and 90.9% for the femoral component. If the survival free of revision is defined as the end point of surveillance, the 16-year survival was 92.3% for the acetabular and 95.6% for the femoral component. Of particular significance was a strong correlation between acetabular failure and a higher than normal early wear rate (Fig 7). Given that the typical wear rate is approximately 0.1 mm/year, those with at least 0.2 mm wear per year demonstrated a much higher rate of acetabular loosening.

Conclusions.—In addition to the rapid polyethylene wear rate, another unfavorable prognostic characteristic was the radiographic appearance of the arthritic process. Those that showed little tendency for osteophyte formation as part of their disease expression revealed a statistically higher failure rate. Unfavorable femoral geometries, large canals greater than 17 mm, and a large disparity between metaphyseal and isthmus discussions (canal flare index) were also determined to be risk factors. A correlation between deficiency of cement mantle or cement technique with radiographic failure was not found.

▶ This is an excellent and carefully done study of a relatively large group of individuals (of a young age) with various classifications of degenerative arthritis. These features place this overall population at some risk for mechanical failure. The reader should refer to the original article and review it in detail because this is one of the most comprehensive analyses of implant failure as a function of risk variables that has yet appeared in the literature.

The methodology is compelling, and consequently their results and conclusions, I think, are valid and worthy of note.

The demonstration of rapid wear as a risk factor for cup loosening has been noted in the past. The reason for the rapid wear is not clear but possibly relates to the heterogeneous nature of the ultra-high molecular rate of polyethylene, which is used in the manufacturing of the acetabular component. These authors also clearly demonstrate the morphology of the proximal femur as being a risk factor. Consequently, those individuals with very large femoral canals (measuring more than 17 or 18 mm) should be noted. The so-called *canal flare index*, which is the ratio of the intracortical width 20 mm proximal to the lesser trochanter and the dimension at the isthmus of canal, should also be noted as a predisposing factor to failure.

Finally, the authors' careful documentation of the biologic response with or without hypertrophic changes is worthy of note because the data demonstrate that patients with osteoarthritis and little hypertrophic reaction have a statistically higher likelihood of implant failure. The absence of statistical correlation with radiologic measures of cement quality is of particular note and deserves further assessment.

B.F. Morrey, M.D.

Total Hip Arthroplasty With an Uncemented Femoral Component: Excellent Results at Ten-Year Follow-up

McLaughlin JR, Lee KR (Kennedy Ctr for the Hip and Knee, Neenah, Wis)
J Bone Joint Surg Br 79-B:900–907, 1997   8–3

Objective.—Advances in the design of uncemented prostheses have improved the duration of fixation of femoral components after primary total hip arthroplasty (THA). Clinical outcome, incidence of osteolysis, and efficacy of fixation after 10 years of use of the Taperloc femoral component were reported.

Methods.—Primary uncemented THAs were performed on 145 hips in 138 patients between September 1983 and October 1985. Follow-up averaged 10 years for 107 patients (114 hips). The remaining 31 patients died before 8 years of follow-up. Level of function was determined before surgery and at each follow-up visit, using the Harris hip score. Cortical hypertrophy, stability of the femoral component, subsidence, and stress shielding were assessed, and presence of halo was noted. Kaplan-Meier survival analysis was used to estimate cumulative survival of the femoral component.

Results.—Of the 31 patients who died before the minimum follow-up period, 30 had the femoral component in place. Five of the remaining 114 hips required revision of the femoral stem for aseptic loosening, 3 during acetabular revision, 1 for sepsis, and 1 for aseptic loosening. Of the 109 hips not requiring revision, 94 (87%) were rated good or excellent, 8 (7%) were rated fair, and 7 (6%) were rated poor. The final average Harris hip score increased to 88 from a presurgery score of 48. Fixation by bone ingrowth was observed in 103 hips (94%), and fibrous ingrowth in 3. Three were unstable. Stress shielding was apparent in 106 hips (97%) and heterotopic ossification in 81 (74%). At the final visit, cortical hypertrophy was present in 59 hips (54%), spot welding in 96 (88%), a halo in 53 (49%), a complete pedestal in 20 (18%), and a partial pedestal in 28 (26%). There were 11 intraoperative and postoperative complications. There were findings of major osteolysis in 1 hip and osteolytic involvement in another 6 hips.

Conclusion.—Excellent results of THA were obtained using the Taperloc femoral component. There was a 1% incidence of aseptic loosening at 10 years.

▶ This experience reveals that reliable long-term results can be obtained with an uncemented femoral component. Although this finding is not unique, there is merit in noting that reports are emerging regarding several different designs that reveal the reliability obtainable with uncemented fixation. This, like other series, also highlights the fact that limitations to an ultimately successful procedure continue to relate to the bearing surfaces and problems with the modular acetabular component.

B.F. Morrey, M.D.

Tapered Design for the Cementless Total Hip Arthroplasty Femoral Component

Mallory TH, Head WC, Lombardi AV Jr (Joint Implant Surgeons Inc, Columbus, Ohio; Texas Ctr for Joint Replacement, Plano; Ohio State Univ, Columbus; et al)
Clin Orthop 344:172–178, 1997

8–4

Introduction.—Adaptive bone remodeling determines the long-term outcome of total hip arthroplasty. Prostheses designed for tight distal fit and fill show stress adaptation leading to metaphyseal bone atrophy, which may reflect bone adaptation resolving a conflict between femoral component stiffness and bone flexibility. When tapering prostheses are used, the pattern of bone adaptation may be different. Bone adaptation occurring in response to the placement of tapered prostheses was analyzed.

Methods.—Four studies in which cementless, tapered femoral components were placed were reviewed. The studies included a total of 748 arthroplasties, with an average follow-up of 58 months. The studies used different types of prostheses, but all emphasized avoidance of a tight diaphyseal fit and fill. Although the studies used differing definitions and measurement criteria, the review focused on the incidence of reactive bone modeling of the proximal femur.

Results.—The incidence of revision for aseptic loosening was only 0.4%, while the rate of significant thigh pain was 0.5%. Six percent of cases showed radiographic evidence of proximal bone atrophy, which was never severe or extensive. The amount of cortical hypertrophy varied, occurring in up to one half of the cases in 1 series. Overall, most cases showed no bone remodeling.

Conclusions.—The use of tapered femoral components in total hip arthroplasty does not appear to cause severe bone loss. The results indicate that stiffness of the femoral component may not be the only factor affecting reactive bone adaptation. The design of the femoral component may also be a significant factor. Tapered femoral components can achieve good clinical results without problems related to bone resorption of the proximal femur.

▶ These authors, each from a different institution, offer a reasonable case for the increasing awareness of a tapered implant as being a valuable design concept not just for the cemented but also for the cementless femoral component replacement. The tapered design allows better and more rigid fixation with increasing axial load. The clinical experience with all such designs has shown an aseptic loosening rate of less than 2% and, importantly, thigh pain typically less than 1%. Our own experience with a short-stemmed, double-tapered design is very similar to these authors' observations and this appears to be an important design characteristic. The double taper does allow a shorter implant to be employed because fixation occurs in the more proximal metaphyseal rather than the more distal diaphyseal region of the femur. This may account for the decreased amount of thigh pain noted with these patients.

B.F. Morrey, M.D.

Total Hip Arthroplasty Performed With Insertion of the Femoral Component With Cement and the Acetabular Component Without Cement: Ten to Thirteen-Year Results

Smith SE, Harris WH (Massachusetts Gen Hosp, Boston)
J Bone Joint Surg Am 79-A:1827–1833, 1997   8–5

Background.—A hybrid total hip prosthesis that combines an acetabular component inserted without cement and a femoral component inserted with cement was developed to lower the rate of aseptic loosening associated with cemented acetabular components and to retain the longevity of cemented femoral components. The hybrid total hip prosthesis used in this study is no longer manufactured, the acetabular component having been redesigned.

Methods.—One surgeon performed 52 total hip arthroplasties in 47 unselected, consecutive patients. The average patient age was 57 years. The prosthesis consisted of a hemispherical, porous-coated acetabular component inserted with screws through 3 peripheral flanges, but without cement, and a femoral component inserted with cement.

Results.—The clinical result was known in all patients. Of the 47 patients, 4 died for reasons unrelated to arthroplasty and 1 hip was revised, leaving 42 patients with 47 nonrevised hips who had a minimum follow-up of 10 years. Clinical follow-up of these 42 patients ranged from 10.8 to 13.3 years. Radiographic follow-up was 10.0–13.0 years. The 1 hip revision was performed for late recurrent dislocation without loosening 9.7 years after the initial arthroplasty. There was a relatively high rate of dislocation (13%), which may have been related to the shallow-chamber acetabular design and small femoral head. At the last follow-up examination, no femoral component was loose. Of the 52 acetabular components, 1 was loose, according to radiographs, but the hip was functioning well 12.4 years after arthroplasty. Pelvic osteolysis was seen in 1 hip, femoral osteolysis was seen in 8 hips, and distal femoral osteolysis was seen in 3 hips. For the 47 nonrevised hips, the average Harris hip score increased from 48 points before arthroplasty to 89 points at the last follow-up. Of the 47 hips, the result was good or excellent in 40, fair in 5, and poor in 2.

Discussion.—In these patients, primary total hip arthroplasty using a hybrid total hip prosthesis resulted in very good functioning at 10–13 years, although there was a high rate of dislocation. Although the surgical technique and design of the acetabular component were different in this study from those in other shorter studies of hybrid total hip arthroplasty, the longer follow-up of the current study adds value to the results. Hybrid total hip arthroplasty provides good functioning over an intermediate period.

▶ This carefully done study gives additional information regarding the expected clinical outcome from the so-called hybrid implant. The 12-year follow-up is impressive, but the sample is small. Although there were few revisions in this experience, the extremely high instability rate is of some concern, and it is not that clear, in my opinion, whether this is truly the result of the design or of other features of the technique. The fact that a posterior approach was used would seem to enhance the likelihood of instability and might be considered a factor as much as the cup design.

The overall incidence of osteolysis approached 25%, and although it is concluded that the hybrid represents a reliable and efficient surgical strategy, the implication of the 23% incidence of osteolysis is not clear without additional surveillance. This was a relatively challenging group of patients in that the mean age was 57 years and half the patients were male. The presence of a modular acetabular component correlating with the development of osteolysis remains, in our opinion, an unsolved problem.

B.F. Morrey, M.D.

Hybrid Total Hip Replacement: A 5–10-Year Follow-up Study of 106 Patients

Sarafis KA, Karatzas GD, Feroussis JC, et al (Asklepieion Hosp, Athens, Greece)
Acta Orthop Scand 68:21S–26S, 1997   8–6

Introduction.—Improved cement techniques have enhanced duration of stem fixation, but similar results have not been observed in cup fixation for patients undergoing hip surgery. Of 124 patients (83 women) who underwent 135 hybrid total hip replacements (THR), 106 patients (74 women) with 113 hybrid hips were followed from 5 to 10 years to determine the outcome of this surgical approach.

Methods.—The mean age of the patients was 63. Three types of acetabular components were used: the 2-peg porous coated PCA in 21 cases, the Universal porous coated PCA in 62, and the Kirschner integrity cup in 30. Anatomical PCA stems were used in 83 cases, and Kirschner dimension PC stems were used in 30. The mean preoperative Harris Hip Score (HHS) was 47. The position of the acetabular and femoral components was measured, and the condition of the cement mantle and the bone-cement interface was assessed at 6 months, 12 months, and yearly thereafter.

Results.—Postoperatively, 92% of patients were pain free and satisfied with their operation. The overall mean HHS was 89. Three of 113 hips required revision; 2 for wear or migration of the acetabular component, and 1 for loosening of the femoral stem. The remaining hips were stable, although 3 had signs of future loosening. Clinical outcome did not differ between the 3 types of prostheses used.

Conclusions.—At a follow-up of 55–116 months, hybrid hip replacements were clinically and radiographically satisfactory. All 3 types of acetabular components were uncemented with press-fit fixation. Longer follow-up is needed to accurately determine the prognosis of uncemented cup prostheses in hybrid hips.

▶ Any information regarding the long-term or even intermediate-term results of the hybrid replacement is worthwhile. In this study of 106 patients followed between 5 and 10 years, satisfactory results were observed in 92% of patients. The data are a little hard to interpret because 3 different cup designs were used. It should be noted that the distribution of the patients was not what might be termed "high risk," that is, approximately two thirds were women and the mean age was 63 years.

The average surveillance was just over 6 years. The overall success rate of 92% is certainly acceptable but is not significantly improved over other reports using other fixation modalities. Although the use of the hybrid may protect the cemented femoral component, in this series 4% showed radiographic signs of failure on both the femoral and the acetabular side, which is not an appreciable improvement compared with cemented implants with the same age and gender distribution. In my opinion, the data provided by this study does not demonstrate a superiority of hybrid fixation.

B.F. Morrey, M.D.

Femoral Revision

The Cement Mantle in the Exeter Impaction Allografting Technique: A Cause for Concern
Masterson EL, Masri BA, Duncan CP (Vancouver Hosp and Health Sciences Centre, BC)
J Arthroplasty 12:759–764, 1997   8–7

Background.—Many sources report that the longevity of a cemented total hip arthroplasty is improved when an adequate cement mantle is achieved circumferentially. It is also believed that a thin cement mantle has a higher risk of fragmentation, particle generation, and osteolysis. The authors have been using the femoral impaction allograft technique since 1994 and have been concerned about various cases of early rapid subsidence of the femoral component associated with fractures of the cement mantle.

Methods.—There were 35 patients who had revision arthroplasty with impaction allografting with a cemented stem for revision of the femoral component because of proximal femoral bone loss. The mean patient age was 62 years; there were 16 men and 19 women. Demographic and other preoperative data were reviewed, as well as surgical reports, postoperative data, and postoperative radiographs.

Results.—Radiographs showed that nearly 40% of the Gruen zones that could be clearly visualized had areas with absent cement. Cement voids were often seen, even in cases of an adequate mantle. A series of cadaveric impaction allografting procedures confirmed these cement mantle deficiencies, which seemed to result partly from an inadequate differential between trial and actual component sizes. Within 6 months of surgery, 4 additional patients had significant component migration secondary to radiographically visible cement mantle fractures.

Conclusion.—These results indicate that the cement mantle produced by the Exeter impaction allograft technique is often incomplete and associated with voids in the cement mantle. This surgical technique needs to be modified to achieve a more consistent cement mantle and to improve outcome.

Impaction Bone-grafting Before Insertion of a Femoral Stem With Cement in Revision Total Hip Arthroplasty: A Minimum Two-Year Follow-up Study

Meding JB, Ritter MA, Keating EM, et al (Ctr for Hip and Knee Surgery, Mooresville, Ind)
J Bone Joint Surg Am 79-A:1834–1841, 1997

8–8

Background.—Revision total hip arthroplasty is complicated by loss of bone stock secondary to particles of debris and mechanical instability. The best means to a successful outcome has not been determined. One technique that has been described involves cancellous allograft impacted to reconstitute a deficiency of the proximal femoral bone stock before a collarless, polished, tapered stem is inserted with cement. Early reports of partial restoration of the proximal femoral bone stock have been documented histologically and radiographically. To clarify the role of impaction bone grafting in revision hip operations, early clinical results and complications—as well as the degree of radiographic changes in the proximal part of the femur—were reported.

Methods.—There were 34 patients who had impaction bone grafting before insertion of a collarless, polished, tapered femoral stem with cement in 34 revision total hip arthroplasties performed because of aseptic loosening. In 28 patients, the procedure was the initial revision; 22 patients

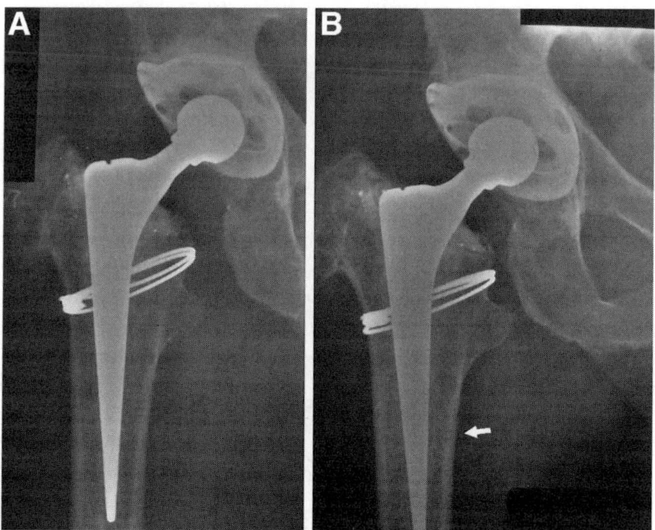

FIGURE 1.—**A,** initial postoperative radiograph of a 57-year-old man who had impaction bone grafting before insertion of the femoral stem with cement. Cerclage wires were placed prophylactically before impaction. **B,** 26 months postoperatively, stress-oriented trabeculae (*arrow*) have formed, especially medially and about the middle of the stem. (Courtesy of Meding JB, Ritter MA, Keating EM, et al: Impaction bone-grafting before insertion of a femoral stem with cement in revision total hip arthroplasty: A minimum two-year follow-up study. *J Bone Joint Surg Am* 79-A:1834–1841, 1997.)

also had revision of the acetabular component. The average follow-up was 30 months.

Results.—There were 4 intraoperative and 2 postoperative fractures of the femur and 1 dislocation. Repeat revision of the femoral stem was performed in 2 patients because of aseptic loosening at 26 and 36 months. These 2 patients had an associated fracture of the femur. Subsidence occurred in 38% of patients, averaging 10.1 millimeters. Although this sample was small, with the numbers available, subsidence was not found to be associated with preoperative or postoperative hip scores, segmental or cavitary femoral defects, femoral ectasia, intraoperative fracture of the femur, strut grafting, trochanteric osteotomy, or varus position of the femoral component. Radiographs showed incorporation of the allograft into the trabecular bone in 94% of patients and secondary remodeling in 41%, often within 1 year (Fig 1). Although follow-up was short, there was no localized resorption of the allograft. Cortical repair was seen in 1 patient at 3 years. At the last follow-up, Harris hip scores had improved from an average of 51 points preoperatively to an average of 87 points. Of the 34 patients, 28 reported no pain or only slight pain.

Discussion.—Although the early clinical results were satisfactory, the high rate of fracture of the femur and the rate and extent of subsidence of the femoral component are areas of concern. On the basis of the worrisome findings after 2 years, it is recommended that impaction bone grafting be used only in cases of severe proximal femoral osteopenia when stability cannot be achieved with insertion of a long-stemmed femoral component without cement. In such cases, impaction bone grafting may be considered an alternative to implantation of a massive proximal femoral allograft combined with insertion of a femoral component with cement.

▶ These 2 papers (Abstracts 8–7 and 8–8) report similar clinical experiences with the popular impaction bone grafting as a means of revising the femoral component after aseptic loosening. The study from Indiana is meticulous in defining the patient population and appropriately emphasizes the high rate of fracture and subsidence. Although some degree of subsidence is expected—and possibly even desirable—with a polished, tapered stem, the amount of subsidence reported by Ritter's group is of some concern. We would concur with their conclusion that this particular strategy is probably best reserved for those with significant proximal femoral osteopenia and for those in whom a long-stem implant would, otherwise, not be considered appropriate.

The study by Masterson et al. also provides a possible explanation for the high degree of subsidence. The difficulty of obtaining a uniform cement mantle is pointed out in this study and certainly may be implicated in the clinical failures. In spite of these shortcomings, we continue to favor this technique as a means of reconstituting the proximal femur but would emphasize that which is clearly pointed out in these papers: Appropriate patient selection and technique are critical for the success of this procedure.

B.F. Morrey, M.D.

The Cement Mantle in Femoral Impaction Allografting: A Comparison of Three Systems From Four Centres
Masterson EL, Masri BA, Duncan CP, et al (Univ of British Columbia, Vancouver)
J Bone Joint Surg Br 79-B:908–913, 1997   8–9

Objective.—In a number of instances, the cement mantle used with the Exeter impaction allografting system has shown evidence of fracture and fragmentation, particularly around the distal end of the prosthesis. Results of a study to distinguish the difficulties of an individual unit from problems produced by the design of the system were presented for 3 systems in 4 hospitals.

Methods.—Mantles from the Exeter impaction allografting system, the Harris Precoat system, and the CPT impaction allografting system were compared using anteroposterior and lateral radiographs taken within 3 months after surgery. The mantle was described as unclear, adequate, or deficient, depending on the thickness in any of 7 Gruen zones. Stem alignment, use of intramedullary plugs, management of the acetabular component, and use of cerclage wires, cortical strut allografts, and wire mesh were noted. Measurements of each component were also recorded.

Results.—Examinations were performed on 187 femoral impaction allografting procedures in 185 patients. With uncertain Gruen zones excluded, cement in the Exeter system was absent or deficient in 46.1% of zones in 1 hospital and in 50.4% of zones in the second hospital. Cement was absent or deficient in 20.7% of zones in the CPT system and in 18.3% of zones in the Harris Precoat system. The proximal impactor of the CPT system and the allograft impactor of the Harris Precoat system allow more space for cement around the length of the prosthesis.

Conclusion.—The cement mantle of the Exeter system is more often deficient or absent than in the CPT or Harris Precoat systems, possibly because of lack of sufficient space for the cement mantle to form around the length of the prosthesis. A functional study was not performed.

▶ Since the initial enthusiasm for this technique of revision—at least for certain types of femoral loosening—increased knowledge with regard to technique and patient selection have emerged. This report addresses the issue of an adequate cement mantle as 1 of the many variables that must be addressed when using this type of revision technique. While demonstrating that a continuous cement mantle is necessary for a reliable outcome, 2 different implants were used, yet the results of these 2 are relatively similar, differing by only a few percentage points. The take-home message of this paper is one that is emerging in the literature, that is, that whereas impaction grafting is a viable alternative for femoral revision, a properly designed femoral component, meticulous impaction, and careful cement technique are all required for a predictable and reliable outcome.

B.F. Morrey, M.D.

Acetabular Revision and Issues

Treatment of Pelvic Osteolysis Associated With a Stable Acetabular Component Inserted Without Cement as Part of a Total Hip Replacement
Maloney WJ, Herzwurm P, Paprosky W, et al (Barnes-Jewish Hosp, St Louis)
J Bone Joint Surg Am 79-A:1628–1634, 1997   8–10

Objective.—Osteolysis is a frequent occurrence in patients with uncemented total hip replacement. Revision of the acetabular component can result in destruction of bone pods, which can compromise the reconstruction, and result in a defect of the medial wall of the acetabulum and extensive damage to the anterior and posterior columns or even pelvic discontinuity. The clinical and radiographic results of a revised approach of replacing the acetabular liner, débriding the osteolytic lesion, and, in some cases, packing allograft bone chips into the lesion but leaving the original metal shell in place were reviewed.

Methods.—A retrospective review of all anteroposterior pelvic radiographs and lateral radiographs of the hip identified pelvic osteolysis in 35 (12 women) age 29–85 of 162 patients who underwent revision hip replacements between January 1991 and June 1994. The average length of time to revision was 5.5 years. Osteolytic lesions were located in the ilium, ischium, or pubis. At revision, a capsulectomy was performed, and the hip was dislocated to assess stability of the femoral component. Unstable components were removed. Stable components were revised according to the new approach. Bone grafts were used in 34 lesions of 26 patients. Preoperative and follow-up Harris hip scores were determined. Patients were followed up for at least 2 years.

Results.—All but 2 femoral heads were eccentric within the metal shell. A total of 46 lesions were found, and only 2 patients had no lesions in the ilium. Average lesion size was 2.4 by 1.7 cm. All ischial and pubic lesions were filled with bone graft. At last follow-up, all revisions were stable and no new osteolytic defects had formed. Of the 34 filled lesions, 22 had regressed and 12 had resolved completely. Preoperatively 14 patients had hip pain scores of at least 40 out of a possible 44 (slight, occasional, or no pain), 15 patients had a mean pain score of 18 probably as a result of a loose femoral component, and 4 patients had an average pain (in the groin) score of 23 despite stable components. The average hospital stay was 3.5 days, and patients were able to walk unassisted by 3 weeks. Patients with groin pain had less pain after surgery but were not pain-free. The mean pain score of 18 before surgery was 38 after revision.

Conclusion.—Preliminary results indicate that replacement of the liner and débridement of the lesion, with or without bone graft, when the metal shell is not damaged is an effective treatment for pelvic osteolysis after total hip replacement without cement.

▶ Today, when more and more hip replacement procedures are being revised because of the consequences of wear, several presentations or possible treatment scenarios must be considered. These authors have specifically addressed the question of reoperation primarily based on selection factors relating to the radiographic appearance of osteolysis. A metal-backed porous-coated acetabular component, which is known to be the one common denominator in the development of wear debris, was used in all patients. Thus, the common presentation of a worn high-density polyethylene liner and osteolysis was shown to be successfully treated at least in the short term by replacing the high-density polyethylene and bone grafting the defects. The reader must be particularly sensitive, however, to the admonition of the authors that this does represent relatively short-term follow-up, averaging just over 3 years, which, although successful, does not necessarily indicate that this will prove to be effective in the long-term.

B.F. Morrey, M.D.

Isolated Revision Acetabuloplasty Using a Porous-coated Cementless Acetabular Component Without Removal of a Well-fixed Femoral Component: A 3- to 9-Year Follow-up Study
Moskal JT, Danisa OA, Shaffrey CI (Roanoke Orthopaedic Ctr, Va; Univ of Virginia, Charlottesville; Naval Med Ctr, Portsmouth, Va)
J Arthroplasty 12:719–727, 1997   8–11

Background.—About 15% of revision hip arthroplasties are done for isolated failure of the acetabular component. Removal of the femoral component has been recommended to provide adequate acetabular exposure when a significant reconstruction is necessary. Combined femoral and acetabular revision is associated with a higher complication rate, longer surgical time, more blood loss, and higher cost compared with isolated revision acetabuloplasty. Because the long-term clinical results of revision femoral arthroplasty are inferior to femoral components of primary total hip arthroplasty, it would be preferable to maintain an original, well-fixed femoral prosthesis if it did not compromise the revision acetabuloplasty.

Methods.—Isolated acetabular revision was performed in 32 hips in 31 patients. Follow-up was 3–9 years. The average patient age was 66 years; there were 11 men and 20 women. At the time of the index procedure, all femoral components were well fixed and not removed or revised. Four hips had little or no acetabular bony defect, 2 hips had segmental defects, 10 hips had cavitary defects, 15 hips had combined segmental cavitary defects, and 1 hip had pelvic discontinuity.

Results.—The procedures consisted of 4 grade I reconstructions, 16 grade II reconstructions, and 12 grade III reconstructions. At the last follow-up, 94% of the cups were considered to be stable. A second revision acetabuloplasty was performed in 2 hips because of loss of fixation of the cup; these were performed without removal of the femoral component. There was evidence of rotational migration in 1 acetabular component, but this stabilized and remained nonprogressive. No cases of femoral component radiographic or clinical failure were seen. The mean hip scores were 44 preoperatively and 83 postoperatively. The mean pain scores were 12 preoperatively and 42 postoperatively.

Conclusion.—The results seen in these patients indicate that isolated revision acetabuloplasty with a porous-coated hemispheric cup without cement can be performed without removing or revising a well-fixed femoral stem and without compromising final outcome.

▶ This paper addresses a common question and one for which, to date, there is not a well-accepted position. Most surgeons generally accept the tenet that a well-fixed, unworn implant should remain intact if the opposite side of the joint is being revised. This paper does offer some insight with the demonstration that leaving well-fixed femoral components does not result in a high frequency of reoperation for subsequent problems or loosening. Technically it must be recognized, however, that leaving the femoral head and neck in place does pose some difficulties with regard to exposure, and the surgeon should be careful not to allow this to interfere with an adequate reconstruction of the acetabulum.

The femoral head should be removed in those implants with modular heads and necks, particularly if adequate exposure is otherwise not possible. The greater question for most surgeons is what to do with the acetabular component when revising the femur. To our mind, this is a much more vexing question than is the management of the femoral side, as reported here.

B.F. Morrey, M.D.

Bone Grafting in Total Hip Arthroplasty for Insufficient Acetabulum

Xenakis T, Koukoubis T, Hantes K, et al (Univ of Ioannina, Greece)
Acta Orthop Scand 68:33–37, 1997   8–12

Background.—Congenital hip disease (CDH) is associated with insufficient acetabulum for good bone coverage of the cup. Thus, most surgeons believe that bone graft supplementation is needed when performing arthroplasties in such patients. However, there continue to be some doubts about bulky cortical cancellous bone grafts, especially their long-term behavior. The long-term behavior of 3 types of bone grafts was examined.

Methods.—Two groups of patients with CDH were studied. Thirty-three patients, with a mean age of 54, underwent arthroplasty with a threaded ceramic conical acetabular cup without cement (group 1). Another 85 patients, with a mean age of 55, underwent arthroplasty with a threaded, noncemented, titanium cup (group 2). Bone grafts were used to supplement these procedures in 3 ways: intrapelvic application using the cotyloplasty method, as bone chips to cover small defects around the upper and lateral part of the cup, and as a bulky corticocancellous graft secured with screws. The mean follow-ups for groups 1 and 2 were 11 and 9 years, respectively.

Findings.—All grafts in group 1 consolidated within 6 months. Only 2 partial absorptions occurred: 1 intrapelvic graft and 1 corticocancellous graft. Two revisions were performed in these patients; the revisions were unrelated to bone graft resorption. In group 2, 63 of the 85 patients had consolidated bone grafts by the end of 6 months. Three of 16 patients with intrapelvic cotyloplasty had complete graft absortion, and 1 had a partial graft absorption. Three cup revisions were done in the patients with complete graft absorption.

Conclusion.—Autologous bone grafts provide satisfactory fixation of total hip arthroplasty in patients with CDH. The ceramic threaded cup was better than the titanium threaded cup in bone graft consolidation and the number of revisions needed.

▶ The value of this work is in the large number of patients followed for a long period. The data are stratified according to 2 acetabular designs and 3 bone grafting techniques. Unfortunately, the presentation of the data makes the 2 central questions for most orthopedic surgeons somewhat difficult to answer, that is, the long-term results of the autologous bulk grafting technique and issues relative to wear. What information is provided suggests that the ceramic screw-in cup was associated with a better clinical result than the titanium screw-in cup. As such, this information adds relatively little value for the North American surgeon as neither is frequently used. Nonetheless, the issue of wear debris as a confounding variable associated with graft resorption is worthy of consideration.

B.F. Morrey, M.D.

2- to 10-Year Follow-up Study of Acetabular Revisions Using Allograft Bone to Repair Bone Defects

Avci S, Connors N, Petty W (Univ of Florida, Gainesville)
J Arthroplasty 13:61–69, 1998   8–13

Objective.—High failure rates have been reported with revised acetabular components. Some studies have reported good long-term success with particulate allografts with large-diameter prosthetic cups for correction of bone deficiencies with at least 30% to 50% host-cup contact. The long-term results of complex acetabular revisions with at least 50% contact between the allograft bone and prosthetic cup were reported.

Methods.—The series included 47 hips undergoing revision total hip arthroplasty with massive allograft reconstructions of the acetabulum during an 8-year period. In most hips, aseptic loosening of a cemented cup was the reason for revision. All hips had a graft-cup contact area of at least 50%. All hips were managed with placement of various types of prosthetic cups and bone allografting. Thirty-four hips had particulate allografts, 1

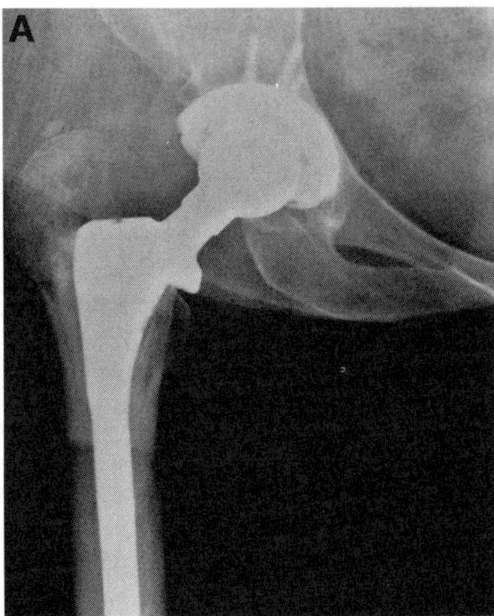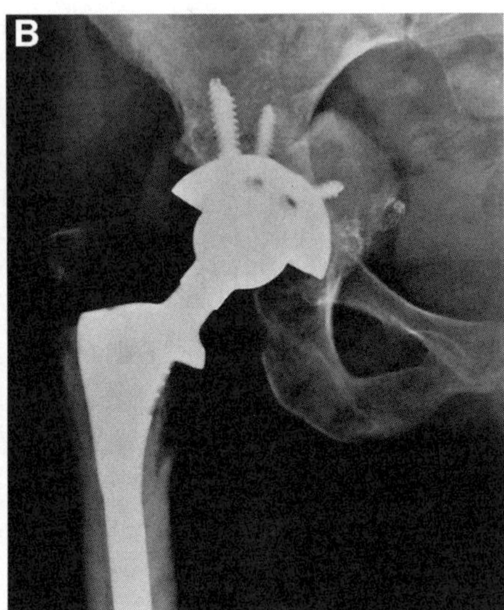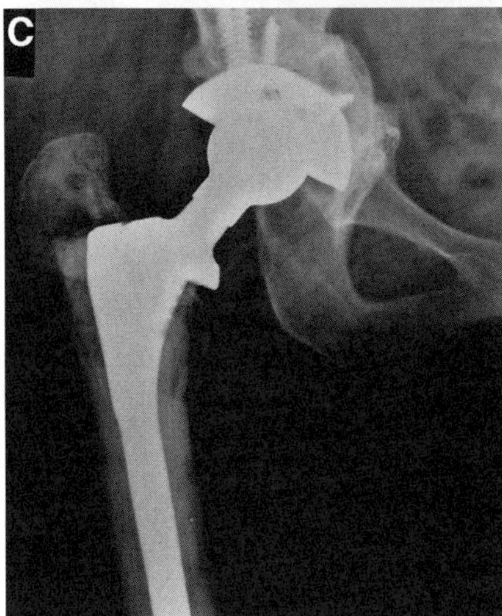

FIGURE 3.—Preoperative, postoperative, and follow-up radiographs of the hip of a 58-year-old woman with recurrent dislocations. **A,** preoperative radiograph shows the medial deficient bone. **B,** immediate postoperative radiograph shows reconstitution with a mushroom structural allograft and particulate allograft. **C,** radiograph taken at 5-year follow-up examination indicates that the cup is stable and bone graft is incorporated. Note the remodeling of the medial portion of the allograft. (Courtesy of Avci S, Connors N, Petty W: 2- to 10-year follow-up study of acetabular revisions using allograft bone to repair bone defects. *J Arthroplasty* 13:61–69, 1998.)

had a structural allograft, and 16 had both types of allografts. The hips were followed up clinically and radiographically for a mean of 5 years.

Results.—The results were graded as excellent in 37% of hips, good in 26%, fair in 17%, and poor in 19%. The mean overall Harris hip score was 82.5. Three hips showed migration of the prosthetic cups; however, 2 of these stabilized within 1 year (Fig 3). Complete radiolucent lines, without migration, were noted in 2 cups. This finding was unrelated to the location of the allografts.

Conclusions.—Good results were reported with complex acetabular revisions with at least 50% contact between the allograft bone and prosthetic cup. This procedure is effective in restoring the center of rotation of the hip and, if the allograft is supported, in providing bone stock for immediate and long-term stability. It is unclear whether there is bone ingrowth from the allograft into porous surfaces.

▶ Conflicting reports are beginning to appear regarding the effectiveness of allograft reconstruction of acetabular defects. One reason for the disparity is the numerous variables that must be considered. The most significant of these is the issue of whether a structural or cancellous type of grafting technique is required. Furthermore, the type of implant used in conjunction with the grafting technique is also an important variable with regard to the long-term success of the reconstruction. That 3 different cups were used during the study period makes interpretation of the findings somewhat more difficult because this results in a stratification of relatively small numbers with different types of grafts as being an additional variable. A total of only 17 structural allografts were used, making the interpretation that massive allograft reconstruction can provide long-term stability and restore bone stock somewhat questionable, given that more than a third of these patients had outcomes rated as fair or poor. Nonetheless this does provide additional data that, at least in some instances, both particulate and structural allografts can be effective in restoring osseous integrity, as well as in providing substrate on which a stable acetabular reconstruction can be performed.

B.F. Morrey, M.D.

Replacement of Deficient Acetabulum Using Burch-Schneider Cages: 22 Patients Followed for 2–10 Years
Symeonides P, Petsatodes G, Pournaros J, et al (Univ of Thessaloniki, Greece)
Acta Orthop Scand 68:30–32, 1997   8–14

Background.—A major problem in revision hip arthroplasty and primary arthroplasty for congenital dislocation of the hip (CDH) is the absence of good bone stock with massive acetabular deficiency. Replacement of deficient acetabulum using Burch-Schneider antiprotrusio cages was reported.

Methods.—Twenty-two patients with 24 affected hips were treated. The patients, aged a mean of 58 years, had substantial bone loss. Twenty-one revisions and 3 primary replacements were performed. Surgery involved preparing the acetabulum, filling the defect with bone autografts, and placing the cage with its flanges. Fixation was then performed with screws on the lateral wall only, and placement of a cement and plastic cup.

Outcomes.—Only 1 patient had radiographic loosening with screw breakage. After 2–10 years of follow-up (mean, 8 years), stability was found to be good in all patients. There were no mechanical failures.

Conclusion.—The use of Burch-Schneider antiprotrusio cages in this series of patients with CDH yielded satisfactory outcomes in almost all.

Antiprotrusio cages can be combined with pelvic grafting or allografts. In this study, pelvic bone autografts were used successfully.

▶ This is a worthwhile addition to the literature because the American Academy of Orthopaedic Surgeons–Classification of Acetabular Deficiency is used, allowing comparison with other, more contemporary reports. The mean follow-up of 8 years is also of value as is the relatively large sample of 22 patients all treated with a single device. The indications for the use of this or other acetabular cages is referable to acetabular deficiencies similar to those of other reports in the literature. The success rate of over 90% is consistent with experience with this device at our institution as well as other reports. This experience indicates that the effectiveness of this particular design is reproducible by a spectrum of surgeons in various orthopedic practices.

B.F. Morrey, M.D.

Complications

The Effect of Active Movement of the Foot on Venous Blood Flow After Total Hip Replacement

McNally MA, Cooke EA, Mollan RAB (Univ of Oxford, England; Musgrave Park Hosp, Belfast, Northern Ireland)
J Bone Joint Surg Am 79-A:1198–1201, 1997   8–15

Introduction.—The use of mechanical devices for prophylaxis against deep-vein thrombosis has been shown to be effective in patients undergoing hip surgery. There are no known reports on the effects of active exercise on the venous system in the orthopedic literature. The hemodynamic effects of active movements of the ankle and foot on the venous system during the early postoperative period after surgery for hip replacement was evaluated in 38 patients.

Methods.—Twenty patients were randomized to an exercise group, and 18 were randomized to a nonexercise control group. The actual venous flow was determined at baseline by using venous occlusion strain-gauge plethysmography. A controlled protocol was used for the exercise group that consisted of maximum active plantar flexion and dorsiflexion of the ankle, foot, and toes at a rate of 30 cycles per minute for 1 minute. Controls rested for 1 minute. Venous outflow was measured again for all participants at 2, 7, 12, and 30 minutes.

Results.—Venous outflow in the control group remained close to baseline values throughout all tests. An increase in venous outflow was detectable 2 minutes after exercise in the exercise group and became significantly greater than baseline at 7 minutes ($P < 0.04$). There was a greater increase in outflow at 12 minutes ($P < 0.002$). This level returned close to baseline by 30 minutes ($P < 0.2$) after exercise. Movement of the foot produced a mean maximum venous outflow in patients who exercised that was 22% greater than the baseline value. In 4 patients, this rate was 50%, and there was a significantly greater value at 30 minutes compared with controls.

Conclusion.—Findings confirm the beneficial hemodynamic effects of active movement of the foot during the postoperative period in patients undergoing major orthopedic surgery of the lower limbs.

Clinical Significance.—Patients should continue to be instructed to move their feet and toes regularly as part of a prophylactic regimen after undergoing hip operations.

▶ Realizing that simple active ankle motion can significantly alter the local circulation of the extremity is a very important observation. It helps not only to offer this simple exercise to the postoperative patient but it helps to explain and justify the more controlled sequential compressive devices, specifically providing some basis for using the below-knee variety of these devices.

B.F. Morrey, M.D.

Update on Nerve Palsy Associated With Total Hip Replacement
Schmalzried TP, Noordin S, Amstutz HC (Orthopaedic Hosp, Los Angeles; Harbor-Univ of California at Los Angeles Med Ctr, Torrance)
Clin Orthop 344:188–206, 1997   8–16

Introduction.—Close intraoperative attention to the sciatic nerve (Fig 1) has reduced the incidence of nerve palsy after total hip replacement. However, this complication can still occur. A comprehensive review of the previous literature on nerve palsy associated with total hip replacement was done.

Findings.—The English-language literature on nerve palsy associated with total hip replacement was reviewed. The findings were based on 32 studies including a total of 34,335 hip replacements. The overall prevalence of this complication was approximately 1%. About 80% of the palsies involved the sciatic nerve or its peroneal division. Women were at higher risk than men, as were patients with developmental dysplasia and those undergoing revision surgery. The origin of the palsy was unknown in most cases; unrecognized compression may have been involved. The degree of nerve damage determined the chances for neurologic recovery. About 41% of patients had complete or near-complete recovery, whereas 44% were left with only a mild deficit. The outcome was poor for the remaining 15% of patients, with weakness that interfered with walking ability, persistent dysesthesia or both. The chances for recovery were good for patients who had some motor function in the immediate postoperative period and for those who had some return of motor function within 2 weeks postoperatively. Femoral nerve palsies showed more consistent recovery than sciatic nerve palsies.

Conclusions.—Review of the literature on nerve palsy as a complication of total hip replacement indicates that these palsies most often affect the sciatic nerve, though the cause is generally unknown. Risk factors include female sex, developmental dysplasia, and revision surgery. The medical

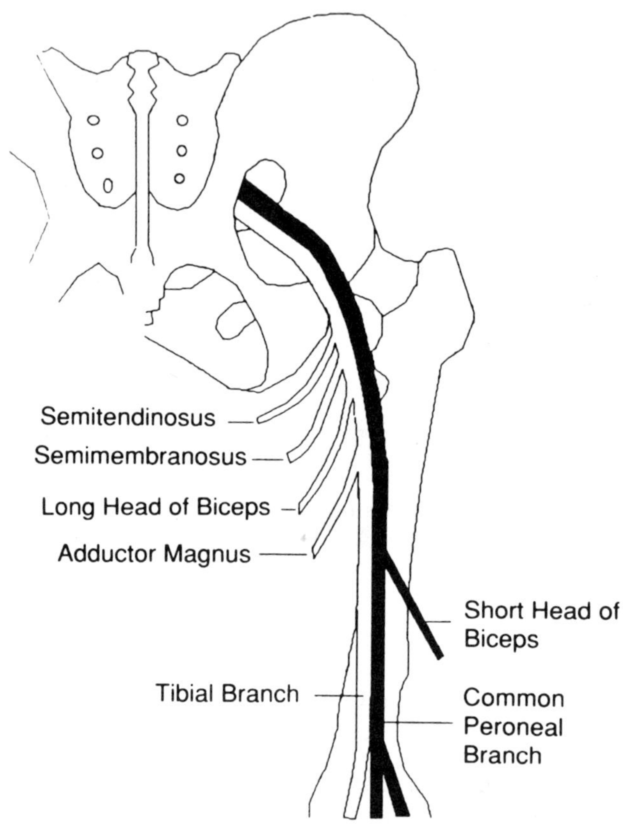

FIGURE 1.—Diagram of the sciatic nerve and serial order of muscle innervations. Note that innervation to the short head of the biceps is derived from the peroneal division. (From Schmalzried TP, Noordin S, Amstutz HC: Update on nerve palsy associated with total hip replacement. *Clin Orthop* 344:188–206, 1997. Courtesy of Nuwer MR, Schmalzried TP: Nerve palsy: Etiology, prognosis, and prevention, in Amstutz HC (ed): *Hip Arthroplasty.* New York, Churchill Livingstone, 1991, pp 415–427.)

record should include a notation that the patient was informed about the possibility of complications, and that care was taken during the procedure to avoid injury to the sciatic and other major nerves.

▶ This is an excellent contribution to the literature, not so much because it provides new information but because it reviews a large clinical experience as well as providing a significant review of the literature, allowing the clinician to have a better appreciation of the incidence and expectation of nerve injuries associated with hip replacement. The 1% prevalence is worth keeping in mind, particularly when discussing risks and benefits with the patient before surgery. Should a nerve injury ensue, the awareness that 40% to 45% will spontaneously and completely recover and another 40% to 45% will have only a mild deficit, leaves only 10% to 15% with a poor outcome of this event. It is also worth emphasizing that the recovery period is prolonged, and that it may well exceed a year. Finally, that the femoral nerve palsy is less frequent but typically more likely to completely recover is worth noting. The vulnerability of the peroneal portion of the sciatic nerve during retraction for hip replacement is again noted, helping to explain the high incidence of peroneal type of deficiency as the presentation for sciatic nerve injury.

B.F. Morrey, M.D.

Randomized Trial Comparing Early Postoperative Irradiation vs. the Use of Nonsteroidal Antiinflammatory Drugs for Prevention of Heterotopic Ossification Following Prosthetic Total Hip Replacement

Kölbl O, Knelles D, Barthel T, et al (Univ of Würzburg, Germany; Orthopedic Clinic König-Ludwig-Haus Würzburg, Germany)
Int J Radiat Oncol Biol Phys 39:961–966, 1997   8–17

Introduction.—The development of heterotopic ossification (HO) between the periacetabular pelvis and the proximal femur is a common complication after total hip replacement (THR). Methods reported to prevent the development of HO include postoperative irradiation and administration of nonsteroidal anti-inflammatory drugs (NSAIDs). A randomized trial was conducted to compare the efficacy of these therapies.

Methods.—Enrolled in the trial were 301 patients, 259 women and 142 men, who received THR. The median age of the group was 67 years; 23.1% were considered at high risk for the development of HO. Patients were randomized to postoperative irradiation (95 patients to a single 7-Gy fraction and 93 to a single 5-Gy fraction within 4 days after surgery) or to NSAIDs (113 patients to indomethacin, 2 × 50 mg/day for 1 week). An historical control group included 100 patients with THR who received no prophylactic therapy against HO. Results were assessed by 4 experts who compared preoperative and postoperative hip x-ray studies obtained immediately after surgery and at 3 and 12 months.

Results.—The incidence of HO was 15.9% in the NSAID group, 30.1% in the 5-Gy group, and 11.6% in the 7-Gy group. In historical controls, the incidence of overall HO was 65%. Compared with the untreated historical control group, all treated groups had a significantly lower incidence of HO (Table 2). Although the 7-Gy and indomethacin groups did not differ significantly in the overall incidence of HO, the 7-Gy group had a significantly lower incidence of HO that can result in functional impairment (Brooker Score II and III).

Conclusion.—Functional impairment occurs in about 30% of patients in whom HO develops after THR. Both irradiation and the use of NSAIDs reduce the incidence of HO compared with no prophylactic treatment, but the most effective modality was a single 7-Gy fraction.

▶ The issue of HO remains a matter of controversy within the orthopedic community. However, a number of recent studies have suggested that radiation is one of the most effective modalities for controlling this problem.

TABLE 2.—Incidence of Heterotopic Ossification

Treatment	Number of patients	Grad 0 in %	Grad I in %	Grad II in %	Grad III in %	Grad IV in %	Grad I–IV in %
Indometacin	113	84.1	8.0	6.2	1.7	0	15.9
7 Gy	95	88.4	11.6	0	0	0	11.6
5 Gy	93	69.9	24.7	4.3	1.1	0	30.1
Historical control group	100	35.0	26.0	15.0	19.0	5.0	65.0

Note: The modified Brooker grading system is used.

(Reprinted with permission of Elsevier Science from Kölbl O, Knelles D, Barthel T, et al: Randomized trial comparing early postoperative irradiation vs. the use of nonsteroidal antiinflammatory drugs for prevention of heterotopic ossification following prosthetic total hip replacement. *Int J Radiat Oncol Biol Phys* 39:961–966. Copyright 1997, Elsevier Science.)

This particular study is worthwhile in that it provides a threshold of 7 Gy, below which radiation is less effective. The prospective nature of the study and the large number of subjects provide significant support for the establishment of the effectiveness of this threshold level.

One finding that we found particularly interesting but which was not emphasized in the abstract is that indomethacin was also statistically significantly more effective than the control treatment and was, in fact, statistically more effective than the 5-Gy dose ($P = 0.015$). This study, therefore, substantiates the well-recognized effectiveness of radiation, places the effective threshold at 7 Gy, and also reopens the issue of NSAIDs, such as indomethacin, as having some prophylactic value.

B.F. Morrey, M.D.

Avascular Necrosis

The Trapdoor Procedure Using Autogenous Cortical and Cancellous Bone Grafts for Osteonecrosis of the Femoral Head

Mont MA, Einhorn TA, Sponseller PD, et al (Good Samaritan Hosp, Baltimore, Md; Boston Univ)
J Bone Joint Surg Br 80-B:56–62, 1998   8–18

Objective.—Osteonecrosis of the femoral head can be a difficult problem to treat, with a high rate of failure of total hip arthroplasty. Many different procedures have been proposed in the attempt to avoid total hip replacement. One approach is the so-called trapdoor procedure, in which dead bone is removed and replaced by autograft bone. An experience with the trapdoor procedure for advanced osteonecrosis of the femoral head was evaluated.

Patients.—The experience included 30 hips of 23 patients with osteonecrosis of the femoral head. All patients had stage III or early stage IV disease, according to the classification of Ficat and Arlet and the combined necrotic angle. There were 16 men and 7 women, mean age 26 years; the series included only patients younger than 50 years. All were treated with the trapdoor procedure. An opening was made in the articular cartilage and subchondral bone, through which dead bone was removed and autogenous cortical and cancellous bone was placed (Fig 1). The bone grafts stimulated bone formation while supporting the femoral head subchondral bone and articular cartilage. The patients were followed up for a mean of 56 months, with the results assessed using the Harris hip scoring system.

Results.—The results were graded good or excellent in 83% of hips with stage III disease vs. 33% of hips with stage IV disease. Of 21 hips with a combined necrotic angle of 200 degrees, 86% had good or excellent clinical results. Of 9 hips with a combined angle of greater than 200 degrees, only 44% had good or excellent results. Three fourths of the hips with fair or poor results were in patients treated with corticosteroids; most of these hips had a combined necrotic angle of greater than 200 degrees

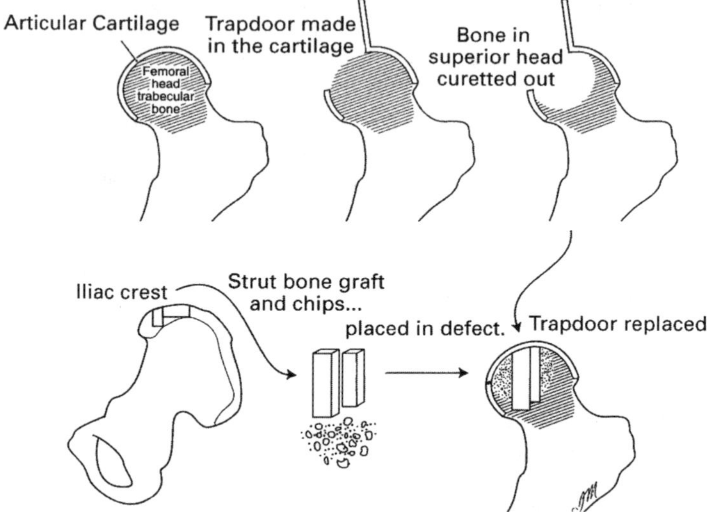

FIGURE 1.—Diagram of the trapdoor procedure. (Courtesy of Mont MA, Einhorn TA, Sponseller PD, et al: The trapdoor procedure using autogenous cortical and cancellous bone grafts for osteonecrosis of the femoral head. *J Bone Joint Surg Br* 80-B:56–62, 1998.)

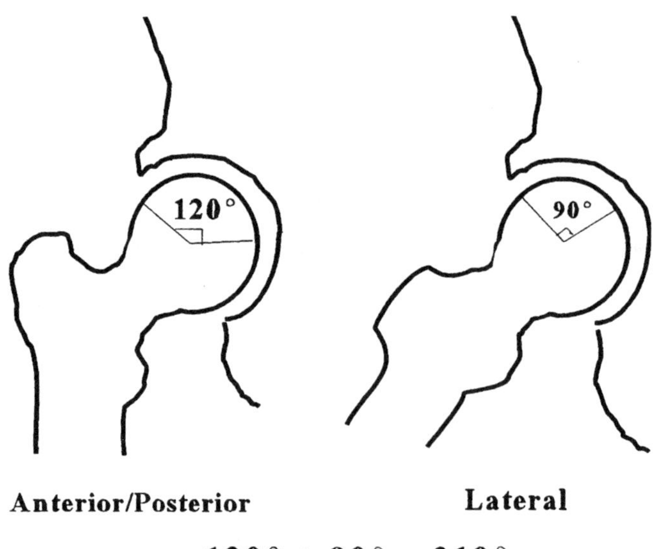

FIGURE 3.—Diagram of combined necrotic angle. (Courtesy of Mont MA, Einhorn TA, Sponseller PD, et al: The trapdoor procedure using autogenous cortical and cancellous bone grafts for osteonecrosis of the femoral head. *J Bone Joint Surg Br* 80-B:56–62, 1998.)

(Fig 3) or were in stage IV. None of the patients had intraoperative complications or fracture.

Conclusions.—The trapdoor procedure, with autogenous cortical and cancellous bone grafting, provides good results in patients with small- to medium-size stage III osteonecrosis of the femoral head. Although later reconstruction may be necessary, this procedure appears to have arrested the progress of disease. The results are not as good in patients with stage IV disease, i.e., acetabular involvement.

▶ The concept of dislocating the hip and elevating the cartilage under which the necrotic bone resides is not unique. However, this is the most extensive report of the so-called trapdoor procedure yet presented in the literature. It is certainly impressive that more than 80% of patients with type III lesions had a satisfactory result even with follow-ups averaging over 50 months with this technique. It is less surprising that only one third of the patients with type IV lesions had a satisfactory result. It is possible that the specific surgical technique is important to the success. However, the operation is difficult and this is well described in the article. It is, furthermore, somewhat difficult to know the precise role and efficacy of this procedure because a control group is not reported. However, the literature does serve as a reasonable control with the recognition that type III lesions are well known to progress to the point of requiring hip joint replacement in a relatively short period of time. Finally, the radiographic changes over time are not extensively documented, making the ability to distinguish between clinical and radiographic results somewhat difficult. Nonetheless, this is an important additional contribution, allowing the consideration of possible treatments for the more advanced avascular necrosis short of joint replacement arthroplasty.

B.F. Morrey, M.D.

Rotation Osteotomies for Osteonecrosis of the Femoral Head
Langlais F, Fourastier J (Univ Hosp Sud, Rennes, France)
Clin Orthop 343:110–123, 1997   8–19

Purpose.—For young patients with idiopathic necrosis of the femoral head, rotation osteotomies have been proposed to reduce strain on the necrotic zone. The results have been promising, though with complications related to insufficient resistance of fixation by screws. Most of these complications were eliminated by the introduction of a new technique, in which rotation and fixation were obtained with a nail plate. Thus, the results depended on the clinical conditions, including stage and volume of necrosis and type of operation. The results of 20 rotation osteotomies performed for idiopathic necrosis of the femoral head were assessed.

Experience.—The operations were performed in 19 patients, average age 35 years. Anterior extension Sugioka osteotomy was performed in 16 hips, with an average rotation of 52 degrees; the other 4 hips were treated with posterior flexion Kempf osteotomy, with an average rotation of 77 degrees. All operations were done using a nail plate for rotation and fixation of fragments, providing precise rotation and osteotomy fusion, without mechanical or vascular complications. Eighteen patients were followed up for at least 5 years. Evaluation included radiographic measurement of the relative positions of the necrosis and of the major weight-bearing zone of the acetabulum. The results were judged satisfactory in 9 cases, fair in 2, and failed in 7.

Discussion.—For properly selected young patients with idiopathic osteonecrosis, rotation osteotomy of the proximal femur can successfully delay joint deterioration. Sugioka's anterior rotation should be used only in Ficat stage 2 nonflattened hips, because the necrotic zone is usually in contact with the acetabular major bearing zone while the hip is in flexion. Kempf's posterior rotation can be performed in stage 3 hips, because the necrotic zone is unloaded with the hip in extension and flexion. Hips with necrosis extending beyond the proximal one third of the femoral head should not be treated by osteotomy, as overloading of the healthy part of the femoral head could produce mechanical deterioration.

▶ Because there remains no universally accepted or reliable treatment for avascular necrosis, any contribution that furthers our knowledge or offers some hope for avoiding joint replacement is attractive to the orthopedic community. In this context, these authors discuss and introduce posterior rotational osteotomy as potentially effective in presenting more normal cartilage by rotating the necrotic segment of the femoral head away from the weight-bearing surface. Although the procedure is eloquently documented, the relative infrequency of posterior lesions that would be amenable to such surgery makes the application relatively limited in most surgeons' practice. The authors also offer a new way of measuring the extent of involvement, which is particularly useful according to this study in determining whether or not a patient is a candidate for the rotational osteotomy. The one question one might ask is whether or not the classification can be reliably made on plain films and whether or not the use of MRIs would lessen or enhance the value of this classification scheme of percentage of head involvement.

B.F. Morrey, M.D.

9 Knee

Introduction

Topics relating to the ligament and meniscus continue to dominate literature regarding the diagnosis and management of pathology of the knee. The use of some intermediate-term follow-up data regarding meniscal-bearing knees is also contained in the recent literature, as is the management of complications following arthroplasty. Alternative management of early arthritis, including osteotomy and visco-enhancing agents, are also presented, which complements joint replacement as options for the younger patient with early arthrosis. Overall, this year's literature significantly expands our knowledge of knee pathology in addition to the management options for some of the more difficult problems.

Bernard F. Morrey, M.D.

Reconstruction/Arthritis

OUTCOMES

Health-related Quality of Life After Knee Replacement: Results of the Knee Replacement Patient Outcomes Research Team Study
Hawker G, Wright J, Coyte P, et al (Women's College Hosp, Toronto; Hosp for Sick Children, Toronto; Univ of Toronto; et al)
J Bone Joint Surg Am 80-A:163–173, 1998   9–1

Introduction.—Previous studies of knee replacement have focused on improvements in joint mechanics, postoperative complications, and revision rates. Such outcomes as pain and physical function have been neglected. These studies have also been done largely at high-volume, tertiary care centers, whereas most knee replacements are done at nonteaching hospitals. Patient-relevant outcomes of knee replacement—including pain, physical function, and long-term satisfaction—were assessed in a representative sample of patients.

Methods.—A random sample of 1,750 Medicare patients were studied. All patients were at least 65 years old and had undergone unilateral or bilateral primary or revision knee replacement between 1985 and 1989. Three separate surveys were performed in a national sample and 2 regional samples to assess the validity of the results in the national sample. The patients were stratified by race, age, urban vs. rural residence, and year of surgery. Using valid and reliable survey instruments, the researchers asked for the patients' assessments of pain, physical function, and satisfaction 2–7 years after operation.

Results.—The final analysis included 1,193 patients: 71% were women and 71% were white, and their mean age was 73 years. At follow-up, the patients reported little or no knee pain. This finding was independent of age at the time of surgery, body mass index, or time since surgery. Factors associated with better physical function, after adjustment for potential confounders, included lack of problems in the other knee, primary rather than revision knee replacement (in 1 of the regional samples), and lower body mass index (in both of the regional samples). In the national sample, the satisfaction rate was 85%.

Conclusions.—This community-based study finds that most elderly patients undergoing knee replacement have lasting pain relief, significant improvements in function, and high levels of satisfaction. Age and obesity do not appear to have a negative impact on pain and physical function. These good results should promote appropriate referrals for knee replacement surgery, thus reducing the prevalence of osteoarthrosis-related pain and disability.

▶ This analysis once again is primarily generated by the nonorthopedic community and is important because as it represents a large community-based study. The methodology is sound and clearly articulated, with representative samples stratified by age and geographic region. The dramatic improvement in the quality of life is well recognized by orthopedic surgeons performing these procedures, and these types of analyses particularly when initiated by the nonorthopedic community are very important to provide objective information when cost-benefit issues are continually being addressed and emphasized. This study, therefore, demonstrates what is obvious to the orthopedic surgeon. Hip and knee replacements dramatically improve the patient's quality of life and, therefore, are a cost-effective intervention.

B.F. Morrey, M.D.

Health-related Quality of Life After Elective Surgery: Measurement of Longitudinal Changes
Mangione CM, Goldman L, Orav EJ, et al (Brigham and Women's Hosp, Boston; Harvard Med School, Boston)
J Gen Intern Med 12:686–697, 1997 9–2

Purpose.—Recent research has included efforts to assess patients' perceptions of health-related quality of life (HRQL), in addition to traditional medical outcomes. The 36-item Short Form Health Survey (SF-36) is a practical, valid, and reliable measure supported by population-based data. This instrument was used to assess changes in HRQL in patients undergoing certain elective surgical procedures, including total hip arthroplasty (THA).

Methods.—The prospective cohort study included 528 patients hospitalized for THA, thoracic surgery for non–small-cell lung cancer, or repair of abdominal aortic aneurysm. Information on preoperative health status was available for 454 of these, and follow-up interviews were conducted in 390. The patients were evaluated for changes in health status at 1, 6, and 12 months postoperatively by the SF-36, the Specific Activity Scale, validated health transition questions, and a global health scale. The data were analyzed to determine the responsiveness of the SF-36 to clinical changes, and to assess changes in HRQL over time.

Results.—At the 1-month evaluations, physical function and role limitations caused by physical health problems were significantly worsened in all 3 surgical groups. However, significant gains were apparent at 6 months and sustained at 12 months. Factors positively associated with changes in SF-36 scores over time included responses to the health transition questions, changes on the Specific Activity Scale, global health rating, and clinical indicators for patients undergoing aneurysm repair. The data suggested that the SF-36 was a valid instrument that responded to changes in HRQL anticipated with surgery. At baseline, SF-36 scores for patients undergoing THA were significantly lower than scores in an age- and sex-adjusted population-based sample for 7 of 8 subscales. At 6 and 12 months, scores for the THA group were at least as good as in the population-based sample for all 8 subscales. For patients undergoing THA , the SF-36 was most responsive on scales measuring physical constructs. For the other 2 groups, the responsiveness of the SF-36 depended more on the type of surgery and the timing of follow-up.

Conclusions.—The SF-36 appears to be responsive to changes in HRQL after THA and other types of major elective surgery. Particularly for patients undergoing THA, HRQL is reduced at 1 month, but subsequently shows a persistent improvement. The results support the validity of the SF-36 as an outcome measure after elective surgery.

▶ It is increasingly important to document the objective and subjective value of surgical intervention, particularly for elective conditions. This is another one of a series of studies demonstrating the value of hip joint replacement, but in this instance comparing it with other surgical procedures. The important feature of this particular article is that it is not written primarily by the orthopedic community. In spite of this, the findings are that hip replacement was the most successful in relieving pain and improving function and in fact benefited all 8 subjective domains of the SF-36 questionnaire. The significant benefit of quality of life as documented by this article is extremely important to the orthopedic surgeon, not only as it relates to discussions with the patient, but also, sadly, relating to reimbursement issues and it goes directly to the cost-effectiveness question.

B.F. Morrey, M.D.

TOTAL KNEE ARTHROPLASTY

St Georg Sledge for Medial Compartment Knee Replacement: 461 Arthroplasties Followed for 4 (1–17) Years

Ansari S, Newman JH, Ackroyd CE (Baylor Univ, Dallas; Avon Orthopaedic Ctr, Bristol, England)
Acta Orthop Scand 68:430–434, 1997   9–3

Background.—Various survival outcomes for total knee replacements have been reported. Revision is the most commonly used indicator of failure. Pain has rarely been used in the criteria of failure in survival assessment. Long-term survival after medial compartment knee replacements was determined using revision and the presence of moderate-to-severe pain, or revision as 2 end-point criteria for failure.

Methods and Findings.—Data on 461 medial compartment knee arthroplasties were analyzed. Objective scores indicated a good or excellent result in 92%. Mean range of motion was 112 degrees. Twenty arthroplasties were revised or recommended for revision at an average of 5.5 years. The incidence of failure from arthrosis progression in the unreplaced compartment was less than 2%. Loosening or wear occurred in 1.5% of the patients. Two of these 6 patients had implant fracture. When revision alone was used as the end point for failure, the 10-year survival rate was 87%. Using pain or revision as the end point, the survival rate was 74% at 10 years.

Conclusions.—This survival analysis included moderate-to-severe pain as an end point for determining the success of unicompartmental knee arthroplasty. This procedure provides long-term pain relief in elderly patients with medial compartment arthrosis.

▶ This is one of the largest clinical experiences reporting a long-term practice of unicompartmental replacement. The information in this article attempts to substantiate the generally recognized indication that unicompartmental replacement is best reserved for the older rather than younger individual. The functional and clinical results also are quite good in this as in other series. However, as with previous reports of other designs, the failure rate of the unicompartmental remains higher than the preponderance of reports for condylar-type knees. Thus we continue to be left with the option of providing an excellent result in a discreet patient population but with known higher likelihood of reoperation, generally because of loosening.

B.F. Morrey, M.D.

Reduction of Polyethylene in a Congruent Meniscal Knee Prosthesis: Experimental and Clinical Studies
Tsakonas AC, Polyzoides AJ (Hippokratio Gen Hosp, Thessaloniki, Greece; Sollihul Hosp, Birmingham, England)
Acta Orthop Scand 68:127S-131S, 1997   9–4

Background.—The longevity of knee prostheses is governed by infection and mechanical failure. Wear has become a major concern in new prosthetic designs. Polyethylene wear was evaluated in the Rotaglide congruent meniscal bearing total knee prosthesis and a partial congruent total knee prosthesis with fixed bearing polyethylene tibial platform and a posterior stabilizer mechanism.

Methods and Findings.—The 2 prostheses were tested using a special wear test rig under a compression load of about 4 times the mean body weight and continuous 0- to 70-degree flexion-extension motion at a rate of 1 cycle per second. There was a lack of measurable wear on the Rotaglide mensical bearing up to 3.5 million cycles, whereas the other prosthesis started to show wear from the first million cycles, progressing to 0.38 mm at about 3.5 million cycles. At 11 million cycles, equivalent to about 20 years of wear, penetration wear of 0.35 mm was noted in the Rotaglide, compared with 2.1 mm in the other prosthesis. Seven meniscal bearings retrieved at postmortem or reoperation showed no measurable penetration wear after 3 years of placement. Only 1 prosthesis, obtained 5 years after implantation, demonstrated 0.23 mm penetration wear or about 0.05 mm per year.

Conclusions.—Although component wear in total knee replacement is unavoidable, the optimization of the prosthesis design should attempt to maximize the contact area while minimizing the yield region of the post. The current data suggest that congruency provides these qualities.

▶ This study offers additional and emerging information about the wear characteristics of the mobile bearing knee. Overall the results are consistent with both clinical statements as well as simulated wear studies done in the past. The combination of a congruent articular joint and a polished platform seems to offer substantive and significant theoretical advantages that are certainly worthy of consideration. The retrieval data as mentioned in this paper, however, offer too few examples with too short of follow-up to really substantiate the hypothesis. Finally, the methodology of simulated wear continues to emerge, and there remains uncertainty as to the accuracy of such measurement methodology.

B.F. Morrey, M.D.

Blood Loss in Sequential Bilateral Total Knee Arthroplasty

Bould M, Freeman BJC, Pullyblank A, et al (Southmead Hosp, Bristol, England)
J Arthroplasty 13:77–79, 1998   9–5

Objective.—Many patients with bilateral osteoarthritis of the knees require 2 total knee replacements. The replacements are often done at the same operation, either simultaneously or sequentially. Some reports have indicated that blood loss is similar when the arthroplasties are done as staged vs. simultaneous procedures; however, other surgeons' experience suggests otherwise. Blood loss was compared between knees in patients undergoing sequential bilateral total knee arthroplasties (TKAs).

Methods.—Two groups of patients were studied: 28 patients undergoing sequential bilateral TKAs and 28 age- and sex-matched patients undergoing unilateral TKA. Blood drainage from each knee was measured in vacuum bottles. In a subsequent series of 13 patients undergoing bilateral sequential TKAs, clotting studies were performed.

Results.—Tourniquet times were similar in the 2 groups, but blood loss in the second knee averaged 323 mL greater than in the first knee. Blood loss in the first knee in the bilateral group was similar to that in the unilateral knee group, average 875 mL. Both groups had a mean postoperative hemoglobin drop of 2.3 g/dL, yet only the bilateral TKA group required intraoperative infusion. Mean transfusion requirement was more than twice as high in the bilateral group, 3.9 vs. 1.4 U. Clotting studies revealed that prothrombin time, activated partial thromboplastin time, and thrombin time were significantly increased after the first tourniquet was released.

Conclusions.—In patients undergoing bilateral sequential TKAs, bleeding is significantly greater from the second operated knee than from the first. Clotting factors appear to be reduced at the time of the second arthroplasty. The mechanism of this effect is unknown; surgical trauma, tourniquet application, and hypothermia may all play a role.

▶ Most surgeons would not consider there to be a different qualitative process that could account for increased blood loss after the second replacement. These authors nonetheless do show a statistically significant increase in blood loss after the second joint replacement, thus accounting for the somewhat surprisingly elevated blood loss in these patients undergoing bilateral replacement. This further accounts for the slightly higher than might be anticipated need for transfusion. This simple but informative article helps explain this clinical phenomenon.

B.F. Morrey, M.D.

Continuous Passive Motion After Primary Total Knee Arthroplasty: Does it Offer Any Benefits?
Pope RO, Corcoran S, McCaul K, et al (Royal Adelaide Hosp, Australia)
J Bone Joint Surg Br 79-B:914–917, 1997   9–6

Objective.—Postoperative management of total knee arthroplasty (TKA) with continuous passive motion (CPM) is controversial. Whether CPM plus physiotherapy soon after TKA improved fixed flexion or maximal flexion or functional score compared with physiotherapy alone was examined prospectively.

Methods.—Total knee arthroplasty was performed on 57 knees in 53 patients aged 64–75. Patients were randomly assigned to receive no CPM ($n = 19$), CPM with a range of 0–40 degrees, ($n = 18$), and CPM with a range of 0–70 degrees ($n = 20$). Continuous passive motion was performed for 48 hours, and all patients received identical physiotherapy regimes. Patients were evaluated at baseline, and at 3, 6, and 12 months postoperatively. The number of cemented and cementless TKAs were evenly distributed among the 3 groups.

Results.—At 1 year there were no significant differences between groups for mean flexion, overall range, fixed flexion deformity, or function. Complications included 1 patient in the no CPM group who required anesthesia for manipulation for poor range of motion, 2 in the 0- to 40-degree CPM group who needed revision for patellar dislocation, and 1 in the 0- to 70-degree group who died of pulmonary embolism.

Conclusions.—At 1 year after TKA, patients with CPM plus physiotherapy did not have improved range of motion when compared with patients receiving physiotherapy only.

► This is another of the emerging and controversial studies relating to CPM in the postoperative period. Although the sample sizes are very small, these investigators actually found a deleterious impact particularly as it relates to analgesia and blood loss. The fact that this was observed in the group with greater motion (0–70 degrees) is worrisome because most surgeons who use CPM prefer the largest and most aggressive arc of motion in the earliest postoperative period. This would favor the development of these untoward events. It is unlikely that this specific study will alter physicians' clinical practice because most either have preconceived ideas or have a sense of what works for them clinically. However, efforts to objectively look at our clinical practice are valuable, and these findings must be placed in this context.

B.F. Morrey, M.D.

The Use of Cold Compression Dressings After Total Knee Replacement: A Randomized Controlled Trial

Webb JM, Williams D, Ivory JP, et al (Nuffield Orthopaedic Centre, Oxford, England; Princess Margaret Hosp, Swindon, England)
Orthopedics 21:59–61, 1998

9–7

Purpose.—In the early postoperative period after total knee replacement (TKR), patients have pain, swelling, and blood loss, which may be reduced by cold and compression. However, recent studies of cold compression after TKR have yielded conflicting results. In a prospective, controlled trial, the efficacy of cold compressive dressings in the postoperative period after TKR was examined.

Methods.—The study included 40 patients undergoing TKR. One group was randomized to receive cold compression in the postoperative period, achieved with application of an Aircast Cryo/Cuff. The control group received a wool and crepe dressing. The 2 groups were compared for total suction drainage, analgesic requirements, pain scores, range of motion of the knee, and swelling.

Results.—Total blood loss suction drainage was significantly reduced in the cold compression group, 768 vs. 982 mL. Patients in the cold compression group were also less likely to require postoperative blood transfusion. Mean opiate requirement was 0.57 mg/kg per 48 hours in the cold compression group vs. 0.71 mg/kg per 48 hours in the control group. Early range of motion and swelling were similar between groups.

Conclusions.—In patients undergoing TKR, cold compression in the early postoperative period can help to reduce blood loss and pain, compared with conventional compressive dressings. Cold compression has no effect on swelling or return of motion. To maximize the benefits of cold compression, the Cryo/Cuff should be refilled every hour.

▶ Any prospective study helping to document the utility of standard and generally accepted practice is of value. This study is a prospective one, although the sample size is relatively small. Nonetheless, the experimental design was effective in demonstrating that cold compressive dressings of the Cryo/Cuff variety were statistically effective in decreasing pain as well as blood loss. The authors were not, however, able to demonstrate a lessening in the hemarthrosis as measured by the knee circumference nor was the intermediate or late or long-term range of motion significantly altered by the cold compressive dressing. The surgeon, therefore, is free to determine whether or not a modality that does decrease pain and blood loss is of value in the routine practice. In our instance, we do use this precise product for elbow surgery but do not use it routinely for the knee.

B.F. Morrey, M.D.

COMPLICATIONS AND RELATED ISSUES

Results of 2-Stage Reimplantation for Infected Total Knee Arthroplasty

Hirakawa K, Stulberg BN, Wilde AH, et al (Cleveland Clinic Found, Ohio)
J Arthroplasty 13:22–28, 1998
9–8

Objective.—Several different types of treatment of infection after total knee arthroplasty (TKA) have been reported, but the optimal approach remains unknown. Each option, including antibiotic suppression, alone or combined with aggressive débridement, or 1-stage revision, has advantages and disadvantages. The results of a series of patients managed with 2-stage reimplantation for infected TKA were evaluated.

Methods.—The 13-year experience included 66 infected TKAs in 64 patients treated with 2-stage reimplantation of the TKA. At the first stage, the knee was débrided, the prosthesis was removed, and a spacer with antibiotics was placed. The patient also received systemic antibiotics, based on infectious disease consultation. When cultures of knee aspiration were negative, an average of 6 weeks later, a new prosthesis was implanted. The follow-up results were evaluated using the Hospital for Special Surgery knee score. Data were available on 55 knees of 54 patients with an average follow-up of 62 months.

Results.—The initial diagnosis in 41 knees was osteoarthritis originally, and in 14, it was rheumatoid arthritis. There were 29 women and 25 men, with an average age of 67 years. There were 14 recurrent deep infections, most developing within 24 months after reimplantation. The success rate of reimplantation was 80% in knees with such low-virulence infections as coagulase-negative *Staphylococcus* or *Streptococcus*; 71% for those with

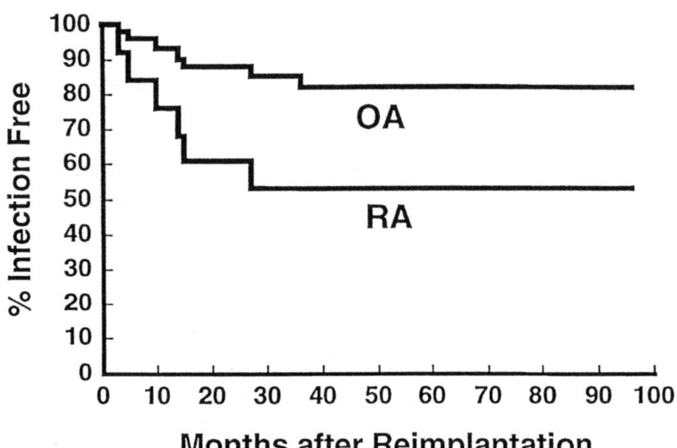

FIGURE 2.—Infection-free analysis comparing initial diagnoses of osteoarthritis (OA) and rheumatoid arthritis (RA). Kaplan-Meier analysis with log-rank test shows patients with OA had a higher infection-free rate of success ($P = 0.02$). (Courtesy of Hirakawa K, Stulberg BN, Wilde AH, et al: Results of 2-stage reimplantation for infected total knee arthroplasty. *J Arthroplasty* 13:22–28, 1998.)

polymicrobial infections; and 67% for those with high-virulence infections, such as methicillin-resistant *Staphylococcus aureus*. The success rate was 82% in patients with an initial diagnosis of osteoarthritis vs. 54% in those with rheumatoid arthritis (Fig 2). Two-stage reimplantation was successful in 92% of patients infected after primary arthroplasty, vs. 41% for those with multiple previous knee surgeries.

Conclusions.—In most knees with infected TKAs, 2-stage reimplantation with appropriate antibiotics is an effective treatment strategy. However, the success rate is lower for infections with highly virulent or multiple organisms, in patients with rheumatoid arthritis, and in patients with multiple previous knee operations. With these caveats, the protocol for 2-stage reimplantation presented provides predictable success in patients with infected TKAs.

▶ This article provides yet another input to the growing body of evidence that clearly demonstrates the enhanced value of infection-free replacement by using a 2-staged strategy. The article reviews the technique in detail and stratifies the various confounding variables such as type and virulence of organism, underlying diagnosis, duration of interval before reimplantation, and the like. There is merit in recognizing that the expectations of patients with rheumatoid arthritis are significantly lower than those with osteoarthritis. It is also of interest to note that these authors report almost the identical success rate that was reported by Hanssen et al. from our institution.[1]

B.F. Morrey, M.D.

Reference

1. Hanssen AD, Rand JA, Osmon DR: Treatment of the infected total knee arthroplasty with insertion of another prosthesis: The effect of antibiotic impregnated bone cement. *Clin Orthop* 309:44, 1994.

Shelf Life and In Vivo Duration: Impacts on Performance of Tibial Bearings
Currier BH, Currier JH, Collier JP; et al (Dartmouth College, Hanover, NH; Dartmouth Hitchcock Med Ctr, Lebanon, NH; Brigham and Women's and New England Baptist Hosps, Boston)
Clin Orthop 342:111–122, 1997   9–9

Background.—Polyethylene has long been used as a bearing material in orthopedic implants. Recent studies have looked at the early failure that occurs with some of these bearings, which is sometimes related to gamma radiation sterilization in an air environment. However, not all gamma-sterilized bearings show the characteristics that lead to early component failure. The effects of shelf life and in vivo duration on the performance of tibial bearings were analyzed.

Methods.—A database of retrieved tibial components was searched to identify 2 groups of polyethylene components: those that failed prema-

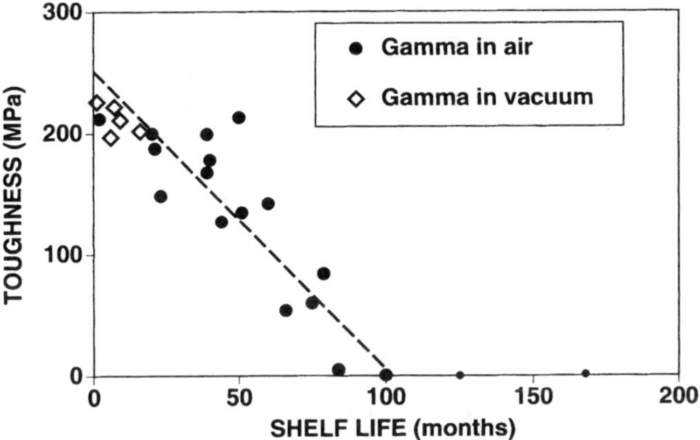

FIGURE 3.—Mechanical toughness (representing a combination of mechanical strength and ductility of the polyethylene) vs. length of time on the shelf after gamma sterilization in air for never-implanted tibial bearings. Bearings have less than the minimum toughness required for implantable polyethylene after 5 years on the shelf. (Courtesy of Currier BH, Currier JH, Collier JP, et al: Shelf life and in vivo duration: Impacts on performance of tibial bearings. *Clin Orthop* 342:111–122, 1997.)

turely and those that were long-term successes. A total of 17 bearings from 8 manufacturers, with an in vivo duration of 1–134 months, were evaluated for damage. Twenty-seven never-implanted bearings with shelf lives of 2–84 months were also studied to determine the shelf oxidization rate. This information permitted estimates of in vivo oxidization for retrieved bearings on known sterilization.

Findings.—The results showed often dramatically different outcomes in pairs of retrieved bearings from the same manufacturer, for the same time, same material and design, same sterilization technique, and similar patient variables. The never-used bearings showed evidence of oxidization over

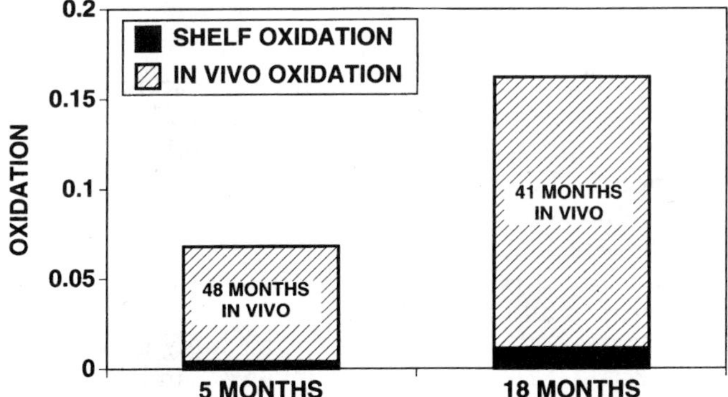

FIGURE 9.—Estimated shelf and in vivo oxidation for retrieved tibial bearings of the same design, same manufacturer, and similar duration in vivo. Bearing with a shelf life of 5 months before implantation shows oxidation lower in vivo. Bearing with a shelf life of 18 months before implantation shows much higher in vivo oxidation after shorter duration. (Courtesy of Currier BH, Currier JH, Collier JP, et al: Shelf life and in vivo duration: Impacts on performance of tibial bearings. *Clin Orthop* 342:111–122, 1997.)

time. Oxidization occurred slowly for the first 5 years of shelf life, but increased by an order of magnitude thereafter. Along with oxidation occurred a decrease in toughness, i.e., strength and elongation of the polyethylene (Fig 3). Analysis of retrieved bearings suggested that those stored for less than 1 year after gamma sterilization had lower in vivo oxidation and better in vivo performance than those stored for longer times (Fig 9).

Conclusions.—In polyethylene tibial bearings gamma-sterilized in air, preimplantation storage time appears to have a major impact on in vivo performance. Bearings with a shelf life of longer than 1 year may be prone to accelerated oxidation in vivo. This causes accelerated loss of mechanical toughness, thus leading to polyethylene failure.

▶ This is an extremely important contribution as it provides yet additional and carefully studied information regarding gamma sterilization in the air and the adverse effect on the material property of the tibial implant. The figures included in the abstract show dramatically the toughness decreasing as does the shelf life when gamma radiation is performed in the air compared to a vacuum. Possibly even more dramatic is the estimated shelf and in vivo oxidation in the retrieved specimens demonstrating that those patients whose implants have longer shelf life also have a more pronounced in vivo oxidation response. The take-home message is clear: inventory should be purged periodically to avoid this phenomenon.

B.F. Morrey, M.D.

Sports

ARTHROSCOPY

A Prospective Study of the Accuracy of Clinical Examination Evaluated by Athroscopy of the Knee
Yoon Y-S, Rah J-H, Park H-J (Yonsei Univ, Wonju, Korea)
Int Orthop 21:223–227, 1997   9–10

Introduction.—The accuracy of clinical examination for the diagnosis of intra-articular injuries of the knee was evaluated by arthroscopy.

Study Design.—During 1994, a prospective study was carried out on 200 injured knees in 122 men and 73 women. Of these 200 injuries, 65 were acute and 135 were chronic. Every patient had a history, physical examination and standard radiographs. In 50 knees, MRI was performed. Each patient was evaluated to determine whether the preoperative clinical diagnosis was correct and complete.

Findings.—Of the 200 injured knees in the study group, clinical diagnosis was correct in 52%, incomplete in 35%, and incorrect in 13%. When there was only 1 lesion, the clinical diagnosis was correct in 70%, but accuracy decreased as the number of lesions increased. For medial meniscal tears, the sensitivity of clinical examination was 87%, specificity was 93%, and the overall accuracy was 90%. For anterior cruciate liga-

TABLE 2.—Sensitivity, Specificity, and Accuracy of the Clinical Knee Examination for Intra-articular Lesions

Type of Lesion	Preoperative diagnosis				Sensi-tivity (%)	Speci-ficity (%)	Accu-racy (%)
	Lesion present		Lesion absent				
	ARTH + (T+)	ARTH − (F+)	ARTH + (F−)	ARTH − (T−)			
Medial meniscal tear	84	7	13	96	87	93	90
Lateral meniscal tear	47	10	11	132	81	93	90
ACL tear	38	4	12	146	76	97	92
Degenerative joint disease	46	0	3	151	94	94	99
Plica	23	2	10	165	70	99	94
Loose body	10	3	5	182	67	98	96
Chondral Fracture	5	2	32	161	14	99	83
Fat pad Fibrosis	2	1	2	195	50	99	98

Abbreviations: ARTH, arthroscopy; T+, true positive; T−, true negative; F+, false positive; F−, false negative.
(Courtesy of Yoon Y-S, Rah J-H, Park H-J: A prospective study of the accuracy of clinical examination evaluated by arthroscopy of the knee *Int Orthop* 21:223–227. Copyright 1997, Springer-Verlag.)

ment tears, the diagnostic sensitivity was 76%, specificity 97%, and accuracy 92%. There was a significant association between partial tears and difficulty of clinical diagnosis. For chondral fractures, sensitivity was 14%, specificity 99%, and accuracy 83% (Table 2). Chronic injuries were more difficult to diagnose than acute injuries. There was no correlation between diagnostic difficulty and age, sex, or additional diagnostic studies.

Conclusions.—The diagnostic accuracy of clinical examination for intra-articular injuries of the knee was assessed by arthroscopy. Clinical diagnosis was correct in 70% of single lesions, but accuracy decreased with increasing lesion number. The most difficult lesions to detect clinically were chondral fractures, loose bodies and partial tears of the anterior cruciate ligament. Chronic lesions were more difficult to diagnose than acute lesions.

▶ With the increased incidence of arthroscopy there is a concurrent decreased focus on the clinical examination. This prospective study clearly reveals the value of a clinical assessment demonstrating the accuracy in excess of 90% for intraarticular lesions. The difficulty of diagnosing chondral fractures on clinical examination is the most notable exception to the ability to accurately diagnose intraarticular knee pathology by clinical examination. Whereas this study in no way lessens the value of arthroscopy, it should be viewed as a stimulus to continue the careful assessment if for no other reason than to assure the accurate correlation of the findings of arthroscopy with the clinical features and findings at examination.

B.F. Morrey, M.D.

Arthroscopic Repair of Meniscal Tears That Extend Into the Avascular Zone: A Review of 198 Single and Complex Tears

Rubman MH, Noyes FR, Barber-Westin SD (Deaconess Hosp, Cincinnati, Ohio)

Am J Sports Med 26:87–95, 1998   9–11

Background.—It has been suggested that meniscal excision, rather than repair, is indicated for meniscal tears extending into the avascular zone, or for complex tears with multiple components in more than 1 plane. Some studies have described the repair of tears in the avascular zone, but none have included a large group of patients with exclusively avascular tears. The results of arthroscopic repair of single or complex meniscal tears involving the avascular zone were evaluated.

Methods.—A total of 177 patients, with a mean age of 28 years, who had 198 meniscal tears with a major segment in the central avascular zone were studied. The meniscal injuries occurred during sports in 82% of cases, and anterior cruciate ligament reconstruction was required in addition to meniscal repair in 71%. All tears were repaired by the arthroscopically assisted inside-out technique. The results were assessed by clinical examination (180 cases at a mean follow-up of 42 months) and/or arthroscopic evaluation (91 cases at a mean of 18 months).

Results.—At follow-up, 80% of knees were free of tibiofemoral joint symptoms, and 20% had undergone repeat arthroscopic surgery for such symptoms. In the arthroscopically evaluated cases, the repair was judged healed in 25% of cases, partially healed in 38%, and failed in 36%. Overall, 64% of injured menisci were retained.

Conclusions.—Arthroscopic repair of meniscal tears extending into the avascular zone is recommended for properly selected patients, i.e., those in their second and third decades of life, and competitive athletes. The 20% reoperation rate reflects the high incidence of tibiofemoral joint symptoms, rather than the rate of meniscal healing. Although relatively high, the risk of reoperation is justified to obtain a potentially functional meniscus.

▶ Because repair of meniscal lesions in the avascular zone is controversial, this extensive experience is of particular value. Modest mean follow-up of 42 months is sufficient to determine whether healing in this compromised anatomical region of the meniscus had taken place, at least from the perspective of the absence of retear or recurrence of symptoms. The reassessment of 91 such repairs arthroscopically further validates the conclusions. Although more than one third of these efforts failed, the recommendation that patients should undergo such repairs if they are 20 or 30 years of age and are physically active seems reasonable. The alternative is to remove this meniscus, which potentially increases the risk of degenerative changes in the future. Thus, the relatively high failure rate would seem to be justified considering the implications of the alternative surgical decision.

B.F. Morrey, M.D.

Spinal, Epidural or Propofol Anaesthesia for Out-patient Knee Arthroscopy?

Dahl V, Gierløff C, Omland E, et al (Bærum Hosp, Oslo, Norway; Ullevål Univ, Oslo, Norway)

Acta Anaesthesiol Scand 41:1341–1345, 1997   9–12

Objective.—There is no general agreement on the ideal anesthetic technique for outpatient arthroscopy of the knee. Spinal anesthesia, epidural anesthesia, and general anesthesia were compared with respect to preoperative time spent, postoperative pain experienced, costs, and side effects.

Methods.—Average and maximal pain levels, assessed on Visual Analogue Scales were determined before and after elective arthroscopy in 91 patients in American Society of Anesthesiologist's class I–II. Patients were premedicated with 10 mg of diazepam and 500 mg of naproxene orally and then given spinal anesthesia with 50 mg/mL lidocaine in 7.5% glucose (group S, $n = 32$), a lumbar epidural block with 20 mg/mL of mepivacaine and 5 µg/mL of epinephrine (group E, $n = 29$), or propofol anesthesia beginning with a bolus of 2 mg/kg IV and followed by a continuous infusion of 10 mg/kg/hr for the first 10 minutes, 8 mg/kg/hr for the next 10 minutes, and then 6 mg/kg/hr, thereafter (group P, $n = 30$). Group P were also premedicated with 0.5–1.0 mg IV alfentanil. Pain, patient satisfaction, and costs were compared.

Results.—Preparation time was significantly lower for group P than for groups S and E (7.4 vs. 23.0 vs. 31.0 minutes). Operative times varied between 33 and 37 minutes. Time from end of operation to recovery room entry was significantly longer for group P than for group S (15.0 vs. 10.0 minutes) and longer than for group E (13.0 minutes). Times from end of operation to discharge and incidences of postoperative nausea were similar between groups. Although postoperative pain levels were low, they were significantly higher in group P than in either group E or S on arrival in recovery and at 60, 120, and 180 minutes thereafter. Costs of drugs and disposables were $6.50 for group S, $22 for group E, and $30 for group P.

Conclusion.—Whereas the time for outpatient arthroscopic knee surgery using propofol is shorter than for epidural or spinal anesthesia, postoperative pain and perioperative costs are significantly higher. Spinal anesthesia is the low cost method.

▶ The relative merits, both immediate and intermediate term, of different forms of anesthesia, continue to be of interest to the orthopedic surgeon. This prospective study is of particular interest in that it demonstrates clearly that the agent that is most effective in the short-term, propofol, is, in fact, associated with a greater amount of postoperative pain and a higher cost of administration. Thus, the careful analysis negates the initial impression of it having a clear advantage over the other 2 techniques. To date, there is clearly no universally accepted method for outpatient anesthesia, but this and similar such studies do provide stepping stones to the ultimate goal.

B.F. Morrey, M.D.

ANTERIOR CRUCIATE LIGAMENT

Reconstruction of the Anterior and Posterior Cruciate Ligaments After Knee Dislocation: Use of Early Protected Postoperative Motion to Decrease Arthrofibrosis

Noyes FR, Barber-Westin SD (Cincinnati Sportsmedicine and Orthopaedic Ctr, Ohio; Deaconess Hosp, Cincinnati, Ohio)
Am J Sports Med 25:769–778, 1997   9–13

Objective.—Because most knee dislocations result in rupture of both the anterior cruciate ligament (ACL) and the posterior cruciate ligament (PCL) and can lead to partial or total impairment and even to amputation, most surgeons recommend primary repair of the ligaments and cast immobilization. Few studies have evaluated knee stability after surgery. Objective data and a critical rating of operative treatment using allogenic tissues and immediate protected knee motion for combined ACL and PCL ruptures after complete knee dislocation were presented.

Methods.—Seven male patients (group 1) underwent operative reconstruction of both ligaments for acute injuries within 14 days after injury, and 4 patients (1 woman) (group 2) were treated for chronic cruciate ligament and lateral and posterolateral complex deficiency. Group 2 patients were treated with allograft reconstructions in 3 cases and a bone-patellar tendon-bone autogenous PCL reconstruction in 1 case. All patients were given immediate knee motion exercises and had postoperative rehabilitation. Knee flexion was assessed preoperatively and at an average of 4.8 years later.

Results.—One group 1 ACL repair failed reconstruction. At follow-up at 20 degrees of flexion, 1 group 1 patient had 3 mm of difference in anteroposterior displacement testing compared with the contralateral knee. At 70 degrees of flexion, 1 group 1 patient had less than 3 mm of difference in displacement. In group 2, 2 PLC and 1 posterolateral split biceps tendon transposition failed. At follow-up, all patients had less than 3 mm of displacement at 20 degrees of flexion, and 2 had more than 6 mm of difference at 70 degrees of flexion. Five group 1 patients and 3 group 2 patients had no limitations on daily or sports activities. Five group 1 patients required additional surgery for motion limitations. In group 1, outcome was rated as excellent for 1 patients, good for 2, fair for 1, and poor for 3.

Conclusion.—Complete reconstruction and repair of the ACL and PCL ligaments and of collateral damage after knee dislocation restores satisfactory function, although some patients may require additional procedures for motion restriction problems.

▶ Fortunately, this is a relatively uncommon injury and, therefore, information regarding the optimum management of these patients is relatively limited. Thus, this sample, although small, shows that contemporary reconstruction techniques applied to the unstable knee—particularly in the acute

BUSINESS REPLY MAIL
FIRST-CLASS MAIL   PERMIT NO 135   ST LOUIS MO

POSTAGE WILL BE PAID BY ADDRESSEE

SUBSCRIPTION SERVICES
MOSBY–YEAR BOOK, INC.
11830 WESTLINE INDUSTRIAL DRIVE
ST. LOUIS   MO 63146-9988

BUSINESS REPLY MAIL
FIRST-CLASS MAIL   PERMIT NO 135   ST LOUIS MO

POSTAGE WILL BE PAID BY ADDRESSEE

 **Mosby**

PAT NEWMAN
11830 WESTLINE INDUSTRIAL DRIVE
PO BOX 46908
ST. LOUIS   MO 63146-9934

Want to speed up the process?

**To order the *Year Book*,
you also may call 1-800-426-4545**

**To subscribe to the journal today,
call toll-free in the U.S.:
1-800-453-4351
or fax 314-432-1158
Outside the U.S., call: 314-453-4351**

Visit us at:
www.mosby.com/Mosby/Periodicals

Mosby–Year Book, Inc.
Subscription Services
11830 Westline Industrial Drive
St. Louis, MO   63146 U.S.A.

Mosby

setting—offer improved overall results compared with nonsurgical treatment. Although this tenet may be well accepted, there has been concern regarding acute reconstruction and arthrofibrosis. This has been effectively addressed by early motion and arthroscopic debridement, if necessary. Thus, overall, this paper appears to provide a reasonable surgical strategy for the patient sustaining an acute knee dislocation.

B.F. Morrey, M.D.

Reconstruction of the Anterior Cruciate Ligament in Patients Who Are At Least Forty Years Old: A Long-term Follow-up and Outcome Study
Plancher KD, Steadman JR, Briggs KK, et al (Steadman Hawkins Clinic, Vail, Colo; Steadman Hawkins Sports Medicine Found, Vail, Colo; Univ of Nebraska, Omaha)
J Bone Joint Surg Am 80-A:184–197, 1998   9–14

Background.—The best treatment of a torn anterior cruciate ligament in patients older than 40 years has not been determined. Most such patients are treated nonoperatively because of concern that operative reconstruction of the anterior cruciate ligament in this population is associated with a higher rate of arthrofibrosis and a decreased arc of motion. Studies have suggested that patients who are managed nonoperatively have a high rate of reinjury after they return to preinjury activity levels and that use of a brace does not lower reinjury rates.

Methods.—The long-term results for 72 patients who had a bone-patellar ligament-bone intra-articular reconstruction of the anterior cruciate ligament in 75 knees were reviewed. The mean patient age was 45 years. A questionnaire, functional results, and objective clinical data were analyzed. The clinical examination included range-of-motion evaluation, Lachman and pivot-shift tests, and measurements with a KT-1000 arthrometer. The Lyshom and Gillquist scale, The Hospital for Special Surgery scale modified by Insall et al., and the International Knee Ligament Standard Evaluation Form were used.

Results.—The main causes of injury were skiing, tennis, and soccer. Follow-up was 26–117 months. At the last follow-up examination, 3 patients had pain or swelling. There were no reports of giving-way or symptoms related to the patellofemoral joint. The mean range of extension was −8 to 42 degrees preoperatively and −12 to 6 degrees at the last postoperative examination. The mean range of flexion was 52–154 degrees preoperatively and 112–150 degrees postoperatively. In one patient, flexion was limited to 112 degrees, but this was 5 degrees greater than in the unaffected knee. Pivot-shift test results were negative in 80% of knees, and 13% of knees had a grade of 1+. Testing with the KT-1000 arthrometer at maximum manual pressure showed that the mean difference between the injured and uninjured knees improved by 5.1 mm.

On the International Knee Ligament Standard Evaluation Form, 96% of knees had a grade of C or D preoperatively, and 93% of knees had a grade

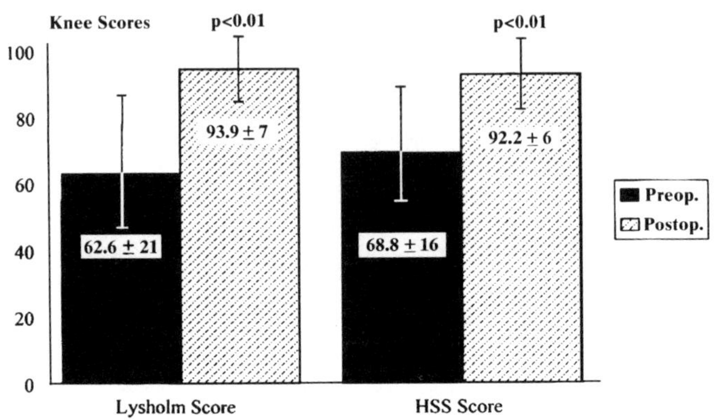

FIGURE 4.—Graph shows the results of the modified Hospital for Special Surgery (*HSS*) and Lysholm and Gillquist knee-rating scales. *I-bars* indicate 95% confidence intervals; *p* values indicate a significant difference between preoperative and postoperative scores. (Courtesy of Plancher KD, Steadman JR, Briggs KK, et al: Reconstruction of the anterior cruciate ligament in patients who are at least forty years old: A long-term follow-up and outcome study. *J Bone Joint Surg Am* 80-A:184–197, 1998.)

of A or B postoperatively. Mean scores on the Hospital for Special Surgery scale were 69 points preoperatively and 92 points postoperatively. Mean scores on the Lyshom and Gillquist scale were 63 points preoperatively and 94 points postoperatively (Fig 4). All patients were pleased with their results. Bicycling was resumed at a mean of 4 months, jogging at a mean of 9 months, skiing at a mean of 10 months, and tennis at a mean of 12 months.

Discussion.—These patients older than 40 years had a satisfactory outcome after reconstruction of the anterior cruciate ligament. The range of active and passive motion was excellent. There was no arthrofibrosis, and reinjury rates were lower than those reported in studies of younger patients treated nonoperatively. A satisfactory outcome after operative treatment is very likely when strict patient selection criteria are followed.

▶ There is relatively little information with regard to this topic because degenerative changes of the knee tend to be correlated with age, and there are relatively few individuals over the age of 40 who are considered candidates for ligament reconstruction. Nonetheless, this paper represents a large experience with just such a population.

It is important to emphasize that the outcome of this group of patients, using objective standards, is comparable with that reported for younger, more ideally suited individuals. The fact that several different surgical procedures were used reflects the time period over which these patients were treated but does serve as a noncontrollable weakness of the study.

Although an appropriate amount of analysis was given to objective and subjective functional improvement, there is very little information regarding to the status of the articular cartilage of the knee. This is, in my judgment, an important issue with regard to the selection of patients in this age group who may or may not be candidates for anterior cruciate ligament reconstruction. Although 15 knees had chondral lesions, 6 of which were rated a grade IV defect, it is difficult to determine the influence of these findings in the final follow-up.

B.F. Morrey, M.D.

Anterior Cruciate Ligament Reconstruction: Bone-Patella Tendon-Bone Versus Semitendinosus Anatomic Reconstruction
Feagin JA Jr, Wills RP, Lambert KL, et al (Duke Univ, Durham, NC)
Clin Orthop 341:69–72, 1997   9–15

Introduction.—Options for anterior cruciate ligament (ACL) reconstruction include semitendinosus anatomic reconstruction and bone-patellar tendon-bone reconstruction with interference kit fixation. However, it remains unclear which of these options gives better results, or whether either gives lasting results. A long-term follow-up study comparing these 2 approaches is presented.

Methods.—Over a 10-year period, 1 of the 2 ACL reconstructive techniques was used by 4 orthopedic surgeons in nearly 1,000 patients. Two-to 10-year follow-up data were available on 137 patients: 76 males and 52 females, average age 31 years. The semitendinosus procedure was used in 68 knees; patellar tendon autografting with interference screw fixation was used in 69 knees. The results were assessed by subjective questionnaire, KT-1000 arthrometric testing, and isokinetic dynamometric testing. Mean follow-up was nearly 5 years.

Results.—The 2 groups were similar in their subjective results and level of physical activity. Manual testing showed no significant differences. On KT-1000 testing, the manual maximum failure rate in the semitendinosus group was 17%, compared with 11% in the patellar tendon group. There was no deterioration in arthrometric stability; however, patients undergoing meniscectomies reported lower satisfaction.

Conclusions.—This analysis suggests that the semitendinosus anatomic and bone-patellar tendon-bone techniques give comparable results in ACL reconstruction. Long-term follow-up finds satisfactory results with both approaches. However, of the 2 techniques, the patellar tendon offers a somewhat stiffer construct, and is thus preferred for patients with compromise of the secondary restraints.

▶ Clinical results following intra-articular ACL reconstruction using a patellar tendon appear comparable to those following semitendinosus autograft. Reproducible anatomic positioning of the graft is the most critical component for success. The slightly higher failure rate with the semitendinosus graft by arthrometer testing suggests that the stiffer patellar tendon is a better choice for the chronic ACL-deficient knee. This recommendation is based on a small sample (137 out of 1,000 procedures) of the results of 4 different surgeons over a 10-year span. These deficiencies, along with the changes in fixation techniques and postoperative rehabilitation during the course of the study period, do not allow firm conclusions.

M.J. Stuart, M.D.

Anterior Cruciate Ligament Reconstruction With Autogenous Patellar Tendon Graft Followed by Accelerated Rehabilitation: A Two- to Nine-Year Followup
Shelbourne KD, Gray T (Thomas A Brady Clinic, Indianapolis, Ind)
Am J Sports Med 25:786–795, 1997   9–16

Background.—The authors have previously reported good short-term results of anterior cruciate ligament (ACL) reconstruction using an autogenous patellar tendon graft and accelerated rehabilitation program. They report the long-term follow-up results of this approach, including return to athletic activity.

Methods.—The 7-year experience included 1,057 patients undergoing ACL reconstruction with an autogenous bone-patellar tendon-bone graft. Surgery was followed by an accelerated rehabilitation program that focused on prevention of complications, rehabilitation of the donor site, restoration of normal motion, and return of normal knee function. The patients were permitted to return to athletic participation once certain criteria were met. Prospective follow-up was attempted in all patients. At a mean of 4 years after surgery, objective physical examination data were available on 806 patients and subjective data on 948 patients.

Results.—The patients had a mean final range of motion of 5/0/140 degrees, with a mean manual maximum KT-1000 arthrometer score of 2.0 mm. Postoperative isokinetic quadriceps muscle strength testing suggested that ACL reconstruction restored a mean of 94% strength in acute cases and 91% in chronic cases. According to International Knee Documentation Committee evaluation of acute cases, 42% of knees were normal, 47% near normal, 10% abnormal, and 1% severely abnormal. In chronic cases, 41% of knees were normal, 44% near normal, 14% abnormal, and 1% severely abnormal. Radiographs showed no joint space narrowing in 94% of acute and 89% of chronic cases. The mean score on a subjective modified Noyes questionnaire was 93 points. Mean time to return to sport-specific activity was 6 weeks, and time to return to competition at full capacity was 6 months (Fig 4).

Conclusions.—The authors' approach to ACL reconstruction—with autogenous patellar tendon grafting and accelerated rehabilitation—offers good long-term results. The reconstructed knees show full range of motion, excellent stability, and good strength, permitting the patient to return to full activity in most cases. The autogenous patellar tendon appears able to cope with demands of accelerated rehabilitation, and may be enhanced by an optimal amount of stress.

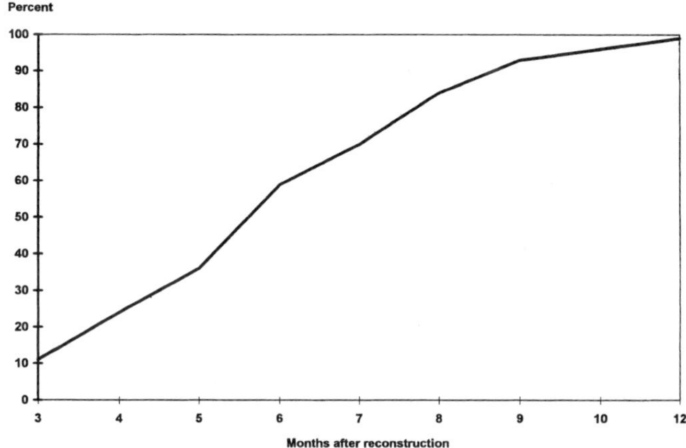

FIGURE 4.—The percentage of patients returning to athletic competition at 100% capability at different times postoperatively. (Courtesy of Shelbourne KD, Gray T: Anterior cruciate ligament reconstruction with autogenous patellar tendon graft followed by accelerated rehabilitation: A two- to nine-year followup. *Am J Sports Med* 25:786–795, 1997.)

▶ This large prospective series of patellar tendon autograft ACL reconstruction patients sheds some valuable light on the specific surgical technique and the postoperative rehabilitation protocol. All of the procedures were performed by a single surgeon using an identical graft source, tensioning technique, and method of fixation. Clear-cut goals are provided, including the importance of limiting knee swelling and restoring full terminal knee extension in the first week after surgery. Mid-term results (4 years after surgery) are promising, despite the accelerated rehabilitation program and return to full competition at approximately 6 months postoperatively.

M.J. Stuart, M.D.

ARTHRITIS

The Effects of Hyaluronan on the Meniscus and on the Articular Cartilage After Partial Meniscectomy

Sonoda M, Harwood FL, Wada Y, et al (Univ of California San Diego La Jolla; Chiba Univ, Japan)
Am J Sports Med 25:755–762, 1997   9–17

Background.—Meniscectomy—even arthroscopic partial meniscectomy—is followed by articular cartilage degeneration. After partial meniscectomy, meniscal remodeling occurs within the avascular region; however, the mechanism of this remodeling process is unclear. Hyaluronan, a component of proteoglycan aggregate with a molecular weight of 8×10^5d, inhibits articular cartilage degeneration and preserves glycosaminoglycans in the lateral meniscus after medial total meniscectomy. The meniscal and articular cartilage effects of hyaluronan after partial meniscectomy were studied in rabbits.

Methods.—Morphologic, histologic, vascular, and biochemical studies were performed after partial meniscectomy in rabbits. Some knees were injected with sodium hyaluronate for several weeks after surgery, whereas others were injected with vehicle. The animals were killed for examination after 12 weeks.

Results.—Remodeled tissue—which was translucent and looked newly synthesized—appeared in both groups of menisci. The remodeled tissue showed glycosaminoglycans on safranin O staining, although mature collagen architecture was lacking. Menisci from hyaluronan-treated knees were significantly less hydrated than those from vehicle-treated knees. The treated knees exhibited a greater degree of collagen remodeling, as evidenced by an increase in the reducible collagen cross-link dihydroxylysinonorleucine. On in situ hybridization, the hyaluronan-treated menisci showed high expression of type I procollagen messenger RNS (mRNA) but minor expression of types II and III mRNA. Expression of the type I collagen gene was also increased in the hyaluronan-treated group. Mild cartilage fibrillation was noted in the tibial plateaus after surgery, although the osteoarthritic changes were not sufficiently advanced for the difference between groups to be significant.

Conclusion.—After partial meniscectomy in rabbits, hyaluronan treatment appears to enhance collagen remodeling and reduce meniscal swelling in the avascular region. Extrinsic hyaluronan incorporated into the synovial tissues and menisci may stimulate synovial cells to upregulate synthesis of intrinsic hyaluronan, which plays key roles in cell movement and regulation of extracellular matrix aggregation and synthesis. More study is needed to establish the benefits and risks of using hyaluronan after meniscectomy.

▶ As greater clinical interest in and experience with hyaluronan emerges, enhanced value is placed on understanding the mechanism of action and the spectrum of indications for its use. Although this report concerns an animal model, it does suggest that hyaluronan enhances collagen remodeling of the menisci and, thus, serves as a possible explanation of the mechanism of effectiveness in the knee with articular degeneration as well.

B.F. Morrey, M.D.

Fresh Osteochondral Allografts for Post-Traumatic Osteochondral Defects of the Knee

Ghazavi MT, Pritzker KP, Davis AM, et al (Mount Sinai Hosp, Toronto)
J Bone Joint Surg Br 79-B:1008–1013, 1997   9–18

Introduction.—Fresh osteochondral allografts have been used successfully in the experimental and clinical settings. Fresh osteochondral allografts have been used for the reconstruction of joint defects resulting from injury at the Mount Sinai Hospital in Toronto, Canada since 1972.

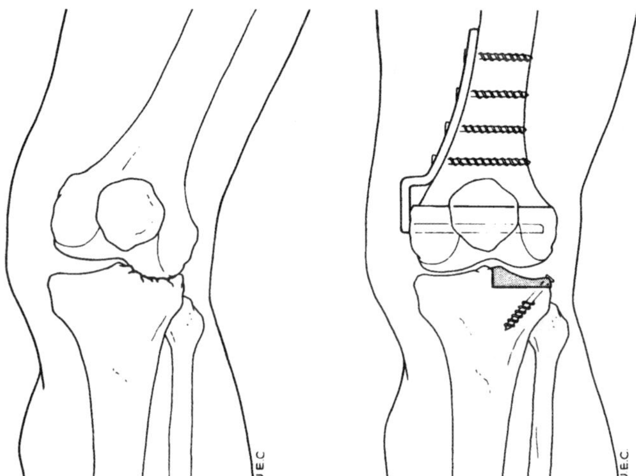

FIGURE 1.—Diagram showing fracture of the lateral tibial plateau with secondary valgus deformity treated by allograft of the lateral tibial plateau and distal femoral varus osteotomy. (Courtesy of Ghazavi MT, Pritzker KP, Davis AM, et al: Fresh osteochondral allografts for post-traumatic osteochondral defects of the knee. *J Bone Joint Surg Br* 79-B:1008–1013, 1997.)

The long-term clinical and radiologic findings and survival of these allografts were assessed.

Methods.—The average age of 123 patients (126 knees) with osteochondral defects after injury was 35 years. All donors were 30 years or younger. Ninety-seven knees had 1 or more prior surgeries. Defect sites were: 63 tibial plateau, 50 femoral condyle, 8 bipolar tibial and femoral, and 2 patellofemoral. An osteotomy was added in 68 knees. Valgus deformity secondary to an old fracture of the lateral plateau was treated by a distal femoral varus osteotomy with an allograft of the lateral tibial plateau (Fig 1). Varus deformity secondary to an old fracture of the lateral plateau was treated by a high tibial valgus osteotomy and an allograft of the medial femoral condyle. Knees were evaluated using a modified hospital Special Surgery Knee scoring system and radiographic assessment.

Results.—The average follow-up was 7.5 years. Treatment in 108 of 126 knees was successful (86%); 18 were failures. The factors related to failure included age older than 50 years, bipolar defects, malaligned knees with overstressing of the grafts, and workers' compensation involvement. In failed grafts, collapse of the graft by more than 3 mm and of the joint space of more than 50% were seen more often in radiographs.

Conclusion.—Fresh small-fragment osteochondral allografts are indicated for unipolar posttraumatic osteochondral defects of the knee in patients who are young and active.

▶ The increasing interest of offering nonreplacement solutions for arthritis has prompted a number of "biological" solutions to the problem of gonarthrosis in the young. This report is probably the greatest experience yet reported in the literature with significant follow-up of almost 8 years of more than 120 patients. The findings, therefore, are as reliable as any available today. The points worth emphasizing are that the small osteochondral grafts work best and all grafts require proper alignment and balancing, thus, concurrent osteotomy is required as emphasized in Figure 1. The fact that histologic viability has been confirmed is an encouraging finding and suggests opportunities for long-term solutions, at least in the properly selected patient.

B.F. Morrey, M.D.

Joint Loading With Valgus Bracing in Patients With Varus Gonarthrosis
Lindenfeld TN, Hewett TE, Andriacchi TP (Cincinnati Sportsmedicine and Orthopaedic Ctr, Ohio; Rush-Presbyterian-St Luke's Med Ctr, Chicago)
Clin Orthop 344:290–297, 1997   9–19

Background.—Some patients with unicompartmental gonarthrosis who are not candidates for total knee arthroplasty will receive a knee brace. Manufacturers claim that these braces unload the degenerative knee compartment, providing the advantages of realignment osteotomy without the expense. Patients do appear to obtain pain relief from valgus knee bracing; however, there are few data to confirm that the braces actually alter knee compartment loads. The effects of valgus knee bracing on adduction moments in the knee, in addition to the effects on pain and function scores, were studied.

Methods.—The study included 11 patients with arthrosis primarily of the medial compartment who were treated with a valgus brace. Before and after wearing the brace, the patients were tested by automated gait analysis, as well as by pain and function scoring instruments. The biomechanical data were analyzed to determine whether the brace truly affected medial compartment loads by decreasing the adduction moment at the knee, compared with the findings in 11 healthy controls.

Results.—Brace wear was associated with a 48% reduction in pain and a 79% increase in activities of daily living. The mean adduction moment decreased by 10%—4.0% vs. 3.6% body weight times height—when the brace was worn. Studies in controls showed a mean adduction moment of 3.5% body weight times height. This suggested that brace wear decreased the mean adduction moment from approximately 1 standard deviation above normal to a near-normal value. Brace wear decreased the adduction moment in 9 patients. Five patients showed a decrease of more than 10%, and 1 as high as 32%.

Conclusions.—In patients with medial compartment arthrosis, wearing a brace designed to unload the medial compartment of the knee actually alters biomechanical knee loading, presumably leading to improved pain and function. Bracing significantly reduces abnormal adduction moments about the knee, reducing medial tibiofemoral load to within the normal range. Thus, valgus knee bracing is a valid approach to treating medial compartment gonarthrosis.

▶ This is one of the few efforts to provide a scientific basis to the clinical practice of therapeutic bracing for gonarthrosis. The investigators do demonstrate a marked decrease in the varus thrust with the brace tested in this study. Although patient compliance may be an issue, the properly constructed brace can effectively unload the medial or lateral compartment and, therefore, assist as a nonoperative adjunct in the patient with unicompartmental arthrosis.

B.F. Morrey, M.D.

Time-dependent Clinical and Roentgenographical Results of Coventry High Tibial Valgisation Osteotomy

Bettin D, Karbowski A, Schwering L, et al (Westfälische Wilhelms Universität Münster, Germany)
Arch Orthop Trauma Surg 117:53–57, 1998   9–20

Background.—Patients with unicompartmental arthrosis of the knee have pain and progressive, irreversible deformity. A valgus producing osteotomy to shift the weight-bearing axis from the medial to the lateral knee compartment has reportedly given good results. Coventry et al. reported that this operation reduced pain, improved joint function, and corrected the weight-bearing axis. The clinical and radiographic results of Coventry osteotomy over time were evaluated.

Methods.—Coventry high tibial valgization osteotomy was performed in 129 knees of 118 patients with unicompartmental osteoarthrosis of the knee. The patients were 59 men and 59 women, with average age 57 years at the time of surgery. Most cases of osteoarthrosis were idiopathic. The clinical and radiographic outcomes were assessed at a median follow-up of 12 years.

Results.—The preoperative total HSS knee score was 33 points. This score improved to 68 points for all 129 cases, with follow-up of longer than 2 years. Scores subsequently declined to 55 points in 41 cases with more than 4 years' follow-up and to 44 points in 15 cases with more than 8 years' follow-up. The improvement began about 5 months postoperatively, and continued for 4 years. Functional knee score improved from 62 to 72 points in the 2-year follow-up group, to 70 in the 4-year follow-up group, to 64 in the 8-year follow-up group. Initial evaluation showed a 6-degree loss in knee flexion and a 1-degree loss in extension. Stability of the anteroposterior ligament decreased from 9 points to 6 points in the longest follow-up group. There was little change in lateral ligament stability, however. There were 6 cases of peroneus paresis, 4 of hematoma, and 1 each of fracture, infection, and pseudarthrosis. Knee angulation decreased from 9 degrees varus to 5 degrees valgus, with some deterioration over time. The distance between the weight-bearing axis and the eminentia intercondylaris decreased from 32 to 1 mm. Knee arthrosis continued to progress despite surgery.

Conclusions.—Coventry tibial osteotomy appears to be an effective treatment for medial compartment gonarthrosis. The technique presented includes rigid standardization, a precise operative technique, and accurate radiographic measurement of the mechanical axis. Their result of failed osteotomy, leading to knee arthroplasty, was only 15%. The technique meets the goal of delaying the need for total knee replacement.

▶ Any contribution that helps us better understand options short of joint replacement is of value. These investigators take great care in revealing the long-term radiographic results after a proximal tibial osteotomy. Their data, however, show that the mean correction of approximately 5 degrees of valgus is in fact undercorrection compared to the usual recommendation of 10 degrees of valgus. This may account for the deteriorating results seen over a period of time. The authors, however, emphasize the recurrence of varus as a cause of failure, also noting the progression of the disease as an additional cause of conversion to joint replacement arthroplasty. Their data are consistent with but their interpretation is different from a study done by Stuart et al. at the Mayo Clinic.[1] It was concluded that recurrence of varus was a rare cause of failure of this procedure, but rather the ongoing and progressive degenerative arthritis was most strongly correlated to surgical failure requiring ultimate joint replacement arthroplasty. These authors' data confirm this observation.

B.F. Morrey, M.D.

Reference

1. Stuart JJ, Kelly M, Morrey BF: Late recurrence of varus deformity after proximal tibial osteotomy. *Clin Orthop* 260:61–66, 1990.

Impact of CT Scan on Treatment Plan and Fracture Classification of Tibial Plateau Fractures
Chan PSH, Klimkiewicz JJ, Luchetti WT, et al (Univ of Pennsylvania, Philadelphia)
J Orthop Trauma 11:484–489, 1997   9–21

Background.—Treating tibial plateau fractures can be challenging. Preoperative planning is very important because of the potential complexity of fracture patterns. Interobserver and intraobserver agreement for treatment planning and fracture classification of tibial plateau fractures using plain films alone and with CT scans were determined.

Methods and Findings.—The plain films and CT scans of 21 patients with tibial plateau fractures were analyzed by 2 orthopedic traumatologists, 2 orthopedic residents, and 2 skeletal radiologists. When using plain films alone, the mean interobserver kappa coefficient for classification was 0.62. This declined to 0.61 when CT scans were added. When plain films alone were used for treatment planning, the mean interobserver kappa coefficient was 0.58. This increased to 0.71 with the addition of CT scans. The mean intraobserver kappa coefficient for fracture classification using plain films alone was 0.70; with plain films plus CT scans, it was 0.80. The mean intraobserver kappa coefficient for the treatment plan based on plain films alone was 0.62 and, with CT scans added, it was 0.82. The addition of CT scans prompted a change in class in an average of 12% of cases. It also changed treatment plans an average of 26% of the time.

Conclusion.—The addition of CT scanning to plain radiography does not increase agreement on fracture class of tibial plateau fractures. However, agreement in treatment planning does increase with the addition of CT scanning, and this is the ultimate goal of any fracture classification system.

▶ This study offers a worthwhile methodology, not just in defining the intraobserver variation of a popular classification system, but, by going a step further, it determines whether the addition of a CT scan significantly alters the treatment plan. This makes it a particularly worthwhile study. As expected, the CT scan offered details demonstrating a greater severity of injury than is typically appreciated on plain films; hence, the direction of the change in treatment plan was almost always more toward a surgical, as contrasted with a nonoperative, intervention. This study would suggest that CT offers little to the classification of the fracture but may help in determining whether surgical intervention would be of value, based primarily on the degree of comminution, displacement, and depression.

B.F. Morrey, M.D.

PATELLA

Recurrence After Patellar Dislocation: Redislocation in 37/75 Patients Followed for 6–24 Years
Mäenpää H, Huhtala H, Lehto MUK (Univ of Tampere, Finland)
Acta Orthop Scand 68:424–426, 1997   9–22

Objective.—The incidence of recurrence after patellar dislocation ranges from 2% to 50%, It is not known whether all recurrences have the same pathogenesis. Clinical and radiographic findings, isokinetic thigh muscle test results, and outcome were compared between patients with and without recurrence to identify variables predictive of recurrence.

Methods.—Of the 75 patients receiving closed treatment for a primary unilateral acute patellar dislocation between 1970 and 1988, 37 patients aged 12–64 years had a recurrence over a median period of 11 years and 38 patients aged 11–47 years, did not. The Cox proportional hazards regression model was used to find predictors for recurrence.

Results.—Patients with Wiberg-Baumgartl unstable patellar type (2/3–5) had an increased risk for recurrence of 2.3. This patellar type occurred in 60% of patients with recurrence and 40% of patients without. Spontaneous reduction of the dislocation increased the risk by 1.8 times. This spontaneous reduction occurred in 60% of patients with recurrence and in 50% of patients without. These risk factors were not associated. The time between dislocation and recurrence varied from 3 weeks to 6.5 years, and 11 patients had repeated recurrences. Outcomes for both groups were similar.

Conclusion.—Outcomes were similar for patients with and without recurrence after patellar dislocation. Spontaneous reduction of the dislocation and Wiberg-Baumgartl unstable patellar type (2/3–5) increased the risk for recurrence, but recurrence did not lead to patellar joint degeneration.

▶ The risk of recurrence after a patellar dislocation is substantial, occurring in nearly 50% of patients in this cohort. The authors attempted to identify predictive variables by comparing the patients with and without a recurrent dislocation. Although the follow-up was performed at a median of 11 years after the injury, true risk factors are difficult to establish because of possible selection bias and confounding variables in the "matched" groups. Nineteen patients with initial closed treatment and no recurrence were not included in the study because of residual complaints that were treated operatively. All patients reviewed received "conservative" treatment without differentiation of the type, extent, and duration of the nonoperative treatment program (strengthening, proprioceptive training, bracing, etc). No strategies are provided for improved functional outcome or preventive management.

M.J. Stuart, M.D.

Operative Versus Closed Treatment of Primary Dislocation of the Patella: Similar 2-Year Results in 125 Randomized Patients
Nikku R, Neitosvaara Y, Kallio PE, et al (Malmi City Hosp, Helsinki; Helsinki Univ; Sugical Hosp, Helsinki)
Acta Orthop Scand 68:419–423, 1997   9–23

Objective.—There is disagreement on whether closed treatment or surgery is preferred for treating primary patellar dislocation. Whether surgical realignment offers any advantage over immobilization after primary patellar dislocation was examined prospectively.

Methods.—Between 1991 and 1992, 125 patients with 180 first-time primary patellar dislocations of 14 days or less duration, who had no previous knee injuries or operations, no ligament injuries, and no osteochondral fractures, were randomly assigned to closed (C) treatment ($n = 55$) or to operative (O) treatment ($n = 70$). All patients had identical after-care and were encouraged to wear an orthosis for 6 months. Patients were followed up for an average of 25 months. Patient opinion, Lysholm II score, and Hughston visual analogue scale (VAS) knee score were recorded and compared statistically.

Results.—Subjective Hughston VAS knee scores were better in group C. The other 2 scores were similar for both groups. Fifteen patients in group

C and 12 in group O had redislocations, and 8 and 10 patients had recurrent subluxations, respectively. Nine patients in group C had 11 knee operations, and 12 patients in group O had 15 reoperations.

Conclusions.—Closed treatment is superior to open treatment for routine management of primary dislocation of the patella. Recurrence of patellar dislocation is more frequent than commonly reported.

▶ This article attempts to address a common dilemma, that is, knowing when to surgically intervene in acute patella dislocations. There is some difficulty accepting the conclusion that surgery is of no value. The study by Cofield and Bryan more than 20 years ago clearly demonstrated merit when risk factors for redislocation were present.[1] Because the groups of the current study were randomly selected, it would be expected that surgery was performed on some individuals for which it would be anticipated to be of no value. A relatively small sample would have a tendency to mute any advantage of surgical intervention on the group that had the high risk factors. In addition, a careful assessment of the results reveals that 23 of 55 (42%) had recurrent instability compared with only 22 of 70 (31%) in the group treated with surgery. The sample size was too small to demonstrate statistical significance, but there would certainly appear to be a difference in stability of the extensor mechanism in those undergoing surgery. It would be our interpretation that an early surgical intervention continues to be of value based on the presence of high-risk radiographic characteristics such as patella alta, dysplastic patella, and high Q angle as reported by Cofield and Bryan.[1]

B.F. Morrey, M.D.

Reference

1. Cofield RH, Bryan RS: Acute dislocation of the patella: Results of conservative treatment. *J Trauma* 17:526–531, 1977.

10 Complications

<hr>

Introduction

This is a small selection of very good articles dealing with a wide range of complications and outcomes. Two particularly important articles (Abstracts 10–4 and 10–5) report morbidity and mortality in comparison with hospital patient volume and surgeon patient volume. There are many databases (without orthopedic surgeon input) currently gathering information, and many more statisticians analyzing the data, that may have an impact on the practice of orthopedics in the future.

I have included two papers (Abstracts 10–2 and 10–9) on antibiotic beads for the treatment of osteomyelitis. The use of soluble media to deliver depot antibiotic has been a long-awaited development. Both papers are excellent and provide encouraging information on the use of these drug delivery systems. The results of failed treatment for the infected implant is also included; the report (Abstract 10–1) provides sobering data on the outcome of these patients' infections.

Two studies (Abstracts 10–11 and 10–12) deal with failure of devices and reconstructive techniques. Both provide support for the need for a national registry for monitoring implant performance and complications.

Christopher P. Beauchamp, M.D.

<hr>

Outcome After Reinfection Following Reimplantation Hip Arthroplasty
Pagnano MW, Trousdale RT, Hanssen AD (Mayo Clinic, Rochester, Minn)
Clin Orthop 338:192–204, 1997   10–1

<hr>

Introduction.—Eradication of infection has been the basic tenet guiding treatment of the infected total hip arthroplasty. Restoration of function and alleviation of pain are the secondary goals. Careful evaluation of the patient's medical status, the specific microorganism isolated, and the status of the prosthesis are involved in selecting the most appropriate treatment plan. Antibiotic suppression, open debridement, resection arthroplasty, arthrodesis, reimplantation of another prosthesis, and amputation are the fundamental management options. Resection arthroplasty has been used for the infected total hip arthroplasty, which eradicates the infection, preserves motion of the hip, but leaves a significant leg length discrepancy. For the knee, arthrodesis after deep prosthetic infection is commonly

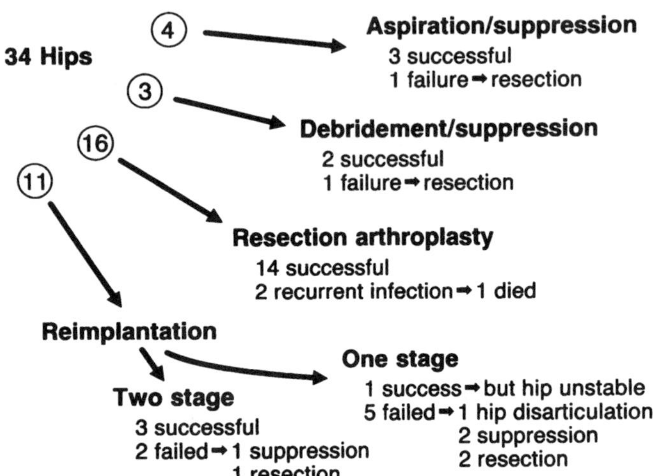

FIGURE 1.—The treatment and subsequent outcome for each of the 34 hips in this series in which re-infection developed after an attempt at reimplantation total hip arthroplasty following deep prosthetic infection. (Courtesy of Pagnano MW, Trousdale RT, Hanssen AD: Outcome after reinfection following reimplantation hip arthroplasty. *ClinOrthop* 338:192–204, 1997.)

recommended. Total hip arthroplasty reimplantation may be recommended for many patients with an infection. Little is known about the specific management and final outcome of those patients with reinfection after reimplantation for the infected total hip arthroplasty.

Methods.—Thirty-four patients were treated during a 16-year period for an infected total hip arthroplasty with removal of the prosthesis and implantation of another prosthesis. These patients had reinfection of their new hip arthroplasty. Eleven hips were infected with *Staphylococcus aureus* and 12 with coagulase-negative staphylococcus. In 23 patients the femoral prosthesis was cemented at the time of reimplantation, and in 11 patients, it was of a proximally coated uncemented design. Seven patients had antibiotic impregnated bone cement used; in 5 of those patients tobramycin alone was used, and in 2 patients, gentamicin alone was used.

Results.—Reinfection was eradicated with resection arthroplasty but led to poor function and was associated with persistent pain (Fig 1). Three patients achieved an excellent result with reimplantation of a third prosthesis. The worst functional results occurred in 8 hips that failed a third reimplantation attempt. Further attempts at a 1-stage reimplantation of another prosthesis are contraindicated when infection recurs after an attempt at reimplantation. Reasonable candidates for an attempt at a 2-stage reimplantation of a third prosthesis may be those patients in whom the same single microorganism has been identified from the failed primary total hip and from the failed first reimplantation, particularly when a deficiency in prior antibiotic therapy or surgical technique can be identified.

Conclusions.—Previous studies have shown success rates of 88.5% when patients are treated with delayed reconstruction, no antibiotic impregnated beads, or spacers but with antibiotic impregnated cement at the time of reimplantation. A successful outcome was found in 93.5% of patients when antibiotic beads or spacers are used in addition to antibiotic impregnanted cement as part of a delayed reimplantation. Reinsertion of another prosthesis is a reliable means of eradicating infection, preserving function, and relieving pain as part of a staged procedure after component removal and treatment with intravenous antibiotics.

▶ The authors report on a small but very important group of 34 patients with recurrent infections after reimplantation of a prosthesis for the management of total arthroplasty infection. The complication of prosthetic infection after joint implantation is a devastating one and a reinfection is even more so. There are few reports in the literature regarding the outcome of these patients. The authors site poor results with attempts at single-stage revision for reinfection. The best results are seen in patients in whom the same organism has been identified. Resection arthroplasty was shown to be a reliable technique in controlling infection, but was associated again with a poor functional outcome. Perhaps the most important step in treating these patients is to determine why the previous treatment plan failed. Only by understanding the mechanism of failure can a subsequent treatment be formulated.

C.P. Beauchamp, M.D.

Treatment of Osteomyelitis With a Biodegradable Antibiotic Implant
Calhoun JH, Mader JT (Univ of Texas, Galveston)
Clin Orthop 341:206–214, 1997   10–2

Introduction.—It is difficult to treat acute and chronic bone infections. Antibiotics are often prescribed for extended periods because of the ischemia and slow healing. Intravenous antibiotic injection with a long-term indwelling catheter and local implant of antibiotic-containing polymethylmethacrylate beads are the 2 methods currently available for the administration of antibiotics. Significant disadvantages are found with both methods. An operation for catheter placement is necessary for the intravenous route. Locally bactericidal levels of antibiotics are found for only 2–4 weeks with the beads, and a second operation is required for their removal. Biodegradable beads may be better in that they provide bactericidal concentrations of antibiotics for a prolonged time; many types of infections may be treated; there is no need for surgical removal; and there is no need for reconstruction. In a localized osteomyelitic rabbit model, a biodegradable antibiotic implant was developed and evaluated.

Methods.—Polylactic acid and poly (DL-lactide):co-glycolide combined with vancomycin were used to create the biodegradable antibiotic implant. *Staphylococcus aureus* was used to develop localized rabbit tibial osteomyelitis. The rabbits were divided into 8 groups and received treatment with or without debridement, systemic antibiotics, or biodegradable beads

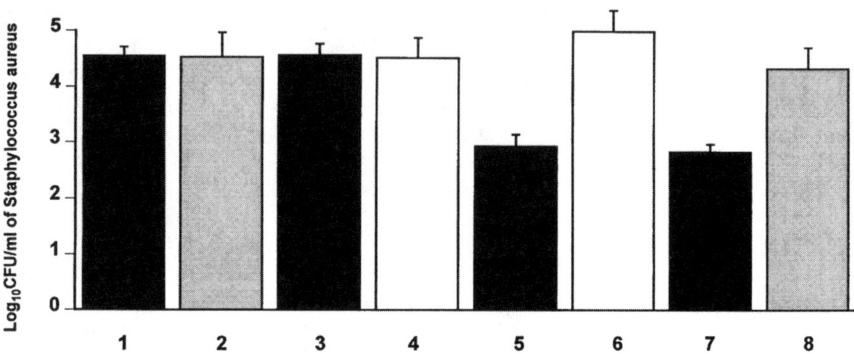

FIGURE 2.—The bar graph shows the mean concentration of *Staphylococcus aureus* present in each of the groups for which different treatments were applied, and the *t symbol* at the top of each bar represents the SEM. *1*, nontreated control rabbits; *2*, rabbits to be treated by debridement only; *3*, rabbits to be treated only with systemic vancomycin; *4*, rabbits to be treated with debridement and systemic vancomycin; *5*, rabbits to be treated with debridement and vancomycin loaded polyactic acid and poly (DL-lactide):co-glycolide (PLA-PL:CG) beads; *6*, rabbits to be treated with debridement and plain (no vancomycin) PLA-PL:CG beads; *7*, rabbits to be treated with debridement, vancomycin PLA-PL:CG beads, and systemic vancomycin; *8*, rabbits to be treated with debridement, plain (no vancomycin) PLA-PL:CG beads, and systemic vancomycin. The lower the concentration of *S. aureus*, the more effective the treatment method. *Abbreviation: CFU,* colony-forming unit. (Courtesy of Calhoun JH, Mader JT: Treatment of osteomyelitis with a biodegradable antibiotic implant. *Clin Orthop* 341:206–214, 1997.)

(Fig 2). Radiographs were obtained of the involved bones after 4 weeks of therapy. They were cultured for concentrations of *S. aureus* per gram of bone.

Results.—Bone colony-forming unit levels of $10^{2.93}$ colony-forming units per gram were found when treatment consisted of antibiotic containing polylactic acid and poly (DL-lactide):co-glycolide beads with systemic vancomycin. Bone colony-forming unit levels of $10^{2.84}$ colony-forming units per gram were found when treatment consisted of antibiotic containing polylactic acid and poly (DL-lactide):co-glycolide beads without systemic vancomycin. When compared with all other treatment groups, these bacterial concentrations were about 100 times lower.

Conclusions.—Extended bactericidal concentrations of antibiotics for the time needed to completely treat the particular orthopedic infection may be provided by a biodegradable antibiotic bead. Surgery is not needed to remove the beads. Other models should be used to test this protocol, such as hardware infection, a joint arthroplasty infection, and an infection prevention model.

▶ The treatment of acute and chronic orthopedic infections is time-consuming, and expensive, and is associated with significant morbidity. Depo administration of antibiotics has gained popularity during recent years. Standard treatment currently consists of debridement, intravenous antibiotics, and often, insertion of polymethylmethacrylate antibiotic impregnated beads. This has been shown to be effective, but the antibiotic beads must be removed. This requires a second surgical procedure. The authors report their experience using an osteomyelitic rabbit model. The study is well designed and clearly demonstrates that biodegradable antibiotic beads can provide extended bactericidal concentrations of antibiotics, and do not require a subsequent surgical procedure to remove them. This has many attractive features for the management of patients with orthopedic infections.

C.P. Beauchamp, M.D.

Complications After Concomitant Bilateral Total Knee Arthroplasty in Elderly Patients

Lynch NM, Trousdale RT, Ilstrup DM (Mayo Clinic, Rochester, Minn)
Mayo Clin Proc 72:799–805, 1997   10–3

Introduction.—Recent reports have documented the safety and cost-efficiency of concomitant bilateral total knee arthroplasty. Historically concomitant bilateral TKA had limited indications but today it is a commonly performed procedure. The risk associated with concomitant bilateral TKA may be acceptably low in younger patients but is unknown for elderly patients. The risk of intraoperative and postoperative medical and surgical complications was evaluated in elderly patients after concomitant bilateral TKA.

Methods.—Ninety-eight patients age 80 or older undergoing concomitant bilateral TKA were matched according to age, diagnosis, surgeon, and year of operative intervention with 98 patients undergoing unilateral TKA. Both groups were similar in medical status. A comparison of preoperative anesthetic risk and type of anesthetic agent was made. Median operative time for the unilateral and bilateral groups was 155 and 185 minutes, respectively; median tourniquet time was 108 and 102 minutes per knee, respectively; estimated blood loss was 250 and 530 mL, respectively; and total hospitalization days were 11 and 15 days, respectively.

Results.—There were 81 and 136 intraoperative, immediate postoperative, and posthospitalization complications (within 1 year after surgery) in the unilateral and bilateral groups, respectively. The American Society of Anesthesiologists (ASA) classification system was not predictive of the total number of complications for either group. Most complications occurred before hospital discharge: 35 of 49 in the unilateral group and 46 of 63 patients in the bilateral group. For both groups, postoperative complications prolonged duration of hospitalization (11 vs. 10 days in the unilateral group and 15 versus 11 days in the bilateral group). Significantly more patients in the bilateral group had complications than did patients in the unilateral group: 1, 2, 3, and 4–8 complications in 34, 14, 9, and 6 patients in the bilateral group, compared with 32, 12, 4, and 1, respectively, in the unilateral group. Postoperative cardiovascular complications occurred in 4 and 22 patients, respectively, in the unilateral and bilateral groups. Congestive heart failure occurred significantly more frequently in the bilateral group, compared with the unilateral group. The risk of developing postoperative cardiovascular complications was significantly correlated with presence of preoperative cardiovascular complications: 24

of 26 patients with cardiovascular complications had a pre-existing condition. Longer anesthesia time was significantly associated with development of cardiovascular complications in patients with unilateral TKA. Significantly more patients in the bilateral group developed neurologic complications, compared with the unilateral group (19 vs. 6); acute delirium was significantly more frequent in the bilateral than in the unilateral group. There was no association between ASA classification, type of anesthesia, operative time, anesthesia time, tourniquet time, or intraoperative complication and the occurrence of postoperative neurological complications. Development of acute delirium was not correlated with specific use of H_2-receptor antagonists. Of 4 patients in the bilateral group who died, 1 died 19 days after surgery and 3 died between 5–12 months after surgery. All patients in the unilateral group were alive at 12-month postoperative follow-up.

Discussion.—Earlier reports regarding similar medical and surgical complications in patients undergoing unilateral and bilateral TKA resulted in expansion of indications for and performance of concomitant bilateral TKA. These reports did not distinguish age-related differences in complication rates. In this comparison of elderly patients who underwent unilateral and bilateral procedures, the overall, cardiovascular, and neurological complication rates were higher in patients who underwent bilateral TKA. The higher rate of congestive heart failure in the bilateral group was probably because of a greater and more rapid fluid shift. This reflects a lack of cardiovascular reserve available to elderly patients to respond to a greater hemodynamic challenge. The higher rate of acute delirium in the bilateral group could be a manifestation of a more frequent fat embolism syndrome in that group.

Conclusion.—Elderly patients undergoing any orthopedic procedure may be at higher risk for complications than are younger patients. Patients in the unilateral and bilateral groups had a similar mortality rate, but it should be noted that 4 patients died within 12 months of operation in the bilateral group, compared with none in the unilateral group. Patients in the bilateral group had a significantly higher incidence of congestive heart failure and acute delirium than did patients in the unilateral group. Elderly patients may not possess the reserve to manage the fluid shifts that occur after a bilateral procedure. Embolic load may be responsible for the higher rate of acute delirium in the bilateral group. It is recommended that elderly patients with symptomatic bilateral gonarthrosis undergo a staged procedure, particularly if they have demonstrable pre-existing cardiac dysfunction.

▶ Concomitant bilateral total knee arthroplasty has enjoyed popularity lately. It is certainly more convenient for patients and has shown to be a cost-effective surgical endeavor. This study from the Mayo Clinic specifically evaluates how well patients over the age of 80 do with bilateral v. unilateral total knee arthroplasties. They have clearly shown a much greater risk of complications in this age group. The group quite rightly points out that the magnitude of surgery, the length of anesthesia, and the significant shifts in fluid volume in these patients are poorly tolerated. Many of these patients are coping adequately medically but cannot endure the additional physiologic loads demanded by such extensive surgery. Patients (of any age) with impaired cardiovascular reserve should be considered for staged bilateral TKA rather than simultaneous bilateral total knee arthroplasties.

C.P. Beauchamp, M.D.

Relationship Between Mortality Rates and Hospital Patient Volume for Medicare Patients Undergoing Major Orthopaedic Surgery of the Hip, Knee, Spine, and Femur

Taylor HD, Dennis DA, Crane HS (HCIA/LBA Health Care Management, Englewood, Colo; Denver Orthopedic Specialists; Rose Inst for Joint Replacement, Denver)
J Arthroplasty 12:235–242, 1997   10–4

Objective.—Whether the relationship between hospital patient volume and patient outcome after major orthopedic surgery is the result of experience or reputation is not known. Because quality-of-care issues all have an impact on mortality, the relationship between mortality and patient volume was investigated.

Methods.—In-house plus 30-day mortality data were compiled and analyzed for Medicare patients undergoing major orthopedic surgery (DRGs 209, 210, and 214) between October 1992 and September 1994.

Results.—Mortality rates declined consistently as volume increased in each procedure category. For DRG 209, low volume hospitals had an in-house mortality rate and an in-house plus 30-day mortality rate of 2.39% and 4.78%, respectively, as compared with high-volume hospitals with rates of 0.88% and 1.77%, respectively. For DRG 210, the low-volume mortality rates were 4.09% and 8.18% vs. high-volume rates of 3.35% and 6.70%, respectively. For DRG 214, the low-volume mortality rates were 1.04% and 2.09% vs. high-volume mortality rates of 0.64% and 1.27%, respectively.

Conclusion.—Patient mortality and patient volume are inversely related. The reasons behind increased patient mortality in hospitals with low patient volume needs to be investigated.

Relationship Between the Volume of Total Hip Replacements Performed by Providers and the Rates of Postoperative Complications in the State of Washington

Kreder HJ, Deyo RA, Koepsell T, et al (Univ of Toronto; Univ of Washington, Seattle)
J Bone Joint Surg Am 79-A:485–494, 1997   10–5

Objective.—The rate of adverse outcomes after surgery may be affected by the experience of the surgeon and hospital, as well as by patient age, disease severity, and co-morbidity. High-volume providers are known to achieve excellent results in total hip arthroplasty, but there are few data on the outcomes of patients treated by lower-volume providers. Any valid comparison of providers must consider variations in case mix. A computerized administrative database was used to determine how provider volume affects the rate of complications after elective total hip arthroplasty.

Methods.—The study used Washington State hospital discharge data on 7,936 patients undergoing 8,774 primary total hip replacements between 1988 and 1991. For each hospital and surgeon involved, the average number of hip replacements performed per year was determined. The complication rate was analyzed in terms of the volume of procedures performed, with adjustment for relevant factors.

Results.—On analysis of case mix, the patients treated by lower-volume providers—those whose volume was below the 40th percentile—had a more adverse risk profile in terms of age, comorbidity, and diagnosis. However, even after adjustment for these factors, outcomes were worse for surgeons who performed an average of fewer than 2 hip replacements per year. Patients of low-volume surgeons had higher mortality, more infections, more revision surgeries, and more serious in-hospital complications. An inverse relationship was noted between length of hospitalization and surgeon's volume, and a direct relationship between length of stay and hospital volume. There was also an inverse relationship between hospital charges and hospital volume, even after adjustment for length of stay, year of operation, and discharge destination.

Conclusions.—The outcome of primary hip replacement surgery appears to be related to provider volume. Patient outcome seems to be influenced by surgeon volume, whereas resource utilization is influenced by hospital volume. The findings must be interpreted cautiously, given the drawbacks of using administrative data sets. However, if confirmed, the results suggest that some types of elective total hip replacements may be best performed at regional centers.

▶ These 2 papers (Abstracts 10–4 and 10–5) represent analyses of data from 2 large databases. Both studies note a relationship between outcomes and patient volume. Both groups of authors quite rightly draw attention to the fact that these conclusions may not necessarily be valid. This is because results come from analyses of data from general databases and not from a specific prospective study. Nonetheless, the implications of these findings are potentially far reaching. A large number of other databases with similar data will be analyzed in similar fashion. This study, therefore, gives further support to the need for a national registry of patients. It is extremely important that we track morbidity, mortality, and outcome rates for commonly performed surgical procedures. If we do not do it, someone else will.

C.P. Beauchamp, M.D.

Prognosis of Dislocation After Total Hip Arthroplasty

Joshi A, Lee CM, Markovic L, et al (Wrightington Hosp, Lancashire, England)
J Arthroplasty 13:17–21, 1998   10–6

Introduction.—The most dramatic complication of total hip arthroplasty (THA) is dislocation. This event can be alarming to the patient and embarrassing and discouraging to the surgeon. Improvement in surgical technique and introduction of the long posterior wall socket in the Charnley THA reduced the dislocation rate in one medical center from 0.8% to 0.4%. Little has been published about the fate of dislocation. The fate of dislocation after Charnley THA and prognosis of recurrent dislocation after further surgery was assessed in 161 dislocations after cemented THA.

Methods.—Patients with hip dislocation after THA and a minimum of 2 years of follow-up were identified by a hospital database. Mean age of 99 females and 62 males was 55 years. Reasons for THA were 106 osteoarthritis, 32 rheumatoid arthritis, 11 congenital dislocation of hip, 6 Perthes' disease, 3 slipped upper femoral epiphysis, 2 Paget's disease, and 1 ankylosing spondylitis. Early dislocation was defined as dislocation within 5 weeks of surgery. Patient records and radiographs were assessed.

Results.—Fifty-nine (57%) dislocations were early dislocations and 102 (63%) were late dislocations. Of late dislocations, 54 (53%) occurred within 2 years after surgery, 43 (42%) occurred in 2–5 years, and 5 (5%) occurred between 5 and 9.5 years after surgery. Five hips underwent open reduction. Of 156 hips that underwent closed reduction, 26 recurred and underwent open reduction. During surgery, these faults were identified: 13 component malposition, 11 trochanteric separation, and 2 combination of faults. These patients had no further recurrence after surgery. Eighty-four percent of dislocations were single dislocations and 16% were recurrent dislocations. The rate of tronchanteric nonunion was 46% for single dislocations and 58% for recurrent dislocations. The significant interaction between factors made identification of individual factors contributing to dislocation difficult to determine.

Conclusion.—The finding of a higher rate of late dislocations is not in agreement with earlier findings. Initial closed reduction was successful in 156 of 161 patients. Excluding the 26 patients with recurrence after closed reduction, 130 (81%) of closed reductions were successful. Closed reduction is recommended as the first line of treatment. All patients with recurrent dislocation had 1 or more faults. Component malposition was the most common fault, then abductor mechanical failure. The prognosis of dislocation after THA is favorable. Understanding by the surgeon of the patient's pelvic and femoral orientation must be well understood. Malposition is definitely a technical failure.

▶ Instability following THA remains an ongoing problem. We are fortunate, as this paper continues to demonstrate, that most patients do not have an ongoing problem following the first dislocation. These patients tend to do well. The problem is identifying this particular group of patients and preventing the rest of the patients from being subject to the most distressing complication of recurrent instability with multiple dislocations. Every effort should be made to identify the patient at risk for recurrent dislocations. My personal belief is that patients undergoing a second dislocation should be carefully evaluated and examined under anesthesia to determine how unstable the hip is, why it is unstable, and whether surgical intervention is necessary. The most important key to the success in the management of patients with recurrent instability is to make the diagnosis as to the etiology of the instability. The results in the literature of surgical intervention for instability are not encouraging, and nearly 25% of patients have persistent instability following surgical attempts at its correction.

C.P. Beauchamp, M.D.

The Addition of Continuous Intravenous Infusion of Ketorolac to a Patient-controlled Analgetic Morphine Regime Reduced Postoperative Myocardial Ischemia in Patients Undergoing Elective Total Hip or Knee Arthroplasty
Beattie WS, Warriner CB, Etches R, et al (McMaster Univ, Hamilton, Ont; St Paul's Hosp, Vancouver, BC; Royal Brisbane Hosp, Australia; et al)
Anesth Analg 84:715–722, 1997   10–7

Introduction.—The rate of the incidence of myocardial infarction postoperatively is twice that of the incidence in the general population. For patients with perioperative ST depression, the relative risk of infarction is 12%. It is believed that decreasing ischemia may diminish the morbid event rate. Strategies include improved postoperative analgesia with epidural or intravenous (IV) narcotics and platelet inhibitors, such as ketorolac. When combined with patient-controlled analgesia (PCA) with morphine, ketorolac produces superior pain scores, narcotic sparing, and decreased antiemetic need. The addition of a nonsteroidal anti-inflammatory drug to a regimen of PCA morphine was assessed for its effect on the degree of ischemia (determined by ST depression) in patients undergoing elective total joint arthroplasty.

Methods.—One hundred thirty patients were randomized to receive either ketorolac 30 mg bolus, then infusion of 5 mg/hr for 24 hours or placebo. Patients were connected to a PCA morphine system. No analgesics were administered preoperatively. Visual analogue pain scores, blood pressure, heart rate, oxygen saturation, and ST segment depression were assessed.

Results.—The addition of ketorolac resulted in morphine sparing of about 40%. At 2 and 6 hours after surgery, visual analogue pain scores were significantly better in the ketorolac group. The postoperative heart rate increased significantly more in the placebo group than the ketorolac group (19 vs. 10 beats per minute). There was no significant between-group difference in the incidence of ischemia (17% ketorolac, 14%

placebo). Ischemia was highest at 3 hours after surgery, then peaked again at 8–12 hours and 18–24 hours.

Discussion/Conclusion.—The duration of postoperative ischemic attacks was shorter in patients who received ketorolac, compared with placebo. Aggressive treatment of postoperative pain with a regimen that includes IV ketorolac decreases postoperative ischemia. The single most important predictor of postoperative ischemia was preoperative use of calcium channel blockers. Analgesia is important in decreasing ischemia. It must be cautioned that ST segment depression is a nonspecific indicator of ischemia. Postoperative pain is a strong initiating factor for ST depression, ischemia, and maybe even subsequent infarction. A recent report showed that ischemia increases with cessation of epidural analgesia. Patients undergoing total hip and knee arthroplasty experienced decreased pain score, arterial blood pressure, heart rate, and duration of ischemia when IV ketorolac was added to a PCA morphine analgesic regimen.

▶ Serious postoperative complications involving pain control following elective total knee and hip arthroplasty are, fortunately, not that common. When they do occur, however, the effects can be catastrophic. Greater efforts at providing satisfactory postoperative analgesia comes with an increased complication rate associated with this goal. These include confusion, hypoxia, cardiovascular compromise, aspiration, overdose, and others. This study very nicely shows the improvement in postoperative patient morbidity with the addition of ketorolac delivered as a continuous IV infusion. Greater efforts must be made to reduce the risk of analgesia complications in surgical patients.

C.P. Beauchamp, M.D.

Early Excision of Heterotopic Ossification About the Elbow Followed by Radiation Therapy
McAuliffe JA, Wolfson AH (Cleveland Clinic Florida, Fort Lauderdale; Univ of Miami, Fla)
J Bone Joint Surg Am 79-A:749–755, 1997   10–8

Introduction.—Heterotopic ossification, characterized by the formation of bone in periarticular regions, can lead to severely limited motion in the affected joint. Excision of heterotopic bone about the elbow is reported to be a successful treatment, but recurrence is common. This review of 8 patients with heterotopic ossification about the elbow demonstrated the benefits of early excision followed by radiation therapy.

Methods.—Heterotopic bone was excised in these patients at an average of 7 months after the initial injury. Five patients had a neurologic injury (the spinal cord in 3 cases and the head in 2), and 3 had a local injury of the elbow. Heterotopic bone was predominantly posteromedial in all patients. Excision was performed under tourniquet control, and the ulnar nerve was transposed anteriorly at the end of the procedure. The nerve was identified so that it could be protected as deeper bone was excised. Radiation therapy consisted of 5 fractions, started on the first postoperative day and administered over a 7-day period. The total dose was 1,000 cGy. Therapist-supervised active and assisted range-of-motion exercises were begun on the first postoperative day.

Results.—The average arc of motion was 103 degrees at latest follow-up (average, 46 months), which compared favorably with that attained intraoperatively (average, 121 degrees). Two patients had residual motor deficits; their arcs of motion were 50 degrees and 70 degrees. When these 2 cases were excluded from analysis, the average arc of motion was 118 degrees in patients with normal motor function. No patient had substantial recurrence of ossification, and no complications resulted from radiation therapy.

Discussion.—Heterotopic ossification occurs in approximately 1% of patients with burn injury, in 3% with local injury of the elbow, and in 11% with head injury. Prophylaxis using pharmacologic agents or radiation therapy has disadvantages, and it is difficult to identify patients in whom heterotopic ossification will develop. Early excision followed by radiation therapy was successful in restoring elbow function in this small series of patients. There appears to be no advantage in delaying treatment for 2–18 months after the injury to allow for maturation of heterotopic bone.

▶ It has long been taught that excision of heterotopic ossification prior to maturation will result in immediate and/or aggressive recurrence. The concept of an evolutionary disorder, beginning with an aggressive inflammatory response and ending with mature bone with marrow elements, is certainly supported pathologically. Does this mean that patients must endure a lengthy wait prior to relief from restricted joint motions secondary to heterotopic ossification? The authors have shown very nicely that early intervention with adjuvant treatment was effective in a series of 8 patients. The success makes sense if the assumption that radiation therapy truly stops heterotopic ossification is correct, an assumption supported in the literature with respect to radiation therapy and total hip arthroplasty. If the mechanical impediment to joint motion can be effectively dealt with, adjuvant radiation therapy should prevent a flare-up of the underlying disorder.

C.P. Beauchamp, M.D.

Treatment of Experimental Osteomyelitis by Surgical Debridement and the Implantation of Bioerodable, Polyanhydride-Gentamicin Beads
Nelson CL, Hickmon SG, Skinner RA (Univ of Arkansas, Little Rock)
J Orthop Res 15:249–255, 1997   10–9

Introduction.—Sequestered, necrotic, infected bone is responsible for the chronicity of osteomyelitis. The granulation tissue that surrounds the infected necrotic area is replaced by relatively avascular fibrous tissue. This stimulates the surrounding tissues and the periosteum permeative mesen-

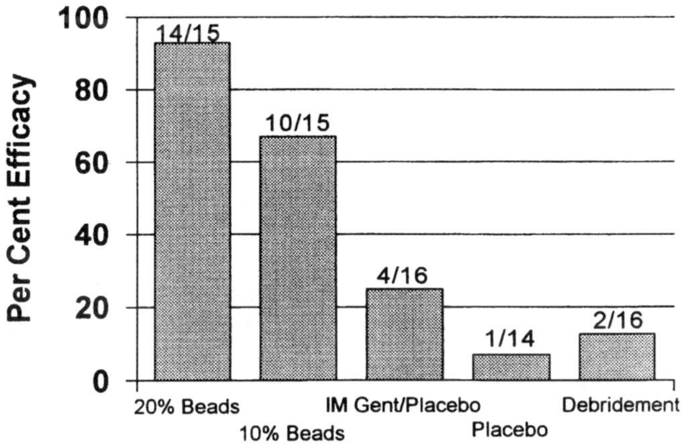

Treatment Group

FIGURE 4.—Efficacy rates for the five treatment groups studied. *Abbreviation: IM Gent,* intramuscular injection of gentamicin sulfate. Fractions represent successful cases out of the total of treated individuals per group. (Courtesy of Nelson CL, Hickmon SG, Skinner RA: Treatment of experimental osteomyelitis by surgical debridement and the implantation of bioerodable, polyanhydride-gentamicin beads. *J Orthop Res* 15:249–255, 1997.)

chymal cells to form new reactive bone to wrap around the sequestered, necrotic, infected bone. Systemic antibiotic therapy is limited by toxicity, need for systemic access for drug delivery, and expense. Various methods of local delivery of antibiotics and surgical debridement have been considered. Outcome of experimental osteomyelitis treated by surgical debridement and implantation of a bioerodable polyanhydride-gentamicin sulfate bead delivery system is reported.

Methods.—Osteomyelitis was induced into the radius of 77 rabbits. Histological examination and culture confirmed infection. Wounds were debrided at 4 weeks and animals were treated with either fatty acid dimer-sebacic acid beads (a bioerodable composite) impregnated with 20% or 10% gentamicin, placebo beads and intramuscular gentamicin sulfate alone, placebo beads alone, or debridement only. Four weeks later, animals were sacrificed and eradication of infection was assessed by histological examination and culture. Fatty acid dimer-sebacic beads were then implanted in noninfected animals, and gentamicin sulfate concentrations were measured in bone, serum, urine, and wound exudate.

Results.—Osteomyelitis was eradicated in 93% of rabbits treated with beads and 20% gentamicin, 67% treated with beads and 10% gentamicin, 25% treated with placebo beads and intramuscular gentamicin, 7% treated with placebo beads alone, and 12.5% treated with debridement alone (Fig 4). Gentamicin sulfate was detectable in bone for up to 8 weeks after implantation. Levels as high as 4,746 µg/mL were seen in wound exudate for the first 7 days after implantation. Serum and urine levels peaked at 1.03 µg/mL and 1.35 µg/mL, respectively.

Conclusion.—These findings offer a comprehensive measurement of antibiotic levels detected in bone, muscle, serum, urine, and wound exudate in the treatment of osteomyelitis induced in a rabbit model. This data provides a substantive background for helping determine the ideal local drug delivery system.

▶ The authors have successfully demonstrated that bioerodable beads have a significant role in the management of rabbits with infections of bone. They have not only demonstrated a positive effect of gentamicin-impregnated beads but also that there is a significant dose response.

C.P. Beauchamp, M.D.

Effect of the Elevated-Rim Acetabular Liner on Loosening After Total Hip Arthroplasty

Cobb TK, Morrey BF, Ilstrup DM (Mayo Clinic and Found, Rochester, Minn)
J Bone Joint Surg Am 79-A:1361–1364, 1997   10–10

Objective.—Whereas elevated-rim acetabular liners improve stability of total hip prostheses, the potential adverse effects of the liner on formation of debris and loosening has not been studied. Data on 5,167 primary and revision total hip arthroplasties performed with an elevated-rim acetabular liner or standard acetabular component were retrospectively reviewed to compare prevalences of revision as a result of loosening.

Methods.—Between September 1, 1985 and December 31, 1991, 2,469 arthroplasties were performed with an elevated-rim acetabular component and 2,698 with a standard component with and without cement. Five-year follow-up data were available on 174 hips with an elevated-rim acetabular liner and 1,063 with a standard component.

Results.—Four percent of hips (108) with an elevated-rim acetabular liner and 7% of hips (179) with a standard liner underwent revision because of loosening. Kaplan-Meier probabilities of survival without revision (91.8% and 92.8%, respectively) were not significantly different. Five-year probabilities of survival were 98.8% for patients with the elevated-rim liner and 98.3% for patients with the standard liner. There were no survival differences with respect to cemented and cementless components, primary and revision arthroplasties, or male and female patients. No studies have assessed the impact of acetabular augmentation in preventing posterior dislocation of the femoral head. The long-term effect of wear on the elevated-rim acetabular component continues to be of concern and has been reported in isolated incidents of osteolysis induced by particles of polyethylene wear debris as a result of a foreign-body giant-cell reaction with intracellular polyethylene.

Conclusion.—Although wear data for this new design will continue to be collected, results of this study do not show any difference in the probability of loosening between the elevated-rim acetabular liner and the standard liner.

▶ It has been shown that the rate of instability after total hip arthroplasty using an elevated rim is less than with a flat liner. The results of this study are important. Unfortunately, every time we correct or make an improvement in 1 problem, we tend to create a different problem. The authors have demonstrated that elevated-rim acetabular liners do not have an effect on loosening after total hip arthroplasty and that their continued use is endorsed. It is important, however, when using an elevated-rim acetabular liner to understand the effects that this device has on the global range of motion permitted by the femoral component. Oftentimes, impingement is added to the equation of instability when an elevated liner is used.

C.P. Beauchamp, M.D.

Massive Early Subsidence Following Femoral Impaction Grafting
Eldridge JDJ, Smith EJ, Hubble MJ, et al (Univ of Bristol, England)
J Arthroplasty 12:535–540, 1997   10–11

Objective.—Loss of femoral bone after aseptic loosening is a major challenge in revision hip surgery. Bone grafting has been used successfully to restore bone stock loss. The incidence of early subsidence associated with femoral impaction grafting is reported.

Methods.—Between December 1991 and August 1994, 86 hips in 84 patients were revised using impacted cancellous allograft and cement for fixation of the femoral component. There were 79 patients (38 women), aged 27–88, (79 hips) followed radiographically for at least 6 months. The CPT (Zimmer, Swindon, England) (n = 48) and Exeter (Howmedica, Staines, England) (n = 31) collarless, polished, double-tapered impaction systems were used. Subsidence of less than 5 mm was defined as *minimal*, 5–10 mm was defined as *moderate*, and 10 mm or more was termed *massive*.

Results.—Patients were followed for an average of 12.6 months. Alignment was neutral in 37 prostheses, valgus in 7, and varus in 35. Subsidence was minimal in 61 hips, moderate in 9, and massive in 9. Five CPT and 4 Exeter prostheses subsided in 7 men and 2 women. Seven of the subsided stems were inserted in the varus position, 1 in the neutral position, and 1 in the valgus position. Alignment changed in 2 stems, 1 into valgus and 1 into varus. Migration was observed on radiographs 3 months after surgery in all hips with massive subsidence and was progressive in 8 hips. Early clinical results show no revision using this technique as opposed to standard cemented and cementless revision hip arthroplasty rates. High re-revision and loosening rate have been observed with poor preoperative bone stock. In the 79 hips reviewed here, distal migration by the femoral component of more than 10 mm in the early postoperative period caused thigh pain in 11% of hips. There was no late subsidence. Subsidence was not correlated with presence or absence of radiolucent lines or any other predisposing factors. All patients with subsidence had thigh pain, an apparent early predictor of failure.

Conclusion.—Massive subsidence occurs after femoral impaction bone grafting, which appears to be potentiated by varus alignment. Additional research needs to be conducted to evaluate risk factor associated with this procedure.

▶ Impaction bone grafting is a technically challenging and demanding surgical technique. It requires meticulous attention to detail. Despite this attention to detail, however, this reconstructive method does carry a significant incidence of complications. Periprosthetic fracture, subsidence, and persistent pain all contribute to the need for subsequent revision arthroplasty. There is a steep learning curve for this procedure, and further reports regarding its success rate will be forthcoming.

C.P. Beauchamp, M.D.

Fatigue Fracture of a Forged Cobalt-Chromium-Molybdenum Femoral Component Inserted With Cement: A Report of Ten Cases
Woolson ST, Milbauer JP, Bobyn JD, et al (Menlo Park, Calif; Marshfield Clinic, Wis; Montreal Gen Hosp, et al)
J Bone Joint Surg Am 79-A:1842–1848, 1997   10–12

Introduction.—Early in the history of total hip replacement with cement, the prevalence of fracture of stainless-steel femoral components was as high as 0.67%, but stems made of high-strength titanium or cobalt-chromium-molybdenum alloys rarely fracture. An unusually high prevalence of fracture of forged cobalt-chromium-molybdenum stems inserted with modern cementing techniques was documented and characterized.

Methods.—Ten patients with a total hip replacement with a forged cobalt-chromium-molybdenum femoral prosthesis inserted with cement had a fatigue fracture of the stem an average of 50 months after the operation. Patients had an average age of 61 years, and an average weight of 96 kg. Osteoarthrosis and rheumatoid arthritis were the diagnoses at the time of the primary hip replacement. Primary total hip replacement was performed on 8 patients, and 2 had a revision with all the acetabular components being inserted without cement. Cement was used to insert the femoral component, and no cement was used in the acetabular component. The femoral component had a 28-mm diameter femoral head, and all were inserted with modern cementing techniques, which involved cleaning the femoral canal with pulsatile lavage, injecting the cement with a cement gun, and reducing the porosity of the cement with vacuum mixing.

Results.—Four of 8 hips that had a primary replacement had radiographs available, and all 4 had evidence of debonding of the cement mantle from the proximal end of the stem, which caused exaggerated cantilever bending stresses on the proximal aspect of the stem as the distal end of the stem was well fixed. There was a nonunion of the greater trochanter in radiographs of both hips that had a revision. A fatigue fracture that began near the anterolateral corner of the prosthesis was seen in scanning electron micrographs of 5 of the 10 fractured prostheses. There were subsurface voids or inclusions under the region that had been etched on the implant with a laser, according to metallurgical analysis, which is consistent with thermal changes to the microstructure of the alloy that may have caused a focal reduction in the material strength. A poor cement mantle was seen in 7 of the 10 stems. Six of these stems were implanted in patients who weighed more than 80 kg, indicating relative undersizing of the prostheses. All fractures occurred near the junction of the middle and distal thirds of the femoral stem. Each of the 10 stems had polymethylmethacrylate precoating on portions of the proximal fragment. At the index operation, the cement inserted into the femoral canal failed to wet and polymerize completely with the precoated layer of cement on the stem, causing the precoated layer to debond from the doughy cement that was injected.

Conclusions.—The risk of fatigue fracture should be explained to patients who have radiographic evidence of a debonded Precoat femoral component, and they should be followed up closely, even though there is no evidence of symptoms of loosening of the femoral component. There was a 2% prevalence of fracture, which was high. Initial debonding of the proximal end of the femoral component from the cement mantle in 4 of 8 patients was the mechanism of failure. The cement mantle at the proximal portion of the stem may have been deficient because the femoral rasp was undersized. In all 10 patients, proximal debonding at the cement-prosthesis interface or a nonunion of the greater trochanter occurred before the fracture of the prosthesis. The surgeon should be warned that a fatigue fracture of a precoat stem may occur if these radiographic signs are seen. A prophylactic revision is recommended because it is easier to revise an intact, proximally debonded, femoral prosthesis, than to revise a fractured prosthesis.

▶ This important paper reports a complication associated with a particular stem design and manufacturing method. It highlights a number of points. First, this is a good example of why long-term studies are needed for new designs, and that new designs are not necessarily better and may introduce new problems or complications. Second, it emphasizes a need for ongoing continual follow up of patients who have had prosthetic joint replacements not only to identify those who are at risk for known problems such as wear and normal aseptic loosening, but to identify new and unrecognized problems. Third, this study is a good example of why an implant registry would be of benefit. We have all had experiences with products and prostheses that have had problems associated with them, and when one goes back through the records, it is can be difficult to find out who has what prosthesis, how many were inserted, who needs to be recalled, etc. Last, in patients in whom we identify this problem, early prophylactic revision is advisable.

The extraction of a firmly incarcerated broken chrome-cobalt-molybdenum stem is extremely difficult. Standard broken-stem technique extractions are difficult because the metal is much harder than stainless steel. Old broken stainless-steel stems were relatively easy to remove in comparison with this particular problem.

C.P. Beauchamp, M.D.

11 Foot and Ankle

Introduction

Contributions to the literature regarding the management of afflictions of the foot and ankle have increased steadily over the years. In this chapter, the common conditions of a sprained ankle and ruptured Achilles' tendon are featured with several significant contributions. Furthermore, the salvage reconstructive procedures of both ankle and subtalar fusion are complemented by discussions involving acute and repetitive trauma which lie at the opposite spectrum of functional impairment. Finally, significant attention is paid to the management of patients with bunion deformity with the increasing popularity of the Chevron osteotomy being balanced by alternate procedures such as cheilectomy or joint fusion. Overall, a full complement of contributions investigating the management options that will hopefully prove to be of value to those involved in both general and specialty practices that include the foot and ankle.

Bernard F. Morrey, M.D.

Ligament Injuries

Effect of Ankle Orthoses on Functional Performance for Individuals With Recurrent Lateral Ankle Sprains

Gross MT, Clemence LM, Cox BD, et al (Univ of North Carolina, Chapel Hill; Shea Physical Therapy, Corpus Christy, Tex; Pitt County Mem Hosp, Greenville, NC; et al)

J Orthop Sports Phys Ther 25:245–252, 1997   11–1

Introduction.—Previous studies have addressed the effects of various approaches to providing ankle support on the restriction of joint motion. The results have suggested that semirigid orthoses are more effective in preventing ankle sprains than are other systems such as taping, elastic supports, and cloth orthoses. Other studies have suggested that semirigid orthoses do not adversely affect functional performance; however, most of these studies were performed in healthy subjects with no history of ankle sprain or instability. Two semirigid ankle orthoses, the DonJoy Ankle Ligament Protector (ALP) and the Aircast Sport Stirrup (AS), were compared for their effects on functional performance in athletes with a history of recurrent unilateral ankle sprains.

Methods.—The study included 23 athletes with at least 2 lateral ankle sprains of 1 ankle, with no sprains of the contralateral ankle. Each subject's most recent sprain had occurred within the preceding 2 years, but not during the preceding 3 months. On the first day of testing, the subjects performed various functional tests, including a 40-m sprint, a figure-of-eight run, and a standing vertical jump, with both ankles unbraced and again wearing the ALP or AS on the recurrently sprained ankle. On a second test day, the same tasks were performed with the ankle unbraced and with the other orthosis on the recurrently sprained ankle. The effects of the 2 orthoses on task performance were compared. The athletes also rated the 2 devices for comfort and support.

Results.—On analysis of variance, task performance was not significantly different between the braced and nonbraced conditions. Neither was their any significant difference between the 2 orthosis conditions. Three fourths of the subjects rated the AS more comfortable than the ALB, and more than 60% thought the AS offered greater support.

Conclusions.—In patients with a history of recurrent unilateral ankle sprain, the AS and ALP semirigid ankle orthoses have no effect on functional task performance. The findings support previous studies in healthy subjects. Patients may differ as to which orthosis they prefer, and these subjective differences may affect compliance with wearing the orthosis and thus in protecting against ankle sprain.

▶ In spite of the widespread use of ankle orthoses after injury to the ligaments, there is relatively little hard objective or controlled clinical data justifying or supporting their use. This prospective study does demonstrate at least the subjective value with the use of ankle orthoses for chronic instability, but there is little selection preference between the two designs that were used, ALP and AS. It appears that neither of the devices altered the functional capabilities of the individual. It should be noted that the selection criterion was chronic instability, and these observations may not necessarily, although they would logically, correlate with the use of the devices in the acute setting as well. Nonetheless, the study confirms the general clinical impression that subjectively most feel benefited from these devices.

B.F. Morrey, M.D.

Tenodeses Do Not Fully Restore Ankle Joint Loading Characteristics: A Biomechanical In Vitro Investigation in the Hind Foot

Rosenbaum D, Bertsch C, Claes LE (Biomechanik Universität Ulm-Klinikum, Germany)
Clin Biomech 12:202–209, 1997   11–2

Background.—The incidence of residual problems is high in patients treated for acute ruptures of the ligaments, independent of type of treatment. The biomechanical consequences of ligament injuries and surgical reconstruction procedures, and their effects on intra-articular loading in the ankle joint complex and Chopart joint line and on the plantar pressure patterns were studied in vitro.

Methods.—Twelve fresh-frozen lower leg specimens were examined. The specimens were freed of soft tissue down to the malleoli and prepared for accessing the talocrural, subtalar, talonavicular, and calcaneocuboid joints. The specimens were then fixed in a loading simulator and loaded axially with 600 N in 1 of 6 conditions: intact; after cutting the anterior talofibular ligament; after cutting the calcanefibular ligament also; and after performing the Evans, Watson-Jones, and Chrisman-Snook procedures.

Findings.—The mean intra-articular pressures were increased, related to either reduced contact areas or increased contact forces in all joints after ligament resections and tenodeses. Plantar loading was increased under the medial aspect of the foot and reduced under the midfoot area.

Conclusions.—Ankle ligament injuries as well as surgical reconstructions by tenodeses affect joint loading characteristics. As a result, joint degeneration may be exacerbated.

▶ The central hypothesis of this project is a legitimate one; specifically to determine whether commonly used ligamentous reconstructive procedures simulate, replicate, or restore the kinematics of the normal ankle and the force distribution associated with imparted loads. The methodology uses pressure-sensitive films, which is known to be less accurate in demonstrating graded contact pressures on curved surfaces. Furthermore, the insertion of pressure-sensitive film does require the ablation of certain portions of the capsule and possibly could disturb the normal anatomy sufficiently as to cause generation of spurious data. The combination of axial load and simulated muscle contracture is a worthwhile concept; however, it is unclear as to the number of degrees of freedom provided by the simulation device. The illustrations suggest that motion about all 3 coordinate axes is possible, which is essential if any valid conclusions are to be drawn. The precise replication of the reconstructive procedures, specifically the placement of the *tunnels in the bone* and the amount of tension that is applied, can be problematic. Furthermore, significant individual variation in the anatomy of individual specimens results in marked variation in experimental results. The relatively small sample size does make interpretation difficult. This is supported by the rather large standard deviations that typically equaled or exceeded 10%, particularly with regard to area and force. The findings that reconstruction by tenodesis causes significant changes in the loading characteristics had been observed clinically, although this clinical material was not cited in the references. Overall, the value of studying the implications of these reconstructive procedures is of value, and further studies such as this should be undertaken.

B.F. Morrey, M.D.

Valgus Stress Radiography in Normal Ankles

Leith JM, McConkey JP, Li D, et al (Univ of British Columbia, Vancouver)
Foot Ankle Int 18:654–657, 1997   11–3

Introduction.—Deltoid ligament injury is believed to be rare. Signs of complete rupture of the deltoid ligament may be difficult to determine or may be interpreted as another injury. There is no standardized method for determining medial ligament insufficiency in acute or chronic laxity. The range of normal (physiologic) talar tilt and the range of asymmetry between ankles when valgus stress is employed has not been investigated and reported. The degree of normal talar tilt in individuals with no history of ankle injuries was assessed. The degree of side-to-side differences in talar tilt were compared.

Methods.—Thirty-two normal male and female research subjects ages 23–42 underwent valgus stress and unstressed radiographs. Twenty-one pairs of ankles acting as controls underwent unstressed radiographs. Two examiners performed 2 different measurements of 3 × 5 radiographs cropped so that only the distal tibia, the malleoli, and the talus were visible.

Results.—Fifty-eight stressed ankles had a mean talar tilt angle of 2 degrees or less (91%) and 6 had a mean talar tilt angle of over 2 degrees but less than 3 degrees (9%). The mean talar tilt angle in 41 unstressed ankles was 2 degrees or less (98%) and 1 ankle had a mean talar tilt angle of over 2 degrees (2%). The mean talar tilt angles for stressed and unstressed ankles were 0.9 degrees and 0.3 degrees, respectively.

Conclusion.—Stress radiography demonstrates a measurable but minimal range of talar tilt on valgus stress in previously uninjured ankles. These findings create the basis for diagnosis of the rare, isolated rupture of the deltoid ligament of the ankle.

▶ It is well known that a significant normal variation exists in the laxity of the lateral ligamentous complex making interpretation of varus stress roentgenograms difficult. There has been very little reported regarding the normal variation of valgus stress radiography testing that would provide the same information referable to the medial ligament complex. As might be expected, there is very little variation. Ninety percent of the ankles had less than 2 degrees of tilt, and there was no ankle exhibiting more than 3 degrees of varus tilt. This provides baseline information indicating that virtually no valgus joint tilt is normally present with the functioning deltoid ligament.

B.F. Morrey, M.D.

Acute Repair and Delayed Reconstruction for Lateral Ankle Instability: Twenty-Year Follow-up Study
Kitaoka HB, Lee MD, Morrey BF, et al (Mayo Clinic and Found, Rochester, Minn; Fort Wayne, Ind; Sioux Falls, SD)
J Orthop Trauma 11:530–535, 1997   11–4

Introduction.—Most patients with lateral ankle ligament injury are successfully treated nonoperatively. There is disagreement about optimal surgical treatment for lateral ankle instability. The long-term results of primary ligament repair and delayed reconstruction for lateral ligament instability were assessed in 48 patients who underwent 53 procedures.

Methods.—Patients treated surgically for acute or chronic gross ankle instability resulting from trauma between 1958 and 1977 were evaluated using a clinical scale and radiologic results based on stress radiographs and plain film radiographs. Twenty-one patients underwent 22 primary repair operations, and 28 patients underwent 31 ankle reconstructive procedures (Evans or Watson-Jones procedures).

Results.—Patients were evaluated at an average of 20 years after surgery (range, 12–33 years). The clinical grading scale showed that results of primary repair were excellent in 20 ankles, good in 1, fair in 0, and poor in 1. For the Evans procedure, results were excellent in 13, good in 3, fair in 0, and poor in 2. For the Watson-Jones procedure, results were excellent in 8, good in 3, fair in 1, and poor in 1. Patient evaluation was 49 satisfied, 2 satisfied with reservation, and 2 dissatisfied. The mean talar tilt with stress testing before surgery was 20.7 degrees and 2.8 degrees after surgery in the primary repair group and 20.7 degrees and 2.8 degrees, respectively, before and after surgery in the reconstruction group.

Conclusion.—Patients in the primary and reconstruction group had similar clinical and radiographic findings. Most severe ankle sprains can be treated nonoperatively. Late reconstruction can yield satisfactory results for persistent residual instability.

▶ The question of whether or not to operate on the acutely-sprained ankle remains unanswered because the unique circumstances for each patient must be considered. This study adds longer term information to previous work that shows high success rates for delayed reconstruction. Therefore, immediate repair is less imperative, except in the situations outlined by the authors. One argument in favor of early treatment is that no patient with an early repair reported an unsatisfactory result, but two patients in the reconstructed group did.

D.C. Campbell, M.D.

Tendon and Related Injuries

Treatment of Acquired Adult Planovalgus Deformities With Subtalar Fusion

Mangone PG, Fleming LL, Fleming SS, et al (Emory Univ, Atlanta, Ga; Marietta Orthopaedic and Sports Medicine, Ga; Blue Ridge Bone and Joint Clinic, Asheville, NC)
Clin Orthop 341:106–112, 1997   11–5

Introduction.—The goals of treatment of acquired planovalgus, posttraumatic, and inflammatory conditions of the hindfoot in adults are to reduce pain and restore function. The traditional surgical approaches have included triple arthrodesis and subtalar arthrodesis, and some recent reports favor the use of isolated subtalar arthrodesis. Although several studies have evaluated triple and subtalar arthrodesis in adults with chronic foot and ankle pain, they have used a wide range of different outcome measurement scales. This study evaluated the effectiveness of isolated subtalar arthrodesis for acquired adult planovalgus, posttraumatic, and inflammatory conditions of the foot and ankle.

Methods.—The retrospective study included 34 isolated subtalar arthrodeses performed in 32 adult patients over a 3-year period. The patients were 16 men and 16 women, average age 53. Fusion was achieved with a single large cannulated lag screw placed through the talar neck, usually via a sinus tarsi approach. The surgical results were evaluated using the American Orthopaedic Foot and Ankle Society rating system for the ankle and hindfoot. Subjective outcomes based on this scoring system were evaluated as well. Clinical and radiographic follow-up examinations were performed.

Findings.—The patients were followed up for an average of 31 months. Subjective results were available in 24 patients, producing an average score of 47, with a maximum of 60. Clinical data from 17 patients revealed an average objective score of 30, with a maximum of 34. On a combined subjective/objective scale, the average score was 77, with a maximum of 94. Improvement was rated as 100% for 42% of patients, 75% for 42%, and 50% for 16%. When asked whether they would undergo the surgery again, 83% of patients responded that they definitely would.

Conclusions.—For adult patients with painful and disabling inflammatory, posttraumatic, and planovalgus conditions of the hindfoot, subtalar arthrodesis is an effective treatment. The authors recommend isolated subtalar arthrodesis over triple arthrodesis in this situation. Their findings suggest that the American Orthopaedic Foot and Ankle Society ankle and hindfoot rating system corresponds well to the clinical results of subtalar arthrodesis.

▶ One of the most impressive features of this report is the incredibly large number of patients (32) operated on in the 3-year period for prior planovalgus deformity. Of value, the surgical technique is described in the report. Although a significant effort to provide objective measurements is presented, the most salient finding is that 83% indicated that they would definitely have the procedure again, placing the satisfaction rate at approximately this percent. The authors additionally demonstrate the objective that the American Orthopedic Foot and Ankle Society rating system reliably correlates to that of other measurements of clinical outcome and offers growing support for the use of these objective measurements in reporting results. While the selection criteria are not clearly documented, this paper also provides increasing support for limited arthrodesis. Indications are expanding for a number of conditions, including traumatic and inflammatory etiologies.

B.F. Morrey, M.D.

Functional Bracing for Rupture of the Achilles Tendon: Clinical Results and Analysis of Ground-Reaction Forces and Temporal Data

McComis GP, Nawoczenski DA, DeHaven KE, et al (Univ of Rochester, NY)
J Bone Joint Surg Am 79-A:1799–1808, 1997   11–6

Introduction.—Classic treatment for rupture of the Achilles tendon is surgery or immobilization in a plaster cast. Surgery is associated with a lower rate of repeat rupture but also increased risk of morbidity associated with an open procedure and higher cost. The functional brace is a nonoperative approach that allows immediate weight-bearing, active plantar flexion of the ankle, and limited dorsiflexion. Clinical and functional performance was compared in 15 patients who were managed with a functional bracing protocol for treatment of ruptured Achilles tendon and 15 age- and gender matched normal controls.

Methods.—Patients were studied for a mean of 31 months. Participants were given numeric scores (100-point scoring system) based on subjective responses to a questionnaire, clinical measurements of the range of motion of the ankle and the circumference of the calf, and results of the Thompson squeeze test and a single-limb heel-rise test. Ground-reaction forces and temporal data were evaluated during functional dynamic activities, including walking, a single-limb power hop, and a 30-second single-limb heel-rise endurance test.

Results.—Results of functional testing were: 3 excellent, 9 good, 2 fair, and 1 poor. The only significant difference between the treatment group and normal controls was an increase in passive dorsiflexion of the treated ankle. The increase in dorsiflexion was associated with vertical force output between the midstance and terminal-stance phases of gait. There were no significant between-group differences in kinetic or temporal variables measured during functional dynamic activities. Patients who had less peak vertical force and vertical height during the single-limb power hop test were likely to have poorer clinical scores.

Conclusion.—Nonoperative functional bracing may be a viable alternative to surgery or plaster casting for treatment of acute rupture of the Achilles tendon. This approach may reduce the time needed for rehabilitation, facilitate an early return to work and preinjury activities, and offer a feasible alternative for patients not able to undergo surgical intervention.

▶ This report provides consideration of a somewhat intermediate position from the 2 accepted treatment options for Achilles rupture, surgery and casting. The use of the functional bracing allows earlier weight-bearing and appears to lessen the likelihood of atrophy. Careful functional evaluation of gait including the use of the force-plate allows accurate determination of the functional recovery with this mode of treatment. The authors were not able to detect any significant difference between the treatment group and a control group during functional dynamic activities. The exact selection criteria are yet to be determined, however, it does appear as though the functional bracing may be an effective means of treating the acute Achilles tendon rupture without the concern of significant functional residual.

B.F. Morrey, M.D.

Primary Repair Without Augmentation for Early Neglected Achilles Tendon Ruptures in the Recreational Athlete
Porter DA, Mannarino FP, Snead D, et al (Methodist Sports Medicine Ctr, Indianapolis, Ind; Orthopedic Inst, Dayton, Ohio; Write State Univ, Dayton, Ohio; et al)
Foot Ankle Int 18:557–564, 1997   11–7

Background.—Rupture of the Achilles tendon is common in active, middle-aged adults. It has been reported that up to 25% of persons with this injury delay treatment, sometimes because of an incorrect diagnosis. The senior author has used primary repair without augmentation for neglected Achilles tendon ruptures for more than 7 years, with excellent results.

Methods.—The outcomes of 11 patients who had surgical repair of neglected Achilles tendon rupture were analyzed. Repair was done between 4 and 12 weeks after injury. The patients were between 20 and 60 years of age. The ankle was placed in a non–weight-bearing short leg cast in 20 degrees of plantarflexion for 3 weeks. All skin closures were primary, and minimal follow-up was 18 months.

Technique.—All patients had proximal release of the gastrocsoleus complex by blunt dissection of the adhesion and sharp release of the superficial posterior compartment medially and laterally. This release allowed apposition of the tendon ends without cutting muscle or tendon, and obliteration of the tendon gap. The 2 ends were imbricated using existing fibrinous scar as local reconstruction tissue after apposing the ruptured, freshened tendon ends. Three to 5 No. 0 Vicryl sutures were used to augment the repair (Fig 1).

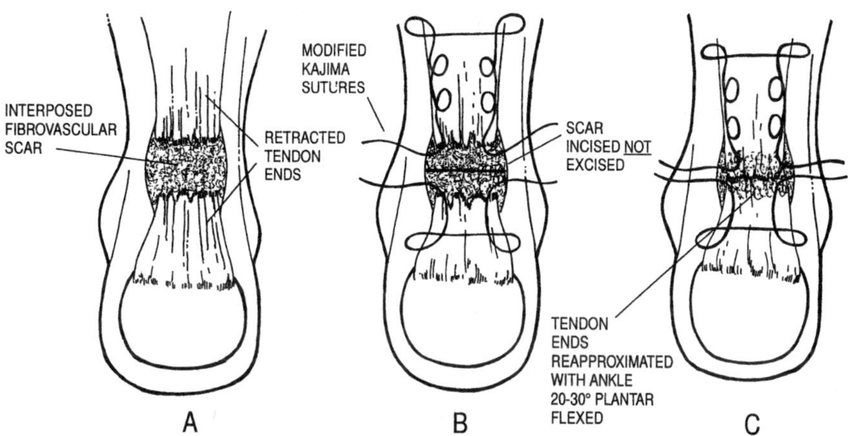

FIGURE 1.—Surgical technique for primary repair without augmentation for neglected Achilles tendon ruptures in recreational athletes. **A,** neglected tear with retracted tendon ends and interposed fibrovascular scar. **B,** neglected tear noting incising of fibrovascular scar and placement of modified Kajima sutures. **C,** neglected tear demonstrating reapproximation of tendon ends with imbrication of fibrovascular scar with ankle in 20 degrees to 30 degrees of plantarflexion. (Courtesy of Porter DA, Mannarino FP, Snead D, et al: Primary repair without augmentation for early neglected Achilles tendon ruptures in the recreational athlete. *Foot Ankle Int* 18[9]:557–564, 1997.)

Results.—At 3 weeks, weight-bearing as tolerated was begun in the short leg cast, and at 6 weeks, the cast was removed. Physical therapy consisted of range of motion exercises and closed kinetic exercises. These exercises progressed to functional exercises as swelling, strength, and pain permitted. At follow-up, there had been no subsequent ruptures. At a mean of 5.8 months, all patients had returned to their preinjury level of activity. The total range of motion was similar in the involved and uninvolved ankles. Plantarflexion loss of strength in the uninvolved ankle was similar to that seen after acute repair at all speeds tested. Pain scores as reported on a visual analogue scale were a mean of 0.7 during activities of daily living and 1.0 during sports activity. There were no skin sloughs, nerve damage, or other complications.

Conclusion.—This is the first report of primary repair without augmentation for neglected Achilles tendon rupture. This management approach and repair 4–12 weeks after injury produced excellent clinical and functional outcomes, a low rate of subsequent rupture, and a high rate of return to sports in these recreational athletes.

▶ The management of Achilles tendon ruptures in the subacute stage is controversial. Although it is recognized that the acute injury may be reliably fixed with a percutaneous technique by those familiar with such a procedure, the use of this approach for the neglected injury is much less recognized. The authors present an impressive experience with such a technique in a very selected population. Although it is not possible to specifically compare this technique with others described, it would seem that this experience justifies the position that a clinically acceptable outcome might be anticipated in those who have developed a facility with this technique.

B.F. Morrey, M.D.

Osseous Injuries

Stress Fracture of the Tibia After Arthrodesis of the Ankle or the Hindfoot

Lidor C, Ferris LR, Hall R, et al (Crystal Clinic, Akron, Ohio; Univ of California, Sacramento; Duke Univ, Durham, NC)
J Bone Joint Surg Am 79-A:558–564, 1997   11–8

Purpose.—Ankle or triple arthrodesis may be performed to treat for pain related to posttraumatic osteoarthrosis, degenerative osteoarthritis, rheumatoid arthritis, talar avascular necrosis, or various causes of deformity. A wide range of complications have been reported, but not stress

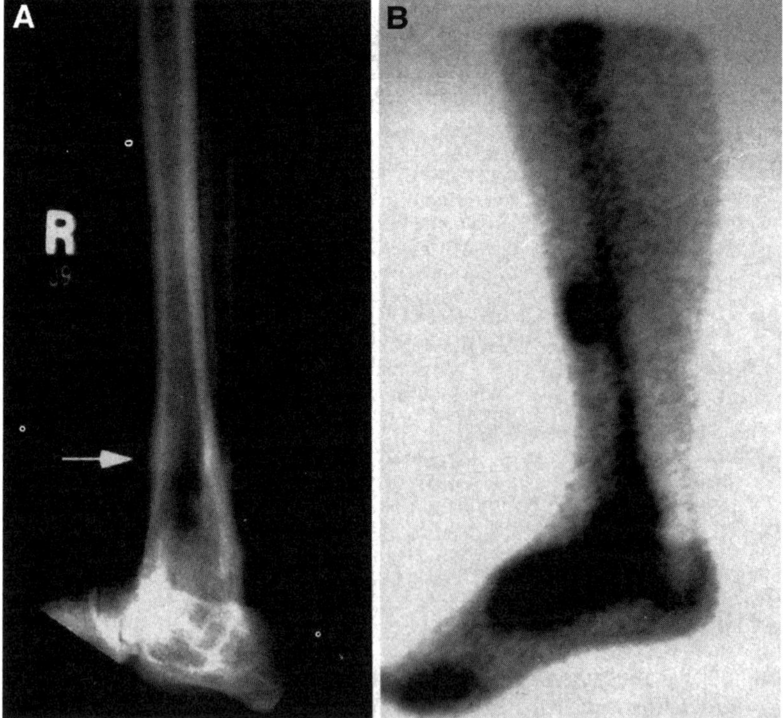

FIGURE 1.—Case 1. A 41-year-old woman had ankle and subtalar arthrodeses performed separately. Two stress fractures occurred in the distal aspect of the tibia. A, lateral radiograph made, with the patient standing, 3 years after the first arthrodesis. There was anterior cortical thickening in the distal third of the tibia (*arrow*). B, lateral technetium-99m bone scan, made 15 years after the first arthrodesis, showing increased uptake of the contrast medium at the junction of the distal and middle thirds of the tibia, indicating a second fracture. (Courtesy of Lidor C, Ferris JR, Hall R, et al: Stress fracture of the tibia after arthrodesis of the ankle or the hindfoot. *J Bone Joint Surg Am* 79-A:558–564, 1997.)

fracture. Thirteen patients with tibial or fibular stress fracture after arthrodesis of the ankle or foot are reported.

Patients.—The patients were identified from a series of 165 patients undergoing ankle or triple arthrodesis over a 14-year period. Follow-up detected tibial stress fracture in 12 patients and fibular stress fracture in 1. Mean time to identification of these fractures was 16 months; 11 were identified on the basis of symptoms and 2 on routine follow-up radiographs. In 2 patients a second stress fracture developed subsequently (Fig 1).

Outcomes.—In 11 patients, the stress fractures were treated nonoperatively and eventually healed. The exceptions were in a patient who required below-knee amputation to treat painful nonunion of a tibial fracture, and in another who required interlocking intramedullary nailing of a displaced fracture. Of the total 15 fractures, only 1 developed before the arthrodesis site had fused. When stress fracture occurred after ankle arthrodesis, it was always located in the middle and distal aspects or in the distal aspect of the tibia. Those following triple arthrodesis occurred in the distal aspect of the fibula or the medial malleolus. In 6 patients, the arthrodesis did not lead to correct alignment or deformity. However, stress fractures could occur even in the presence of optimal alignment.

Conclusions.—Stress fracture is a potential complication after ankle or triple arthrodesis. Such fractures can occur months or even years after solid fusion of the arthrodesis site, and should be considered in any patient with pain developing after arthrodesis. Nonoperative treatment is successful in most cases, but recurrent stress fractures can still develop later.

▶ This information is of particular value in demonstrating the existence of the entity and appropriately emphasizes the need to consider this in the patient with continued or increasing pain after a solid arthrodesis of the ankle or hindfoot. Like most stress fractures of the lower extremity, displacement is uncommon; however, because of the lack of compensatory motion distal to the stress fracture, and since the insufficiency fracture typically occurred with relatively little activity, the etiology may be implicated as primarily associated with the lack of compensatory motion. This would suggest that the traditional "conservative" treatment may not be sufficient, and in fact this was demonstrated by these authors who noted 2 of 12 patients required surgery, 1 of whom even went to amputation. The points worth emphasizing therefore are a high level of suspicion for the diagnosis in this clinical setting and awareness that in some instances a displacement can occur, resulting in significant and problematic treatment with an unpredictable outcome of surgery.

B.F. Morrey, M.D.

Preoperative and Postoperative Evaluation of Intra-Articular Fractures of the Calcaneus Based on Computed Tomography Scanning

Song KS, Kang CH, Min BW, et al (Keimyung Univ, Daegu, Korea)
J Orthop Trauma 11:435–440, 1997   11–9

Background.—Calcaneal fractures are the most common tarsal bone fracture and among the most difficult to treat. Delineating the fracture line is difficult, and the anatomy is complex. Opinions on the outcomes of such fractures vary widely. The relationship between postoperative congruency of the articular surface of posterior facet and clinical results through CT scanning was determined.

Methods.—Twenty-five patients with 29 displaced fractures were included in the prospective analysis. All patients underwent open reduction and internal fixation without bone grafting. Computed tomography scans were obtained before and after surgery.

Findings.—The reduction state of the more comminuted fractures was worse after surgery, as evidenced by preoperative and postoperative CT scans. Eighty-eight percent of the fractures with anatomical reduction and 87% with nearly anatomical reduction had excellent or good clinical outcomes. By contrast, none of the fractures with an approximate reduction had an excellent outcome (Table 2).

Conclusion.—Clinicians generally believe that most displaced fractures of the calcaneus, especially with comminution, are very difficult to reduce anatomically in a blind closed technique. These findings suggest that the more precise open reduction method yields better results. Excellent or good clinical results can be expected when the postoperative displacement of the posterior facet of the subtalar joint is less than 2 mm.

▶ This report is from a very active trauma center seeing over 50 calcaneal fractures in a 2-year period. The high percentage of patients lost to follow-up is not uncommon with this type of study. Although a number of reduction and fixation techniques were used, the objective rating scale provides a reasonable standard for comparing the overall results. The classification of pain from the CT assessment appears to be a worthwhile prognostic tool.

B.F. Morrey, M.D.

TABLE 2.—Preoperative CT Classification and Clinical Results

	Excellent	Good	Fair	Poor
Type I	1	0	0	0
Type II	5	14	2	0
Type III	0	3	2	0
Type IV	0	0	1	1

(Courtesy of Song KS, Kang CH, Min BW, et al: Preoperative and postoperative evaluation of intra-articular fractures of the calcaneus based on computed tomography scanning. *J Orthop Trauma* 11:435–440, 1997.)

Fractures of the Calcaneus: Open Reduction and Internal Fixation From the Medial Side. A 21-Year Prospective Study
Burdeaux BD Jr (Baylor College of Medicine, Houston; Twelve Oaks Hosp, Houston)
Foot Ankle Int 18:685–692, 1997   11–10

Introduction.—Most open reductions for treatment of intra-articular fractures of the calcaneus are performed from the lateral side. Some are done from both the lateral and medial sides. Reported are results of a modified McReynolds medial approach.

Methods.—Sixty-one patients with displaced fractures of the calcaneus underwent a modified medial approach technique for fracture reduction. Fifty-three patients were followed for a mean of 4.4 years (range, 1–21 years).

Modified Surgical Technique.—A 5-cm incision was made posterior to the neurovascular bundle and a single 4-mm threaded pin was passed longitudinally through the tuberosity fragment and into the sustentacular fragment. This produces a stable fixation and the need for a large incision, and retraction of the neurovascular bundle is avoided.

Results.—Reduction of depressed posterior facet fragments was done from the medial side in 77% (47 fractures) of patients, with occasional assistance from fluoroscopy. Twenty-three percent (14) of fractures needed supplemental lateral incision. At follow-up, there were 49 (80.3%) successful surgeries and 12 (19.7%) unsuccessful surgeries. The mean American Orthopedic Foot & Ankle Society Scoring System score was high (94.7). Patients returned to work after an average of 4.9 months.

Conclusion.—The modified medial approach technique may be used for all displaced fractures of the calcaneus. A stable reduction is achieved when the medial wall of the calcaneus is restored. This approach allows early weight bearing at 4 weeks after surgery.

▶ This is a large series of 61 displaced intra-articular calcaneal fractures which were treated by 1 surgeon using a medial approach similar to the McReynolds technique. The author is an expert at this operation, and there are few reports of the results of the medial approach to calcaneus fractures that have been published. Most of the patients were located, and the average follow-up was 4 years. There was an effort to correlate the clinical results with the fracture type. Interestingly, two thirds of the patients had more than 50% movement of the subtalar joint and one third had less than 50%. More than one third of the patients continued to have pain, but in spite of this, 87% were satisfied. One quarter of the patients had less than anatomic reduction of the fracture. Surprisingly, only 6 patients had any evidence of subtalar arthritis. The overall clinical results were also quite favorable toward 46 of the 61 patients that had good or excellent results. The report suggested that, in the author's hands, the McReynolds approach to open reduction and internal fixation of intra-articular calcaneus fractures had successful clinical and radiologic results.

H.B. Kitaoka, M.D.

Biomechanical Study of Stress in the Fifth Metatarsal

Arangio GA, Xiao D, Salathe EP (Lehigh Valley Hosp, Allentown, Pa; Lehigh Univ, Bethlehem, Pa)
Clin Biomech 12:160–164, 1997   11–11

Background.—Stress fractures are a major cause of foot injury. Proximal fifth metatarsal stress fractures are among the most common. To better understand the causes of fractures to this bone, stress throughout the fifth metatarsal was assessed under various loading conditions.

Methods and Findings.—Cross-sections of bone were created by slicing a mould containing bone at various intervals. Analytic expressions describing each cross-section were then obtained by fitting a Fourier series to points along the boundary. The maximum stress in the fifth metatarsal resulted from an oblique load. This stress had a lower magnitude than would occur in an individual during normal walking.

Conclusions.—The magnitude of the stress found in the current study was submaximal. Thus, these findings support the clinical observation that the diaphyseal fracture is a stress fracture.

▶ The authors provide a methodology of analyzing stress distribution across the fifth metatarsal both in compression and tension and then correlate this with the loading pattern during gait. The conclusions are relevant in that the loading of the fifth metatarsal that occurs during inversion may predispose to the insufficiency fracture. This being the case, methods to treat the lesion or even prevent its occurrence would be directed principally at compensating for the inversion loading pattern, such as with a slight medial sole wedge.

B.F. Morrey, M.D.

Arthritis/Arthrodesis

A Prospective Study of Prognostic Factors Concerning the Outcome of Arthroscopic Surgery for Anterior Ankle Impingement

van Dijk CN, Tol JL, Verheyen CCPM (Academic Med Ctr, Amsterdam)
Am J Sports Med 25:737–745, 1997   11–12

Introduction.—The causes of anterior ankle pain are soft tissue and bony obstruction. Bony obstruction may be caused by osteoarthritic changes or spurs from repetitive minor trauma, commonly seen in athletes. Painful anterior ankle bone spurs may be classified according to their size and location. Sixty-two consecutive patients with painful, limited dorsi-

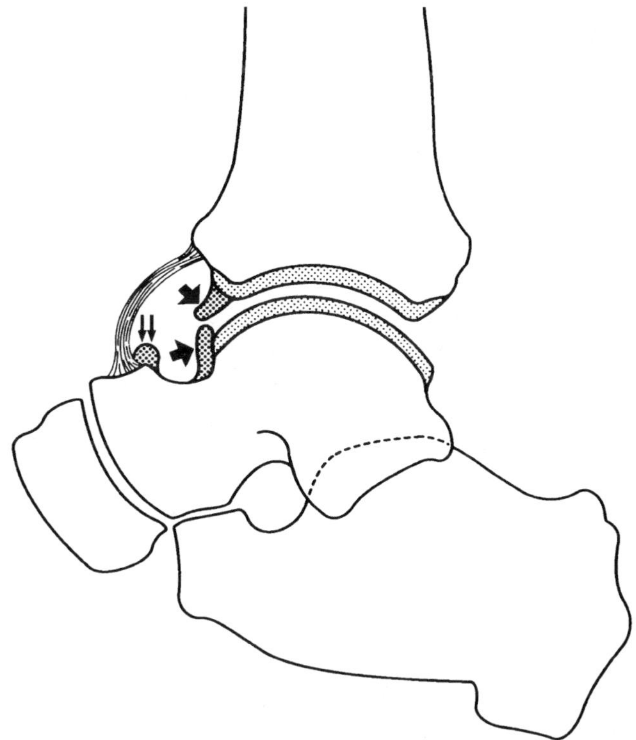

FIGURE 6.—Anatomic location of the anterior joint capsule. Note that the common location of the osteophytes (*arrows*) is well within the capsule. (Courtesy of van Dijk CN, Tol JL, Verheyen CCPM: A prospective study of prognostic factors concerning the outcome of arthroscopic surgery for anterior ankle impingement. *Am J Sports Med* 25:737–745, 1997.)

flexion of the ankle refractory to nonoperative treatment were evaluated to define prognostic factors for outcome of arthroscopic surgery for anterior ankle impingement.

Methods.—Forty-two males and 20 females (average age, 31 years) with anterior ankle impingement underwent arthroscopic surgery. Preoperative radiographs were scored using osteoarthritic and impingement classification systems. Patients were evaluated at baseline and 4 months and 1 and 2 years after surgery.

Results.—The degree of osteoarthritic changes was a better prognostic factor for arthroscopic surgical outcome than were size and location of spurs. At 2 year follow-up, 73% of patients had excellent or good results. Fifty percent and 90%, respectively, of patients with and without joint space narrowing had significantly better scores 2 years postoperatively than preoperatively in pain, swelling, ability to work, and engagement in sports. Patients with less than 2 years of ankle pain before surgery and spurs located anteromedially were more pleased with their surgical results than were patients with longer periods of preoperative pain and spurs located anterolaterally (Fig 6).

Conclusion.—The degree of osteoarthritic changes is a good prognostic factor for outcome of arthroscopic surgery for anterior ankle impingement. Outcome was less desirable in patients with joint space narrowing, a 2 year or longer history of ankle pain, an anteromedial versus anterolateral impingement, or a combination of these factors.

▶ This is a prospective study of prognostic factors concerning outcome of arthroscopic surgery for anterior ankle impingement. The authors reported a large series of patients who underwent arthroscopic surgery for anterior ankle impingement and who had failed nonoperative treatment. Of the 62 patients, the best clinical results were achieved in patients who had a spur without joint space narrowing. The results also suggested that patients who had symptoms less than two years before surgery had greater satisfaction and those who had spurs anteromedially had a greater satisfaction. Those who had longer periods of preoperative pain or spurs anterolaterally had lower satisfaction rates. This report is consistent with other publications concerning arthroscopic treatment for ankle impingement. It provides useful information regarding prognostic factors for surgery for anterior ankle impingement in a large group of critically-studied patients.

H.B. Kitaoka, M.D.

Arthroscopic Treatment of Anterior Ankle Impingement

Branca A, Di Palma L, Bucca C, et al (Sondalo Hosp, Italy)
Foot Ankle Int 18:418–423, 1997   11–13

Purpose.—Ankle impingement is a common cause of anterior ankle pain, particularly among athletes whose sport involves repeated stress on the ankle in dorsiflexion. Treatment is usually surgical. With the availability of ankle arthroscopy, less invasive techniques for the treatment of anterior ankle impingement have been described. A 7-year experience with arthroscopic management of anterior ankle impingement is reported.

Patients.—The experience included 58 patients: 37 men and 21 women, mean age 28.5. All underwent tibiotalar arthroscopy after failure of nonsurgical treatment of ankle impingement. Twenty-seven patients were athletes whose sports involved abnormal stresses on the ankle, most frequently cross-country skiers and soccer players. Preoperatively, according to a modified McGuire scoring system, 50 cases were rated as poor and 8 as fair. Therapeutic arthroscopy included resection of adhesions, cartilage shaving, and removal of impinging bone using powered instruments, curettes, or small osteotomes. The patients were followed up for a mean of 21.5 months.

Outcomes.—After arthroscopic treatment, McGuire ratings were good in 37 patients, fair in 13, and poor in 8. When lateral radiographs were graded according to the classification of Scranton and McDermott, 15

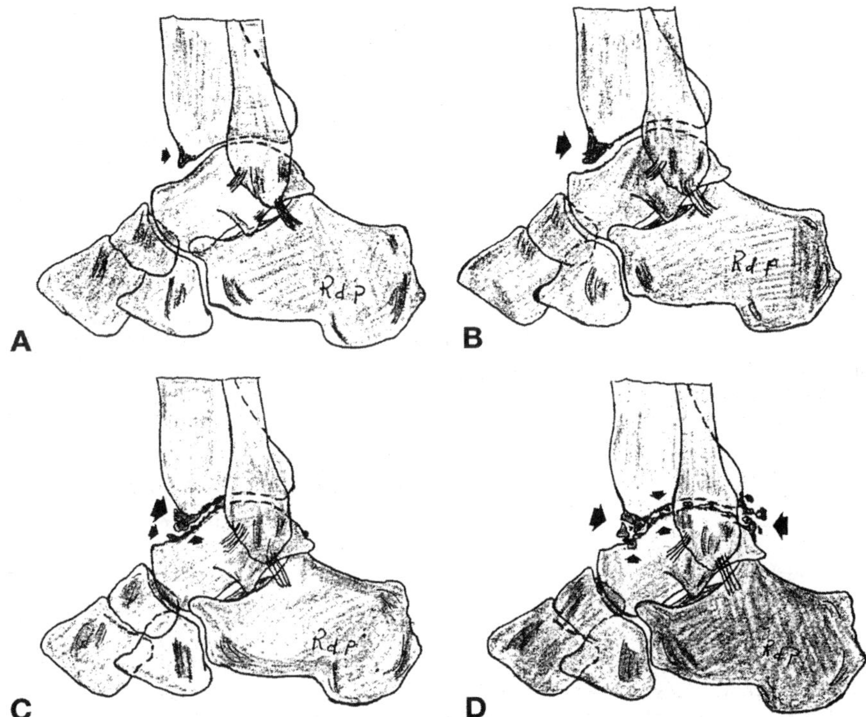

FIGURE 1.—McDermott's radiological classification. (Courtesy of Branca A, Di Palma L, Bucca C, et al: Arthroscopic treatment of anterior ankle impingement. *Foot Ankle Int* 18[7]:418–423, 1997.)

cases were stage I (Fig 1, A), 23 stage II (Fig 1, B), 13 stage III (Fig 1, C), and 7 stage IV (Fig 1, D). There were no neurovascular or infectious complications. Four patients with stage III and IV abnormalities had recurrent impingement. Thirteen of the 27 athletes were able to return to their previous level of sports competition.

Conclusions.—Arthroscopy is a viable option for the treatment of anterior ankle impingement. The results depend on the radiologic stage of the abnormality, early diagnosis, and the presence of widespread cartilage damage. Even in severe cases, however, arthroscopy can serve a useful role in delaying the need for definitive arthrodesis.

▶ This review does provide an extensive experience with anterior ankle impingement treated arthroscopically. Unfortunately, the surveillance is relatively limited, averaging less than 2 years. Nonetheless, the authors document the expectation that reliable relief of pain may be observed in approximately 80% of instances. One concern with this, as with any arthroscopic procedure in this type of setting, is the long-term effectiveness of the procedure. Nonetheless, the relatively low complication rate and the low morbidity rate justifies its use in the selected patient. The technique does require distraction of the joint, but if this is carried out the procedure is relatively straightforward for an experienced arthroscopist.

B.F. Morrey, M.D.

Subtalar Distraction Bone Block Fusion: An Assessment of Outcome
Bednarz PA, Beals TC, Manoli A II (Wayne State Univ, Detroit; Univ of Utah, Salt Lake City; Univ of South Alabama, Mobile)
Foot Ankle Int 18:785–791, 1997   11–14

Introduction.—Subtalar distraction bone block arthrodesis may be performed in patients with painful subtalar arthrosis that has not responded to conservative management. Previous studies have documented the results of this approach, but have not used a standard outcome instrument to document the intermediate-term improvement. An experience with subtalar distraction bone block arthrodesis in 28 patients is reported.

Methods.—The experience included 29 feet with subtalar deformities associated with symptomatic arthrosis refractory to nonoperative treatment. The patients were 18 men and 10 women, mean age 44. Arthrodesis was performed on average 34 months after the injury. The arthrosis followed traumatic injury in 27 feet: os calcis fracture in 19, subtalar dislocation in 5, and talar fracture in 3.

Subtalar distraction bone block fusion was performed according to the technique of Carr et al. At an average postoperative follow-up of 33 months, the results were assessed with use of the American Orthopaedic Foot and Ankle Society (AOFAS) Ankle-Hindfoot Scale score. In an additional analysis, the possible link between subtalar nonunion and smoking was assessed.

Results.—With subtalar distraction bone block fusion, the mean AOFAS Ankle-Hindfoot Scale score improved from 25 to 75. All but 1 patient was satisfied with the results, and 64% of patients returned to full-time or part-time work. On standing lateral radiographs, hindfoot height on average by 8 mm, lateral talocalcaneal angle by 9 degrees, and lateral talar declination by 11 degrees. There were 4 cases of nonunion, 2 of varus malunion, 1 of metatarsal stress fracture, and 1 of medial plantar nerve paresthesia. The rate of nonunion in smokers was 29%, whereas union occurred in all patients who did not smoke.

Conclusions.—Subtalar distraction bone block fusion produces good results in patients with refractory subtalar arthrosis. The results are documented by a standard outcome instrument, as well as by subjective measures. The procedure is technically difficult and demands strict attention to detail. More study is needed to confirm the relatively high nonunion rate among patients who smoke.

▶ Increasing focus is being applied to limited fusions about the foot and ankle. This report is of value for 2 reasons. First, it documents an interposition fusion technique that would have a tendency to correct angular deformities, particularly valgus hindfoot angulation. Second, it documents a relatively short-term follow-up of a moderately large series of patients with a fairly homogeneous diagnosis and treatment. As pointed out by the authors, an additional characteristic is that this report uses an established instrument to evaluate outcome. The satisfaction rate (96%) is quite high and somewhat surprising, given the nature of the soft tissue injuries that might be anticipated with this patient sample. It is less surprising that the 4 nonunions were associated with patients who smoked, once again implicating this as a major problem in reconstructive procedures requiring osseous integration. One deficiency of this report is the lack of a clear definition of the hindfoot deformity before and after surgery. Nonetheless, this does provide worthwhile information regarding this particular treatment modality for posttraumatic hindfoot arthrosis.

B.F. Morrey, M.D.

Subtalar Arthrodesis With Internal Compression for Post-traumatic Arthritis

Dahm DL, Kitaoka HB (Mayo Clinic and Found, Rochester, Minn)
J Bone Joint Surg Br 80-B:134–138, 1998   11–15

Background.—Hindfoot arthrodesis is the treatment of choice for symptomatic subtalar arthritis when nonoperative management has failed. Although triple arthrodesis is the standard in this situation, complications may lead some surgeons to consider subtalar arthrodesis. An experience of subtalar arthrodesis with internal compression in 24 patients with posttraumatic arthritis is reported.

Patients.—Over a 4-year period, subtalar arthrodesis with internal compression was performed in 25 feet of 24 patients with posttraumatic subtalar arthritis. The patients were 15 men and 9 women, mean age 43. The most common precipitating injury was calcaneal fracture; the mean time to arthrodesis was 4 years. In each case, the pain of subtalar arthritis had failed to respond to various conservative treatments. Subtalar arthrodesis was performed through a standard lateral hindfoot incision over the sinus tarsi (Fig 1). All feet were managed with a single compression screw, and 10 with iliac crest bone grafting.

Outcomes.—Subtalar arthrodesis produced union in 96% of cases. The clinical results were graded as excellent in 10 feet (Fig 2, D), good in 7, fair in 6, and poor in 2. According to the Angus and Cowell score, the results were good in 19 feet, fair in 4, and poor in 2 (1 case of nonunion and 1 of reflex sympathetic dystrophy). The patients reported satisfaction in 18 cases, satisfaction with reservations in 4, and dissatisfaction in 3. For feet without preexisting degenerative changes in the ankle or midfoot, no arthritis developed in these joints.

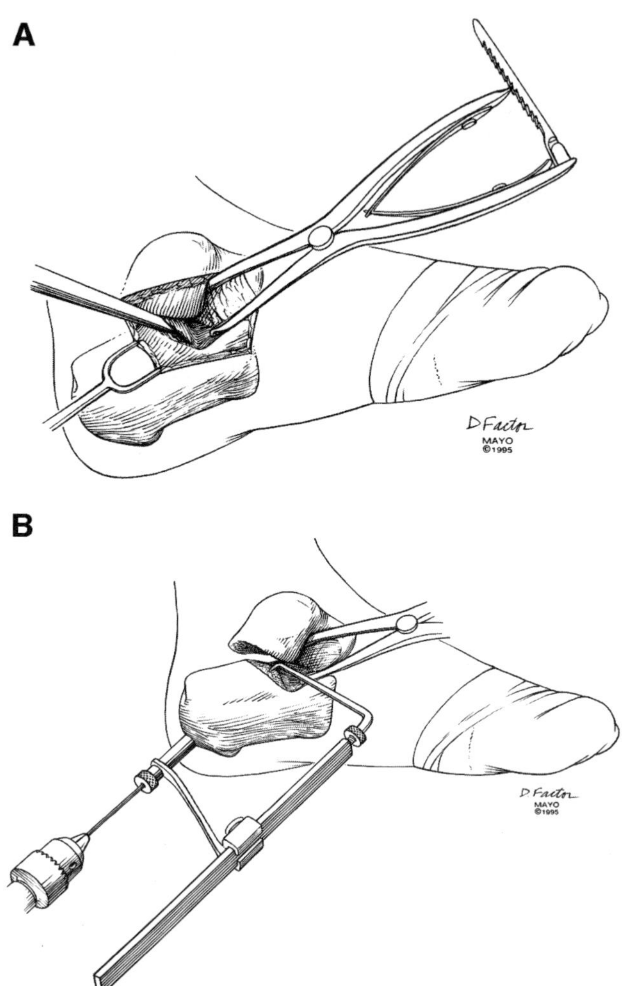

FIGURE 1.—Diagram of the operative procedure. **A,** through a lateral hindfoot incision, remnants of articular cartilage and subchondral bone are removed from the subtalar joint, with preservation of the bony contour. There is a laminar spreader in the sinus tarsi. **B,** using a combined aiming device, a guide pin is introduced through an incision in the heel. The aiming device is removed, and the pin is advanced across the subtalar joint, followed by a cannulated drill and screw. (Reprinted by permission of the Mayo Foundation, from Dahm DL, Kitaoka HB: Subtalar arthrodesis with internal compression for posttraumatic arthritis. *J Bone Joint Surg Br* 80-B:134–138, 1998.)

Conclusions.—The authors report good results with isolated subtalar arthrodesis with internal compression for feet with posttraumatic subtalar arthritis. This procedure offers a high rate of union, a low complication rate, and few problems with progressive arthritis in adjacent joints. Iliac crest bone grafting, and its attendant complications, can be averted in many patients.

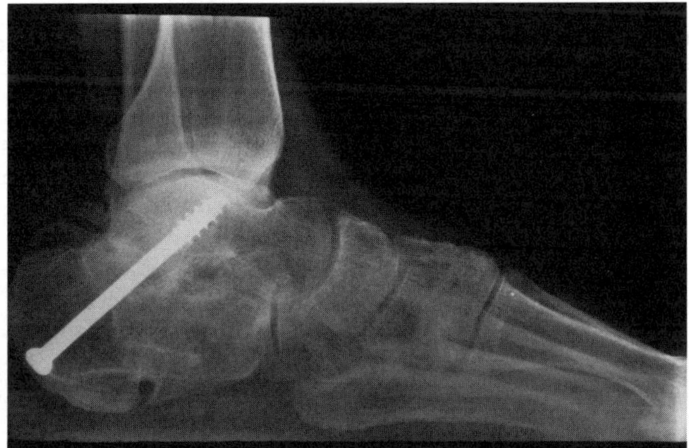

FIGURE 2, D.—Radiograph of a 49-year-old man after calcaneal fracture. Lateral view 3 years after operation. The result is excellent, with improved alignment, no impingement, and a normal joint space. (Reprinted by permission of the Mayo Foundation, from Dahm DL, Kitaoka HB: Subtalar arthrodesis with internal compression for post-traumatic arthritis. *J Bone Joint Surg Br* 80-B:134–138, 1998.)

▶ This valuable contribution provides insights with regard to a surgical technique that, as described, has resulted in a very high fusion rate exceeding 95%. This is of particular value since there is very little in the literature regarding isolated subtalar arthrodesis, and the rationale as explained by the authors is very sound, that is, avoiding some of the functional limitations of a triple arthrodesis. The authors also very carefully document the fact that, depending on whether or not objective or subjective schedules are emphasized, the satisfactory results are only 67% to 75%. This is relatively low for an elective reconstructive procedure. Thus, although the complication rate is very acceptable, there is a significant question referable to the selection factors and the reasons for this somewhat disappointing overall patient satisfaction rate. It may well be that these patients were so disabled that this might be considered very acceptable, however, the authors do not clearly state the inclusion criteria. The strength, therefore, in this contribution is the documentation of a high fusion rate with a straightforward technique not typically requiring supplemental bone grafting. The questions that remain to be answered is the long-term impact on the associated joint, since the mean follow-up was only 4 years. It does appear as though hindfoot alignment was not severely altered preoperatively, and the postoperative values were also quite acceptable, averaging 8 degrees of valgus.

B.F. Morrey, M.D.

Salvage of Pseudoarthrosis After Tibiotalar Arthrodesis

Levine SE, Myerson MS, Lucas P, et al (Union Mem Hosp, Baltimore, Md)
Foot Ankle Int 18:580–585, 1997   11–16

Background.—Treatment for pseudoarthrosis after ankle arthrodesis has not been well documented. An experience with revision of pseudoarthrosis of ankle arthrodesis in patients with no complicating features of systemic disease, infection, or avascular necrosis was reported.

Methods and Findings.—Twenty-three patients underwent revision arthrodesis 4 months to 17 years after the initial unsuccessful procedure. Fourteen had isolated revision tibiotalar arthrodesis and 9 had an additional hindfoot arthrodesis at the time of the procedure. When possible, rigid internal fixation with screws was performed. An external fixator was used in patients with poor bone quality. In 14 patients with bone loss, autogenous bone grafting was done. Union was successful in 21 of the patients, occurring at 6–48 weeks (mean, 14 weeks). The remaining 2 patients had persistent nonunion; it produced no symptoms in 1 patient and symptomatic subtalar arthritis in the other. In 2 patients, arthrodesis was successful but pain persisted from reflex sympathetic dystrophy. Overall, 19 patients were satisfied with the outcomes of surgery.

Conclusion.—Revision arthrodesis for tibiotalar pseudoarthrosis is beneficial. Surgeons must try to achieve bone-to-bone apposition and avoid large interposition grafts. Autologous bone graft is placed in defects remaining between the bleeding bone surfaces. Positioning the foot plantigrade and performing simultaneous arthrodesis of any symptomatic arthritic joints should produce satisfactory outcomes.

▶ This is yet another contribution to the literature presented over the last several years in which the issue of a reoperation for failed ankle arthrodesis is discussed. These authors confirm previous experience, including that reported from our institution, that failure is largely caused by infection and inadequacy in fixation. Addressing these 2 features can result in a high probability of success with the revision operation. In this instance, approximately 90% of the patients were satisfied with the procedure.

It is, however, worthy of note that some patients, even after obtaining a solid union with the additional surgery, will have persistent pain and discomfort, because of either the underlying disease or the multiple procedures. We currently also favor the multiple cancellous screw fixation. It has been successful, in our experience, when this mode of fixation can be used.

B.F. Morrey, M.D.

Revision

An Anatomical Basis for the Degree of Displacement of the Distal Chevron Osteotomy in the Treatment of Hallux Valgus

Badwey TM, Dutkowsky JP, Graves SC, et al (Univ of Missouri—Kansas City; Univ of Tennessee, Memphis; Inst of Bone and Joint Disorders, Phoenix, Ariz)

Foot Ankle Int 18:213–215, 1997   11–17

Background.—The chevron distal metatarsal osteotomy is recommended for patients with symptomatic hallux valgus and an intermetatarsal 1 to 2 angle of 15 degrees or less. This study was performed to determine the maximal amount of lateral shift of the capital fragment, which would equal 50% of the metatarsal shaft width.

Methods.—The first metatarsal was obtained from 72 cadavers. A point was located on the medial surface of the metatarsal 15 mm from the osteochondral junction. A measurement was taken at this point, perpendicular to the metatarsal shaft, and recorded as the metatarsal width. The average metatarsal width was calculated separately for males and females.

Results.—The mean male metatarsal width was 15.3 mm, with a range of 13–18 mm. The mean female metatarsal width was 14.5 mm, with a range of 11–18 mm. This difference was statistically significant. There was no significant difference between left and right side. The width of the metatarsal was independent of age. The maximal amount of lateral displacement possible when performing a chevron osteotomy to displace the capital fragment 50% of its diameter was calculated to be 6 mm in males and 5 mm in females, with a confidence level of 97.5%.

Conclusions.—The results of this study indicate that if lateral displacement of more than 6 mm in males or 5 mm in females is necessary to correct the metatarsus primus valgus deformity, then alternative approaches to the chevron osteotomy should be considered.

▶ This study is of value giving the expected anatomic limitations to displacement of the distal portion of the Chevron osteotomy. It is documented that the majority of patients do allow 50% translation of the diameter which is equivalent to 5–6 mm. This simple observation is of use in determining the limits of potential correction in preoperative planning.

B.F. Morrey, M.D.

Fixation With Bioabsorbable Pins in Chevron Bunionectomy

Gill LH, Martin DF, Coumas JM, et al (Miller Orthopaedic Clinic, Charlotte, NC)

J Bone Joint Surg Am 79-A:1510–1518, 1997   11–18

Objective.—Fixation of distal chevron bunionectomy with Kirschner wires increased stability but can cause pain and lead to infection. Fixation with bioabsorbable pins reduces the discomfort and infection risk of wires but can lead to osteolysis and increased failure because the implants are weaker. The comparative risks associated with fixation with a bioabsorbable pin and those associated with Kirschner wires in chevron bunionectomy were evaluated.

Methods.—Chevron bunionectomies were performed on 114 patients (144 feet) who had fixation with Kirschner wires and 59 patients (74 feet) who had fixation with bioabsorbable (poly-p-dioxanone) pins. Outcome was evaluated radiographically.

> *Technique.*—A Y-shaped incision is made into the joint capsule and the medial prominence is exposed. The medial exostosis is removed, and a chevron-shaped osteotomy is constructed in the metatarsal neck with a 35-degree angle at the apex of the proximal fragment. The fragment is fixed in place with 2 pins. The proximal bone fragment is shaved flush, and the medial aspect of the capsule is shortened and repaired to correct the hallux valgus. Fixation is accomplished with two 0.062-inch stainless-steel Kirschner wires or one 1.3-mm bioabsorbable pins.

Results.—The prevalence of osteolysis and complications were similar in both groups. None of the feet fixed with bioabsorbable pins showed formation of a sinus.

Conclusions.—Bioabsorbable implants are less expensive and more comfortable than Kirschner wires and related hardware. The implants provide a safe and reliable fixation method for a distal chevron bunionectomy that does not increase the risk of osteolysis or sinus formation.

▶ Although most surgeons recognize the reaction that can occur with bioabsorbable pins, this has not been shown to be the case or an issue with use of poly-p-dioxanone pins in this study. This study is of particular value in that it did use a stainless-steel Kirschner wire as control. The experience supports the use of either mode of fixation, which would be determined based on cost and surgeon preference.

B.F. Morrey, M.D.

The Role of Cheilectomy in the Treatment of Hallux Rigidus

Mackay DC, Blyth M, Rhymaszewski LA (Stobhill Hosp, Glasgow, Scotland)
J Foot Ankle Surg 36:337–340, 1997   11–19

Background.—The role of cheilectomy in the treatment of Regnauld's grade 2 hallux rigidus has not been clearly defined. The outcomes of cheilectomy were assessed against the radiologic grade of disease in 1 practice.

Methods.—Thirty-nine patients with grades 1, 2, or 3 hallux rigidus were assessed at a mean of 3.8 years after cheilectomy. Pain, activity level, footwear problems, tiptoe walking, and metatarsophalangeal joint range of motion were documented before and after surgery.

Findings.—Patients with all grades of hallux rigidus had significant improvement in pain, activity level, tiptoe walking, and range of motion. Footwear selection was also improved significantly in patients with grades 1 and 2 hallux rigidus, although not in those with grade 3 disease.

Conclusion.—These outcomes compare favorably with previously reported results. Cheilectomy outcomes were considered satisfactory in 94% of the patients with grade 1 disease, in 100% with grade 2 disease, and in 66% with grade 3 disease.

▶ The attractiveness of a simple procedure, such as cheilectomy, justifies an analysis of its outcome. A number of studies have discussed simple cheilectomy, with the major point of contention being the improvement to be anticipated as a function of the severity of involvement. Although there is general, if not universal, agreement that simple cheilectomy is effective for early (grade 1) changes and to be discouraged in severe (grade 3) changes, this paper attempts to address the issue of cheilectomy in the grade 2 intermediate stage. This, unfortunately, is a retrospective study; nonetheless, the numbers presented are equal to or greater than most other such reports in the literature.

Although I do not believe this report can be considered conclusive, it does tend to justify and document the value of the simple cheilectomy, even in those with grade 2 involvement. The surgical technique is detailed, and it is possible that the specifics of this surgical technique account for the greater number of good results in type 2 disease than have been previously reported. Regardless of this, the authors have adequately demonstrated that a good result can be expected with this type of problem and, thus, do contribute to the decision-making process.

B.F. Morrey, M.D.

Hallux Valgus in the Elderly: Metatarsophalangeal Arthrodesis of the First Ray
Tourné Y, Saragaglia D, Zattara A, et al (Hôpital Sud, Grenoble, France)
Foot Ankle Int 18:195–198, 1997   11–20

Objective.—Successful metatarsophalangeal (MTP) arthrodesis of the great toe eliminates pain on weight-bearing and results in stable fixation. There is no general agreement on the preferred angle of fixation that produces the highest biomechanical and functional success. An experience with hallux valgus was presented.

Methods.—Between May 1982 and October 1994, 42 arthrodesis procedures were performed in 33 patients (3 men), aged 57–78 years. Average preoperative hallux valgus, intermetatarsal, and metatarsal spread angles were 43, 15, and 33 degrees, respectively. A silicone elastomer ball-shaped spacer was used for 20 MTP dislocations or subluxations and an interphalangeal arthroplasty fixed with temporary pins for 13 hammertoes. Postoperative nerve blocks were used. Flat-footed weight-bearing in a special shoe was permitted on the first postoperative day. Regular walking was not permitted until day 45. Walking with heeled shoes was allowed at 3 months.

Results.—Complications included 1 inflammatory scar, 1 deep venous thrombosis, and 1 nonhemorrhagic gastritis. Data were available on 41 arthrodeses. Bone consolidation occurred an average of 60 days after surgery. Interphalangeal joint arthritis developed in 2 patients. Valgus angle was between 10 and 20 degrees in 76% of toes, and dorsiflexion angle ranged from 25 to 35 degrees in 80% of toes. Postoperatively, there was a significant decrease in hallux valgus angle from 43 to 17 degrees, in the intermetatarsal angle from 15 to 11 degrees, and in the degree of metatarsal spread from 33 to 28 degrees. Four (10%) patients had first ray pain. Gait was normal in 35 patients, whereas 3 patients had restrictions on uneven surfaces, and 3 had difficulties on flat surfaces. Patients were very satisfied in 28 cases, satisfied in 11, and dissatisfied in 2. Overall results, including effects on the first ray, functional results, and patient satisfaction were excellent in 25 toes, good in 13, fair in 1, and poor in 2. Surgical results were good or excellent in 93% of toes.

Conclusions.—First ray arthrodesis in elderly patients with moderate-to-severe-hallux valgus provides good surgical and functional results. The stability of the first ray is improved and patient satisfaction is high.

▶ Although the management of bunion deformity has numerous options, most attempt to salvage the joint and still allow motion at the MTP joint or at the resected joint. Whereas fusion is a well-recognized option, limited long-term experience with a large patient sample has been reported. The authors outline the indications for the use of this procedure in their practice, which includes salvage of failed previous procedures. The sliding rating scale resulted in over 90% being considered satisfactory, with surveillance ranging from 2 to 15 years. Both intramedullary cancellous screw and a 4-hole dynamic compression plate were the treatment of choice and appeared to be effective.

B.F. Morrey, M.D.

Miscellaneous

Clinical Characteristics and Outcome in 223 Diabetic Patients With Deep Foot Infections
Eneroth M, Apelqvist J, Stenström A (Univ Hosp, Lund, Sweden)
Foot Ankle Int 18:716–722, 1997   11–21

Objective.—Foot infections in diabetic patients result in amputation rates of 25% to 50%. Clinical characteristics and outcome prospectively evaluated in consecutive diabetic patients with deep foot infections treated by a multidisciplinary foot care team were presented.

Methods.—Laboratory tests were performed at baseline and at least every 3 months thereafter until healing in 223 diabetic patients (61% males), age 28–94, with a primary deep foot infection. The mean duration of diabetes was 19 years; 96% of patients had peripheral neuropathy, 49% had retinopathy, 36% had nephropathy, 50% had hypertension, 28% has ischemic heart disease, 16% had congestive heart failure, and 18% had had a cerebrovascular lesion. The outcome was healing, amputation, or death.

Results.—Fever and inflammation were frequently absent in these patients. Of the 86 patients (39%) who healed without amputation, 60 had surgery and 26 healed without surgery. Of the 94 patients (42%) who healed after amputation 79 had a minor amputation, and 18 had a major amputation. Of the 36 patients (16%) who died without healing, 8 patients had had a minor amputation and 4 a major amputation. There were 7 patients (3%) unhealed at the end of the observation period. Factors related to healing without amputation included diabetes for less than 14 years, the presence of a palpable popliteal artery pulse, a toe pressure of more than 45 mm Hg, an ankle pressure of more than 80 mm Hg, absence of exposed bone, and a white blood cell count of less than 12×10^9/L.

Conclusion.—Most diabetic patients with a deep foot infection required surgery. Although only 10% had a major amputation, almost one third required a minor amputation. Such patients should be admitted to hospital for a thorough evaluation because fever and inflammation are frequently absent, making early diagnosis difficult.

▶ This careful analysis of a large group of patients provides evidence that a foot ulceration need not eventuate in major amputation. The large cohort allowed correlation with clinical and laboratory data to assist in determining prognosis and the likelihood of success with more limited procedures. It is not surprising that a duration of diabetes of less than 14 years, palpable pulses, a toe pressure of greater than 45 mm Hg and an ankle pressure of greater than 80 mm Hg without systemic evidence of infection is correlated with a better result. However, it does provide an objective basis for clinical impression. The fact that these investigators and surgeons avoided major amputation in 90% of these patients is quite encouraging. It should be noted, however, that the health care workers involved in the study and in the care of the patients were quite experienced and were part of a well-developed foot care team. Thus, the experience reported here may not be readily replicable in all orthopedic practices.

B.F. Morrey, M.D.

Neuropathic Ulcerations Plantar to the Lateral Column in Patients With Charcot Foot Deformity: A Flexible Approach to Limb Salvage

Rosenblum BI, Chrzan JS, Giurini JM, et al (Harvard Med School, Boston)
J Foot Ankle Surg 36:360–363, 1997   11–22

Background.—In diabetic patients, neuroarthropathy of the midfoot may result in a structural deformity that predisposes to skin breakdown and ulceration. Conservative management is not sufficient in some patients, necessitating surgical intervention. One group of patients requiring surgical intervention for a specific pattern of neuroarthropathy were studied retrospectively.

Methods.—Thirty-one patients with 32 affected feet undergoing surgery during a 2.5-year period for nonhealing neuropathic ulcerations beneath the lateral column of Charcot feet were reviewed. Exostectomy was performed in all feet. Seventeen underwent excision of the ulcer with primary closure; 8, closure via rotational fasciocutaneous flap with transpositional intrinsic muscle; and 6, through an incision adjacent to the ulcer. The incision was placed directly over the prominence in a patient whose ulcer had healed by the time of surgery.

Outcomes.—Functional limb salvage was achieved in 29 feet. This included 8 feet in patients needing revisional surgery by resection of more bone or creation of a local flap for coverage. The overall success rate, according to life-table analysis, was 89%.

Conclusions.—A flexible approach to skin and soft tissue coverage is needed in patients with nonhealing neuropathic ulcerations beneath the lateral column of Charcot feet. Attention must be directed to the underlying bony prominence.

▶ The value of this paper is its detailed discussion of surgical technique, the results of which are discussed as an alternative to an ablation procedure such as amputation. However, the exact selection criteria are unclear because they are not identified in the manuscript. This deficiency is heightened by the recognition of a spectrum of clinical findings that the patients had, including variable peripheral pulses, severity of diabetes, duration of symptoms, whether there had been attempts at revascularization, and even the duration of ulceration varying from 1 to 48 months. Given this broad spectrum of variables, some of which may alter the outcome, it is somewhat difficult to know which patients would benefit from this procedure. In general terms, however, it is clear that midfoot lateral column ulceration can be effectively managed by debulking the prominent bone and mobilizing the soft tissue in any one of several ways. The authors suggest but the data do not necessarily prove that the major problems with the surgical approach, and or the complication rate, are associated with an inadequate removal of bone or mobilization of the soft tissue. Overall this does provide added insight into a salvage procedure for this difficult patient population.

B.F. Morrey, M.D.

Tarsal Tunnel Syndrome: Diagnosis, Surgical Technique, and Functional Outcome
Bailie DS, Kelikian AS (Ctr for Sports Medicine and Orthopedics, Phoenix, Ariz; Northwestern Univ, Chicago)
Foot Ankle Int 19:65–72, 1998   11–23

Objective.—Patients with tarsal tunnel syndrome (TTS) have pain, paresthesias, or numbness in the foot and ankle, caused by compression neuropathy of the posterior tibial nerve in the tarsal tunnel. There are few large studies of TTS, which has many different causes and can be difficult to diagnose. There is disagreement as to whether treatment should be surgical or nonsurgical. The results of surgery in 47 patients with TTS are reviewed.

Patients.—Over a 10-year period, 1 orthopedic surgeon saw 126 patients with TTS. Forty-seven patients were treated surgically with decompression of the tarsal tunnel, after nonoperative treatments had failed to resolve the patients' symptoms. Follow-up data, including questionnaire and physical examination results, were available on 36 feet of 34 patients. Medical record data were available on another 10 patients. The patients were 24 males and 20 females, mean age 38 years. Average duration of nonoperative treatment before surgery was 16 months; average follow-up was 35 months.

Outcomes.—All patients had pain related to the tarsal tunnel along the course of the posterior tibial nerve or one of its branches. The most frequent clinical picture was a triad of pain, numbness, and paresthesias. Tinel's sign and a nerve compression test at the tarsal tunnel were positive in all patients. Eighty-one percent of feet had abnormal results on electrodiagnostic studies. The average reduction in 2-point discrimination was 6.7 mm.

At follow-up, 2-point discrimination had increased by an average of 3.8 mm. Tinel's sign and the nerve compression test remained positive in 18 feet. The patients reported satisfaction in 72% of cases, with corresponding improvements in the Symptom Severity Score and Functional Foot Score. The satisfaction rate was somewhat better in non-worker's-compensation cases. Thirteen percent of patients had significant perioperative complications, such as wound infections and sterile abscesses. Including cases of sensitive and nonsensitive hypertrophic scarring, the complication rate was 30%.

Conclusions.—A surgical experience with TTS is reviewed. This condition is diagnosed mainly on the basis of history and clinical findings, with electrodiagnostic studies being supportive in more than 80% of cases. Surgery is indicated after a trial of nonsurgical treatment has failed. To ensure complete surgical release of compressed nerve, it is essential to divide the deep portion of the abductor hallucis fascia.

▶ TTS remains an enigma for many clinicians. This thoughtful retrospective analysis of a 10-year experience of 47 patients confirms the triad of pain, paresthesia, and numbness as the most common clinical presentation, found in 81% of patients by electrodiagnostic studies. This is worth emphasizing since patient selection is the most important factor in a satisfactory outcome after surgical intervention. The surgical intervention was offered to 47 of 126 patients, indicating that the majority (approximately two thirds) do not come to surgical treatment. It is, therefore, particularly relevant that given the careful selection factors and the more than 80% of patients who had electrodiagnostic evidence of pathology, only approximately 70% were subjectively satisfied with the outcome. The authors emphasize the release of the deep portion of the abductor hallucis fascia as an important technical point to assure an adequate decompression.

B.F. Morrey, M.D.

Tarsal Tunnel Syndrome: Outcome of Surgery in Longstanding Cases
Turan I, Rivero-Melián C, Guntner P, et al (Huddinge Univ, Sweden)
Clin Orthop 343:151–156, 1997   11–24

Purpose.—Tarsal tunnel syndrome, involving compressive neuropathy of the posterior tibial nerve, is a relatively rare condition. Symptoms include a burning sensation or pain at the medial plantar surface, usually worst at the end of the work day. Early surgical decompression provides good results. An experience with surgical treatment of tarsal tunnel syndrome is reported in a group of patients with longstanding symptoms.

Patients.—The patients were 14 females and 5 males, age range 15–59. All had diffuse burning sensations and exertional pain at the medial surface of the foot. Tinel's sign was positive in 16. The patients had undergone many examinations and received a number of preliminary diagnoses, commonly plantar fasciitis. The median duration of symptoms was 60 months; 1 patient had had symptoms for 16 years. Three patients had undergone previous surgery for tarsal tunnel syndrome, without success. Magnetic resonance imaging was performed in 10 patients, with positive findings in only 2.

Outcomes.—Surgery was performed with spinal anesthesia and a tourniquet through a medial skin incision over the tarsal tunnel. Entrapment of the posterior tibial nerve or one of its branches was observed in 15 patients. Nerve entrapment was isolated or associated with varicose veins, fascial septa, scar tissue, neuroma, and abductor hallucis muscle. No entrapment was apparent in 3 patients. At a median follow-up of 18 months, 61% of patients were symptom free, 22% had decreased symptoms, and 17% had no change. The latter group included patients with very long duration of symptoms or with previous direct trauma.

Conclusions.—For most patients with tarsal tunnel syndrome, surgery can eliminate or reduce symptoms, even for patients with a long duration of symptoms. Treatment failure may be more likely for patients with very longstanding symptoms or direct trauma. The diagnosis should be suspected in any patient with a burning sensation at the medial plantar surface of the foot. At surgery, it is important to remember that compression can occur anywhere along the course of the nerve.

▶ This experience continues to illustrate the problematic diagnosis and treatment of tarsal tunnel syndrome. While clinically this entity is relatively straightforward in the majority of instances, objective studies are not particularly helpful. Magnetic resonance imaging was considered to be of value in only 2 of 10 patients, and this is an important point because the success of surgery is reported in the literature to be variable and there were 17% failures in this group. This implies that the selection factors are particularly important. In the final analysis, this would appear to place a major burden on the clinician to accurately establish the diagnosis, clearly understand the patient, particularly be aware of any secondary motivational characteristics, and finally, successfully execute the decompressive procedure.

B.F. Morrey, M.D.

Intermittent Pneumatic Pedal Compression and Edema Resolution After Acute Ankle Fracture: A Prospective, Randomized Study

Thordarson DB, Ghalambor N, Perlman M (LAC+USC Med Ctr, Los Angeles)
Foot Ankle Int 18:347–350, 1997   11–25

Objective.—In some acute ankle fractures, severe edema may lead to delays for surgery. A prolonged period of recumbency with the ankle elevated increases the risk for serious complications and can compromise fracture fixation. Intermittent pneumatic pedal compression (PPC) has been studied for use in the treatment of edema in the foot and ankle region, but not in preoperative patients. The ability of intermittent PPC to hasten resolution of posttraumatic edema after acute ankle fracture was evaluated.

Methods.—The prospective, randomized trial included 30 patients with acute Weber B or C ankle fracture. Half of the patients were assigned to a control group, in which posterior splinting, ice, and elevation were prescribed before surgery. The other group received the same treatment plus full-time use of intermittent PPC before surgery. Volumetric measurements of the injured foot were performed at baseline and then every 24 hr until surgery. The 2 groups were compared for time to resolution of posttraumatic edema.

Results.—In the first 24 hr, volume measurements decreased by 88 mL in the PPC group, compared with a 33-mL increase in the control group. In the first 48 hr, volume decreased by 31 mL in the PPC group, compared with a 32 mL increase in the control group. Most patients went to surgery by the third day. Only 1 patient could not tolerate the use of PPC because of pain.

Conclusions.—In patients with acute ankle fracture, intermittent PPC appears to reduce preoperative edema significantly, compared with conventional management. Intermittent PPC could be a useful adjunct in helping to reduce edema before surgery for ankle fracture. Pneumatic pedal compression is well tolerated by most patients.

▶ Any insight with regard to controlling swelling after ankle fractures is of value. This nicely done prospective study clearly demonstrates the value of a well-tolerated, relatively inexpensive device that controls the swelling in the preoperative period. The major implication of this finding is that the timing for surgery may be optimized, possibly lessening the need to rush into a procedure in the middle of the night under less than ideal circumstances. If edema can be controlled in this fashion, then more elective surgical intervention may be offered. The logical question is whether or not this approach can be used in some fashion in the postoperative period to continue to control edema and facilitate soft tissue rehabilitation. This question was not addressed in this report.

B.F. Morrey, M.D.

Combination Chevron Plus Akin Osteotomy for Hallux Valgus: Should Age Be a Limiting Factor?
Tollison ME, Baxter DE (Baylor College of Medicine, Houston)
Foot Ankle Int 18:477–481, 1997   11–26

Background.—The chevron osteotomy is a V-shaped osteotomy of the distal first metatarsal, useful for the correction of mild to moderate hallux valgus deformity. The literature restricts the use of this procedure to patients younger than age 50. To determine whether this limitation was necessary, results with patients older than age 55 who had undergone a double chevron-Akin osteotomy for the correction of hallux valgus were studied.

Study Design.—A retrospective review was performed of 47 patients with 73 bunions who were older than age 55 at time of chevron-Akin osteotomy. Each participant returned for follow-up including standing radiographs and questionnaire. There were 44 women and 3 men, age 55–81 in this study group. The average period of follow-up was 4.5 years.

Findings.—The overall patient satisfaction rate was 95%. Pain or stiffness in the first metatarsophalangeal joint was no worse than that experienced with other bunion procedures. Radiographic results were better in those patients with a preoperative intermetatarsal angle of less than 15 degrees and a tibial sesamoid position less than or equal to 2.

Conclusions.—A review of results of patients older than age 55 who underwent chevron-Akin osteotomies did not support the age limitation of chevron procedures in the literature. This procedure is useful for mild-to-moderate bunion deformity even in elderly patients.

▶ This article offers an alternative to the generally accepted dictum that Chevron osteotomy be reserved for patients under the age of 50. There is a modest average follow-up of over 4 years with a wide range of patient age of up to 81. The follow-up did involve direct examination including standing radiographs and clinical assessment. The high subjective rate of satisfaction as well as the low complication rate would seem to offer some justification that the age limits for osteotomy be reassessed.

B.F. Morrey, M.D.

12 Spine

Introduction

The field of spinal disorders is evolving at a rapid pace, and this year significant contributions to the literature were made in an array of disciplines. We are approaching the long-awaited time when bone graft substitutes will relegate donor site morbidity to the history books. Health care "reform" has transformed the terms *coding, documentation,* and *guidelines* from stale to stimulating. Spinal cages have had a dramatic impact on the implant marketplace, but time will tell if our patients will reap similar benefits from the technology. Solid basic science studies have added critical pieces of information about the pathophysiology of sciatica, and we are nearing the stage when we can expect to have new therapeutic options for patients with herniated disks. New insights on the old topics of infection, degenerative conditions, and surgical techniques round out this group of articles, the highlights of 1998.

Bradford L. Currier, M.D.

Bone Graft Substitutes

In Vivo Evaluation of a Resorbable Osteoinductive Composite as a Graft Substitute for Lumbar Spinal Fusion

Boden SD, Schimandle JH, Hutton WC, et al (Emory Univ, Atlanta, Ga; VA Med Ctr, Atlanta, Ga)
J Spinal Disord 10:1–11, 1997   12–1

Objective.—Osteoinductive bone graft substitutes have been suggested as alternatives to autogenous iliac crest bone graft for posterolateral intertransverse process arthrodesis. The efficacy of a resorbable coral particulate as a carrier with several doses of a bovine-derived osteoinductive bone protein mixture was tested in vivo in the rabbit model.

Methods.—A single-level posterolateral intertransverse process lumbar arthrodesis was performed at L5-L6 using a 0, 100-, 300-, or 1,000-µg dose of an osteoinductive bone protein extract in a biocoral/collagen carrier as a bone graft substitute in 4 groups of 16 adult female New Zealand rabbits. Fusion rates were assessed by posterolateral radiographs, manual palpation, and biomechanical testing or light microscopy. Two

TABLE 2.—Summary of Results

Graft material	Fuson rate	Relative strength	Relative stiffness
Biocoral alone	0% (0/14)	1.4 ± 0.1	1.1 ± 0.1
BP (100 µg)* Biocoral	31% (4/13)	1.5 ± 0.1	1.2 ± 0.1
BP (300 µg)* Biocoral	100% (14/14)*	2.1 ± 0.2†	1.4 ± 0.1†
BP (1,000 µg)* Biocoral	100% (13/13)*	1.9 ± 0.1†	1.5 ± 0.1†

*Significantly different from Biocoral alone (Fisher exact test. $P < 0.05$).
†Significantly different from Biocoral alone (analysis of variance, Bonferoni test, $P < 0.05$).
Abbreviation: BP, bone protein extract.
(Courtesy of Boden SD, Schimandle JH, Hutton WC, et al: In vivo evaluation of a resorbable osteoinductive composite as a graft substitute for lumbar spinal fusion. *J Spinal Disord* 10:1–11, 1997.)

rabbits from each group were killed at 2 and 5 weeks for undecalcified histology. Fusion rates were compared using Fisher's exact test.

Results.—Two rabbits died perioperatively, and 6 had infections when they were killed. Seromas that developed in 16 rabbits between days 3 and 7 resolved spontaneously. Fusion rates were highest at doses of 300 and 1,000 µg of bone protein extract (Table 2). Fusions at these doses also appeared to be more homogeneous. In rabbits without bone protein extract, there was no evidence of bone formation, and early resorption of coral was apparent on radiographs.

Conclusion.—Biocoral/collagen is an effective carrier of bone protein for posterolateral intertransverse process fusion in the rabbit. Bone protein at doses of 300 and 1,000 µg resulted in 100% fusion.

▶ With this paper, we are 1 step closer to the day when we can reliably perform a spine fusion without harvesting the patients iliac crest for graft. In this report, Boden et al. used their well-established rabbit model to demonstrate that a resorbable osteoinductive composite can function as a graft substitute. Although they did not assess the fusion rate with autogenous bone graft in this study, their previous experiments, using the same animal model at the same end point, revealed fusion rates of 62% to 77% with autogenous graft.[1, 2]

In the study abstracted here, the authors were able to demonstrate a clear dose-response curve for the bone protein extract, with solid fusions developing in 100% of the animals receiving the higher dosages. Many more studies will be required before we can send our bone gouges to the museum, but this study proves that the goal is within reach.

We are just beginning to understand the differences between the various bone morphogenetic proteins. More work is needed to determine the most effective protein, the most appropriate dose of the protein, and the best carriers. Studies using higher animal models and, eventually, humans will need to be performed to answer these questions. Biological replacement, using tissue engineering strategies and enhancing repair processes, should be our ultimate long-term goal, but achieving a successful fusion without donor site morbidity will solve many immediate problems.

B.L. Currier, M.D.

References

1. Boden SD, Schimandle JH, Hutton WC: The use of an osteoinductive growth factor for lumbar spinal fusion: Part II. Study of dose, carrier, and species. *Spine* 20:2633–2644, 1995.
2. Boden SD, Schimandle JH, Hutton WC: An experimental lumbar intertransverse process spinal fusion model: Radiographic, histologic, and biomechanical healing characteristics. *Spine* 20:412–420, 1995.

Coding and Documentation

Spinal Range of Motion: Accuracy and Sources of Error With Inclinometric Measurement

Mayer TG, Kondraske G, Beals SB, et al (Univ of Texas, Dallas; Univ of Texas, Arlington)

Spine 22:1976–1984, 1997   12–2

Introduction.—Although several studies have addressed the reliability of inclinometric measurements of lumbar motion, there has been little attention to the sources of error accounting for the observed variability. The clinical applications of range of motion make it particularly important to recognize and correct for factors that limit accuracy of measurement. The accuracy of inclinometric measurements of lumbar spine motion was evaluated, including a progressive analysis of sources of error.

Methods.—Bench testing was performed on a computerized inclinometer to assess possible device error. The inclinometer was then used to measure sagittal lumbar mobility in 38 healthy volunteers. Initial tests were administered by untrained testers, with no controls for human performance or procedural variables. The same tests were performed by trained administrators, who monitored and controlled total motion to control human performance variability. Finally, procedurally trained testers administered the tests without controlling for human performance variability. The sources of error were analyzed to identify those aspects of the measurement process and device that caused the greatest problems in accuracy.

Results.—Various sources of error contributed to progressive degradation in the accuracy of the measurements. Compared to errors related to the test process, device error had little effect on accuracy. The most important sources of error were lack of training of the test administrators and the magnitude of the measurements. The most accurate measurement was combined lumbar flexion, for which worst case accuracy was greater than 95% for the overall test conditions. The least accurate was pelvic extension, with worst case accuracy of 36%.

Conclusions.—Tester training is a major source of error in inclinometric measurements of lumbar spine sagittal motion. Absolute error is relatively constant, so error is greater with measurements of greater magnitude. Device error has little adverse effect on measurement accuracy. Examining sources of error provides a more sophisticated analysis of human performance measurements than is possible with reliability coefficients. These sources of error have been little corrected for or considered in previous studies.

▶ Spinal range-of-motion measurements are a standard part of the physical examination. The information is used to justify treatment, monitor therapy, and rate permanent impairment. Spinal range of motion is an essential element required in a physician's report for reimbursement by the Health Care Financing Administration. Unfortunately, these measurements are extremely inaccurate and imprecise most of the time. It is difficult to separate lumbar spine motion from hip motion clinically. Computerized inclinometers have been marketed to allow accurate measurements, but this study clearly shows that the measurements are subject to several sources of error. Clinicians who choose to use these devices must be certain that the individual performing the test is well trained, otherwise the data will be inaccurate and potentially misleading. The methods used in this study for assessing accuracy and sources of error could be applied to other quantitative musculoskeletal measurements.

B.L. Currier, M.D.

Quality of Data Regarding Diagnoses of Spinal Disorders in Administrative Databases: A Multicenter Study
Faciszewski T, Broste SK, Fardon D (Marshfield Clinic, Wis; Knoxville Orthopedic Clinic, Tenn)
J Bone Joint Surg Am 79-A:1481–1488, 1997   12–3

Objective.—The quality of data in databases affects the validity of the conclusions derived from them. The accuracy of the commonly used *International Classification of Diseases, Ninth Revision, Clinical Modification* (ICD-9–CM) codes for diagnoses related to the spine was evaluated to gain a better understanding of the limitations of conclusions drawn from data in administrative databases.

Methods.—A spine surgeon reviewed clinical data in 189 complete records of patients aged 17–84 years having a lumbar spine procedure. The sensitivity, specificity, positive and negative predictive values, percent agreement, and kappa coefficient were calculated for diagnostic codes applied to 6 categories: herniation of a lumbar disc, a previous operation on the lumbar spine, spinal stenosis, cauda equina syndrome, acquired spondylolisthesis, and congenital spondylolisthesis.

Results.—Records were contributed by 8 institutions, 6 of which were teaching hospitals. Only 10 of 68 hospital coders were certified, and 26% of coders received only on-the-job training. Sensitivity, the percentage of correctly coded diagnoses, ranged from 28% to 100%, and specificity, the percentage of patients who did not have a particular diagnosis and were not coded for it, ranged from 94% to 98% (Table 3). The positive predictive value, the percentage of patients correctly assigned a particular

TABLE 3.—Sensitivity and Specificity of Hospital Coding

Diagnosis	Total No.	Code Correctly Assigned by Hospital Personnel*	Sensitivity (Per cent)	Total No.	Code Correctly Not Assigned by Hospital Personnel*	Specificity (Per cent)
		Code Assigned by Physician Reviewer			Code Not Assigned by Physician Reviewer	
Herniation of a disc	84	79	94	105	99	94
Previous spinal op.	61	17	28	128	126	98
Spinal stenosis	87	65	75	102	100	98
Cauda equina syndrome	2	2	100	187	184	98
Acquired spondylolisthesis	45	32	71	144	140	97
Congenital spondylolisthesis	0	0	—	189	180	95

*Given as the number of times that the code was assigned.

(Courtesy of Faciszewski T, Broste SK, Fardon D: Quality of data regarding diagnosis of spinal disorders in administrative databases: A multicenter study. *J Bone Joint Surg Am* 79-A:1481–1488, 1997.)

diagnostic code, ranged from 0% to 97%, and the negative predictive value, the percentage of patients who did not have a particular diagnosis and who were not coded for that diagnosis, ranged from 74% to 100% (Table 4). Only 28% of previous spinal operations were coded correctly. The sensitivity of hospital coding, ranging from 62% to 75%, was similar for all hospitals. There were too few false codes to allow comparison of specificities among hospitals.

Conclusions.—Few studies have examined the quality of data in administrative databases. Random misclassification, improper training or supervision, and other nonrandom sources of error such as reimbursement regulations favoring 1 code over another or hospital regulations limiting the number of codes that can be assigned, are responsible for coding errors. Administrative data should be validated before it is published.

▶ Health-care policy is being influenced by studies that rely on administrative databases. The validity of the conclusions reached in these studies depends on the quality of the data. Faciszewski et al. have proved the old axiom of "garbage in, garbage out." These authors have established a new standard that should be required of any future study using an administrative database: the accuracy of the codes used in the study must be determined to judge the validity of the conclusions.

The investigators recognize that the major limitation of their study is that the opinion of a single physician reviewer was considered to be the gold standard for judging the accuracy of the hospital coders. A small sample of records were reviewed by another physician and there was good interobserver agreement, suggesting that this was not a major source of error. The physician who was the primary reviewer of the records, Dr. Faciszewski, is also a recognized authority in coding. In future studies, if one of the inves-

TABLE 4.—Positive and Negative Predictive Values of Hospital Coding

Diagnosis	Code Assigned by Hospital Personnel			Code Not Assigned by Hospital Personnel				
	Total No.	True Positives*	Positive Predictive Value (Per cent)	Total No.	True Negatives*	Negative Predictive Value (Per cent)	Per Cent Coded Correctly	Kappa Coefficient
Herniation of a disc	85	79	93	104	99	95	94	0.88
Previous spinal op.	19	17	89	170	126	74	76	0.32
Spinal stenosis	67	65	97	122	100	82	87	0.74
Cauda equina syndrome	5	2	40	184	184	100	98	0.56
Acquired spondylolisthesis	36	32	89	153	140	92	91	0.73
Congenital spondylolisthesis	9	0	0	180	180	100	95	0.00

*According to the physician reviewer.

(Courtesy of Faciszewski T, Broste SK, Fardon D: Quality of data regarding diagnosis of spinal disorders in administrative databases: A multicenter study. *J Bone Joint Surg Am* 79-A:1481–1488, 1997.)

tigators is not well versed in coding, a Certified Coding Specialist may be used for determining the correct codes.

This study did not evaluate the accuracy of coding comorbidities or the relative accuracy of coders with different educational backgrounds. Future studies could address these important variables.

B.L. Currier, M.D.

Degenerative Conditions

Degenerative Lumbar Spondylolisthesis With Spinal Stenosis: A Prospective, Randomized Study Comparing Decompressive Laminectomy and Arthrodesis With and Without Spinal Instrumentation
Fischgrund JS, Mackay M, Herkowitz HN, et al (William Beaumont Hosp, Royal Oak, Mich)
Spine 22:2807–2812, 1997   12–4

Objective.—Whether spinal instrumentation is beneficial in the operative management of patients with degenerative spondylolisthesis and spinal stenosis is controversial. The results of decompression and arthrodesis alone were compared prospectively with those of decompression and arthrodesis combined with instrumentation at the level of the arthrodesis in patients with single-level degenerative spondylolisthesis associated with lumbar spinal stenosis.

Methods.—Patients aged 53–86 years, were randomly assigned to decompressive laminectomy and single-level autogenous bilateral lateral intertransverse process arthrodesis with (7 men and 28 women) and without (6 men and 27 women) transpedicular instrumentation. Patients were followed up for 2 years.

TABLE 1.—Data on the 68 Patients

	Instrumentation (N = 35)		No Instrumentation (N = 33)	
	Preoperative	Postoperative	Preoperative	Postoperative
Result				
Excellent		20 (57%)		16 (49%)
Good		7 (21%)		12 (36%)
Fair		4 (12%)		1 (3%)
Poor		4 (12%)		4 (12%)
Mean scores for pain (points)				
Back	4	1	4	2
Lower limbs	4	1	4	1
Mean olisthesis (mm)	8	6	7	7
Mean sagittal motion on flexion and extension (mm)	3	1	3	2
Mean angulation (°)	9	1	9	5

(Courtesy of Fischgrund JS, Mackay M, Herkowitz HN, et al: Degenerative lumbar spondylolisthesis with spinal stenosis: A prospective, randomized study comparing decompressive laminectomy and arthrodesis with and without spinal instrumentation. *Spine* 22:2807–2812, 1997.)

TABLE 2.—Factors Affecting Fusion Rate

	Successful Arthrodesis	Pseudarthrosis
Instrumentation	29 (83%)	6 (18%)
No instrumentation	15 (45%)	18 (55%)
Preoperative		
Olisthesis (mm)	8	7
Angulation (°)	8	11
Motion (mm)	3	4
Postoperative		
Olisthesis (mm)	7	7
Angulation (°)	1	8
Motion (mm)	1	3

(Courtesy of Fischgrund JS, Mackay M, Herkowitz HN, et al: Degenerative lumbar spondylolisthesis with spinal stenosis: A prospective, randomized study comparing decompressive laminectomy and arthrodesis with and without spinal instrumentation. *Spine* 22:2807–2812, 1997.)

Results.—Patients in the instrumented group had 4 pedicle screws implanted. Clinical outcomes were excellent or good in 78% of the instrumented group and in 85% of the noninstrumented group (Table 1). There was no significant difference in results between the 2 groups. After surgery, leg and back pain were rated 0 or 1 (on a visual analog scale, ranging from 0 [no pain] to 5 [severe pain]) by 64% and 58%, respectively, of the instrumented group. In the noninstrumented group, 75% and 53%, respectively, rated leg, and back pain at 0 or 1 after surgery. Arthrodesis was significantly more successful in the instrumented group than in the noninstrumented group (83% vs. 45%) (Table 2).

Conclusions.—Although the pedicle screws used in the instrumented group may have accounted for the significantly higher arthrodesis rate, there was no difference in back and leg pain between the instrumented and noninstrumented groups.

▶ In 1991, Herkowitz and Kurz[1] published a classic article showing that patients with degenerative lumbar spondylolisthesis with spinal stenosis have a better outcome if a fusion is performed at the time of decompression. The present study is a logical extension of the earlier report, and it was performed with the same careful, prospective, randomized methodology. In both papers, the authors have found that a pseudarthrosis does not necessarily lead to a poor clinical outcome. The authors propose that a fibrous pseudarthrosis provides enough stability to prevent progressive spondylolisthesis, a phenomenon that has been shown to correlate with increased back pain. Long-term follow-up of the patients in Fischgrund's series will show whether the good results in patients with pseudarthrosis hold up over time. The disparity between radiographic and clinical success with spinal fusions has been reported since at least 1968.[2] Other authors[3] have documented a positive correlation between clinical outcome and a solid fusion, and therefore the issue has not been resolved. Fischgrund's study confirmed Zdeblick's findings that instrumentation clearly improves the rate of fusion.

The low rate of complications in this series is impressive; no patients had an infection and the only hardware failure occured in a patient with a solid fusion and an excellent clinical result. Other papers show a definite increase in complications when instrumentation is used, and that factor as well as cost and efficacy should be considered when deciding which cases require instrumentation.

B.L. Currier, M.D.

References

1. Herkowitz HN, Kurz LT: Degenerative lumbar spondylolisthesis with spinal stenosis. *J Bone Joint Surg Am* 73A:802–807, 1991.
2. DePalma AF, Rothman RH: The nature of pseudarthrosis. *Clin Orthop* 59:113–118, 1968.
3. Zdeblick TA: A prospective, randomized study of lumbar fusion. *Spine* 18:983–991, 1993.

Epidural Corticosteroid Injections for Sciatica Due to Herniated Nucleus Pulposus
Carette S, Leclaire R, Marcoux S, et al (Laval Univ, Quebec City; Univ of Montreal)
N Engl J Med 336:1634–1640, 1997   12–5

Objective.—Whether epidural corticosteroid injections are effective for sciatica caused by a herniated nucleus pulposus is controversial. The efficacy of up to 3 epidural corticosteroid injections vs. epidural saline injections in patients with sciatica as a result of a herniated nucleus pulposus was evaluated in a double-blind, placebo-controlled trial.

Methods.—Either 3 epidural injections of methylprednisolone acetate (80 mg in 8 mL of isotonic saline; $n = 78$) or of isotonic saline (1 mL; $n = 80$) were administered to 158 patients (103 male) with sciatica lasting for a minimum of 4 weeks and Oswestry disability scores of greater than 20. Patients were evaluated at 3, 6, and 12 weeks after treatment.

Results.—One patient in each group received only 1 injection. Twelve patients in the treatment group and 20 in the placebo group did not complete the study because of lack of efficacy. Nine and 8 of these patients, respectively, underwent back surgery, with 14 having marked or very marked improvement at 3 months. The average number of injections per patient was 2.1. Patients in the placebo group used more acetaminophen at all time points than did patients in the treatment group. Drugs other than acetaminophen were used by 27 patients in the treatment group and 32 in the placebo group. Oswestry scores improved by -8.0 in the treatment group and by -5.5 in the placebo group, and 33% and 29% of patients, respectively, reported marked or very marked improvement. Differences in improvements between groups were not significant, except that the treatment group had greater improvement in the finger-to-floor distance and fewer patients had sensory deficits. Results at 6 weeks were similar to those at 3 weeks except that leg pain was significantly improved in the treatment group. At 3 months, there was no difference between groups in any outcome measure. Cumulative probabilities of undergoing back surgery based on survival analysis were 25.8% for the treatment group and 24.8% for the placebo group.

Conclusions.—Epidural corticosteroid injections for sciatica caused by a herniated nucleus pulposus is effective for a short time only, providing mild-to-moderate improvement in leg pain and sensory deficits, and reducing the need for analgesics. The injections did not influence function or the need for surgery.

▶ Although this paper doesn't show a significant long-term benefit of epidural corticosteroid injections, the short-term improvement in leg pain and sensory deficits is justification to consider epidural injections for symptomatic relief of pain. The natural history of sciatica caused by herniated lumbar disks is favorable, and if patients can be made comfortable during the early stages of the condition, the pain may resolve spontaneously without the need for surgery.

To be eligible for this study, patients had to have had symptoms for at least 1 month. It is possible that epidural steroid injections administered earlier in the evolution of the condition would have had more effect. Future studies should focus on the treatment of patients with acute and subacute sciatica.

This study was not intended as a comparison of surgery and epidural injections, but the response of the patients who withdrew from the study and had surgery is noteworthy. Nine of the 12 patients in the methylprednisolone group that withdrew from the study because of lack of efficacy, and 8 of the 20 patients in the placebo group that withdrew, eventually underwent surgery. Fourteen of these 17 patients reported marked or very marked improvement at the 3-month evaluation. Their mean leg-pain score decreased from 72.7 at baseline to 21.2 compared with 38.9 and 39.5 for the methylprednisolone and placebo groups, respectively. Patients with sciatica from a herniated disk should be referred to a surgeon if they have a significant neurologic deficit or have not improved substantially after 6–12 weeks of conservative care.

B.L. Currier, M.D.

Failed Anterior Cervical Discectomy and Arthrodesis: Analysis and Treatment of Thirty-five Patients
Zdeblick TA, Hughes SS, Riew KD, et al (Univ of Wisconsin, Madison; Wake Forest Univ, Winston-Salem, NC; Washington Univ, St Louis; et al)
J Bone Joint Surg Am 79-A:523–532, 1997   12–6

Objective.—Rates of nonunion after anterior cervical arthrodesis range from 4% to 50%. Thirty-five patients were studied; after a failed anterior cervical arthrodesis they underwent a repeat anterior approach for decompression and bone grafting.

Methods.—The 35 patients (17 men) ranged in age from 31 to 68 years. The mechanisms of failure included failure of arthrodesis without deformity but with neck pain and/or radiculopathy ($n = 23$), migration of the graft ($n = 4$), or kyphotic deformity ($n = 8$). Failure to fuse was defined as greater than 2 mm of motion between the tips of the spinous processes with the spine in flexion, and a radiolucent line or space apparent at the involved disk level. Methods of treatment included anterior block dissection and autogenous bone grafting at the level of failure in 22 patients, and anterior cervical corpectomy with autogenous strut grafting to yield more decompression of the spinal canal and nerve roots and to correct kyphosis in 13. Fusion was defined as solid when the graft bridged the disk space anteriorly on lateral radiographs, and no motion was detected with the spine in flexion and extension. Patients were followed up for an average of 44 months.

Technique.—For nonunion or compression at 1 level, a hemi-corpectomy was performed at adjacent levels. Angular kyphosis was reduced with skeletal traction and extension of the head and neck after decompression was complete. The graft was inserted beneath the anterior cortices leaving 3 mm between it and the posterior longitudinal ligament. Compression of adjacent levels or treatment of vertebral collapse with kyphosis was treated with corpectomy. If more than 2 vertebrae were resected, a fibular graft was required. A 2-poster rigid orthosis or a halo vest was worn for 8 weeks by patients who had had a laminectomy or disruption of the posterior ligament.

Results.—Fusion was achieved in 34 patients with excellent results in 29, good in 1, fair in 4, and poor in 1. Complications included recurrent laryngeal nerve palsy in 1, prolonged drainage from the incision in 2, and leakage of cerebrospinal fluid in 1 treated by reoperation, muscle grafting, and closure with a shunt. Anterior migration occurred with multilevel Robinson-type arthrodesis, primarily because heights of bone grafts were excessive. Posterior migration of the graft into the spinal canal resulted after Cloward arthrodesis. Collapse of the graft with kyphosis occurred mainly after Cloward arthrodesis, particularly in patients with a previous laminectomy or with frozen allograft bone used as graft material.

Conclusions.—A well-prepared graft and graft bed, a graft inserted with good osseous apposition of the opposing vascular bone surfaces, and rigid immobilization can lead to a good outcome in patients with failed cervical discectomy and arthrodesis.

▶ Anterior cervical discectomy and fusion (ACDF) is a commonly performed procedure for radiculopathy and myelopathy. Some surgeons advocate discectomy without fusion for the treatment of radiculopathy, but the persistent neck pain and kyphosis that can be associated with that procedure have led most surgeons to perform a fusion at the time of discectomy. Pseudarthrosis occurs in 4% to 20% of single-level ACDFs and between 27% and 50% of multiple-level procedures. Although a satisfactory result can be achieved despite a pseudarthrosis, several recent studies suggest that a solid fusion increases the likelihood of a good outcome, and a successful fusion should be a goal of the procedure. The excellent results after refusion reported by Zdeblick et al. confirm that many pseudarthroses are painful. Phillips et al.,[1] in a related study from the same institution as the present report, described the natural history of patients with pseudarthrosis. Thirty-three percent of the 48 patients with a pseudarthrosis remained asymptomatic at a mean of 5.1 years after the ACDF. Interestingly, they found that 9 of the 32 symptomatic patients in their series were asymptomatic for at least 2 years after the ACDF was performed and then redeveloped pain after a traumatic episode.

There are several reports of successful management of symptomatic pseudarthroses with posterior foraminotomies and fusion. This paper demonstrates that excellent results can be achieved through an anterior approach. The advantage of operating anteriorly is obvious when treating a pseudarthrosis associated with a kyphotic deformity. Avoiding neck pain caused by extensive posterior dissection is a theoretical advantage that must be weighed against the risk of complications related to operating through scar tissue.

B.L. Currier, M.D.

Reference

1. Phillips FM, Carlson G, Emery SE, et al: Anterior cervical pseudarthrosis: Natural history and treatment. *Spine* 22:1585–1589, 1997.

Infection

Pyogenic Vertebral Osteomyelitis
Carragee EJ (Stanford Univ, Calif)
J Bone Joint Surg Am 79-A:874–880, 1997   12–7

Objective.—The demographics of pyogenic vertebral osteomyelitis have changed, and the infecting organisms found today are not the usual organisms isolated in the past. The records of all patients who had the disease between 1988 and 1993 were reviewed retrospectively at 3 teaching hospitals.

Methods.—Medical records of 111 patients were reviewed for demographic information and findings at the latest follow-up, an average of 4 years. The patients (40% women) ranged in age from 18 to 84 years; 55% were 60 years of age or older. There were 145 segments involved, predominantly those of the lumbosacral and thoracolumbar spine. The immune system was impaired in 40% of patients as a result of illness or the medications used to treat an illness.

Results.—Back pain was present in 101 patients. Thirty-seven had muscle weakness, 18 were febrile, 3 had sepsis, and 2 were paraplegic. White cell counts were elevated in 44 of 108 patients, and the erythrocyte sedimentation rate was elevated in 98 of 103 patients. The infecting organism was *Staphylococcus aureus* in 40 patients, *Staphylococcus epidermidis* in 18, group B hemolytic streptococcus in 11, and *Escherichia coli* and *Streptococcus viridans* in 7. In 21 patients, the urinary tract was suspected as the source of infection, and in 13 patients, this was confirmed as the source. Outcome depended on age, infection with *Staphylococcus aureus*, immune status, and change in erythrocyte sedimentation rate. Thirty-nine patients were treated nonoperatively, and 42 were treated operatively, including 14 who had instrumentation of the spine. Eighteen patients had died at the latest follow-up. Seven of the 89 survivors had chronic severe back pain at the latest follow-up, and most had minor neurologic symptoms.

Conclusion.—The clinical features of pyogenic vertebral osteomyelitis are changing. Whereas *S. aureus* was the most common infecting organism, uncommon pathogens or low-virulence organisms were isolated in 40% of patients. The outcome at 2 years was good, although residual neurologic symptoms remained for most patients.

The Clinical Use of Erythrocyte Sedimentation Rate in Pyogenic Vertebral Osteomyelitis
Carragee EJ, Kim D, van der Vlugt T, et al (Stanford Univ, Calif; Orthopaedic Spine Ctr. at Stanford, Calif)
Spine 22:2089–2093, 1997   12–8

Objective.—Pyogenic vertebral osteomyelitis (PVO) can usually be treated conservatively. The infection must be carefully monitored during the critical first month to avoid neurologic sequelae, spinal instability, progressive or intractable sepsis, and death. Use of erythrocyte sedimentation rate (ESR) to diagnose and manage the infection has not been established. The course of the ESR during the first month of treatment in a cohort of conservatively treated patients with PVO was examined.

Methods.—Charts of 44 conservatively treated patients with PVO (15 women) age 18–84 were retrospectively reviewed. Seventeen (38.6%) were taking immunosuppressive drugs, 14 (13.6%) were IV drug abusers, and 5 (6.3%) were suspected IV drug abusers. Measurement of ESR was performed before or immediately after beginning antibiotic therapy and at least 2 follow-up tests were performed during the month (Table 3).

Results.—All patients had at least 1 month of conservative treatment, including 7–29 weeks of antibiotic therapy. Twelve patients required surgery or died of complications of their disease. The ESR fell by more than 25% in 26 patients during the first month, and in 3, conservative treatment ultimately failed. In the remaining 18, conservative treatment ultimately failed in 9. At mid month, ESR levels for most patients were not significantly lower, and were actually higher than baseline values in 16 patients. Age, immune status, and ESR levels were predictors of response to con-

TABLE 3.—Erythrocyte Sedimentation Rate at Start, Mid-Month, and End-Month Testing

	Mean ESR	% Starting ESR at Week 2–3*	% Starting ESR at Week 4–5†
Success (n = 32)	99.1 (range, 56–125)	89.0%	60.4%
>100%		9	3 (9.4%)
≥75% ≤100%		10	6 (18.6%)
<75%		11	23 (71.9%)
<50%		2	8 (25%)
Failure (n = 12)	86.9 (range, 45–123)	83.4%	77.0%
>100%		7	3 (25%)
≥75% ≤100%		4	5 (41.7%)
<75%		1	4 (33.3%)
<50%		0	2 (16.7%)

*Success vs. failure for ESR at 2 wks., 0.08.
†Success vs. failure for ESR at 4 wks., 0.06.
(Courtesy of Carragee EJ, Kim D, van der Vlugt T, et al: The clinical use of erythrocyte sedimentation rate in pyogenic vertebral osteomyelitis. *Spine* 22:2089–2093, 1997.)

servative treatment. Level of ESR during the first month is an inconsistent predictor of response to conservative treatment.

Conclusion.—Whereas a falling ESR during the first month of conservative treatment for PVO is a good sign, 40% of patients with high or rising ESR also responded to conservative treatment. Levels of ESR must be evaluated as one of a number of clinical signs.

The Clinical Use of Magnetic Resonance Imaging in Pyogenic Vertebral Osteomyelitis

Carragee EJ (Stanford Univ, Calif)
Spine 22:780–785, 1997   12–9

Introduction.—Delays in diagnosis have been common in pyogenic vertebral osteomyelitis (PVO) because of the lack of specificity in symptoms and radiographic features. In some cases with clinical indications suggestive of PVO, MRI is reported to facilitate an earlier diagnosis. A retrospective chart review of 103 cases was conducted to describe the clinical use of MRI in PVO.

Methods.—Spinal MRI scans were performed in all patients before or at the time of diagnosis; 19 additional scans were obtained as follow-up within the first 6 months of treatment. Data recorded were the suggested primary diagnosis based on MRI and the listing of spinal infection as an alternative or differential diagnosis. The impact of scans on subsequent diagnosis was reviewed.

Results.—Patients were 62 men and 41 women, with an average age of 61.5 at the time of diagnosis. Sixty-two had a serious concomitant illness and 44 were immunocompromised in some way. The most common organism identified was *Staphylococcus aureus* (39% of cases). Nearly 75%

of patients had an MRI scan within the first month of illness. After 2 weeks of symptoms, MRI findings provided a correct diagnosis of PVO in 76% of cases and a possible diagnosis in 20%. The MR scans obtained during follow-up suggested progressive disease in some cases that showed clinical improvement.

Discussion.—Most series have reported a 2- to 6-month delay in diagnosis of PVO, but MRI led to diagnosis within 1 month in most cases. The MRI scan suggested vertebral osteomyelitis or discitis as a primary or alternative diagnosis in 93.2% of patients. Although scans obtained within the first 2 weeks of symptoms onset were less specific, MR images obtained this early suggested infection as a primary or alternative diagnosis in 90% of cases. The inflammatory reaction in the marrow of patients with PVO creates abnormal signal on both T1-weighted (decreased signal) and T2-weighted (increased signal) images throughout the involved vertebrae. Paravertebral involvement usually appears as a cuff around the involved vertebrae and disc.

▶ These 3 articles (Abstracts 12–7, 12–8, and 12–9) by Carragee et al. highlight several important concepts regarding the evaluation and treatment of patients with pyogenic vertebral osteomyelitis. The bacteriology of spine infections is changing. Only 36% of the patients in the series were infected with Staphylococcus aureus, the organism that accounted for nearly 100% of spine infections in 1931 and 55% in 1979.[1] Low virulence organisms like Staphylococcus epidermidis and Propionibacterium were as common as Staphylococcus aureus, occurring in 37% of the cases. These organisms should not be dismissed as contaminants in patients clinically suspected to have a spine infection. The use of posterior instrumentation is gaining acceptance in the management of patients with severe kyphotic deformity or instability from major bony destruction. The author's experience with 17 cases treated with instrumentation is describd in more detail in a separate article.[2] These patients should have long-term follow-up and the possibility of late hardware removal should be discussed.

The erythrocyte sedimentation rate is increased in more than 90% of patients with pyogenic vertebral osteomyelitis. An increased erythrocyte sedimentation rate is not sensitive or specific for infection but it is a good screening test and it is also useful for following the response to treatment. As the author states, however, the sedimentation rate must be interpreted in the context of the patient's symptomatic response and other clinical factors, since it is far from 100% accurate at predicting the outcome of treatment. The C-reactive protein has been shown to be helpful in the diagnosis of postoperative discitis[3] and may prove to be beneficial in the diagnosis of vertebral osteomyelitis and in following the response to treatment. These studies must be interpreted in light of the normal rise and fall that occur after any spinal procedure.[4]

Carragee confirmed the report of Gillams et al.[5] concerning the characteristic MRI findings during the temporal evolution of vertebral osteomyelitis. Magnetic resonance scans should not be used to follow the response to treatment, since they are too expensive, return to normal slowly, and may even show increasing enhancement patterns despite clinical improvement.

B.L. Currier, M.D.

References

1. Currier BL, Eismont FJ: Infections of the spine, in Rothman RH, Simeone FA (eds): *The Spine*, ed 4. Philadelphia, WB Saunders, in press.
2. Carragee EJ: Instrumentation of the infected and unstable spine: A review of 17 cases from the thoracic and lumbar spine with pyogenic infections. *J Spinal Disord* 10:317–324, 1997.
3. Schulitz KP, Assheuer J: Discitis after procedures on the intervertebral disc. *Spine* 19:1172–1177, 1994.
4. Thelander U, Larsson S: Quantitation of C-reactive protein levels and erythrocyte sedimentation rate after spinal surgery. *Spine* 17:400, 1992.
5. Gillams AR, Chaddha B, Carter AP: MR appearances of the temporal evolution and resolution of infectious spondylitis. *Am J Roentgenol* 166:903–907,1996.

Instrumentation

Threaded Titanium Cages for Lumbar Interbody Fusions
Ray CD (Spinal Research & Education Found, Norfolk, Va)
Spine 22:667–680, 1997   12–10

Objective.—The safety and efficacy of the Ray-titanium fusion cage (TFC) device in producing solid lumbar fusions in patients with severe, disabling low back pain was investigated in a multicenter, prospective trial. The device was developed and patented by the author who has an indirect financial interest in the product.

Methods.—Ten patients involved in a pilot study were followed up for an average of 78 months. The remaining 236 patients, with severe disabling back pain (96%) as a result of major annular degeneration (74%), herniations (57%), osteophytes (21%), and reduced disk height (43%), were enrolled later in the Investigational Device Exemption (IDE) study at 9 centers with 13 surgeons. Whereas 45% of patients had had previous spinal surgeries, none had posterior lumbar interbody fusions. Patients were followed up at 6 weeks, at 3, 6, 12, 18, and 24 months, and yearly thereafter. Patients were followed up for an average of 32 months.

Results.—All 10 patients in the pilot study had fusion solidity. Six had an 80% or better improvement, and 3 had 60% or better improvement. No patient had a poor result. In the IDE study, 57% of implants were performed at the L5-S1 level, 40% at the L4-5 level, and 3% at the L3-4 level. Eight patients received a single cage only. No space settled around a cage more than 1.5 mm. There was no displacement, dislodgement, or removal, although 3 were readjusted. Half of the patients received hydroxylapatite-coated titanium cages, and half received uncoated cages. There were no serious complications after 6 weeks. Transient temporary foot weakness occurred in 10% of patients. Seven wound infections resolved before the 6-week visit. Fusion was rapid, and at 2 years, 96% of the 208 patients available for follow-up had fusion. Functional improvement was excellent in 40%, good in 25%, fair in 21%, and poor in 14%.

Conclusions.—The Ray-titanium TFC device is safe and effective and yields rapid lumbar interbody fusions. Functional outcome at 2 years is good or excellent in 65% of patients, and complications are few and not serious.

▶ Interbody fusion cages have swept the spinal implant market over the past 2 years. Fortunately the device manufacturers have complied with the Food and Drug Administration (FDA) IDE study requirements, and the spine community may be spared from the wave of litigation caused by the use of pedicle screws.

The author claimed that no serious complications occurred in this series. Although the FDA did not consider complications to be serious if they resolved in less than 6 weeks, most surgeons would consider a 10% rate of temporary foot weakness or numbness and a 3% infection rate significant complications when treating low back pain. Two patients wore an ankle-foot orthosis for up to 6 or 12 months and had permanent 20% motor deficits. The author also stated that "follow-up studies, to date, have failed to show any case of fusion transition syndrome." None of the 5 references cited in support of that statement involved procedures using cages. Two of the author's own first 10 patients (the group with the longest follow-up) required subsequent fusions at adjacent levels. The author's explanation that in those 2 cases "moderately degenerated discs were erroneously not included in the original single-level procedure" may or may not be valid.

The TFC device and other cage designs may prove to be safe and effective treatment options for low back pain, but until long-term follow-up data and corroborative studies are available, caution is advised. Patient selection will always be the most important determinant of outcome, and the allure of new options should not change the indications for surgery.

B.L. Currier, M.D.

Pedicle Screw Fixation for Nontraumatic Lesions of the Cervical Spine
Abumi K, Kaneda K (Hokkaido Univ, Sapporo, Japan)
Spine 22:1853–1863, 1997   12–11

Objective.—Recent studies have demonstrated that pedicle screw fixation is biomechanically superior to lateral mass fixation in the cervical spine. Results of pedicle screw fixation with and without fusion in 45 patients with nontraumatic lesions in the cervical spine were described, as well as the surgical technique.

Methods.—Between 1990 and 1994, reconstructive surgery including pedicle screw fixation and fusion was performed in 45 patients (22 men), aged 22–76 years, who had vertebral tumors ($n = 13$), rheumatoid arthritis ($n = 11$), ossification of the posterior longitudinal ligament or cervical spondylosis ($n = 10$), spinal cord tumor ($n = 5$), destructive spondyloarthropathy as a result of long-term hemodialysis ($n = 3$), and infectious spondylitis ($n = 3$). Previous operations had failed in 13 patients. Plain radiographs, anteroposterior and lateral tomography, CT, and MRI were performed. There were 191 screws inserted into the cervical pedicles.

> *Technique.*—A small pedicle probe was inserted into the pedicle to confirm direction and depth, and a hole was tapped, not drilled, for the screw. Trajectory at each level was determined using preoperative CT scans. A simultaneous laminectomy (after screw insertion) or laminoplasty with posterior fixation was performed in 27 patients. Bone grafting was performed in 37 patients but not in 8 with metastatic tumors. Plates and rods were used. As many as 9 spinal segments were fixed, with the average being 3 or 4. Patients were immobilized after surgery depending on the number of fixed segments, the patient's condition, and the extent of osteoporosis. Rigid external supports were not used. Patients were followed up for an average of 43 months except for 9 who died of metastatic disease. Fusion was assessed radiographically. Screws were located using CT.

Results.—Neurologic deficits did not increase. At last follow-up, solid bony union was achieved in 37 patients, no implant had failed, and 4 patients with severe preoperative kyphotic deformity had maintained the correction. Eleven screws (all in pedicles from C3 to C7) that had penetrated the pedicle were assumed to be at risk for causing injury, but no screws at the C2 pedicle were at risk. One case of radiculopathy caused by a screw penetrating upward from the pedicle spontaneously resolved. Complications included cerebrospinal fluid leakage in 3 patients, and a deep infection in 1. Pedicle screw fixation in the cervical spine, except at the C2 level, has been criticized as risky for neurovascular structures. Several cases of screw loosening have been reported in lateral mass screw procedures. Use of pedicle screws appears to provide more rigid internal fixation than lateral mass screws, except in those patients where pedicle diameter is too small. The technique is particularly helpful in patients with rheumatoid arthritis or spondyloarthropathy, where lateral mass screw fixation does not provide sufficient stability.

Conclusions.—Pedicle screw fixation is safe and effective for reconstructing nontraumatic lesions of the cervical spine.

Cervical Pedicle Screws *Versus* Lateral Mass Screws: Anatomic Feasibility and Biomechanical Comparison
Jones EL, Heller JG, Silcox DH, et al (Emory Univ, Atlanta, Ga)
Spine 22:977–982, 1997   12–12

Objective.—The pull-out strengths of lateral mass and pedicle screws in the human cervical spine were compared, and pull-out strength and bone density, screw length, and vertebral level were correlated. Cervical morphometry was tabulated to facilitate development of a viable screw insertion technique.

Methods.—Ten fresh, normal human cervical spine specimens (56 vertebrae) were disarticulated. Mean pedicle height and width were recorded, and angle with respect to midline was determined by CT. A 3.5-mm cortical screw was placed by the method of An et al. into the lateral mass on one side and into the pedicle on the opposite side. The tip of the unicortical pedicle screws were advanced to the inner edge of the cortex. A coupling device pulled on the axis of each screw with a loading rate of 2 mm/min.

Results.—The mean load-to-failure was significantly higher for cervical pedicle screws than for lateral mass screws (677 N vs. 355 N). The 13 2.7-mm pedicle screws had pull-out strengths similar to those of the 3.5-mm pedicle screws. There were no correlations between pull-out strengths and bone density, screw length, or vertebral level for either type of screw. Seven minor pedicle wall breaches were found.

Discussion.—This study confirms a biomechanical study in the bovine model showing the superiority of pedicle screw fixation over lateral mass fixation in the cervical spine. Care must be exercised when using cervical pedicle screws because of the important anatomical structures that surround the pedicle. Transpedicle screw placement must be individualized because of the variation in pedicle dimensions.

Conclusions.—The force required to pull out cervical pedicle screws was significantly higher than the force needed to pull out lateral mass screws.

▶ Instability of the cervical spine can be caused by a variety of conditions including trauma, neoplasms, inflammatory disorders, and spondylosis. Numerous internal fixation techniques are available to stabilize the cervical spine, including wire constructs and plates or rods secured to the spine with screws placed in the lateral masses or pedicles. The more rigid systems decrease the need for postoperative halos and collars, but that advantage must be weighed against a higher complication rate. In addition to superior stability, lateral mass and pedicle screw fixation can be achieved in situations where the laminae and spinous processes are deficient. Pedicle screws have been widely used in the lumbar spine for more than a decade because of their biomechanical advantages over other fixation methods. Jones et al. (Abstract 12–12) have demonstrated that the pull-out strength of pedicle screws is significantly greater than lateral mass screws. Kotani et al. have also shown that cervical spine pedicle fixation is biomechanically superior to lateral mass plates. They demonstrated that pedicle screw constructs have comparable stability to anterior plates combined with posterior wiring.[1] Since 1990, Abumi (Abstract 12–11) has been successfully using pedicle screws to stabilize the cervical spine. Despite careful preoperative planning with radiographs and CT scans and precise surgical technique, 6.9% of the screws inserted in C3-C7 by Abumi were outside of the pedicle and placed the spinal cord, nerve root, or vertebral artery at risk. Fortunately the rate of clinical sequelae was much lower than that, with only a single case of radiculopathy.

In the study using cadaveric specimens, Jones et al. noted that 13% of their pedicle screws, placed under direct vision in disarticulated specimens denuded of soft tissues, violated the pedicle walls. Several recent studies, including the one by Jones et al., have documented the variability that exists in pedicle morphology.

The following principles have emerged from all of these studies:

1. Choose the simplest, least risky procedure that is capable of providing adequate stability.

2. Before attempting any procedure, have a thorough understanding of the anatomy, obtain adequate training, and plan the procedure preoperatively using appropriate imaging studies (including CT).

3. Use precise surgical technique with intraoperative imaging.

4. Be aware that none of the techniques that rely on screw fixation in the posterior cervical spine have been "approved" by the Food and Drug Administration.

B.L. Currier, M.D.

Reference

1. Kotani Y, Cunningham BW, Abumi K, et al: Biomechanical analysis of cervical stabilization systems: An assessment of transpedicular screw fixation in the cervical spine. *Spine* 19:2529–2539, 1994.

Radiological and Anatomical Evaluation of the Atlantoaxial Transarticular Screw Fixation Technique
Madawi AA, Casey ATH, Solanki GA, et al (Natl Hosp for Neurology and Neurosurgery, London; Natl Inst of Traumatology, Budapest, Hungary)
J Neurosurg 86:961–968, 1997   12–13

Objective.—Little is known about the early and late complications of the atlantoaxial transarticular screw fixation technique. Risk factors for technique-related complications were analyzed radiologically, and the optimum screw trajectory and its safety margin were determined using dry C-2 human vertebrae.

Methods.—Radiologic studies (plain films and plain CT scanning in all patients and MRI and MR angiography in patients with residual neurologic deficits) were performed on 61 patients (18 male), aged 7–77 years. The patients underwent C1-2 transarticular screw fixation for spinal instability to evaluate screw position, stability, and fusion and to identify risk factors for technique-related complications. Pedicle and lateral mass parameters were measured in 25 dry C-2 vertebrae (Fig 1). Patients were followed for an average of 26 months.

Results.—Patients were given a diagnosis of rheumatoid arthritis (37 patients), traumatic atlantoaxial instability (15 patients), and miscellaneous indications (9 patients). Previous anteroposterior atlantoaxial surgery had been performed in 4 patients; a lateral C1-2 procedure in 1;

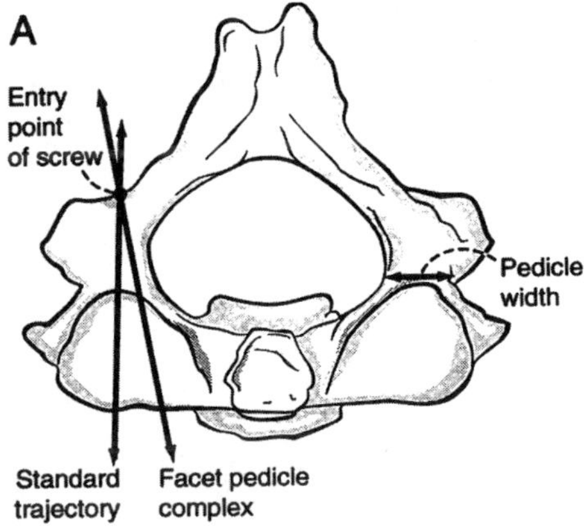

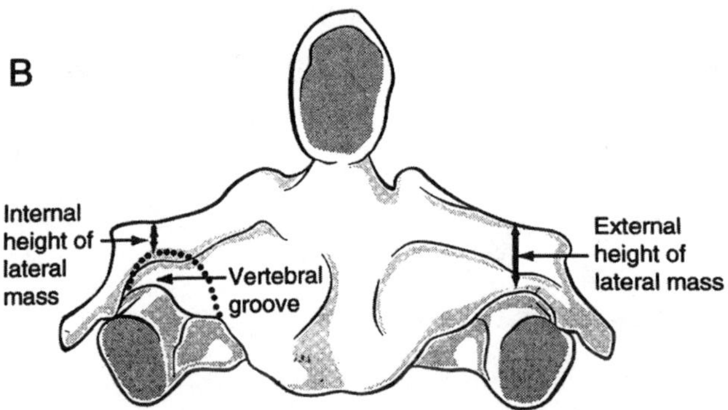

FIGURE 1.—Drawings show the C-2 vertebra (**A**, top view; **B**, frontal view) and the measured anatomical parameters in this study. (Courtesy of Madawi AA, Casey ATH, Solanki GA, et al: Radiological and anatomical evaluation of the atlantoaxial transarticular screw fixation technique. *J Neurosurg* 86:961–968, 1997.)

posterior procedures in 5; and transoral dens resection, dens screw, or transoral plate procedures in 11. No patients died. Complications included 9 malpositioned screws, 5 screw breakages as a result of incorrect placement, 8 nonunions, 4 instability problems, 5 vertebral artery (VA) injuries, and 1 cranial nerve injury that resolved. Anatomical findings revealed significant morphologic variations including an asymmetrical anatomical course of the VA through the lateral mass in 52% of vertebrae and a significant VA groove in 20% of vertebrae, reducing the width of the C2 pedicle sufficiently to interfere with safe passage of a 3.5-mm screw (Figs 4 and 5). Incomplete reduction before screw placement was a risk factor that accounted for two thirds of screw complications and all VA injuries. Prior transoral surgery with removal of the anterior tubercle or the arch of the atlas and lack of awareness of the size of the VA groove in the C-2 lateral mass accounted for most of the remaining complications. There was an 87% fusion rate.

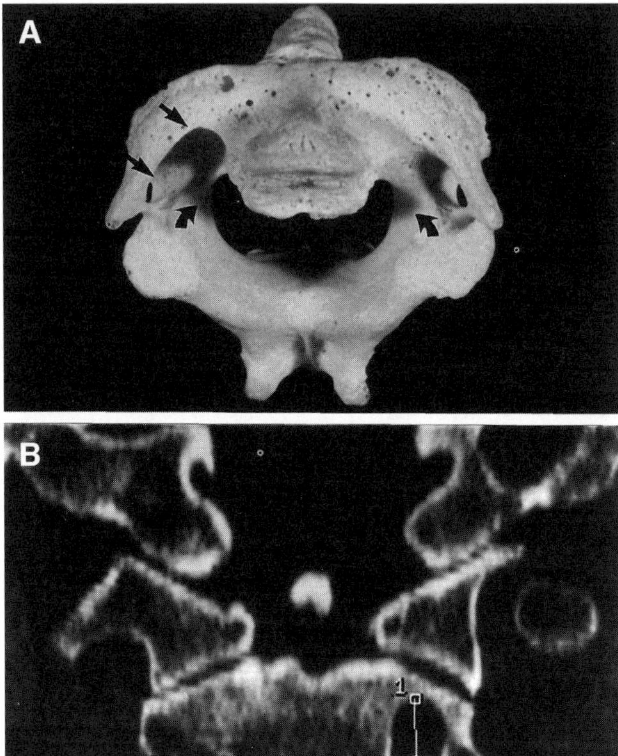

FIGURE 4.—Anatomical and radiologic appearance of an enlarged vertebral artery (VA) groove. **A,** A photograph depicting anatomy; C-2 viewed from below showing large VA groove nearly eroding most of the C-2 lateral mass and pedicle (*left curved arrow*). The right pedicle is normal (*right curved arrow*). In these circumstances transarticular screw fixation would not be recommended. **B,** spine CT reformat shows enlarged left VA groove. (Courtesy of Madawi AA, Casey ATH, Solanki GA, et al: Radiological and anatomical evaluation of the atlantoaxial transarticular screw fixation technique. *J Neurosurg* 86:961–968, 1997.)

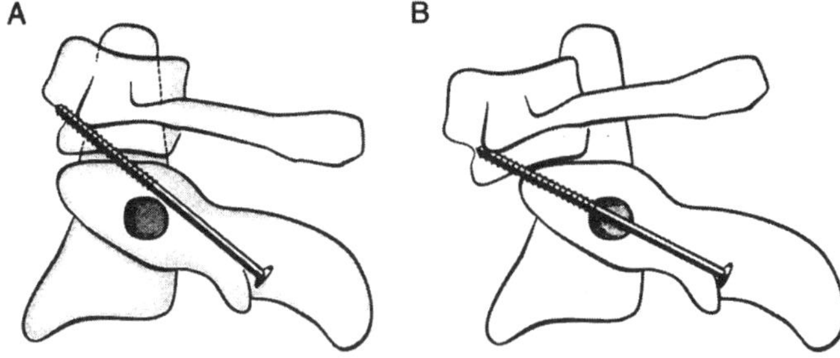

FIGURE 5.—Drawings depict a lateral view of the C1-2 joint. **A,** drawing shows normal position with normal screw trajectory. **B,** drawing shows the effect of incompletely reduced displacement and the segment in full flexion; with screw trajectory aiming to the anterior tubercle of C-1, the screw will be low enough to transect the VA underneath the C-2 lateral mass. A VA injury would be inevitable in these circumstances. (Courtesy of Madawi AA, Casey ATH, Solanki GA, et al: Radiological and anatomical evaluation of the atlantoaxial transarticular screw fixation technique. *J Neurosurg* 86:961–968, 1997.)

Conclusion.—The atlantoaxial transarticular screw fixation technique provides a good outcome provided detailed CT scans are performed preoperatively and careful attention is paid to anatomical landmarks and individual variations in the C1-2 vertebrae.

Unilateral Posterior Atlantoaxial Transarticular Screw Fixation

Song GS, Theodore N, Dickman CA, et al (Mercy Healthcare Arizona, Phoenix; Pusan Natl Univ, Korea)
J Neurosurg 87:851–855, 1997

12–14

Objective.—Whereas bilateral posterior atlantoaxial transarticular screw placement is the most effective technique for achieving C1-2 stability, unilateral anomalies prevent placement of a screw across the C1-2 facet in some patients. Long-term results were reported for unilateral posterior atlantoaxial transarticular screw placement with supplemental bone graft wiring.

Methods.—Between March 1992 and July 1995, unilateral posterior atlantoaxial transarticular screw placement with interspinous bone graft wiring was performed in 19 patients (9 men), aged 19–78 years, given a diagnosis of progressive myelopathy (9 patients), rheumatoid arthritis (7 patients), and os odontoideum (2 patients). Unilateral surgery was performed to avoid neural or vertebral artery injury and to produce C1-2 stability. Autogenous iliac crest bone grafts were used in 18 patients and banked bone was used in 1. Patients wore Philadelphia collars for an average of 8 weeks after surgery.

Results.—Unilateral C1-2 arthrodesis was performed for a high-riding transverse foramen of the C-2 vertebra in 13 patients, poor purchase in 2, screw malposition in 1, severe degenerative arthritis in 1, neurofibroma in 1, and C-1 lateral mass fracture in 1. There were 3 complications. In 1 case, screw fracture and bone subluxation redeveloped at 6 weeks; it was treated with occipitocervical fusion with a Steinmann pin and wire cable from the occiput to the C-3 vertebra. The other 2 cases involved 1 wound dehiscence and 1 donor site infection at the iliac crest bone donor site. Fusion was achieved in all patients. Eighteen patients were followed for an average of 31 months. There were no delayed failures.

Conclusion.—Unilateral posterior atlantoaxial transarticular screw fixation is a satisfactory alternative for patients in whom the bilateral procedure is contraindicated. There were no long-term neurologic or vascular complications.

▶ The transarticular screw fixation technique has gained rapid acceptance since its introduction in 1987.[1] Grob et al.[2] demonstrated the biomechanical superiority of the technique over a Gallie type posterior C1–C2 arthrodesis. Many authors now consider the technique to be the procedure of choice in patients with rheumatoid arthritis and other unstable conditions for avoiding postoperative halo immobilization.

The rate of vertebral artery injuries and hardware failures is sobering, however, and the need for careful preoperative planning and precise surgical technique cannot be overemphasized. Madawi et al. (Abstract 12–13) report a 20% incidence of clinically significant unilateral vertebral groove anomalies, and this finding was confirmed by the authors in a larger anatomical study of 50 specimens.[3] The report by Song et al. (Abstract 12–14), showing an excellent fusion rate when only a single transarticular screw was used, mandates avoidance of the second screw if the preoperative CT demonstrates a unilateral anomaly that would increase the risk to the vertebral artery.

The study also raises the question, Is a single screw always enough? Finally, the enthusiasm for an elegant new technique should not make us loose sight of the fact that a Brooks fusion is as stable as the transarticular screw technique except in rotation[2] and that the complications and inconvenience of a halo pale in comparison with an inury of the vertebral artery.

B.L. Currier, M.D.

References

1. Magerl F, Seemann PS: Stable posterior fusion of the atlas and axis by transarticular screw fixation, in Kehr P, Weidner, A (eds): *Cervical Spine I*. Vienna, Springer-Verlag, 1987, pp 322–327.
2. Grob D, Crisco JJ III, Panjabi MM, et al: Biomechanical evaluation of four different posterior atlantoaxial fixation techniques. *Spine* 17:480–490, 1992.
3. Madawi AA, Solanaki GA, Casey ATH, et al: Variation of the groove in the axis vertebra for the vertebral artery: Implications for instrumentation. *J Bone Joint Surg Br* 79-B:820–823, 1997.

Outcomes of Surgical Management

Single-Level Posterolateral Arthrodesis, With or Without Posterior Decompression, for the Treatment of Isthmic Spondylolisthesis in Adults: A Prospective, Randomized Study
Carragee EJ (Stanford Univ, Calif)
J Bone Joint Surg Am 79-A:1175–1180, 1997   12–15

Objective.—Whether decompression and arthrodesis or arthrodesis alone is recommended for patients who fail conservative management of isthmic spondylolisthesis is controversial, particularly because clinical reviews have involved mixed groups. Patients who had a primary posterolateral arthrodesis at the fifth lumbar and first sacral vertebral levels, and a laminectomy were compared with outcomes in patients not having decompression. Only patients who smoked were managed with transpedicular instrumentation.

Methods.—Between 1989 and 1992, 42 patients with grade I or II isthmic spondylolisthesis and persistent pain were randomly assigned to treatment with posterolateral arthrodesis only (24 patients) or to treatment with posterolateral arthrodesis and decompression (18 patients). Both groups had placement of autogenous bone graft from the iliac crest.

TABLE 2.—Clinical Results at the Latest Follow-up Evaluation

	Arthrodesis with Instrumentation			Arthrodesis without Instrumentation		
	With Decompression	Without Decompression	P Value	With Decompression	Without Decompression	P Value
No. of patients	8	12		10	12	
Pseudarthrosis *(no. of patients)*	1	0	0.2	3	0	0.04
Score on visual-analog scale* *(points)*						
Back pain	2.2 (0–8)	1.1 (0–3)	NS	3.8 (0–8)	1.6 (0–4)	NS
Pain in lower extremities	3.1 (0–6)	0.9 (0–3)	0.1	4.4 (0–10)	1.9 (0–4)	0.06
Activity level	7.3 (3–10)	7.6 (6–10)	NS	6.2 (1–10)	7.5 (6–9)	NS
Satisfaction	8.6 (5–10)	8.9 (7–10)	NS	6.9 (2–10)	8.0 (6–10)	NS
Use of medication*† *(points)*	7.1 (2–10)	8.4 (5–10)	NS	5.3 (0–10)	8.3 (5–10)	NS
Over-all score†‡ *(points)*	7.6 (3.3–10)	8.5 (6.1–10)	NS	6.1 (1–10)	8.0 (5.8–9.8)	NS
Clinical result *(no. of patients)*						
Excellent or good (6–10 points)	6	12	0.07	6	11	0.06
Fair or poor (0–6 points)	2	0		4	1	

*The values are given as the mean, with the range in parentheses.

†Rated as none (10 points), occasional use of non-narcotic medication (8 points), daily use of non-narcotic medication (5 points), occasional use of narcotic medication (2 points), or daily use of narcotic medication (0 points).

‡Calculated as ([satisfaction] + [medication] + [activity] + [10-pain scale/2])/4.

Abbreviation: NS, not significant.

(Courtesy of Carragee EJ: Single-level posterolateral arthrodesis, with or without posterior decompression, for the treatment of isthmic spondylolisthesis in adults. *J Bone Joint Surg [Am]* 79-A:1175–1180, 1997.)

Twenty smokers had posterolateral arthrodesis with instrumentation. Four patients who had decompression and 3 who had arthrodesis also had only an allogenic bone graft. Pain was assessed perioperatively on a 10-point visual analogue scale, and duration of symptoms, pain medication, work status, and other medical problems were recorded. Patients were followed for an average of 4.5 years; the follow-up rate was 98%.

Results.—Four patients managed with decompression had a pseudarthrosis, and 6 had an unsatisfactory outcome. The 24 patients managed without decompression had successful fusion (Table 2). Twelve smokers managed without decompression had a pseudarthrosis, and 1 managed with decompression had a pseudarthrosis. Twelve nonsmokers managed without decompression had a pseudarthrosis, and 1 had an unsatisfactory result. Three nonsmokers with decompression had a pseudarthrosis, and 4 had an unsatisfactory result. Two patients managed with instrumentation and decompression had a pseudarthrosis; none of the 12 managed without decompression had a pseudarthrosis.

Conclusion.—The outcome of patients with low-grade isthmic spondylolisthesis (and no serious neurological deficit) did not improve after the addition of decompression to arthrodesis, performed with or without instrumentation. The decompression increased the rates of pseudarthrosis and failure.

▶ This excellent, prospective, randomized study addresses 2 of the many controversies dealing with the operative treatment of grade I or II isthmic spondylolisthesis in adults. Dr. Carragee concluded that decompression is not necessary and may be deleterious for the treatment of low-grade isthmic spondylolisthesis without significant neurologic deficit. The study did not address the need for a decompression when treating patients with a major neurologic deficit or high-grade slip, but it did show that when a decompression is performed, instrumentation enhances the fusion rate.

Peek et al.[1] demonstrated, in a small series (8 patients), that neurologic improvement can occur with in situ arthrodesis without decompression in adults with a high-grade slip and severe leg pain. The neurologic recovery was good but relatively protracted in some cases; the lower limb pain resolved in 0.5–3.5 months. Schoenecker et al.[2] raised awareness of the risk of cauda equina syndrome after in situ arthrodesis of severe spondylolisthesis. Most surgeons now recommend a decompression with arthrodesis when treating high-grade isthmic spondylolisthesis or when the patient has a significant neurologic deficit.

The use of instrumentation was not randomized in Carragee's study because it was considered unethical to deny instrumentation to smokers as they have a higher pseudarthrosis rate and instrumentation has been shown to enhance the rate of fusion. Despite this limitation, the data suggest that instrumentation should be used in all patients requiring a decompression regardless of their smoking history.

B.L. Currier, M.D.

References

1. Peek RD, Wiltse LL, Reynolds JB, et al: In situ arthrodesis without decompression for grade-III or IV isthmic spondylolisthesis in adults who have severe sciatica. *J Bone Joint Surg Am* 71-A:62–68, 1989.
2. Schoenecker PL, Cole HO, Herring JA, et al: Cauda equina syndrome following in situ arthrodesis of severe spondylolisthesis of the lumbosacral junction. *J Bone Joint Surg Am* 72-A:369, 1990.

Vertical Translocation: Part II. Outcomes After Surgical Treatment of Rheumatoid Cervical Myelopathy

Casey ATH, Crockard HA, Stevens J (Natl Hosp for Neurology and Neurosurgery, London)
J Neurosurg 87:863–869, 1997

12–16

Objective.—A surgical approach to vertical translocation in patients with rheumatoid arthritis and the clinical and radiologic factors that influence outcome were described.

Methods.—A prospective observational study was conducted with 116 patients (24 men), with an average age of 62 years, with rheumatoid cervical myelopathy who underwent cervical spine surgery. The Ranawat neurologic classification, American Rheumatism Association functional grading system, Stanford Health Activity Questionnaire disability index for rheumatoid arthritis, and the Myelopathy Disability Index were used to measure outcomes. Morbidity and mortality rates were calculated. Patients were followed for an average of 45.3 months.

Results.—There were 67 transoral decompressions performed and 33 patients received a bone graft. Nine patients required reoperation at an average of 16 months. There were 45 complications including 23 respiratory, 12 cardiovascular, and 5 transoral. There were also 1 posterior cervical wound infection, 3 meningitis infections, 11 peptic ulcers, and 5 pressure sores or decubitus ulcers. The 30-day mortality was 10.3%. There was improvement by at least 1 Ranawat class in 45% of patients. Younger age and good preoperative muscle power were associated with good neurologic outcome. All scoring systems were significant predictors of outcome. Vertical translocation as measured by the Redlund-Johnell method and spinal cord area were significant predictors of outcome. Neither degree of transgression in the foramen as measured by the McRae method nor anterior or posterior atlantodens interval were predictive of neurologic outcome.

Conclusion.—Preoperative neurologic function, spinal cord area, and degree of vertical translocation were predictive of neurologic outcome after surgical treatment of rheumatoid cervical myelopathy.

▶ In part I of their series, Casey et al.[1] showed that vertical translocation (cranial settling) is caused primarily by collapse of the C1 lateral masses and is associated with a progressive decrease in the anterior atlantodens interval

(ADI). This condition, termed pseudostabilization, was recently investigated by Fujiwara et al.[2] and their findings were similar. Casey et al. found that the ADI is not a reliable predictor of neural compromise in the presence of vertical translocation. This confirms the findings of Boden et al.[3] who noted that the posterior atlantodens interval, not the anterior ADI, correlated with the presence and severity of neurologic compromise.

There are several notable findings in part II of the series by Casey et al. The 30-day mortality rate was 10.3% and the rate was highest in the patients with the poorest preoperative neurologic grades. The authors measured the degree of vertical translocation by the Redlund-Johnell method. This is a particularly effective technique because many of the other methods are difficult to measure on routine radiographs, and in the Redlund-Johnell method, unlike Ranawat's method, the degree of occiput-C1 settling as well as C1-C2 settling can be appreciated. The final neurologic grade was influenced most by the level of preoperative neurologic function, area of the spinal cord, and degree of vertical translocation.

These findings highlight the need to follow patients with rheumatoid arthritis carefully, using reliable radiographic measurement techniques and offering surgery early before significant myelopathy develops. If patients undergo early prophylactic posterior stabilization, they can avoid transoral decompressions as performed in over 50% of the patients in this series.

B.L. Currier, M.D.

References

1. Casey AT, Crockard HA, Geddes JF, et al: Vertical translocation: The enigma of the disappearing atlantodens interval in patients with myelopathy and rheumatoid arthritis: Part I. Clinical, radiological, and neuropathological features. *J Neurosurg* 87:856–862, 1997.
2. Fujiwara K, Yonenobu K, Ochi T: Natural history of upper cervial lesions in rheumatoid arthritis. *J Spinal Disord* 10:275–281, 1997.
3. Boden SD, Dodge LD, Bohlman HH, et al: Rheumatoid arthritis of the cervical spine. A long-term analysis with predictors of paralysis and recovery. *J Bone Joint Surg Am* 75-A:1282–1297, 1993.

Pathophysiology of Sciatica

The Effects of Normal, Frozen, and Hyaluronidase-digested Nucleus Pulposus on Nerve Root Structure and Function

Olmarker K, Brisby H, Yabuki S, et al (Univ of Gothenburg, Sweden; Fukushima Med College, Japan)
Spine 22:471–476, 1997

12–17

Purpose.—Animal studies have shown that the presence of autologous nucleus pulposus in the epidural space can cause nerve root injury. The pathophysiologic mechanisms induced by the nucleus pulposus are unknown, as are which substances from the nucleus pulposus might be involved. This study examined the effects of modifying the nucleus pulposus—either by freezing it, by heating it, or by digesting it with hyaluronidase—on its nerve root-damaging effects.

Methods.—Nucleus pulposus from the lumbar disks of pigs was either frozen, heated, or digested by hyaluronidase. Freezing was to eliminate the effects of living cells; hyaluronidase digestion to remove the proteoglycan matrix. The nucleus pulposus was then applied to the cauda equina. In some cases, freshly harvested nucleus pulposus was applied as a control. Nerve conduction velocity studies and blinded light microscopic assessments were performed after 7 days.

Results.—Nerve conduction velocity was significantly reduced, to an extent similar to that noted in previous studies, when the nucleus pulposus was applied just after harvest, or after heating, or after hyaluronidase digestion. No such change was noted when the nucleus pulposus was frozen. Histologic examination showed no apparent differences among groups. Microscopic staining studies demonstrated cell lysis in the frozen nucleus pulposus specimens, compared with little change in the heated or hyaluronidase-digested specimens.

Conclusions.—Since freezing prevents the damaging effects of autologous nucleus pulposus on nerve root function, these effects appear to be related to cell population. The cell population of nucleus pulposus includes chrondrocytes, fibrocytes, notochordal cells, and secretory stellate cells, the main function of which is to produce the nucleus pulposus matrix. The nucleus pulposus cells may also produce substances that have direct or indirect immunologic, inflammatory, or other effects on nerve tissue.

The Role of Phospholipase A$_2$ and Nitric Oxide in Pain-related Behavior Produced by an Allograft of Intervertebral Disc Material to the Sciatic Nerve of the Rat

Kawakami M, Tamaki T, Hashizume H, et al (Wakayama Med College, Japan; Univ of Iowa, Iowa City; Procter & Gamble Company, Cincinnati, Ohio)
Spine 22:1074–1079, 1997   12–18

Background.—Previous animal studies have shown that applying nucleus pulposus to the lumbar epidural space produces mechanical hyperalgesia, whereas application of anulus fibrosis material to the same location produces thermal hyperalgesia. The 2 phenomena are associated with distinct histologic changes. The mechanism of these effects involves phospholipase A$_2$ in mechanical hyperalgesia and nitric oxide in thermal hyperalgesia. However, the link between hyperalgesia and the activation and involvement of phospholipase A$_2$ and the production of nitric oxide is unclear. This study sought to determine whether the application of intervertebral disk material to the sciatic nerve would produce hyperalgesia, and if this effect could be altered by inhibitors of phospholipase A$_2$ and nitric oxide synthase.

Methods.—Five groups of rats were studied. A control group received no treatment, and a sham group underwent exposure of the sciatic nerve only. The other 3 groups received allografts of either fat, nucleus pulposus, or nucleus pulposus plus anulus fibrosus, onto the sciatic nerve. Before and after the various treatments, the animals underwent testing of withdrawal threshold and latency in response to mechanical pressure and radiant heat applied to the hind paws. These responses were re-evaluated after local sciatic nerve administration of inhibitors of phospholipase A_2 and nitric oxide synthase—N^ω-nitro-L-arginine methyl ester and mepacrine, respectively.

Results.—Mechanical hyperalgesia was apparent only in rats treated with nucleus pulposus. However, after inhibition of phospholipase A_2, animals treated with nucleus pulposus plus anulus fibrosus showed evidence of mechanical hyperalgesia as well. Both of these groups returned to normal after nitric oxide synthase inhibition. None of the 5 groups showed signs of thermal hyperalgesia.

Conclusions.—Phospholipase A_2 produced in peripherally applied intervertebral disk material appears to play a significant role in the development of mechanical hyperalgesia. The findings suggest that both phospholipase A_2 and nitric oxide, produced in or around herniated disk materials, are involved in the mechanism of radicular pain after lumbar disk herniation. The study suggests some possible clinical uses for effective phospholipase A_2 inhibitors in patients with back and radicular pain.

▶ These articles (Abstracts 12–17 and 12–18) add to the authors' long lists of excellent publications on the pathophysiology of sciatica secondary to a herniated nucleus pulposus. In 1993, the group from the University of Gothenburg published their classic article[1] showing that nerve root injury may occur in the presence of autologous nucleus pulposus without mechanical compression. In their recent study, they altered the nucleus pulposus before application of the tissue to the cauda equina to determine which component of the material is responsible for the neurophysiologic changes. The resulting demonstration that the cells are the source of the effects will help to focus research efforts on this important area.

Kang et al.,[2] have shown that cultured human disc cells produce a number of substances, including matrix metalloproteinases, nitric oxide, interleukin-6, and prostaglandin E2. In 1996, Kawakami et al.,[3] reported that mechanical and thermal hyperalgesia result from placing allograft nucleus pulposus and anulus fibrosus with nucleus pulposus into the epidural space. In addition, these authors showed that phospholipase A2 (PLA2) was present in the applied nucleus pulposus and anulus fibrosus, whereas nitric oxide synthase was seen in the granulation tissue around the transplanted anulus fibrosus. Other studies suggest that PLA2 is involved preferentially in mechanical hyperalgesia, and that nitric oxide synthase is involved in thermal hyperalgesia. In their recent study, these authors suggest that nitric oxide production may reduce the mechanical hyperalgesia caused by the PLA2 produced in the intervertebral disc. Future studies will eventually lead to more specific and potent pharmacological treatment strategies for sciatica and back pain.

B.L. Currier, M.D.

References

1. Olmarker K, Rydevik B, Nordborg C: Autologous nucleus pulposus induces neurophysiologic and histologic changes in porcine cauda equina nerve roots. *Spine* 18:1425–1432, 1993.
2. Kang JD, Georgescu HI, Larkin L, et al: Herniated lumbar and cervical intervertebral discs spontaneously produce matrix metalloproteinases, nitric oxide, interleukin-6, and prostaglandin E2. *Spine* 21:271–277, 1996.
3. Kawakami M, Tamaki T, Weinstein JN, et al: Pathomechanism of pain-related behavior produced by allografts of intervertebral disc in the rat. *Spine* 21:2101–2107, 1996.

Practice Guidelines

Primary Care Physicians' Use of Lumbar Spine Imaging Tests: Effects of Guidelines and Practice Pattern Feedback

Freeborn DK, Shye D, Mullooly JP, et al (Kaiser Permanente Ctr for Health Research, Portland, Ore)
J Gen Intern Med 12:619–625, 1997   12–19

Purpose.—Physicians vary in their pattern of care for low back pain, with particularly wide variations in their use of imaging studies. This variation may have implications for quality of care. The ability of a clinical practice guideline and practice pattern feedback to reduce variability in the use of imaging studies for back pain by primary care physicians was evaluated.

Methods.—The study included 67 internists and 28 family physicians in a large HMO. Physicians in one administrative area were assigned to an intervention group. They received a clinical practice guideline on the management of low back pain, followed by 3 feedback reports on the use of lumbar spine radiographs and CT and MRI scans. The remaining physicians served as controls. The effects of this intervention on variability in the use of imaging studies for back pain were assessed by automated radiology utilization data. The ability of the intervention to reduce use of the 3 procedures was examined as well.

Results.—Neither component of the intervention produced any consistent reduction in variability or the rate of use of imaging studies. Family physicians did show some reduction in their rate of use for all 3 imaging procedures. The absence of significant change occurred despite evidence of good dissemination of the intervention tools.

Conclusion.—The study intervention—a clinical practice guideline plus practice pattern feedback—did not reduce variability in or the rate of use of imaging studies for patients with low back pain. Such measures may fail to meet their goals if they do not consider the practice setting and the expectations and behavior of patients. Success of the measures may be enhanced by including them as part of system-wide, organizationally sponsored, quality-improvement initiatives.

► The cost of low back pain in the United States has been estimated to be a staggering $100 billion. The Agency for Health Care Policy and Research (AHCPR) guidelines[1] on acute low back pain, published in 1995, recommended ordering lumbar spine imaging tests only when certain "red flags," indicating serious underlying conditions, were present or when the patient had failed weeks of conservative care. Presumably, following these guidelines would limit unnecessary tests and decrease the cost of evaluating patients with acute low back pain. A recent study performed by Suarez-Almazor et al.[2] in Alberta showed that in Canada, following the guidelines would actually increase utilization!

Freeborn et al. demonstrated that changing physicians' practice patterns is more complex than providing a guideline and limited feedback on performance. This study has some flaws in addition to those recognized by the authors. The practice patterns before dissemination of the guideline should be assessed, as the paper by Suarez-Almazor et al. highlights. The authors had no way of looking specifically at the utilization of tests for a specific diagnosis, and they could not differentiate acute from chronic low back pain. Despite these limitations, their study points out that clinical practice guidelines may not be effective without global quality improvement efforts. Although not stated by the authors, medicolegal factors and societal expectations may also need to change for physicians to practice in a scientifically based, efficient manner.

B.L. Currier, M.D.

References

1. AHCPR Low Back Pain Guideline Panel: Acute low back pain problems in adults, Clinical Practice Guideline No. 14. AHCPR publication No 95–0644. Washington, DC, Department of Health and Human Services, Public Health Service, Agency for Health Care Policy and Research, 1995.
2. Suarez-Almazor ME, Belreck E, Russell AS, et al: Use of lumbar radiographs for the early diagnosis of low back pain: Proposed guidelines would increase utilization. *JAMA* 227:1782–1786, 1997.

Spinal Cord Injury

Administration of Methylprednisolone for 24 or 48 Hours or Tirilazad Mesylate for 48 Hours in the Treatment of Acute Spinal Cord Injury: Results of the Third National Acute Spinal Cord Injury Randomized Controlled Trial

Bracken MB, for the National Acute Spinal Cord Injury Study (Yale Univ, New Haven, Conn; et al)
JAMA 227:1597–1604, 1997   12–20

Objective.—Methylprednisolone is known to suppress lipid peroxidation and hydrolysis, which destroy membranes after acute spinal cord injury. Recoveries after a 24-hour vs. a 48-hour maintenance dose of methylprednisolone were compared, and whether tirilazad mesylate has fewer complications than high-dose 48-hour methylprednisolone was investigated. The effects of early vs. late initiation of treatment within the 8-hours-of-injury window, and of treatment in patients with initial complete vs. incomplete neurologic function were investigated.

Methods.—All 499 patients, mainly white males aged 14–34 years, received a bolus of open-label methylprednisolone before being randomly assigned within 6 hours of injury to receive treatment within 8 hours of injury. Almost half (49.7%) had complete spinal cord injuries and 77.2% had spinal fractures, including 50.7% with fracture dislocations. Treatment consisted of an infusion of methylprednisolone (5.4 mg/kg/hr) administered continuously over 24 or 48 hours, tirilazad (2.5 mg/kg) given as an intravenous bolus over a period of 15–20 minutes every 6 hours for 48 hours, or placebo. Motor and sensory function were evaluated before treatment and at 6 weeks and 6 months after injury, and function independence was evaluated at 6 weeks and 6 months after injury by physicians blinded to treatment.

Results.—Tirilazad patients had significantly worse motor function than methylprednisolone patients. Whereas the difference between the 2 methylprednisolone groups was not significant, those treated for 48 hours had more motor function recovery at 6 weeks and 6 months than those treated for 24 hours. Patients receiving treatment less than 3 hours after injury had the same rates of motor recovery. Of patients receiving treatment between 3 and 8 hours of injury, those in the 48-hour methylprednisolone group had significantly more motor recovery than those in the 24-hour group at 6 weeks and 6 months. Patients with incomplete injuries had significantly greater neurologic recovery than did patients with complete injury. Recovery for the tirilazad group was intermediate between the 2 methylprednisolone groups. Recoveries of sensory function paralleled those of motor function but tended to be smaller and not to be significant. Functional independence scores at 6 months were highest for the 48-hour methylprednisolone group, intermediate for the tirilazad group, and lowest for the 24-hour methylprednisolone group. Complication rates at 6 weeks were similar except for severe sepsis in 2.6% of the 48-hour methylprednisolone group, 0% in the tirilazad group, and 0.6% in the 24-hour methylprednisolone group, and severe pneumonia in 5.8%, 0.6%, and 2.6%, respectively.

Conclusions.—Patients with acute spinal cord injury who receive methylprednisolone within 3 hours of injury should be maintained on the therapy for 24 hours. Patients who receive methylprednisolone within 3–8 hours of injury should receive therapy for 48 hours.

▶ Neuroprotection (limiting the severity of secondary injury) is a well-recognized strategy for enhancing neurologic recovery after spinal cord injury. Bracken and colleagues reported the preliminary results of the landmark second National Acute Spinal Cord Injury Study in 1990[1] and the 1-year follow-up data in 1992.[2] That study immediately influenced the treatment of spinal cord injury worldwide. Although the study has been criticized, the recommendations of the authors have become standard practice: administration of high-dose methylprednisolone (30 mg/kg bolus followed by 5.4 mg/kg per hour for 23 hours) to patients seen within 8 hours of spinal cord injury. Likewise, the recommendations put forth in the current study will become routine practice.

The biggest disappointment of this study is that tirilazad mesylate did not perform as well as the more toxic drug, methylprednisolone. Tirilazad lacks the glucocorticoid effect of methylprednisolone and, as expected, it was responsible for the fewest side effects. The most significant flaw of this study is that the patients randomly assigned to receive tirilazad had significantly lower pretreatment motor scores than the 2 methylprednisolone groups ($P = 0.006$). It is possible (as suggested by the authors) that the tirilazad dose or regimen was inadequate as well, or that methylprednisolone may work by additional mechanisms, but the tirilazad arm never had a chance in this study. The investigators admit that further study of the drug is warranted.

B.L. Currier, M.D.

References

1. Bracken MB, Shepard MJ, Collins WF, et al: A randomized, controlled trial of methylprednisolone or naloxone in the treatment of acute spinal cord injury: Results of the second National Acute Spinal Cord Injury Study. *N Engl J Med* 322:1405–1411, 1990.
2. Bracken MB, Shepard MJ, Collins WF, et al: Methylprednisolone or naloxone treatment after acute spinal cord injury: 1 year follow-up data: Results of the second National Acute Spinal Cord Injury Study. *J Neurosurgery* 76:23–31, 1992.

13 Orthopedic Oncology

Introduction

I have grouped selected articles in this chapter under the categories of reconstruction, chemotherapy, metastatic disease, radiology, Ewing's sarcoma, soft tissue sarcoma, and a miscellaneous group comprising other interesting papers. It is distressing to report that problems related to the workup and biopsy of tumors still exist. A number of articles note errors in diagnosis and treatment. This troublesome issue just will not go away.

We are continuing to evaluate the many reconstructive techniques for patients with musculoskeletal neoplasms. These surgical procedures are complex and, accordingly, have a high complication rate. Our experience with these procedures has reached a degree at which the evaluation of results will hopefully one day better define which reconstructive procedure is best suited to a particular situation. The sequelae of limb salvage surgical procedures are not being reported, and some authors are reporting encouraging results for revisions of massive reconstructions. This is certainly a problem with which we will all be dealing in the future. Limb salvage surgery is again shown to be a cost-effective procedure when compared to amputation.

The management of pelvic disease is always challenging. When lesions are resected and the reconstruction is uncomplicated, patients do well. However, local recurrence, infection, instability, neurovascular injury, and other complications impart significant morbidity on an already difficult situation. Understanding the functional outcomes of the various reconstructive procedures can help in treatment selection.

A number of articles report the results of chemotherapy protocols. Improved survival for patients is always welcome information; however, the long-term effects of treatment causing second malignancies are again reported. Surgery is again supported for the treatment of Ewing's sarcoma, and it is desirable to avoid radiation therapy if possible.

I have included an excellent paper (Abstract 13–22) discussing the systemic effects of phenol. Phenol is used infrequently and at widely variable concentrations. While I am not aware of any reports regarding systemic side effects from its application, this paper may provide cause for concern—particularly among those who use very concentrated solutions of phenol for tumor ablation. It is a must-read article for anyone who uses this agent.

Christopher P. Beauchamp, M.D.

Chemotherapy

Neoadjuvant Chemotherapy for High Grade Malignant Fibrous Histiocytoma of Bone

Bacci G, Picci P, Mercuri M, et al (Istituto Ortopedico Rizzoli, Bologna, Italy)
Clin Orthop 346:178–189, 1997

13–1

Introduction.—High-grade malignant fibrous histiocytoma (MFH) of the bone is a rare neoplasm with an aggressive biologic behavior and high malignant potential. It has a propensity for local recurrence and hematogenous spread. Neoadjuvant chemotherapy has been beneficial in other bone tumors similar to MFH of bone. Outcome of 65 patients with MFH of bone located in the extremities and treated between 1983 and 1994 with 4 different regimens of neoadjuvant chemotherapy is reported.

Methods.—Median patient age was 30 years (range, 8–59 years). During postoperative chemotherapy, patients underwent clinical and radiographic evaluations every 2 months. Cumulative probability of disease-free survival and overall survival of a function of time were determined.

Results.—A clinical and radiographic tumor response was observed in 50 patients (77%). Thirteen patients (20%) experienced no significant changes, and 2 patients had tumor progression. Fifty-eight patients (89%) underwent limb salvage, and 7 patients underwent amputation. The histologic response rate ranged from 17% to 33% with the four regimens, with no significant differences in rates. At a mean of 7 years, 25 patients

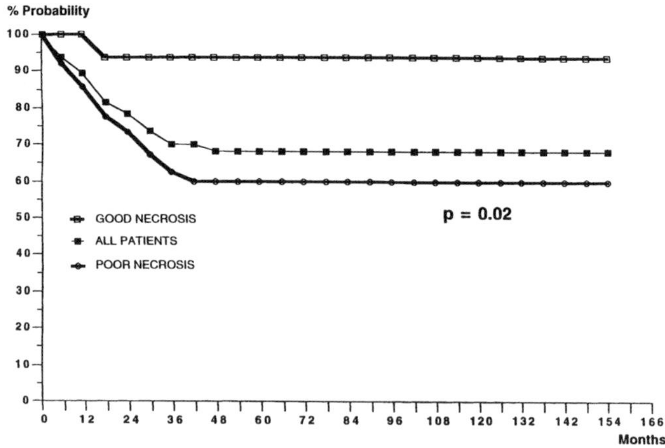

FIGURE 5.—Comparison of disease-free survival curves for patients who had a good necrosis response (16 cases) and patients who had a poor necrosis response to chemotherapy (49 cases). (Courtesy of Bacci G, Picci P, Mercuri M, et al: Neoadjuvant chemotherapy for high grade malignant fibrous histiocytoma of bone. *Clin Orthop* 346:178–189, 1997.)

(69%) were continuously disease free and 20 had relapse (18 metastases and 2 local recurrences). The average time to relapse was 19 months (no significant differences in treatment regimens). Five-year disease-free survival and overall survival were 68% and 76%, respectively (Fig 5). Treatment compliance was good with all 4 regimens. Grade 4 toxicity was observed in about 20% of all chemotherapy cycles. Hospital admission was needed for treatment 62 times. This resulted in a dose reduction from 15% to 30% of scheduled dose in 15% of cycles. Bone marrow depletion caused delays of over 7 days in 13% of cycles.

Conclusion.—Outcomes in these patients treated with neoadjuvant chemotherapy were significantly better than earlier series of patients treated with surgery alone or surgery followed by adjuvant chemotherapy. Only 2 local recurrences occurred during follow-up in this patient cohort treated with neoadjuvant chemotherapy. This suggests that micrometastases are more chemosensitive than are primary tumors. Neoadjuvant chemotherapy may be considered just as effective as adjuvant chemotherapy in increasing survival and is correlated with increased safety for limb salvage.

▶ This is a large group of patients with MFH of bone in the extremities. The authors have demonstrated a very satisfactory response to chemotherapy. The results echo those obtained in osteosarcoma studies. Particularly those patients who had a good histologic response to preoperative chemotherapy did well. This establishes the role for chemotherapy in patients with high-grade MFH of bone. The observation that in comparison to osteosarcoma, MFH of bone does not respond as well to neoadjuvant chemotherapy is interesting. It may be, perhaps, due to the fact that the patients receive less chemotherapy because MFH of bone tends to occur in a slightly older age group. This was not specifically addressed in the paper.

The study does beg the question as to why does MFH of bone respond better than MFH of soft tissues. Clearly, the biology of these two lesions must be different.

C.P. Beauchamp, M.D.

P-Glycoprotein Expression: Critical Determinant in the Response to Osteosarcoma Chemotherapy
Chan HSL, Grogan TM, Haddad G, et al (Univ of Toronto; Univ of Arizona, Tucson; Univ of British Columbia, Vancouver)
J Natl Cancer Inst 89:1706–1715, 1997   13–2

Introduction.—Adjuvant chemotherapy improves survival among patients who have undergone surgery for osteosarcoma, but more than 90% of those with metastatic disease and up to 40% of those without metastatic disease still relapse and die. A suggested cause for treatment failure is increased expression of P-glycoprotein, which confers resistance of the tumor to chemotherapy. A retrospective study sought to correlate P-glycoprotein expression with poor treatment outcome in osteosarcoma.

Methods.—The study group included 62 consecutive patients aged 4.8 to 20.9 years, who had received a diagnosis of upper or lower extremity osteosarcoma from 1980 through 1989. A consensus on P-glycoprotein expression was reached in 61 cases. Disease was staged by radionuclide bone scan, tumor and lung CT, and/or MRI. Fifty-nine patients were treated surgically, 48 by limb-salvage procedure and 11 by amputation; 2 patients had the primary tumor and bone metastases irradiated. Because the assessment of P-glycoprotein expression is qualitative, 2 observers interpreted the results separately and reached a consensus. Findings were correlated with treatment outcome.

Results.—Before treatment, observers detected P-glycoprotein in 44 tumor samples from 27 patients; 53 samples in the remaining 34 patients were negative for P-glycoprotein expression. The finding of P-glycoprotein expression at diagnosis was highly predictive of a patient's response to chemotherapy. Those with undetectable P-glycoprotein had a relapse-free rate of 87% and a survival rate of 94%. In contrast, all patients with any level of P-glycoprotein positivity relapsed and only 35% survived. At a median follow-up of 8.9 years, the relapse-free rate was 87% in the group with undetectable P-glycoprotein vs. 0% in the group with increased P-glycoprotein. Among patients who received chemotherapy before surgery, 23 had undetectable P-glycoprotein and 23 had increased P-glycoprotein. These groups differed significantly in outcome: relapse-free rates of 84% and 0%, respectively, and survival rates of 91% and 27%, respectively. Outcome in the P-glycoprotein–negative group remained better after stratification by tumor size, degree of differentiation, and metastatic status.

Conclusion.—A correlation between expression of the multidrug-resistant protein P-glycoprotein and treatment failure was confirmed in these patients with osteosarcoma. Findings suggest that inhibiting the action of P-glycoprotein may improve outcome in patients with this tumor.

▶ Tremendous advances have been made over the years, in the treatment of osteosarcoma, and these have, in large part, been the result of improvement in chemotherapeutic regimens. Unfortunately, resistance to multidrug chemotherapy remains the major cause of treatment failure. Expression of the *MDR1* gene has been implicated in poor treatment outcome in osteosarcoma.

This study is a retrospective review of patients treated at the Hospital for Sick Children in Toronto for upper or lower extremity osteosarcoma. The study involves the use of monoclonal anti–P-glycoprotein antibodies. The study noted that P-glycoprotein expression is determined by immunohistochemical techniques and is correlated with treatment failure in patients with osteosarcomas. This clinical information should have relevance in the treatment of these patients, as there are drugs available that can modulate the result of P-glycoprotein expression. Similar studies have been observed at The Rizzoli in Bologna, Italy.

Unpublished data from a prospective, international, multicenter study of 136 patients between 1989 and 1994, however, does not support these results. That study recorded no simple linear relationship between *MDR1* gene expression and systemic relapse in osteosarcoma. The technique differed from the study described here in that the gene expression was measured by a quantitative reverse transcription–polymerase chain reaction assay.

Although the potential to identify patients who will relapse is exciting, further study needs to be done. Whether we are at a stage at which clinical trials involving gene modulation can be introduced remains to be seen.

C.P. Beauchamp, M.D.

Late Mortality of Long-term Survivors of Childhood Cancer

Hudson MM, Jones D, Boyett J, et al (St Jude Children's Research Hosp, Memphis, Tenn; Univ of Tennessee, Memphis)
J Clin Oncol 15:2205–2213, 1997   13–3

Introduction.—With current treatments, two thirds of children with cancer will survive for at least 5 years. However, these children have excess mortality related to late recurrences, second cancers, or treatment complications. The patterns of mortality among survivors of childhood cancer and treatment were analyzed.

Methods.—A total of 2,053 children treated for leukemia, lymphoma, and solid tumors between 1962 and 1983 who survived at least 5 years after diagnosis were studied. The children were treated in a single institution on protocol-based therapy. The patients were grouped into early and late treatment eras—1962–1970 and 1971–1983, respectively—reflecting increased intensity of treatment and improved survival. Causes of death were identified from the medical records. Fifteen-year survival was estimated for the cancer survivors, and their risk of death from nonneoplastic treatment complications was compared with adjusted U.S. population estimates.

Results.—Two hundred fifty-eight of the children died after surviving 5 years after cancer diagnosis. One hundred sixty-nine deaths occurred within 5–10 years and 89 after more than 10 years. Recurrent primary malignancy accounted for 61% of the deaths, second malignancy for 20%, nonneoplastic treatment complications for 10%, and unintentional injury or suicide for 8% of the deaths. Patients treated in the later era were significantly less likely to die of recurrent disease and somewhat less likely to die of second malignancies. Second leukemias occurred only in patients treated during the recent era, during which alkylating agents and epipodophyllotoxins were added to chemotherapy. In both treatment eras, projected 15-year survival was greater than 90%, but higher than expected from adjusted population data. Estimated 5-year survival was 31% in the early treatment era and 52% in the late treatment era, compared with 68% from 1984 to 1989 at the same institution.

Conclusions.—More effective treatments for childhood cancer have reduced the number of late deaths from recurrence. At the same time, there has been no increase in late deaths from nonneoplastic treatment complications. The risk of second malignancies is somewhat higher for patients treated after 1970. Continued improvements in survival from childhood cancer are being realized through intensified treatment for aggressive cancers, combined with judicious use of radiation therapy and chemotherapy drugs.

▶ Great strides have been made in the treatment of patients with childhood malignancy. Modern therapeutic protocols have certainly seen an improvement in long term survival for these patients. We continue, however, to see problems created with long-term survival and that the risk of second malignancies is apparently increasing. Currently, the long-term sequelae of radiation therapy, chemotherapy and reconstructive techniques have our increasing attention. The trade-off for improved survival may be an increased risk of secondary malignancy.

C.P. Beauchamp, M.D.

Randomised Trial of Two Regimens of Chemotherapy in Operable Osteosarcoma: A Study of the European Osteosarcoma Intergroup

Souhami RL, Craft AW, Van der Eijken JW, et al (Univ College London; Royal Victoria Infirmary, Newcastle upon Tyne, England; Onze Lieve Vrouw Gasthuis, Amsterdam; et al)
Lancet 350:911–917, 1997   13–4

Introduction.—Although chemotherapy has been shown to improve survival of patients with operable osteosarcoma, randomized trials have not been conducted to assess the optimum duration of treatment and contributions of the drugs. Two regimens of chemotherapy were tested in a previous trial which compared a short intensive chemotherapy regimen with doxorubicin and cisplatin with the complex and longer-duration drug regimens based on the widely used T10 multidrug protocol. These 2 approaches were compared.

Methods.—There were 407 patients with operable, nonmetastatic osteosarcoma (Fig 1). They were randomly assigned to either a multidrug regimen (preoperative vincristine, high-dose methotrexate, and doxorubicin; postoperative bleomycin, cyclophosphamide, dactinomycin, vincristine, methotrexate, doxorubicin, and cisplatin for 44 weeks) or the 2-drug regimen of doxorubicin, 25 mg/m^2 on days 1–3, and cisplatin, 100 mg/m^2 on day 1, for 18 weeks. For the 2-drug group, surgery was scheduled for week 9. For the multidrug group, surgery was scheduled for week 7. Survival and progression-free survival were analyzed. There was a 4-year follow-up.

Results.—With the 2 regimens, toxic effects were qualitatively similar. There was a higher compliance rate with the 2-drug regimen in which 94%

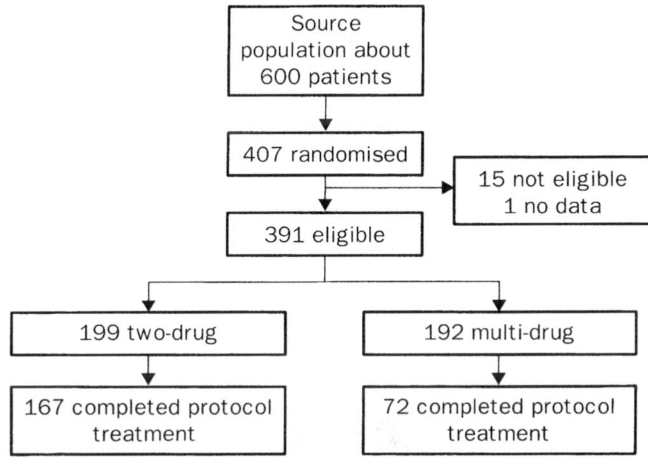

FIGURE 1.—Trial profile (Courtesy of Souhami RL, Craft AW, Van der Eijken JW, et al: Randomised trial of two regimens of chemotherapy in operable osteosarcoma: A study of the European Osteosarcoma Intergroup. *Lancet* 350:911–917. Copyright 1997, The Lancet Ltd.)

of patients completed the cycles, compared with 51% who completed the multidrug regimen. Progression and toxic effects were the most common reasons for termination (Table 3). With both regimens, the proportion showing a good histopathologic response was about 29% (greater than 90% tumor necrosis) to preoperative chemotherapy and was strongly predictive of survival (Fig 5). In both groups, overall survival was 65% at 3 years and 55% at 5 years (Fig 4). Progression-free survival also did not differ between the 2 groups (Fig 3). For the 2-drug group the median time to surgery was 75 days, and for the multidrug group the median time to surgery was 57 days (Fig 2). The types of surgery that patients received included amputation, prosthesis, rotation, or allograft (Table 6).

TABLE 3.—Reasons for Termination of Protocol Chemotherapy

	Two-drug group (n=199)	Multi-drug group (n=192)	
		To cycle 6	After cycle 6
Treatment completed	167 (83·4%)	··	72 (37·5%)*
Treatment terminated			
Progression	14	10	22
Toxic effects	10	5	30
Refusal	3	3	24
Postoperative complications	2	0	3
Change from protocol schedule	2	6	14
Lost to follow-up	1	1	2
Total	32	25	95

*Includes 9 patients who missed 1 or more cycles during treatment period.
(Courtesy of Souhami RL, Craft AW, Van der Eijken JW, et al: Randomised trial of two regimens of chemotherapy in operable osteosarcoma: A study of the European Osteosarcoma Intergroup. *Lancet* 350:911–917. Copyright 1997, The Lancet Ltd.)

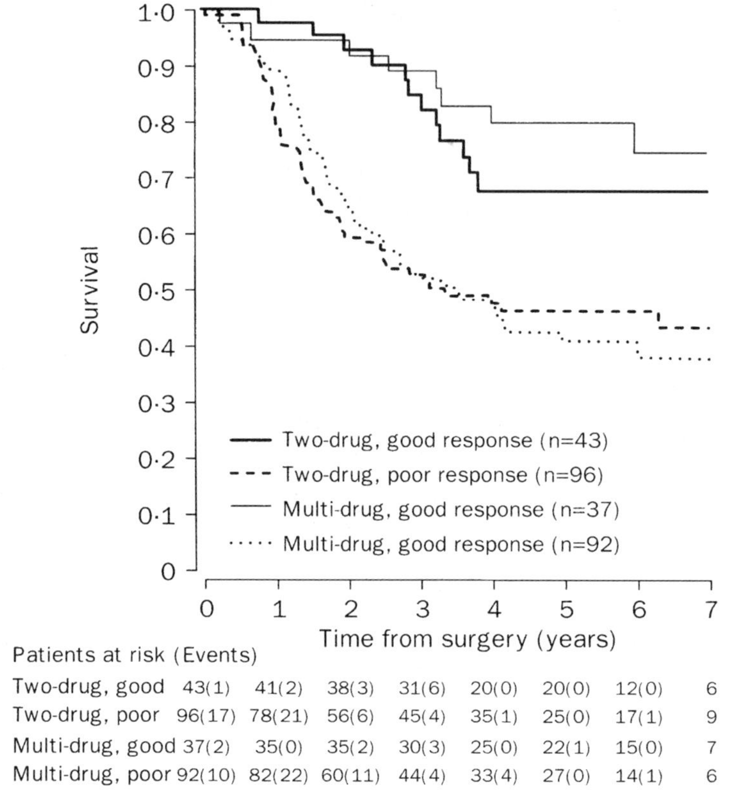

FIGURE 5.—Survival according to histopathological response by treatment group calculated from date of surgery. (Courtesy of Souhami RL, Craft AW, Van der Eijken JW, et al: Randomised trial of two regimens of chemotherapy in operable osteosarcoma: A study of the European Osteosarcoma Intergroup. *Lancet* 350:911–917. Copyright 1997, The Lancet Ltd.)

Conclusions.—In operable, nonmetastatic osteosarcoma treatment, the 2-drug and multidrug regimens showed no difference in survival. The preferred treatment is the 2-drug regimen because it is shorter in duration and better tolerated. To improve results, dose intensification may be necessary because the 5-year survival is still unsatisfactory.

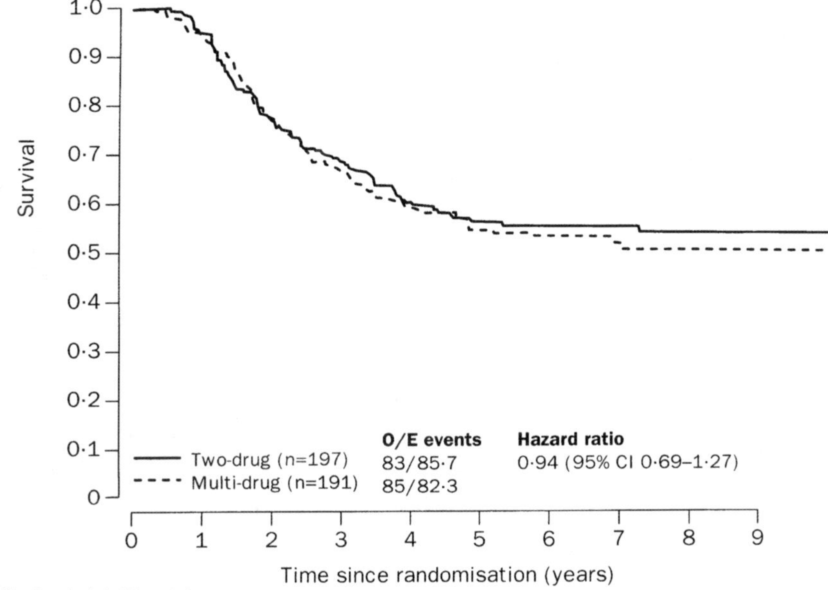

FIGURE 4.—Survival from randomization by treatment group. *Abbreviations:* O/E, observed/expected; CI, confidence interval. (Courtesy of Souhami RL, Craft AW, Van der Eijken JW, et al: Randomised trial of two regimens of chemotherapy in operable osteosarcoma: A study of the European Osteosarcoma Intergroup. *Lancet* 350:911–917. Copyright 1997, The Lancet Ltd.)

▶ This large study comprising more than 400 patients effectively compares multiagent chemotherapy (T10 protocol) with dual chemotherapy. It demonstrated no difference in survival between the 2 treatments. There are significant advantages for 2-drug treatment in terms of cost, morbidity, length of treatment, and probably most important, compliance. Five-year survival with both of these treatments remains disappointing. This study further supports the ongoing randomized trials.

C.P. Beauchamp, M.D.

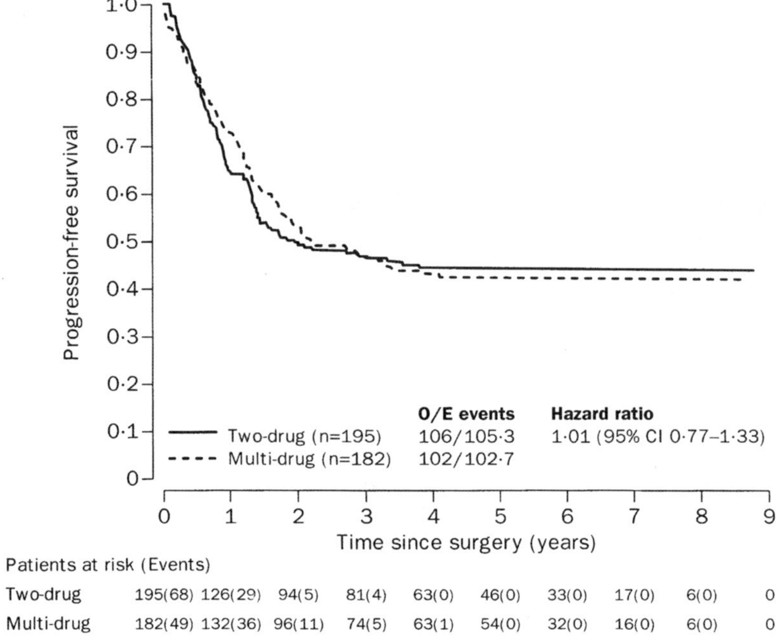

Patients at risk (Events)

Two-drug	195(68)	126(29)	94(5)	81(4)	63(0)	46(0)	33(0)	17(0)	6(0)	0
Multi-drug	182(49)	132(36)	96(11)	74(5)	63(1)	54(0)	32(0)	16(0)	6(0)	0

FIGURE 3.—Progression-free survival by treatment group. *Abbreviations:* O/E, observed/expected; *CI*, confidence interval. (Courtesy of Souhami RL, Craft AW, Van der Eijken JW, et al: Randomised trial of two regimens of chemotherapy in operable osteosarcoma: A study of the European Osteosarcoma Intergroup. *Lancet* 350:911–917. Copyright 1997, The Lancet Ltd.)

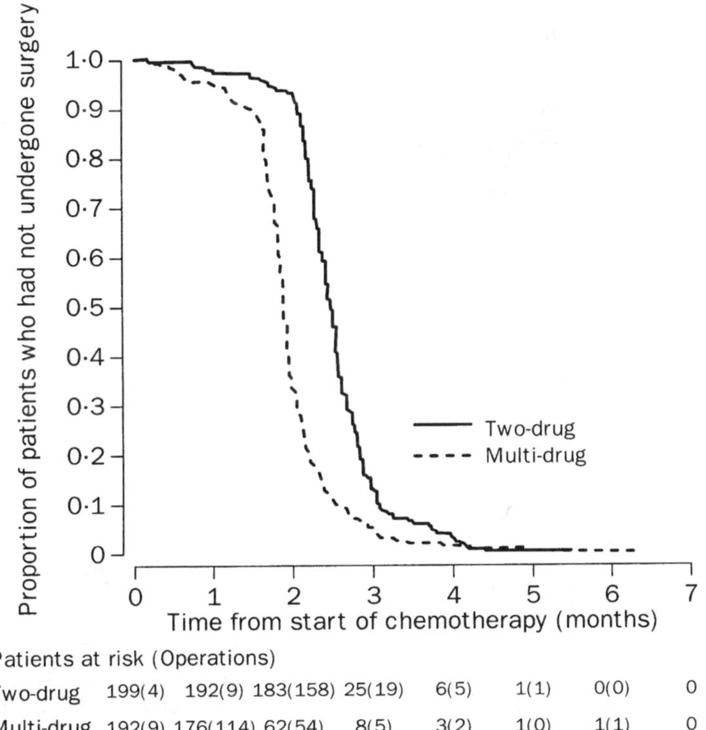

Patients at risk (Operations)

Two-drug	199(4)	192(9)	183(158)	25(19)	6(5)	1(1)	0(0)	0
Multi-drug	192(9)	176(114)	62(54)	8(5)	3(2)	1(0)	1(1)	0

FIGURE 2.—Time from start of chemotherapy to surgery (or date last known to be alive if no surgery done) by randomized treatment group. (Courtesy of Souhami RL, Craft AW, Van der Eijken JW, et al: Randomised trial of two regimens of chemotherapy in operable osteosarcoma: A study of the European Osteosarcoma Intergroup. *Lancet* 350:911–917. Copyright 1997, The Lancet Ltd.)

TABLE 6.—Planned and Actual Surgery Received

Actual surgery	Planned surgery						
	Amputation	Prosthesis	Rotation	Other conservative	Allograft	Unknown	Total
Two-drug regimen							
Amputation	22	19	1	1	0	2	45
Prosthesis	9	106	0	3	0	··	118
Rotation	3	1	2	0	0	··	6
Other conservative	5	13	0	8	1	··	27
Allograft	0	0	0	0	0	··	0
None	1	2	0	0	0	··	3
Total	40	141	3	12	1	2	199
Multi-drug regimen							
Amputation	27	24	1	3	0	1	56
Prosthesis	5	95	0	2	0	··	102
Rotation	0	1	0	0	0	··	1
Other convervative	8	6	1	7	2	··	24
Allograft	0	2	0	0	0	··	2
None	1	6	0	0	0	··	7
Total	41	134	2	12	2	1	192

(Courtesy of Souhami RL, Craft AW, Van der Eijken JW, et al: Randomised trial of two regimens of chemotherapy in operable osteosarcoma: A study of the European Osteosarcoma Intergroup. *Lancet* 350:911–917. Copyright 1997, The Lancet Ltd.)

Radiation and Genetic Factors in the Risk of Second Malignant Neoplasms After a First Cancer in Childhood

Kony SJ, de Vathaire F, Chompret A, et al (Institut Gustave Roussy, Cedex, France)
Lancet 350:91–95, 1997

13–5

Background.—The occurrence of a second malignant neoplasm (SMN) has been associated with radiotherapy and chemotherapy as well as with a familial aggregation. The role of familial factors in the risk of SMN and their potential interaction with treatment effects were investigated.

Methods.—Twenty-five children with an SMN and 96 children without an SMN after cancer treatment were included in the case-control study. The children were selected from a cohort of 649 children treated between 1953 and 1985.

Findings.—Ten family members of the 25 case patients had early-onset cancer, compared with 8 of the 96 control patients. Compared with patients with no family history of early-onset cancer, those with 1 or more affected family members had an odds ratio of 4.7 for SMN. This risk was not affected substantially by adjustment for local radiation dose or by exclusion of paients known to be predisposed to SMN (including *p53* mutation carriers and patients with Recklinghausen's disease).

Conclusions.—Genetic factors and exposure to ionizing radiation independently affect the risk of SMN. Children with a family history of early-onset cancer need especially vigilant follow-up after initial cancer treatment.

▶ This article gives further cause for concern about children who have had radiation therapy as a portion of their treatment for a childhood malignancy. It is clearly shown here that family history is important in determining the prognosis for secondary malignant neoplasms. Treatment for these patients should be modified whenever possible. This has particular implications for patients with Ewing's sarcoma, for which radiation therapy may sometimes be avoided.

C.P. Beauchamp, M.D.

Effect of Cisplatin Chemotherapy on Extracortical Tissue Formation in Canine Diaphyseal Segmental Replacement

Young DR, Shih L-Y, Rock MG, et al (Johns Hopkins Univ, Baltimore, Md; Mayo Clinic and Found, Rochester, Minn)
J Orthop Res 15:773–780, 1997   13–6

Introduction.—Reconstruction of large bone and joint defects after resection of malignant tumors remains problematic. Use of osteo-articular allografts, prosthetic implants, and allographic prosthetic devices are beneficial in limb salvage, but complications continue to cause late morbidity. Chemotherapy has significantly diminished the risk of metastatic disease, but it also has an inhibitory effect on bone healing, bone ingrowth into prosthetic devices, and incorporation of bone grafts. The effects of cisplatin 75 mg/m^2 administered preoperatively or postoperatively were analyzed on the extracortical capsule formation of a canine segmental replacement prosthesis.

Methods.—The prosthetic implant was a bistemmed segmental diaphyseal replacement prosthesis made of titanium alloy. The porous surface was made of commercially pure titanium beads. Implants were secured with intramedullary cement fixation into the left proximal femur. Autograft bone was harvested from the iliac crest and placed around the prosthesis. Eight dogs each received either group 1, no cisplatin; group 2, cisplatin 4 times before surgery; or group 3, cisplatin 4 times after surgery. Animals were sacrificed at 12 weeks after surgery and the left femur was removed and subjected to mechanical testing to determine torsional load.

Results.—All dogs were weight bearing on the treated limb within 5 days after surgery. Specimens tested for torsion usually failed because of fracture of the extracortical bridging callus or shear failure of the extracortical bone and soft-tissue ingrowth into the porous coating. Both types of failure were observed in all 3 treatment groups. The most common site of fracture was through the extracortical bridging bone. Of 7 specimens that failed by obvious fracture, 1, 4, and 2, respectively, were in group 1, 2, and 3. Of 16 specimens with shear failure at the extracortical bone-soft tissue interface with the porous coating of the prosthesis, 6, 4, and 6, respectively, were in group 1, 2, and 3. The prosthesis was completely loose after torsion failure in 8 specimens and remained in position in the other 8 specimens.

Conclusion.—Among the 3 treatment groups, there was no significant difference at 12 weeks in overall clinical outcome, callus size, or mechanical strength of the bone-prosthetic interface. This conflicts with earlier findings of a negative effect on bone formation with chemotherapy. The stronger bone ingrowth into the prosthesis observed with this canine model suggests some kind of acceleration of bone formation after early retardation. The bone graft augmented the formation of the extracortical capsule. Histomorphometric and radiographic findings showed a significant decrease in the cross-sectional area of the perirosthetic callus in the dogs treated with postoperative cisplatin. Other trials have indicated that chemotherapeutic effects on bone formation are dose- and time-dependent. This model needs to be tested against more dose-intensive, multi-agent chemotherapy.

▶ Neoadjuvant and perioperative chemotherapy is certainly advantageous in the management of patients with bone sarcomas. Our ability to achieve satisfactory long-term functional outcome is dependent upon successful reconstructive techniques. These often involve the need for bone graft or host bone healing. Chemotherapeutic agents have been demonstrated to have a deleterious effect on healing, and we have always had long-term concerns of patients undergoing postoperative chemotherapy when elaborate reconstructive techniques have been performed. The authors have demonstrated this effect in a dog model but have noted that the effect on bone healing is temporary. This has the effect of extending the time to union for our patients. Patients reconstructed with utilizing techniques that incorporate allograft host junctions already have a prolonged healing time, and special attention needs to be given to patients for even longer-term fixation when they are going to be receiving postoperative chemotherapy, especially those patients receiving long-term postoperative chemotherapy.

C.P. Beauchamp, M.D.

Ewing's Sarcoma

Ewing's Sarcoma of the Femur: Prognosis in 69 Patients Treated by the CESS Group
Ozaki T, Hillman A, Hoffmann C, et al (Westfälische Wilhelms-Univ, Münster, Germany; Univ of Halle, Germany)
Acta Orthop Scand 68:20–24, 1997   13–7

Objective.—Although the types and results of treatment for Ewing's sarcoma may vary with the anatomical site of the tumor, few studies have examined specific sites. Since 1981, 535 patients have been treated under Cooperative Ewing's Sarcoma Study (CESS) protocols. The outcomes of 69 protocol-treated children and young adults with Ewing's sarcoma of the femur were analyzed.

Methods.—The patients' median age was 14 years. Those with primary distant metastases were excluded, although 4 patients with skip metastases were included. Sixteen patients had pathologic fractures before receiving local treatment. Patients treated on the CESS 81 protocol received 4-drug VACA chemotherapy, consisting of vincristine, actinomycin-D, cyclophosphamide, and adriamycin. Those treated on CESS 86 received VACA if they were at standard risk, i.e., peripheral or small-volume tumor; or VAIA (ifosfamide instead of cyclophosphamide) if they were at high risk, i.e., central or large-volume tumor. High-risk patients treated on the CESS 91P protocol received either VAIA or additional etoposide (EVAIA). Reconstruction was performed in 52 patients, most often with prosthetic replacement or rotationplasty. The patients' median radiotherapy dose was 45 Gy. Survivors were followed up for a median of 60 months.

Results.—Ten-year relapse-free survival was 60%. There were 25 relapses, 19 of which were systemic. Twenty-two patients died of disease and 2 died without relapse. Relapse-free survival was significantly lower in CESS 81 than in CESS 86 or CESS 91P. Local recurrence and survival were unaffected by sex, age, tumor volume, or tumor location. Patients undergoing surgery, with or without radiotherapy, had better local control, combined local/systemic relapse, and relapse-free survival than those undergoing radiotherapy alone. Prognosis was unchanged by the presence of a pathologic fracture. Twelve relapses occurred in 50 patients with adequate surgical margins. Ten-year relapse-free survival was better for patients with a better response to chemotherapy. On multivariate analysis, treatment without surgical resection of the tumor was an independent and unfavorable prognostic factor. Type of protocol was nonsignificant.

Conclusions.—The CESS group reports a 60% 10-year relapse-free survival rate among patients with Ewing's sarcoma of the femur. This is similar to the results reported for Ewing's sarcoma in other sites. Surgery significantly reduces the incidence of local or combined relapse.

► Therapeutic protocols for the management of patients with Ewing's sarcoma of the femur have been evolving over the past 15 years. It has increasingly been shown that surgery is a very important part of the definitive management of patients with Ewing's sarcoma. This study emphasizes the importance of surgery with or without radiation therapy in the treatment of these patients. There is a very high failure rate with radiation therapy alone. This study is particularly important because it is a prospective study, something that has been lacking in this area. Until now, we have made conclusions on the basis of retrospective studies.

An important part of this study is the prospective analysis of a subgroup of patients that had pathologic fractures. They demonstrated no difference in relapse-free survival according to the existence of a pathologic fracture before local treatment.

C.P. Beauchamp, M.D.

Long-term Results From the First UKCCSG Ewing's Tumour Study (ET-1)

Craft AW for the United Kingdom Children's Cancer Study Group, and the Medical Research Council Bone Sarcoma Working Party (Royal Victoria Infirmary, Newcastle Upon Tyne, England; et al)
Eur J Cancer 33:1061–1069, 1997   13–8

Introduction.—In 1978, the Ewing's Tumour Study began to study pediatric and adult oncology patients, and to use radiotherapy and the 4 most effective drugs to maximum potential. The results of that study and late follow-up are reported in patients with Ewing's sarcoma who had multimodal chemotherapy and radiotherapy.

Methods.—One hundred forty-two patients in an 8-year period were part of the Ewing's Tumour Study and were treated with vincristine, doxorubicin, actinomycin D, and cyclophosphamide with radiotherapy plus or minus surgery to the primary tumor. Additional vincristine was given on days 8 and 15 and a second course was administered before local therapy for those who had a good response to the first course. There was a 3-week period for radiotherapy with 45 Gy for tumors of the long bones, 25 Gy for rib primaries, and 30 Gy for pelvic tumors. There was an additional boost of 10–15 Gy for all tumors. Vincristine and cyclophosphamide were given weekly during radiotherapy. Chemotherapy was given for 1 year during the course of the study.

Results.—Forty-five of 120 patients who had no metastases at diagnosis remain alive at a median follow-up of 11.2 years. Only 2 patients with metastases are still alive. Site of disease was the major prognostic factor. The outcome was also influenced by age and serum lactic dehydrogenase at diagnosis. Late effects were documented in 45 of 61 patients who survived 4 years or more. Tumor site, type of local therapy, volume, and dose of radiotherapy influenced the type and extent of the late effects. Second malignancies were found in 4 patients. About one fourth of the patients had surgery, and although these patients had a lower local relapse rate, surgery does not confer survival advantage.

Conclusion.—In patients with Ewing's sarcoma, prospects for long-term survival have improved. In the majority of patients, however, late sequelae are present. About half of patients can be expected to be long-term survivors when treated with these 4 drugs used and radiotherapy with or without surgery. If more patients are to survive, better chemotherapy is needed. Future studies should focus on infusion of doxorubicin rather than bolus injection and on the use of endoprosthetic surgery to minimize the use of radiotherapy.

▶ This article reports the long-term results of patients treated between 1978 and 1986 in a multimodal chemotherapy and radiotherapy program. The article highlights a number of important issues that are slowly being made clear in the literature. Radiation therapy alone yielded an unacceptably high local relapse rate of 32%. Patients who were treated with surgery had a much improved rate of local control, but the authors quite correctly note that patients undergoing surgery generally have more favorable lesions. Patients who were treated with multimodal therapy, chemotherapy, surgery, and radiation therapy had a local relapse rate of 6%. The long-term consequences of treatment in the survivors are concerning in that late sequelae were noted in nearly three fourths of patients.

The article suggests that when surgery is feasible, it is the treatment of choice. When satisfactory surgical margins cannot be obtained, radiation therapy is effective in improving local control. This article confirms the importance of chemotherapy.

C.P. Beauchamp, M.D.

Metastatic Disease

Pain Relief and Quality of Life Following Radiotherapy for Bone Metastases: A Randomised Trial of Two Fractionation Schedules
Gaze MN, Kelly CG, Kerr GR, et al (Western Gen Hosp, Edinburgh, Scotland)
Radiother Oncol 45:109–116, 1997   13–9

Introduction.—Radiotherapy is a well-recognized, effective palliative treatment for metastatic bone pain. There is no consensus regarding optimal radiotherapy regimen. The efficacy, side effects, and effect on quality of life of 2 frequently used radiotherapy schedules were compared in 280 patients with painful bone metastases.

Methods.—Patients excluded were those with prior irradiation of the metastatic area, spinal cord compression, vertebral collapse above the level of the second lumbar, impending or established pathologic fracture, or any prior surgical fixation. Fifteen patients had to be eliminated from analysis, leaving a total of 265 patients for randomization. Patients were randomly assigned to either single 10-Gy treatments or a course of 22.5 Gy admin-

TABLE 3.—Degree of Benefit: The Maximum Level of Benefit Achieved by Patients in Each Arm of the Trial at First or Second Follow-up at 1 Week or 1 Month After Treatment

Degree of benefit	Single treatment (%) ($n = 129$)	Five treatments (%) ($n = 111$)
0	16	11
1	27	32
2	39	37
3	17	19
4	1	2

Note: The values represent the differences in the pain score between the pretreatment score and the follow-up score. For example, 0 represents no change, 1 represents a decrease in pain score from 3 to 2, or 2 to 1, and 2 represents a decrease in pain score from 3 to 1, or 2 to 0 and so on.

(Reprinted from Gaze MN, Kelly CG, Kerr GR, et al: Pain relief and quality of life following radiotherapy for bone metastases: A randomised trial of two fractionation schedules. *Radiother Oncol* 45:109–116, copyright 1997 with permission from Elsevier Science.)

TABLE 4.—Analgesic Use: Analgesic Consumption in Both Arms of the Trial Before and After Treatment

Analgesic score	Initial scores (%)		Scores after treatment (%)	
	Single treatment	Five treatments	Single treatment	Five treatments
0	3	4	17	21
1	5	6	13	12
2	40	35	32	24
3	40	42	33	39
4	10	12	4	5

Note: The values represent the analgesic score. There is no significant difference between the 2 arms of the trial either before or after treatment. After treatment, there is an increase in the proportion of patients who require either no analgesics or simple analgesics. As a result of treatment, there is a corresponding decline in the proportion of patients requiring moderate analgesics, nonsteroidal anti-inflammatory drugs, or opiates.

(Reprinted from Gaze MN, Kelly CG, Kerr GR, et al: Pain relief and quality of life following radiotherapy for bone metastases: A randomised trial of two fractionation schedules. *Radiother Oncol* 45:109–116, copyright 1997 with permission from Elsevier Science.)

istered in 5 daily fractions. They were also stratified according to whether they had uncontrolled disease.

Results.—Only 12 of 245 patients were alive at the time of analysis. The 2 groups were similar in survival time. The overall response rates were 83.7% for patients who received single treatment and 89.2% for patients who received 5 fractions. Complete response rates were 38.8% and 42.3%, respectively, for patients receiving single treatment and 5 fractions (Table 3). The median duration of pain control for patients receiving single treatment and 5 fractions was 13.5 and 14.0 weeks, respectively. None of these were significant differences. Quality of life, performance status, analgesic consumption (Table 4), incidence of acute side effects, and patient assessment of treatment (Table 5) were similar in both groups.

Conclusion.—There are only 3 other trials that have compared single treatment with fractionated course. This and earlier reports have failed to

TABLE 5.—Patients' Assessment of Treatment

	Single treatment	Five fractions
Do you feel better for treatment?		
(number responding)	110	100
Yes (%)	81	89
Was the treatment worthwhile?		
(number responding)	109	98
Yes (%)	84	91
Did you have problems in attending?		
(number responding)	107	98
None (%)	81	77
Minor (%)	16	17
Difficult but worth it (%)	2	4
More trouble than it was worth (%)	1	2

(Reprinted from Gaze MN, Kelly CG, Kerr GR, et al: Pain relief and quality of life following radiotherapy for bone metastases: A randomised trial of two fractionation schedules. *Radiother Oncol* 45:109–116, copyright 1997 with permission from Elsevier Science.)

show any benefit in pain control, toxicity, or other quality-of-life parameters for fractionated course of radiotherapy compared to single treatment. Single treatment is preferred to fractionated course. It is less demanding on the patient and is more cost-effective.

▶ Not being a radiation oncologist, I have often been somewhat uncomfortable discussing the logistics of radiation therapy for palliative management of bone metastases. This typically has occurred after diagnosis or after treatment of a pathologic fracture. I am uncomfortable because I have never been able to predict the treatment regimen under which these patients will be treated. This study outlines the situation very well. There are many different therapeutic options being offered to these patients without a clear consensus as to the best radiotherapy regimen. This is a well-designed, randomized trial and clearly demonstrates no advantage to multiple treatments over a single 10-Gy treatment. This has significant implications to our patients, many of whom are immobile and live at considerable distance from radiation centers. There are certainly many patient morbidity and social advantages to having their therapy done in one session. After all, the goal of palliative care is to minimize symptoms and have the patient visited by family and friends rather than visiting the doctor.

There are times, however, when we as reconstructive surgeons require full-dose radiotherapy for lesions resected and reconstructed. Some circumstances require aggressive local control of bone metastases.

C.P. Beauchamp, M.D.

Giant Cell Tumor of Bone: Prognosis and Treatment of Pulmonary Metastases

Cheng JC, Johnston JO (Univ of Calif, San Francisco)
Clin Orthop 338:205–214, 1997   13–10

Introduction.—Some slow-growing giant cell tumors of bone are discovered only incidentally, whereas other rapid-growing tumors cause destruction of the surrounding cortex and invasion of the adjacent soft tissue. Histologic and radiographic grading systems have been developed in an attempt to predict the clinical behavior of these tumors. The long-term follow-up of 5 patients with pulmonary metastases from an apparently benign giant cell tumor of bone was reported.

Patients.—During a 46-year period, 5 patients with histologically benign giant cell tumors of bone that metastasized to the lung were treated. The radiographs in all cases revealed poor cortical margins and expansile borders within the primary lesions. The tumor filled 75% of the width of the bone in 3 cases. Two lesions located near the knee were associated with pathologic fractures and extraosseous extension. Four patients had local recurrences at an average of 34 months, and 3 had at least 2 such recurrences. Recurrences developed in 3 of 3 patients treated with curettage of the intralesional margins. Two of these patients had repeat curettage with cement or bone grafting.

The average time to pulmonary metastases was 23 months. In each case, the histologic findings of the lung lesion were identical to that of the primary tumor. The metastases were associated with multiple nodules in bilateral lung fields in all patients, and with mediastinal involvement in 2. Four patients underwent resection of the pulmonary metastases. The resection was thought to be complete in 2 cases, although 1 of these patients had a later pulmonary recurrence. In 2 cases, there were too many pulmonary lesions for complete resection; these patients survived without evidence of disease progression for 8 and 38 years, respectively. Two patients with unresectable lesions underwent radiation therapy. One had subsequent disease progression requiring incomplete wedge resection, but then survived without recurrence. At a mean follow-up of 13 years, with annual imaging studies, 4 of 5 patients were alive and without disease progression, despite residual pulmonary lesions in 3 patients. There was 1 death related to complications of systemic chemotherapy, occurring 5 years after diagnosis of the primary tumor.

Conclusions.—Pulmonary metastases from benign giant cell tumors of bone may be more likely in patients with locally aggressive disease and multiple recurrences. The natural history of the pulmonary metastases is unpredictable, just as for the primary tumors. Excellent long-term survival is achieved with excision of pulmonary nodules, even if resection is incomplete.

Giant-cell Tumor of Bone Metastasising to the Lungs: A Long-term Follow-up
Siebenrock KA, Unni KK, Rock MG (Univ of Berne, Switzerland; Mayo Clinic, Rochester)
J Bone Joint Surg Br 80-B:43–47, 1998   13–11

Objective.—Giant-cell tumor (GCT) of bone may sometimes metastasize to the lung. This is a rare condition, occurring in 1% to 9% of cases of GCTs, so little is known about its long-term outcome, risk factors, or treatment. The long-term outcomes of patients with GCT of bone with pulmonary metastases were evaluated.

Patients.—During a 42-year period, 31 patients with GCT of bone that metastasized to the lung were identified. Mean age at diagnosis of the primary tumor was 27 years; the male-to-female ratio was 0.91. The distal radius, distal femur, and sacrum were the most common primary tumor sites. Twenty-three patients were followed up for a mean of 12 years after diagnosis of the primary tumor and 8 years after detection of lung metastases. Nineteen patients were alive at a mean follow-up of 9 years after lung metastases developed. Primary treatment consisted of curettage with bone grafting but without adjuvant therapy in 48% of cases, and marginal-to-wide en bloc resection in 35%. Nineteen patients had local recurrence, with lung metastases detected at the same time in 8 cases or afterward in 11. The local recurrences developed a mean of 3 years after diagnosis of the primary tumor. Two of the remaining 4 patients without local recurrence had pulmonary metastases 6–8 months after treatment of the primary tumors. The other 2 had synchronous bilateral lung metastases with their primary tumors. Treatment for local recurrences consisted of local excision or curettage with bone grafting in 58% of patients, and marginal or wide resection in 32%.

Nineteen patients had multiple lung metastases at presentation. The lung metastases were detected a mean of 4 years after diagnosis of the primary tumor. Of 20 patients for whom complete information was available, 70% were treated by surgical resection alone. All suspicious nodules were resected in 12 patients, 5 of whom had later pulmonary recurrences. One of these patients died of disease. Two patients had long-term survival after incomplete resection. Four patients received chemotherapy, combined with surgery in 2 cases and with radiotherapy in 1. Two of these patients died, 1 from progressive lung metastases. Two patients who refused treatment for their lung metastases were alive at last follow-up.

Outcomes.—Overall, 30% of patients died, 17% of tumor-related causes. Of 16 surviving patients, 81% were free of disease.

Conclusions.—"Benign" GCT of bone can metastasize to the lung. Patients with such metastases seem to have a very high local recurrence rate. Surgical resection of the lung metastases renders many patients disease free, although some will require further operations for subsequent lesions. The authors' series shows 70% long-term survival, suggesting that the prognosis of GCT with lung metastases is not as bad as previously thought.

▶ A benign metastasizing GCT is certainly a curious oxymoron, but this disorder certainly does behave in a different manner than other metastatic lesions. Both of these studies (Abstracts 13–10 and 13–11) had similar observations and conclusions. Certainly those patients that have local recurrence or whose GCTs display aggressive behavior are at increased risk for developing metastatic disease. This is understandable because this truly represents a barometer of the biological nature of the particular lesion. Siebenrock et al. noted a mean interval to presentation of metastatic disease at 4.1 years with an astonishing range from initial presentation to 24 years later. This emphasizes the importance of long-term follow-up in these patients. The overall long-term survival for these patients remains good, but there are still patients who have aggressive, progressive disease that ultimately is fatal. Clearly, we need better methods at predicting tumor behavior.

C.P. Beauchamp, M.D.

A Dose-controlled Study of [153]Sm-ethylenediaminetetramethyl-enephosphonate (EDTMP) in the Treatment of Patients With Painful Bone Metastases

Resche I, Chatal J-F, Pecking A, et al (Centre Rene Gauducheau, Nantes, France; Centre Rene Huguenin, Paris; Univ College Hosp, London; et al)
Eur J Cancer 33:1583–1591, 1997   13–12

Introduction.—The benefits of therapies specifically targeted to treatment of bone metastases can be overshadowed by adverse effects. External beam radiation therapy can offer rapid onset of local pain relief. Bone marrow suppression can occur with treatment of recurrent disease. Hemibody radiation is associated with unacceptable toxicity. Bisphosphonates can be used to prevent certain complications of bone metastases, such as pathological fractures and hypercalcemia. [153]Sm-ethylenediaminetetra-methylenephosphonate (EDTMP) is a radiopharmaceutical composed of samarium-153, a radioisotope that emits beta particles, gamma protons, and the tetraphosphonate ligand ethylenediaminetetramethylenephosphonic acid (EDTMP). The physical and biological characteristics of [153]Sm-EDTMP may render it an effective treatment for the pain of bone metastases. Using data from earlier clinical trials on dose ranges, a dose-controlled clinical investigation was conducted using 0.5 and 1.0 mCi/kg doses of [153]Sm-EDTMP to determine the comparative efficacy and safety of these doses in a large group of patients with bony metastases from a variety of primary tumors.

Methods.—Up to 16 weeks after receiving [153]Sm-EDTMP, patients were evaluated for efficacy, safety, and excretion of the radionuclide. Patients were examined weekly by their physicians for the first 4 weeks, then monthly thereafter. A patient status was rated and the Physician's Global Assessment (PGA) was completed on follow-up visits.

Results.—Of 114 patients, 55 received 0.5 mCi/kg and 59 received 1.0 mCi/kg. Prostate and breast cancer were the most frequent malignancies. Most patients had a history of earlier surgical, hormonal, or radiation therapy for cancer. Concomitant chemotherapy or external radiation therapy was administered to 11 patients in the 0.5 mCi/kg group and 5 patients in the 1.0 mCi/kg group. Patients from both groups experienced alleviation of pain, but patients who received the higher dose had greater reductions in pain (significant at weeks 3 and 4) than did patients who received the lower dose. The proportion of patients with pain most of the time or severe pain causing restriction in activity diminished over the course of the first 4 weeks in both patient groups. Only 33% of patients in each dose group were able to sleep through the night at baseline. By week 4, these values increased to 45% for the 0.5 mCi/kg group and 59% (significant) for the 0.1 mCi/kg group. Weekly pain relief assessments completed by patients indicated increasing levels of pain relief, but mean daily opiate use increased slightly from baseline and week 1 and remained fairly constant thereafter. At week 16, physician assessment indicated that 31% and 39% of patients receiving lower and higher doses, respectively,

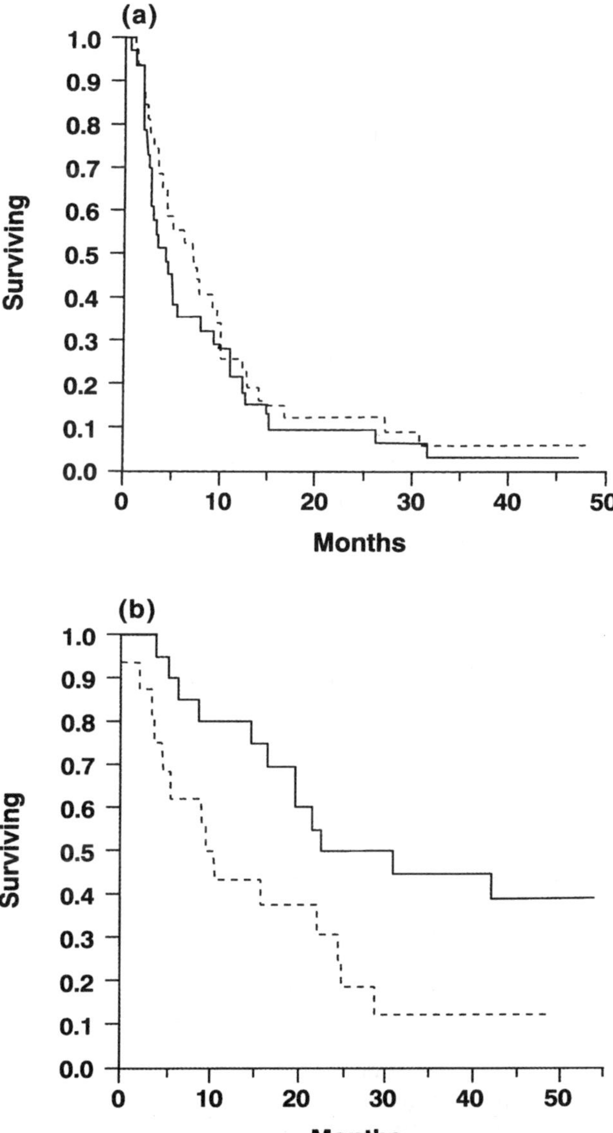

FIGURE 3.—Survival curves for patients with prostate cancer (A) and patients with breast cancer (B). *Solid line* = 0.1 mCi/kg, *broken line* = 0.5 mCi/kg. (Reprinted from Resche I, Chatal J-F, Pecking A, et al: A dose-controlled study of ^{153}Sm-ethylenediaminetetramethylenephosphonate [EDTMP] in the treatment of patients with painful bone metastases. *Eur J Cancer* 33:1583–1591, copyright 1997, with permission from Elsevier Science.)

had experienced some degree of pain relief (24% of patients receiving high dose and 14% of patients receiving low dose treatment were rated either much better or completely better). For both white blood cells and platelets, patients receiving 1.0 mCi/kg had lower mean nadirs and greater changes from baseline than did patients receiving 0.5 mCi/kg. In patients with prostate cancer, survival was not dose-related. Survival in patients with breast cancer was significantly higher in patients who received 1.0 mCi/kg, versus 0.5 mCi/kg (Fig 3).

Conclusion.—The 1.0 mCi/kg dose of ^{153}Sm-EDTMP may be considered safe and effective in the treatment of painful bone metastases. The physical half life of this radionuclide allows it to be administered in a short period of time, which means a greater biological effect may be experienced using high initial dose rates. This translates into rapid onset of pain relief and limited hematological toxicity. The low rate of exposure and rapid clearance and excretion of ^{153}Sm-EDTMP allows patients to be treated on an outpatient basis. This radionuclide may be an appropriate choice for use in early treatment of metastases.

▶ Systemic treatment of painful bony metastasis with radiopharmaceutical agents represents another modality of therapy for patients with metastatic bone disease. Its role is primarily for the patient who has widespread metastatic bone disease with numerous areas of painful metastasis. Focal specific hot spots, impending fractures, or pathologic fractures still require localized radiotherapy treatment or internal stabilization. The observation that patients receiving ^{153}Sm EDTMP have improved survival is encouraging, and certainly further study needs to be done to determine its role in the management of patients with moderately symptomatic skeletal metastases.

C.P. Beauchamp, M.D.

Prosthetic Hip Replacement for Pathologic or Impending Pathologic Fractures in Myeloma

Papagelopoulos PJ, Galanis EC, Greipp PR, et al (Mayo Clinic and Found, Rochester, Minn)
Clin Orthop 341:192–205, 1997   13–13

Objective.—Many fixation devices for fractures of the proximal femur fail in patients treated for malignant myeloma of the hip region. The risk of failure increases with prolonged survival. Because myeloma lesions tend to be more diffuse and extensive than metastatic lesions, more aggressive treatment of myeloma lesions is necessary. The clinical outcome, complications, and patient and implant survival after hip replacement in patients with myeloma were discussed, with special attention to preoperative disease staging and type of bone defects treated.

Methods.—Between 1969 and 1994, 50 patients (22 women), aged 40–85 years, received 53 hip replacements for plasma cytoma (4 lesions) or multiple myeloma (49 lesions). All lesions were lytic, typically circular or

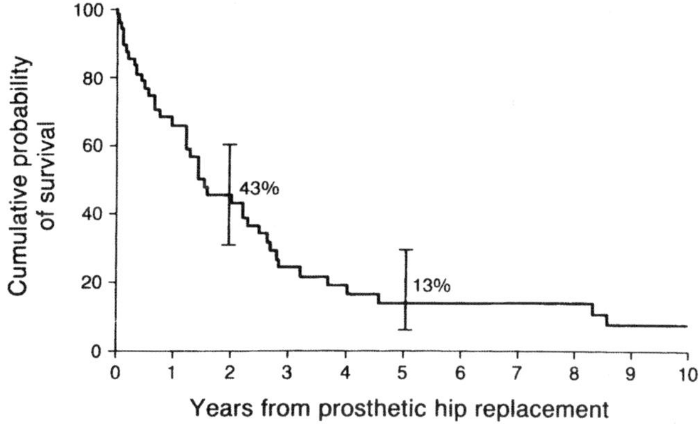

FIGURE 7.—Overall patient survival after prosthetic replacement for pathologic or impending pathologic fractures of the hip. (Courtesy of Papagelopoulos PJ, Galanis EC, Greipp PR, et al: Prosthetic hip replacement for pathologic or impending pathologic fractures in myeloma. *Clin Orthop* 341:192–205, 1997).

elliptical, and extensive with distinct margins. The defects involved the acetabulum and the proximal femur to the cortex. Preoperatively, 49 patients received chemotherapy, and 24 lesions were irradiated with 27–50 cGy. Eleven lesions that progressed were irradiated postoperatively. Fifteen patients had postoperative chemotherapy. A standard femoral component was used for reconstruction in 26 patients, 6 had head and neck replacement, and 13 had proximal femoral replacement.

Results.—Patients were followed for an average of 32.6 months. There were 2 intraoperative and 15 postoperative complications. One patient died intraoperatively, 2 patients died within the first month, and 2 required reoperation during the follow-up period. At follow-up, 41 patients were pain free, 3 had mild pain. and 1 had moderate pain. Six patients occasionally used a cane, and 29 needed no support. At an average of 48 months, there was no radiographic evidence of aseptic loosening. During a follow-up ranging from 7 days to 19.9 years, 1 patient received resection arthroplasty without reimplantation 5 months postoperatively for recurrent dislocation and another patient had resection arthroplasty and reimplantation 5 years postoperatively for deep infection.

The median patient survival was 18.6 months (Fig 7). The 8 patients alive at the time of the study had a median survival of 76 months. Patients with plasmacytoma survived longer than did patients with multiple myeloma (6.3 years vs. 18 months). There was no association between survival and state of disease, age, sex, type or location of myeloma, or type of implant.

Conclusion.—Hip replacement with concomitant irradiation and chemotherapy is effective for patients with multiple myeloma of the hip region not treatable by other means. It provides good function and significant pain relief but with a 28% postoperative complication rate. Patients with plasmacytoma survive longer than do patients with multiple myeloma.

▶ This is a large series of patients with myeloma affecting the hip and periacetabular regions. Patients with myeloma are going to live longer and have more bone pathology that we, as orthopedic surgeons, will have to deal with. The authors advocate reconstructive options with long-term survival in mind. These principals need not necessarily be applied simply to myeloma, but to most other patients with metastatic bone disease. The reconstructive techniques should be designed to allow immediate full weight-bearing, should not rely on assistive devices for ambulation, and should be looking at long-term scenarios for problems in the region that could be addressed during the operative procedure. Such techniques would include the use of such devices as long-stem prosthetic replacements, proximal femoral replacements, and protrusio cage augmentation.

C.P. Beauchamp, M.D.

The Benefits of Surgery in the Treatment of Pelvic Metastases
Giurea A, Ritschl P, Windhager R, et al (Univ of Vienna)
Int Orthop 21:343–348, 1997   13–14

Introduction.—In 40% of patients with bony metastases, the pelvis is affected. The survival time of these patients has been increased from 7 months in the 1960s to 19 months in 1981 by an interdisciplinary approach involving oncologists, orthopedic surgeons, radiologists, and general surgeons. The aim of surgical treatment of pelvic metastases is to maintain or restore mobility and the quality of life. Little is known about the functional outcome and life expectancy of these patients. The outcome of surgery in patients with pelvic metastases was reviewed to determine median survival time, the effect on the quality of life and mobility, and the value of intralesional or extralesional resection on survival time, complications, and local recurrence.

Methods.—There were 43 patients with pelvic metastases (Fig 1) who had 37 intralesional and 6 extralesional resections in a 12-year period. Perioperative adjuvant therapy was performed on 39 patients, which included embolization to reduce blood loss and external radiotherapy, radioiodine therapy, or chemotherapy. Survival time was calculated and a clinical evaluation was conducted.

Results.—Among all patients, the median survival time was 14 months with a range of 2–127 months. There was improvement in the Karnofsky score from 55% before operation to 74% at 3 months and to 77% after 6 months. A median survival time of 13 months, a complication rate of 24%, and a local recurrence rate of 19% were seen in patients with an intralesional resection. Patients with extralesional resection had a median survival of 16 months, a 50% complication rate, and no local recurrences. There were 23 patients who had renal or thyroid carcinoma with metas-

Localisation (according to Enneking)		Resection without stabilisation	Osteo-synthesis	Endoprostheses		
				Saddle	Hip	Pelvis
	involvement					
	single	8	4			
P_1	$+ P_2 + P_3$		2			
	$+ P_2 + P_4$		1			
	single				3	1
P_2	$+ P_1$		3	1		
	$+ P_3$	3		3	1	
	single	5				
P_3	$+ P_2$	2				
	single	3				
P_4	$+ P_1$	1	2			
total 43 patients		22	12	4	4	1

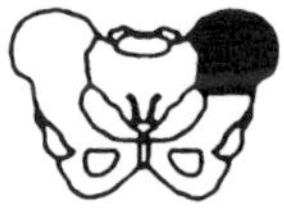

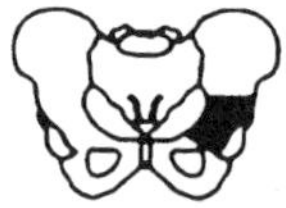

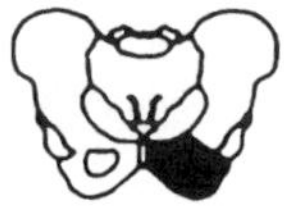

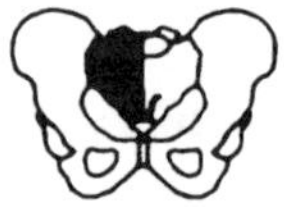

FIGURE 1.—Enneking's localization of pelvic metastases with single and multiple involvement of adjacent regions, and the type of surgical treatment. *Abbreviations: P1*, iliac wing; *P2*, periacetabular; *P3*, pubis and ischium; *P4*, sacrum. (Courtesy of Guirea A, Ritschl P, Windhager R, et al: The benefits of surgery in the treatment of pelvic metastases. *Int Orthop* 21:343–348. Copyright 1997, Springer-Verlag.)

tases (Fig 5). Complications included pelvic vein thrombosis, dislocation of the endoprosthesis, deep infection, superficial infection, and fracture of the pelvis with loosening of a wire after osteosynthesis.

Conclusions.—In most patients, the quality of life was improved by operation, and intralesional resection was preferable. Rapid restoration of function was the aim. There is a good functional outcome, a lower complication rate, and a reduced need for blood with intralesional resections. There should be surgical treatment of metastases that respond poorly to conservative treatment. Regardless of the histologic type, operation is indicated in the periacetabular region because of the difficulty in walking and the danger of fractures. For solitary metastases with a good prognosis, extralesional resection should be considered.

▶ Management of patients with pelvic metastatic disease is, to say the least, challenging. Embarking on a course of surgery for these lesions exposes the patient to a difficult surgical procedure that may carry with it a significant morbidity. The complication rate for this surgery is high, and a complication or poor surgical outcome in this group of patients can be disastrous. It requires a great deal of decision making, planning, and technical skill to design a good surgical procedure for this group of patients.

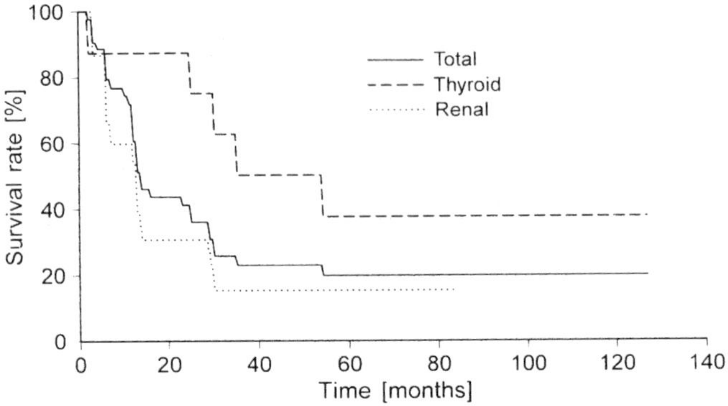

FIGURE 5.—Overall Kaplan-Meier survival curves of patients with pelvic metastases, and patients with renal and thyroid carcinoma. (Courtesy of Guirea A, Ritschl P, Windhager R, et al: The benefits of surgery in the treatment of pelvic metastases. *Int Orthop* 21:343–348. Copyright 1997, Springer-Verlag.)

Long-term survival can be significant for these patients, and the reconstruction should be designed to permit immediate, early full weight-bearing with as much durability built into the reconstruction as possible.

C.P. Beauchamp, M.D.

Posterior Decompression and Stabilization for Spinal Metastases: Analysis of Sixty-Seven Consecutive Patients

Bauer HCF (Karolinska Hosp, Stockholm)
J Bone Joint Surg Am 79-A:514–522, 1997   13–15

Objective.—For patients with vertebral metastases causing epidural compression and neurologic abnormalities, the generally accepted treatment is anterior decompression and stabilization. Anterior decompression carries high morbidity and mortality, however. An alternative approach is posterior decompression plus stabilization with segmental instrumentation. The results of posterior decompression and stabilization for patients with thoracic or lumbar metastases with epidural compression were analyzed.

Methods.—The study included 67 consecutive patients treated for spinal metastases with epidural compression. The thoracic spine was involved in 41 patients and the lumbar spine in 26. The neurologic deficit was assessed as major in 26 patients (grade B or C, according to the system of Frankel et al.), minor in 32 patients (grade D), and absent in 9 (grade E). None of the patients in this series had pathologic vertebral fracture without epidural compression. Through a posterior approach, the patients underwent wide decompression with stabilization. Bone grafts were not used. Stabilization was achieved with a Cotrel-Dubousset device in 32 patients (Fig 3, B), an Olerud posterior fixator in 16, an Isola device in 12, and some other device in 7. The results were analyzed in terms of neurologic function, survival, and rehabilitation.

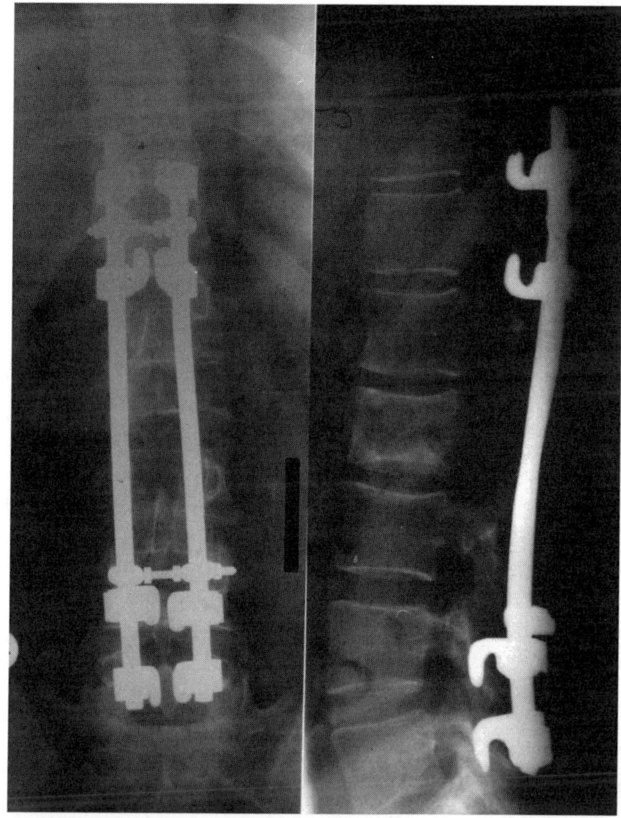

FIGURE 3, B.—Radiographs made after decompression and instrumentation with a Cotrel-Dubousset device. (Courtesy of Bauer HCF: Posterior decompression and stabilization for spinal metastases: Analysis of sixty-seven consecutive patients. *J Bone Joint Surg Am* 79A:514–522, 1997.)

Results.—Eleven patients had wound infection, the most frequent complication. No patient died in the perioperative period or within 14 days after surgery. Survival was 51% at 6 months and 22% at 12 months. Of 58 patients with a preoperative neurologic deficit, 76% experienced complete or partial neurologic recovery within 14 days. All those without neurologic deficits retained normal neurologic function. The percentage of surviving patients who remained able to walk was 86% at 3 months and 85% at 6 months. Reoperation was required in 14 patients: 6 for recurrent epidural compression at another level, 5 for recurrent compression at the same level, and 3 for implant loosening.

Conclusion.—In patients with spinal metastases causing epidural compression, posterior decompression and stabilization is an effective approach to restoring or preserving neurologic function. This experience shows results comparable with those of anterior decompression but with lower morbidity. Posterior decompression offers an alternative technique for patients with extensive metastases in whom an anterior approach is too demanding.

▶ This experience indicates that the decision analysis regarding anterior or posterior decompression and reconstruction can differ in cancer patients from that used in patients with traumatic or degenerative problems. Specifically, the discussion focuses on the selection of posterior decompression and instrumentation in patients whose epidural compression may be primarily anterior and whose anterior spinal elements may be deficient from a mechanical perspective. Forty-four of the 58 patients with preoperative neurologic deficit treated in this manner improved neurologically. None of the patients received bone graft, consistent with the expectation that the posterior instrumentation would provide mechanical stability for the remainder of the patient's life. The study indicates that this group of patients can experience an improved quality of life under difficult clinical circumstances with somewhat less extensive surgery than an anterior procedure would entail.

The study does not address the issue of the selection criteria for surgical decompression. For example, would some of the patients in the study have been candidates for radiation therapy and bracing rather than surgery? The authors do not discuss the role of postoperative bracing in this group of surgically treated patients. Because the instrumentation needs to last for the patient's lifetime, consideration might be given to augmenting the hook and pedicle screw attachment sites with sublaminar wire attachment sites. Although sublaminar wires, of themselves, would not provide resistance to axial translation, they would likely be a useful supplement to screws and hooks as mitigation against implant loosening and failure. Postoperative wound infection was the most frequently reported complication.

The authors have not given data regarding the timing and dosage of any postoperative radiation or chemotherapy given as local treatment for the metastatic focus. These treatments can affect the healing and possible infection of the surgical wound, and a balance between the considerations of tumor control and wound healing needs to be considered in planning their use.

M.J. Yaszemski, M.D.

Miscellaneous

Evidence of the Subperiosteal Origin of Osteoid Osteomas in Tubular Bones: Analysis by CT and MR Imaging
Kayser F, Resnick D, Haghighi P, et al (Veterans Affairs Med Ctr, San Diego, Calif; Baylor Univ, Dallas; Thomas Jefferson Univ, Philadelphia; et al)
AJR 170:609–614, 1998   13–16

Introduction.—Accounting for about 10% of all benign bone tumors, osteoid osteoma occurs most often in the second and third decades of life. The presence of a small, well-defined radiolucent lesion is characteristic, and most osteoid osteomas are intracortical in origin and location. Subperiosteal osteoid osteomas generally occur at the femoral neck and the phalanges and were considered to be rare. To determine the frequency of a subperiosteal site of origin, a large series of patients with osteoid osteomas of tubular bones was reviewed.

Methods.—A total of 38 patients who had the tumor located in a tubular bone had the lesion evaluated by CT scanning or MRI, or both. Categorization of the location of the osteoid osteoma was classified as intracortical, subperiosteal, endosteal, or medullary.

Results.—Imaging was done with CT for 19 patients, with MR for 14 patients, and with both techniques for 5 patients. The tibia was the most commonly affected site (15 patients), followed by the femur (13 patients) and humerus (4 patients). Of the 38 cases, 18 were intracortical, 18 were subperiosteal, and 2 were intramedullary.

Conclusions.—It is not rare to find osteoid osteomas occurring in a subperiosteal or surface location. Many osteoid osteomas that arise in tubular bone may originate in a subperiosteal site and subsequently appear as an intracortical lesion. Continual remodeling of bone with subperiosteal deposition and endosteal erosions appears to be related to the site of origin. Differential remodeling and cortical drift may be another factor.

Subperiosteal Osteoid Osteoma: Radiographic and Pathologic Manifestations
Shankman S, Desai P, Beltran J (Hosp for Joint Diseases/OI, New York)
Skeletal Radiol 26:457–462, 1997   13–17

Introduction.—A benign bone-forming neoplasm, osteoid osteoma usually arises in the cortex or adjacent medullary space. It is believed extremely rare to find any that arise beneath the periosteum. When compared with the more common cortical variety, the radiographic characteristics of these lesions are often atypical, and other diagnoses may be suggested by the radiographic appearance. The radiologic and pathologic manifestations of this unusual lesion were presented.

Methods.—A total of 160 cases of osteoid osteoma occurring during a 30-year period were retrospectively reviewed; of these, 11 were subperiosteal osteoid osteoma, and their radiologic, pathologic, and operative findings were studied. Ranging in age from 13 to 36 years, 8 of the patients were male and 3 were female.

Results.—Four lesions had a reactive periostitis that was atypical and misleading. Features similar to the more common intracortical variety were seen in 4 lesions. On plain radiographs, 3 lesions occurring within the joint, like other intra-articular lesions, were barely seen. Computed tomography and bone scan were virtually diagnostic. These lesions had atypical, but not misleading, histopathology. Occurring within the joint, at the bare area, or outside the confines of the joint capsule, subperiosteal osteoid osteoma may erode into the cortex beneath.

Conclusions.—Subperiosteal osteoid osteoma is a rare lesion that has atypical radiographic and histopathologic features. Other diagnoses may be suggested by the unusual reactive periostitis seen in some extra-articular cases. There is some confusion in the literature in that the terms subperiosteal and intra-articular or juxta-articular are frequently used interchangeably. There is usually less central mineralization and less peripheral reactive bone sclerosis, compared with the conventional intracortical lesion.

▶ It is generally believed that subperiosteal osteoid osteomas are rare. Kayser et al. (Abstract 13–16), in analyzing 38 patients with osteoid osteomas, found that this location was not rare in these patients. They propose an intriguing hypothesis that in fact the reverse may be true; that is, subperiosteal osteoid osteomas may indeed originate in that site and only with time appear in different locations because of remodeling of the new reactive bone formation. Certainly, the radiographic evidence presented does seem to support this, as the intracortical location appears to be a phenomenon created by reactive new bone greatly expanding the size of the cortex.

Shankman et al., in a larger study (Abstract 13–17), provides evidence to the contrary that supports the unusual presentation of a subperiosteal osteoid osteoma. Both of these papers emphasize the importance of CT scanning in the evaluation and diagnosis of patients with osteoid osteomas.

C.P. Beauchamp, M.D.

Idiopathic Necrosis of Skeletal Muscle in Patients Who Have Diabetes: Report of Four Cases and Review of the Literature
Damron TA, Levinsohn EM, McQuail TM, et al (State Univ of New York, Syracuse; Crouse Hosp, Syracuse, NY)
J Bone Joint Surg Am 80-A:262–267, 1998   13–18

Introduction.—An infrequently recognized clinicopathologic entity is infarction of skeletal muscle in patients who have diabetes. The lesion may be misinterpreted radiographically as a soft-tissue sarcoma or infection. Four patients with infarction of skeletal muscle were described. Their mean age was 42 years. They had an exquisitely tender swelling of the anterior aspect of the thigh for 10 days to 4 weeks before their initial evaluation. One patient had diabetes diagnosed at the time of initial evaluation, 1 had a history of non-insulin-dependent diabetes, and 2 had a history of insulin-dependent diabetes. After a mean follow-up of 31 months, 3 patients had no recurrence, but the fourth had a recurrence of the muscular necrosis and died 6 months later.

Necrosis.—In patients who have diabetes, necrosis of skeletal muscle has been called tumoriform focal muscular degeneration and idiopathic diabetic muscle infarction. The differential diagnosis consists of soft-tissue neoplasm, intramuscular hematoma, deep venous thrombosis, and myositis. Mild, nonspecific uptake in the soft tissues in the region of the mass may be seen with radionuclide scanning. To define the extent of the process and to exclude neoplasm, abscess, and hematoma, CT and MRI are frequently useful. The absence of a discrete mass and the involvement of at least 1 major muscle group are characteristic findings of diabetic necrosis of skeletal muscle on MRI. Hemorrhagic necrosis of skeletal muscle and microangiopathy are the histologic findings.

Treatment.—Treatment usually involves alleviation of symptoms and includes administration of analgesics, rest, and immobilization. Some patients require additional insulin to control their diabetes, nonsteroidal anti-inflammatory medications, and nerve blocks. After the initiation of treatment, the symptoms can resolve slowly over 6 weeks to 7 months. Symptoms were exacerbated by early physical therapy.

Conclusions.—In a patient with diabetes mellitus and a mass involving skeletal muscle, necrosis of skeletal muscle must be considered. Its rareness makes it difficult to become familiar with this entity. Involvement of more than 1 muscle group, diffuse swelling within involved muscle, a short duration of symptoms, exquisite tenderness, and a history of long-standing diabetes are the clinical features that are highly suggestive of the diagnosis. Plain radiography and MRI are recommended. The potential risks of delaying the diagnosis of soft-tissue sarcoma outweigh the risk associated with a biopsy.

▶ This is a rare entity. Unless you know about it or have been involved in the care of a patient with this disorder, you will miss this diagnosis. These patients have a fairly characteristic history, physical findings, and in particular have characteristic MR findings. When typical, a biopsy can be avoided in these patients. A biopsy specimen of necrotic muscle can be a difficult diagnostic challenge for the pathologist because the potential for the specimen to be interpreted as a nondiagnostic biopsy may stimulate the need for further, more aggressive biopsy sampling.

C.P. Beauchamp, M.D.

Langerhans' Cell Histiocytosis in Adults: A Clinical and Therapeutic Analysis of 11 Patients From a Single Institution
Giona F, Caruso R, Testi AM, et al (Univ "La Sapienza," Rome)
Cancer 80:1786–1791, 1997   13–19

Introduction.—Langerhans' cell histiocytosis (LCH) is a rare proliferative disorder of unknown etiology observed more frequently in children than adults. Recent reports have indicated that LCH represents a clonal proliferative disorder of cells closely related to Langerhans' cells. Its severity ranges from a curable solitary lytic bone lesion usually seen in adults to a fatal leukemia-like disorder primarily affecting infants. Children and adults with localized disease typically have a good prognosis after remission or surgical or radiotherapeutic treatment. The management of multisystem disease for children and adults is more controversial and challenging. The clinical outcome of 11 adult patients with LCH who were treated and observed for 5 years was assessed.

Methods.—For patients with localized bone lesions with or without soft-tissue involvement, surgery was the preferred treatment. Patients with multifocal bone disease with or without visceral involvement and those with or without lung and lymph node disease were treated with combination chemotherapy.

Results.—All 4 patients with unifocal bone disease were treated surgically. At 29+ -month follow-up, only 1 patient was in complete remission (CR) after initial treatment. Recurrence in the remaining patients occurred at 2, 12, and 30 months. The remaining 3 patients required 1 or more additional treatments and were in CR. Two of 3 patients with multifocal bone disease were treated with combination therapy. Two patients were treated with vinblastine plus high-dose methylprednisolone (HDMP). One patient was in CR at 8 months after surgery and the other patient had progressive disease 11 months after therapy. This patient responded to interferon (INF) therapy. The final patient was in CR at 3 months after treatment with INF and remained so at final follow-up at 35 + months. The 2 patients with bone and visceral disease were treated with etoposide (VP-16) plus HDMP and were in CR after 4 cycles. One patient was still in remission at the 42-month follow-up. Of 2 patients with lung and lymph node disease, 1 was in CR at 30 months after treatment with VP-16 + HDMP. The other patient was in remission at 71+ months after treatment with cyclophosphamine + doxorubicin + vincristine + prednisone. All patients were alive at a median of 34 months after diagnosis.

Conclusion.—Treatment with vinblastine plus HDMP was efficacious in patients with bone disease, especially those with localized disease at diagnosis or recurrence after surgery. The combination of VP-16 and HDMP was used successfully in patients with visceral disease. Treatment with INF was effective in localized and multifocal disease. Long-term follow-up is needed to determine the long-term response duration. Collection of data from international clinical trials would broaden knowledge of the treatment of adults with LCH.

▶ Langerhans' cell histiocytosis is a disorder with multiple clinical forms. Most orthopedists would consider this to be a childhood disorder, and although it does occur more frequently in children, it is present from birth to old age. It has a peak incidence between 1 and 3 years of age. The disease in adults is quite rare and there are few published reports on its outcome. This study unfortunately has a small number of diverse patients. Without multicenter collaboration, it would be extremely difficult to obtain large numbers of this very rare condition. The authors do note that, when necessary, chemotherapeutic agents are effective in the management of these patients. Chemotherapeutic agents used included vinblastine, HDMP, IF, and VP-16. It was noted that surgical treatment alone had a high local persistence rate. Interestingly, the authors did not discuss the role of radiation therapy for these patients. Although this modality is less attractive in children, certainly in adults it could be considered in some of these patients with intercurrent skeletal disease.

All 11 patients were alive and well. There were significant relapses and failures. They all responded to alteration and chemotherapeutic management. This suggests that the lesion in adults, while prone to relapse, does respond to ongoing chemotherapeutic intervention.

C.P. Beauchamp, M.D.

Cementation of Primary Aneurysmal Bone Cysts
Ozaki T, Hillmann A, Lindner N, et al (Westfälische Wilhelms-Univ, Münster, Germany)
Clin Orthop 337:240–248, 1997   13–20

Introduction.—Several treatment modalities have been used for aneurysmal bone cysts. Local relapse rates after resection, curettage and bone graft, and curettage and irradiation, respectively, range from 0% to 19%, 22% to 59%, and 0% to 20%. For irradiation and cryosurgery, rates are 25% and 14% to 18%, respectively. In Germany, one of the most popular treatments for giant-cell tumors is cementation. The effect of cementation for aneurysmal bone cyst is unknown. The effect of curettage and cementation in the treatment of aneurysmal bone cyst was assessed and retrospectively compared with curettage and bone graft in 35 and 30 patients, respectively.

Methods.—For curettage and cementation, bone cement was mixed with gentamycin and packed into the cavity of the bone marrow with digital pressure after curettage of the lesion. The peripheral area of the cavity was packed with cement. Artificial skin patches were used to protect surrounding tissues from the thermal effect of the cement. The central area of the cement was separated into several small fragments by packing it between artificial skin pads for subsequent easy removal.

Results.—Relapses occurred in 6 of 35 patients who underwent cementation and in 11 of 30 patients who underwent bone graft (17% vs. 37%). Relapse-free cumulative 10-year survival was 77% for cementation versus 40% for bone graft. For cementation, local recurrence occurred in 20% of aggressive aneurysmal bone cysts, 20% of active lesions, and 0% of inactive lesions. In the bone graft group, these rates were 50%, 33%, and 28%, respectively. Of 17 local recurrences, 12 underwent cementation. Five and 7 of these patients had prior treatment with cementation and bone graft, respectively. Two of these patients had another local recurrence. One patient with an iliac lesion underwent irradiation and the other patient with a femoral lesion underwent resection and allograft transplantation. There were no third recurrences. One patient experienced a pathologic fracture after cementation because of an extension of a locally relapsed lesion.

Conclusion.—Cementation takes the mechanical stress and prevents fracture with actual increases in mechanical strength. Unlike bone graft, cementation allows early radiographic evidence of local recurrence. Thermal injury of the growth plate or subchondral bone may occur, but this may be prevented by use of artificial skin patches. Late removal of bone cement is recommended. Radiologic follow-up should be performed for a few years after surgery to watch for local recurrence. Local control rates with cementation approximate those of cryosurgery.

▶ Aneurysmal bone cysts can be troublesome lesions to treat. They are unpredictable and can have a high rate of local recurrence. The authors compared 2 groups of patients treated with curettage and bone grafting versus curettage and cementation and have noted a definite superiority in local control with cementation. The protocol the authors used involved removal of the cement and bone grafting as a second surgical procedure. In adults with giant-cell tumors we have generally moved away from this because the morbidity of cement removal and bone grafting was not worth the effort as the long-term sequelae of cementation became less and less of an issue. Whereas there are certainly concerns about using cement in patients with open epiphysts, it certainly has a role in the management of older patients with aneurysmal bone cysts. I do not see an advantage in its removal and subsequent bone grafting.

C.P. Beauchamp, M.D.

Myxoid Chondrosarcoma (Chordoid Sarcoma) of Bone: A Report of Two Cases and Review of the Literature
Kilpatrick SE, Inwards CY, Fletcher CDM, et al (Wake Forest Univ, Winston-Salem, NC; Mayo Clinic, Rochester, Minn; Brigham and Women's Hosp, Boston; et al)
Cancer 79:1903–1910, 1997   13–21

Objective.—Whereas chondrosarcoma of bone is relatively common, morphologically distinct soft tissue choroid sarcoma (CS), or extraskeletal myxoid chondrosarcoma, is relatively rare and has not been completely described. Two cases of skeletal CS were reported, with a discussion of its clinical behavior, and a literature review.

> *Case 1.*—A man, 48, with pain in his right knee of 4 months duration, was given a diagnosis of degenerative joint disease. After he fractured his right femur, radiographs revealed a lesion of the distal femur with extension into soft tissue. He had an above-the-knee amputation. Local recurrences developed. The patient was alive at 13 months, after local radiation therapy and chemotherapy, but had widespread metastatic disease.
> *Case 2.*—Man, 76, with an enlarging right axillary mass of 18 months duration, was found to have destruction of the scapula with extensive soft tissue invasion. He had a right radical forequarter amputation with excision of part of the chest wall. Despite

radiation therapy, local recurrence developed 22 months later. He died 59 months after diagnosis with widespread metastatic disease.

Results.—Both tumors were gray-white, lobulated, and gelatinous, with hemorrhagic and cystic, but no osseous, areas. Microscopically, the tumors resembled CS in soft tissue but with increased cellularity at the edges. Neoplastic cells frequently appeared as lacelike strands within a mucinous matrix and sometimes as aggregates resembling adenocarcinoma. Blood vessels were not prominent in the round-to-spindle-shaped cells. Nuclei were uniform, hyperchromatic, and surrounded by eosinophilic cytoplasm. Vacuolated cells were often visible. Mitotic activity varied from less than 1–10 mitotic figures. Significant bone destruction was observed. Cells in case 1, but not in case 2, were positive for S-100 protein. Case 2 had a reciprocal translocation between chromosomes 2 and 22. Two additional cases were found in the literature.

Conclusion.—Myxoid CS is a rare neoplasm with a worse clinical outcome than typical CS of bone. Whereas wide surgical excision appears to be the most effective treatment, the value of chemotherapy and radiation therapy have yet to be determined.

▶ The authors describe an extraordinary rare tumor of bone that has a distinct histologic appearance. This chondrosarcoma has a distinct predilection for local recurrence and distant metastasis and should be treated as a high-grade chondrosarcoma. Given its behavior, consideration should be given to chemotherapy in these patients.

C.P. Beauchamp, M.D.

Characteristics of Phenol: Instillation in Intralesional Tumor Excision of Chondroblastoma, Osteoclastoma and Enchondroma
Quint U, Müller RT, Müller G (Universitätsklinikum Essen, Germany; Inst of Hygiene and Occupational Medicine, Essen, Germany)
Arch Orthop Trauma Surg 117:43–46, 1998   13–22

Introduction.—Intralesional tumor excision is frequently used to preserve joint function for the treatment of locally aggressive benign tumors. Adjuvant therapy has been preferred to reduce relapses because the procedure leads to a high recurrence. Irrigation of phenol is used for chemical cauterization, and different concentrations of phenol are used at different temperatures. The phenol is quickly absorbed and metabolized because of the bone's good vascularity. It is hard to estimate the risk for the patient because little pharmacokinetic data on the burden to the patient are available. Water and phenol are incompletely soluble because of their physical characteristics. Phenol is easily soluble in ethanol, and the caustic character is reduced by alcohol because of the chemical properties. Phenol is bacteriostatic by denaturing proteins and destroying cell permeability. With concentrations of more than 3%, it is necrogenic, and of 5%, it is

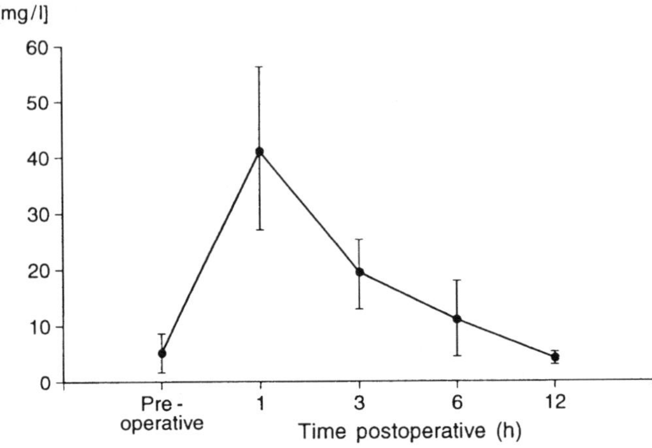

FIGURE 3.—Urinary excretion of phenol according to time after instillation (3 × 34 mL of a 5% solution for 60 seconds each) in the bone cavity. (Courtesy of Quint U, Müller RT, Müller G: Characteristics of phenol: Installation in intralesional tumor excision of chondroblastoma, osteoclastoma and enchondroma. *Arch Orthop Trauma Surg* 117:43–46. Copyright 1998, Springer-Verlag.)

locally anesthetic. Numbness through paralysis of the free nerve endings results after a longer exposure time. By coagulation necrosis, phenol can destroy 1–1.5 mm of tumor tissue. Phenol is well absorbed by the skin, mucosa, and open wounds, and metabolized by sulphatation and glucoronidation. There is a relatively high danger of intoxication, and acute poisoning causes pulmonary insufficiency with lung edema, and paralysis of the CNS with collapse and a decrease in temperature. The acute lethal dose has been observed to be 1–2 g parenterally, 10 g dermally, and 10–30 g orally.

Methods.—The urinary excretion of phenol after the instillation of 102 mL. of a 5% phenol solution was investigated. Urine was collected from 11 patients treated by phenol instillation preoperatively, and at 1, 3, 6, 12, and 24 hours after the operation. Mass spectrometry was used to analyze the urine specimens.

Results.—On average, the value was 5.1 mg/L preoperatively (Fig 3). At 1 hour after instillation, the maximum concentration was 62 mg/L and the average value was 41.5 mg/L. After 3 hours, the concentration was 18.9 mg/L. There was a further rapid decrease in the excretion rate, and after 12 hours normal values were reached. Within 24 hours postoperatively, a maximum of 9% and an average of 2% of the instilled amount of phenol were excreted.

Conclusions.—A relatively low risk of systemic toxicity is found with the instillation of a 5% phenol solution into bony lesions. There might be a potential for serious systemic toxicity in the treatment, depending on the amount of phenol used, because the resorbed phenol is excreted within 24 hours almost completely and the half-life of 1–2 hours is very short. A 5% phenol solution, is effective against dispersed single cells, and higher concentrations yield no significant advantage.

▶ This is an extremely important paper that should be read by all those who use phenol intraoperatively for the treatment of bone neoplasms. There is a tremendous variation in the concentrations used surgically for cauterization of tumor cavities. The authors note that a significant amount of phenol can be absorbed systemically, and that potential serious complications can occur if prolonged exposure or vigorous applications of phenol are used. It is very difficult for surgeons inexperienced with the use of phenol to gain information regarding its use. It is often obtained by word of mouth. It is sometimes often difficult to ignore the rule that more is often not better, and serious harm may occur to patients if too much phenol is used for too long a period. The authors recommend a 5% solution be used.

C.P. Beauchamp, M.D.

Pathologic Fractures Through Nonossifying Fibromas: Is Prophylactic Treatment Warranted?
Easley ME, Kneisl JS (Carolinas Med Ctr, Charolette, NC)
J Pediatr Orthop B 17:808–813, 1997   13–23

Introduction.—Nonossifying fibromas are benign, nonosteroid-producing bone tumors. Usually found in the metaphyses of long bones, these benign fibrous lesions have a predilection for the lower extremities. Pathologic fractures can result from proliferative lesions with extensive cortical involvement. The risk of pathologic fracture has previously correlated with absolute size parameters; the greater the mechanical defect, the larger the lesion and the greater the chance for fracture. Prophylactic curettage and bone grafting of large nonossifying fibromas—defined as demonstrating more than 50% cortical involvement on anterior-posterior and lateral radiographs and a height measurement of more than 33 mm—have been recommended. However, excellent healing potential has been found in fractures through nonossifying fibromas, usually without bone grafting. It may be unnecessary to provide prophylactic curettage and bone grafting, and the previously recommended guidelines may be inappropriate.

Methods.—To evaluate the risk of pathologic fracture, 22 patients with large nonossifying fibromas in weight-bearing bones were studied. There were 14 boys and 8 girls with an average age of 15.8 years. The distal femur, proximal tibia, or distal tibia were the locations of the nonossifying fibroma.

Results.—Despite exceeding the previously established size threshold, 13 large nonossifying fibromas (59%) had not had pathologic fracture. Fractures of the long bone in which the nonossifying fibromas were located, without the fracture involving the lesion, were found in 4 patients. Healing was uneventful after closed reduction and cast immobilization in the 9 patients (41%) in whom pathologic fracture occurred. Nonossifying fibromas that fractured had width-ratio dimensions of 40% to 95% of nonossifying fibroma–involved bone on anterior-posterior radiographs, and 50% to 85% on lateral radiographs. Those that had not fractured had width ratio dimensions of 52% to 92% on anterio-posterior radiographs and 57% to 88% on lateral radiographs. There were no statistically significant differences in the 2 groups with respect to percentage width ratios.

Conclusions.—Although absolute size parameters of nonossifying fibromas may be helpful in predicting a pathologic fracture rate, these parameters do not mandate that prophylactic curettage and bone grafting be performed. Surgical intervention is not necessary for the majority of patients with large nonossifying fibromas; however, these patients need to be monitored. Most fractures can be successfully managed without surgery.

▶ The authors have reviewed 22 patients with large nonossifying fibromas and have questioned the need for prophylactic fixation of these lesions. The lesions at risk for pathologic fracture have been defined as demonstrating greater than 50% of cortical involvement and a height of greater than 33 mm. The authors have shown that these guidelines do not predict risk of fracture in 100% of the individuals. Rather, they chose the positive predictive value of 41%. The authors were not able to demonstrate which patients were at a higher risk for fracture. The conclusion I would reach from this study is that lesions exhibiting the size parameters for which prophylactic curettage and fixation have been recommended do have a very significant risk for fractures. This study provides necessary information to assist patients in decision making regarding surgical intervention.

C.P. Beauchamp, M.D.

Pathology of Disappearing Bone Disease: A Case Report With Immuno-histochemical Study
Pazzaglia UE, Andrini L, Bonato M, et al (Università di Pavia, Varese, Italy; Ospedale Multinazionale, Varese, Italy)
Int Orthop 21:303–307, 1997   13–24

Introduction.—In disappearing bone disease, the bone lesions have thin-walled vessels, like capillaries, filled with blood cells in the marrow spaces and in cortical bone. It is unknown how the massive osteolysis and the replacement of bone by vascular connective tissue occurs, particularly since few osteoclasts have been reported in the bone.

Methods.—A case of disappearing bone disease of the proximal femur was described with histopathologic and immunohistochemical studies. In areas of massive bone destruction, there was a densely packed cellular tissue, positive to endothelial antibodies. Where trabecular cancellous or cortical bone was preserved, a more differentiated vascular tissue was present, with only focal zones of accelerated bone remodeling.

Results.—Two phases of evolution with neoplastic-like proliferation of endothelial cells corresponding to the rapid and massive bone destruction correlated with the self-limited course. There was a later differentiation of the cells in mature vascular structures with accelerated bone resorption that was partly compensated by appositional activity. Massive osteolysis was associated with densely packed cellular tissue. There must have been an earlier phase of intense osteoclastic activity, as was evidenced by the moth-eaten appearance of the surface of remnants of cortical bone.

Conclusions.—The angioma-like or lymphangioma-like tissue is related to the extensive bone destruction in disappearing bone disease. In the first phase, the disease might be successfully treated with radiotherapy or cytotoxic drugs, but in the second phase, no effect could be expected.

▶ This interesting paper puts forward a hypothesis that outlines a biphasic process that results in disappearing bone disease. It appears to be a self-limiting disease that runs a particular course and ultimately stabilizes. This may explain why radiation therapy at times may be of benefit to these patients. The underlying triggering mechanism for this disorder remains unknown.

C.P. Beauchamp, M.D.

A System for Surgical Staging and Management of Spine Tumors: A Clinical Outcome Study of Giant Cell Tumors of the Spine

Hart RA, Boriani S, Biagini R, et al (Univ of Iowa, Iowa City; Ospedale Santa Corona, Pietra Ligure, Italy; Istituto Ortopedico Rizzoli, Bologna, Italy; et al)
Spine 22:1773–1783, 1997   13–25

Purpose.—Surgical staging systems for primary bone neoplasms of the limbs have long been in use. Because of the anatomy of the vertebrae and the difficult of surgical resection in the spine, these systems may have to be modified for use with spinal musculoskeletal tumors. The Weinstein-Boriani-Biagini (WBB) system for classification of spinal tumors was developed to enhance uniform collection of data on these rare tumors. The WBB system was used to evaluate potentially important prognostic factors in giant cell tumors of the spine.

Methods.—The analysis was based on independent review of charts and radiographs of 36 patients with giant cell tumors of the spine from 3 institutions. Each tumor was classified using Enneking's classification system for benign musculoskeletal tumors. Preoperative CT scans were available in 24 cases. These cases were classified by the WBB system, which divides the vertebrae into 12 sectors in a clock-face arrangement and defines 5 tissue layers from the superficial paraspinal soft tissues to the interspinous intradural level (Fig 1). Factors significantly associated with tumor recurrence were evaluated.

Results.—The recurrence rate was 83% for patients who underwent an attempt at surgical excision before referral to a tertiary care center, compared with 18% for those initially treated at a referral center. Tumors involving the vertebral body and posterior elements had a recurrence rate of 24%, compared with no recurrences for those involving only the anterior aspect. The recurrence rate was 21% for tumors with extraosseous

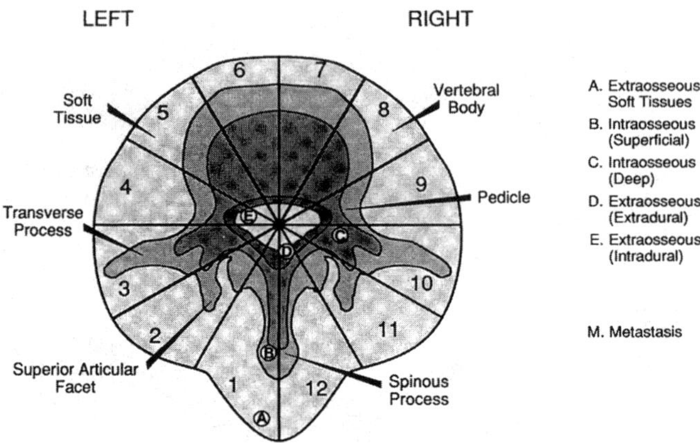

FIGURE 1.—The Weinstein-Boriani-Biagini system used in describing tumor extent for a lumbar vertebra. Vertebrae are divided into 12 sectors in a clock-face arrangement. Five tissue layers are defined, moving from superficial paraspinal soft tissues to interspinous extradural and, finally, to interspinous intradural. (Courtesy of Hart RA, Boriani S, Biagini R, et al: A system for surgical staging and management of spine tumors: A clinical outcome study of giant cell tumors of the spine. *Spine* 22:1773–1783, 1997.)

extension into the spinal canal and paraspinous musculature, compared with 10% for tumors confined to the osseous compartment or extending into the spinal canal or paraspinous planes.

Conclusions.—For patients with rare giant cell tumors of the spine, the WBB classification system may be useful in defining treatment approaches and evaluating outcomes. Enneking's musculoskeletal tumor staging system provides information on the ideal surgical margin and tumor recurrence rate of giant cell tumors. However, the WBB system provides additional information on tumor extent and location, which appears to be relevant to the risk of tumor recurrence. General use of the WBB system would provide for uniform preoperative staging and surgical planning, enhancing the reliability of outcomes evaluation.

▶ The authors have stated that their objective was to seek the correlation between the initial extent of tumor and recurrence for spinal giant cell tumors. Given the rarity of this lesion in the spine, the limitations imposed by the retrospective analysis that it requires, and the uncertainties inherent in any new classification system, I believe that they have achieved their goal. The study takes an important step toward recognition of the unique challenges in surgical management presented by the presence of the spinal cord and nerve roots.

The step has been accomplished by separately considering extraosseous paraspinal extension and extraosseous intracanal extension. In their discussion, the authors combine the intraosseous (superficial) and intraosseous (deep) descriptors. This combination appears reasonable and might be given consideration as a modification to the staging system. There is an "M" descriptor to indicate metastases.

Perhaps additional descriptors, similar to those of the Enneking system, could be given consideration to designate the lesion as benign or malignant, and, if malignant, low or high grade. This system projects 3-dimensional data onto a 2-dimensional grid. This captures all the potential sites of extraosseous extension in a single vertebra, but does not give information concerning the size of the lesion. Perhaps the inclusion of a lesion volume from the CT data would prove a useful addition to the classification system. Much attention is given to the planning and subsequent excision of the biopsy tract in extremity lesions. Perhaps it would be appropriate to emphasize the biopsy in spinal lesions by including a descriptor for the location and nature (open or closed) of the biopsy. In summary, the authors have done an exemplary job in providing a logical format for standardized communication of oncologic information in a difficult anatomical location.

M.J. Yaszemski, M.D.

Chordoma of the Spine Above the Sacrum: Treatment and Outcome in 21 Cases
Boriani S, Chevalley F, Weinstein JN, et al (Università di Bologna, Italy; Centre Hospitalier Vaudois, Lausanne, Switzerland; Univ of Iowa, Iowa City; et al)
Spine 21:1569–1577, 1996   13–26

Objective.—To analyze the relationship of staging, treatment, and outcome in patients with chordoma of the mobile spine.

Background.—Chordoma accounts for 1% to 4% of all malignant bone tumors and is chiefly seen in adults and the elderly. Because of the tumor size at diagnosis and the difficulty of operating around the spine, surgical treatment is often inadequate, and adjuvant radiation therapy is strongly recommended. Metastases occur in up to 5% of cases at onset and are seen in up to 65% of cases at autopsy. Local tumor progression affects survival more often than do metastases. In 63% of cases, death occurs. Five-year survival is 50% and 10-year survival is 28%. The success of treatment largely depends on the size and site of the tumor. CT and MRI have allowed staging systems to be developed.

Methods.—Medical records, radiographs, and images of 21 patients with chordoma of the spine (C1 to L5) were reviewed. Patient age was 38–77, and 17 patients were men. The neurologic status and oncologic results were evaluated by radiography at follow-up.

Results.—Within 137 months of treatment, 10 of the 21 patients died. Four patients have survived with the disease, and 7 patients were symptom-free at final follow up. Conventional radiation therapy did not effectively eradicate the tumor, even when palliative or debulking surgery was also performed. Of 15 patients who had such treatment, 12 had recurrence or progression. Intralesional surgery was equally ineffective in eradicating the tumor. The best results were seen after *en bloc* excision, with or without adjuvant radiation therapy.

Conclusions.—Intralesional incomplete excision and conventional radiation therapy alone or as adjuvant therapy after inadequate surgery are ineffective in treating chordoma of the spine. Even if marginal, *en bloc* resection seemed to be the most effective treatment. Late diagnosis makes treatment difficult.

Clinical Significance.—When possible, *en bloc* excision, or alternatively, a complete excision, is recommended for local control of chordoma of the spine. This treatment cannot be considered definitive because of the slow growth of these tumors and because of the small number of cases reported.

▶ This recent review of 21 cases of chordoma involving the mobile spine reinforces the local aggressiveness and ultimately poor prognosis of this histologic low-grade malignant condition. In an effort to more accurately stage these tumors with possible direction for surgical management, the authors have proposed a somewhat extensive and cumbersome staging system, which is not subsequently validated with locally recurrent or metastatic potential. Although not strictly mentioned, the feasibility of performing wide *en bloc* excision should be predetermined by reconstruction of the MRI and CT, allowing for pre-selection of the patients that could be afforded the only appropriate surgical management of this tumor. Intralesional removal plus adjuvant radiotherapy as recommended by the authors performed to preserve cord or cauda equina function only, needs emphasizing, given the almost universal local recurrence and progression.

M.G. Rock, M.D.

Malignant Bone and Soft Tissue Tumors of the Shoulder Girdle: A Retrospective Analysis of 30 Operated Cases

Meller I, Bickels J, Kollender Y, et al (Tel-Aviv Univ, Israel; Kaplan Hosp, Rehovot, Israel)
Acta Orthop Scand 68:374–380, 1997   13–27

Introduction.—Bone and soft-tissue tumors occur less frequently in the shoulder girdle than in the lower extremity. In the past, amputation was the procedure of choice; limb-sparing surgery now accounts for 85% of operations. A retrospective study of 30 patients with malignant bone and soft-tissue tumors of the shoulder girdle analyzed resection margins, reconstruction techniques, and functional outcome.

Methods.—Patients were 16 men and 14 women with a mean age of 34 years. Twenty-six had primary tumors (21 bone sarcomas and 5 soft tissue sarcomas) and 4 had metastatic lesions. All of those with primary tumors underwent plain radiography of the shoulder girdle and chest, bone scans, CT of the lesion and chest, and MRI of the lesion. The 19 patients with osteosarcoma or Ewing's sarcoma received adjuvant chemotherapy; radiotherapy was administered to those with Ewing's sarcoma, soft tissue sarcoma, and metastatic lesions.

Results.—Five patients underwent major amputation and 25 underwent limb-sparing procedures. Wide resection was performed in 25 patients, radical resection in 4, and marginal resection in 1. Local tumor control was achieved in 28 cases. The 3 amputations were performed because of a lack of response to neoadjuvant therapy or because of invasion of the neurovascular bundle by the tumor. Function was good in 18 patients, moderate in 11, and poor in 1. There was no correlation between reconstruction technique and functional outcome. At the end of follow-up (average, 3 years), 18 patients had no evidence of disease, 2 were alive with disease, and 10 had died (9 because of metastases).

Conclusion.—The rate of postoperative complications was low in this series of patients who underwent surgery for malignant bone and soft-tissue tumors of the shoulder girdle. With properly selected surgical margins, the local recurrence rate was also low (1 patient). The different endoprostheses used did not affect function.

▶ This article adds a great deal to our understanding of the outcome after surgical resection of tumors of the shoulder girdle. The authors were able to assess the oncologic and functional results and compare different techniques of reconstruction by using a standardized classification of the extent of osseous and soft-tissue resection, and the results are compared by means of a uniform functional evaluation system. There are a variety of reconstructive options, and selection of the method of reconstruction of a skeletal defect should be based on the extent of bone and soft-tissue resected and the individual needs of the patient. In our experience, when careful imaging studies of a tumor involving the proximal humerus indicates that an intra-articular resection can be performed with preservation of the axillary nerve and deltoid, function and stability after the reconstruction will be markedly enhanced.[1]

F.G. Sim, M.D.

Reference

1. O'Connor MI, Sim FH, Chao EY: Limb salvage for neoplasms of the shoulder girdle: Intermediate reconstructive and functional results. *J Bone Joint Surg Am* 78:1872–1888, 1996.

Radiology

MR Imaging Based Strategies in Limb Salvage Surgery for Osteosarcoma of the Distal Femur

van Trommel MF, Kroon HM, Bloem JL, et al (Leiden Univ, The Netherlands)
Skeletal Radiol 26:636–641, 1997   13–28

Introduction.—In 32% of patients, osteosarcoma involves the distal femur. Results of limb salvage surgery are equal to those associated with amputation. The method of choice in local staging of most primary malignant musculoskeletal tumors is MRI. No previous studies assessed whether the decisions based on MR observations to perform a specific type of surgical procedure could be made properly. The surgical findings or histopathologic specimens were compared with the preoperative MRI-

TABLE 1.—Involvement of the Nerves at Preoperative MR Imaging Correlated
With the Histopathologic Specimen/Surgical Findings*

| Preoperative | Histopathological specimen/surgical findings | | | |
MR imaging	Not involved	Close	Involved	Total
Not involved	16	0	0	16
Equivocal	8	3	0	11
Involved	0	0	2	2
Total	24	3	2	29

*There were no false negatives. Sensitivity was 100%, specificity 66.7%, positive predictive value 38.5%, and negative predictive value 100%; $P < 0.01$.

(Courtesy of van Trommel MF, Kroon HM, Bloem JL, et al: MR imaging based strategies in limb salvage surgery for osteosarcoma of the distal femur. *Skeletal Radiol* 26:636–641. Copyright 1997, Springer-Verlag.)

based surgical strategy. In determining the surgical procedure in patients
with osteosarcoma, the extent that MR images could be used was evaluated.

Methods.—A total of 34 patients with osteosarcoma were treated in a
7-year period. They had limb salvage surgery or ablative surgery. Low-
grade osteosarcoma was present in 2 patients, and 32 had high-grade
osteosarcoma of the distal femur. The local extent of the tumor as depicted
on MR studies, data from biopsy specimens, age, patient compliance, and
histologic grade were used to plan surgical treatment. All patients were
followed up.

Results.—At subsequent analysis, if no tumor involvement on MRI was
present and this was used as a determining factor, this proved to be correct.
When MR images suggested a close relationship between tumor and nerve,
an oncologically safe plane could be achieved during surgery in 8 of 11
patients (Table 1). A free plane could not be accomplished in 3 patients, as
confirmed at histopathologic examination. Nerve involvement during surgery had to be reassessed and limb salvage surgery reconsidered when
nerve involvement was equivocal on MRI. An oncologically safe plane was
achieved in 6 of 13 patients when vascular involvement was the decisive
factor and tumor involvement was equivocal (Table 2). Except for 1

TABLE 2.—Vascular Involvement at Preoperative MR Imaging Correlated with
Histopathologic Specimen/Surgical Findings

| Preoperative | Histopathological specimen/surgical findings | | | | |
MR imaging	Unknown	Not involved	Close	Involved	Total
Not involved	0	11	0	0	11
Equivocal	2*	6	5	0	13
Involved	0	1	0	3	4
No diagnosis	0	1	0	0	1
Total	2	18	5	3	29

Note: Sensitivity was 100%, specificity 61.1%, positive predictive value 53.3%, and negative predictive value 100%; $P = 0.01$.

*Specimen/MR images not suitable for this question

(Courtesy of van Trommel MF, Kroon HM, Bloem JL, et al: MR imaging based strategies in limb salvage surgery for osteosarcoma of the distal femur. *Skeletal Radiol* 26:636–641. Copyright 1997, Springer-Verlag.)

TABLE 3.—Involvement of the Joint at Preoperative MR Imaging Correlated With Histopathologic Specimen/Surgical Findings

Preoperative MR imaging	Histopathological specimen/surgical findings			Total
	Not involved	Close	Involved	
Not involved	7	0	0	7
Equivocal	2	0	1	3
Involved	1	0	18	19
Total	10	0	19	29

Note: Sensitivity was 100%, specificity 70%, positive predictive value 86.4%, and negative predictive value 100%; $P = 0.25$, not significant.

(Courtesy of van Trommel MF, Kroon HM, Bloem JL, et al: MR imaging based strategies in limb salvage surgery for osteosarcoma of the distal femur. *Skeletal Radiol* 26:636–641. Copyright 1997, Springer-Verlag.)

patient who was assumed to have vascular involvement but was proved to be free, when comprehensive tumor involvement of any structure was noted preoperatively, it proved to be correct at histopathologic examination. In depicting the relationship between tumor and knee joint, MRI is accurate (Table 3).

Conclusions.—Two partially conflicting prerequisites are necessary for successful surgical removal of a primary malignant bone tumor: a surrounding rim of normal tissue must accompany removal of all primary tumor, and sufficient normal tissue must remain to allow as much preservation of limb function as possible. Local staging is vital to find the right balance. In a majority of cases, an oncologically safe plane could be achieved during surgery when MR images suggested a close relationship between tumor and nerve. When nerve involvement was equivocal on MRI, it was valuable to reassess nerve involvement during surgery. The exact borders of tumors were obscured by reactive edema, leading to overestimation. As a decisive argument in planning a surgical procedure, extensive tumor involvement of any structure, as shown by MRI, could be used correctly.

▶ There is no doubt that MRI has provided a tremendous advance in the treatment of patients with osteosarcoma of the distal femur. It certainly is extremely helpful when critical structures are clearly not involved. We have all experienced difficulties in decision making when such studies suggest neurovascular involvement or intra-articular involvement. We have come to the realization that in some instances MRI scans overstate the problem. There still exist situations where intraoperative findings dictate the ultimate surgical procedure. This aspect of orthopedic oncology, involving an "exploration," is unattractive to us because we would like to be able to accurately plan surgical intervention preoperatively.

In this study, when the MR scan indicated a close relationship between the tumor and the nerve, a safe margin could be achieved in the majority of cases (positive predicted value, 38.5%). In 25% of patients whose MRI scans suggested equivocal involvement, the joint was truly involved, thus, making decisions regarding intra-articular involvement in critical situations difficult. (This remains a problem.)

For problematic lesions, it is sometimes helpful to repeat the staging studies with the knee in 35% flexion. Patients in this study are examined supine with the knee in full extension. This draws the neurovascular structures up close against the lesion. With scans performed with the knee in flexion, the neurovascular structures can sometimes be demonstrated to fall away from the lesion with a clear plane of tissue.

C.P. Beauchamp, M.D.

Synovial Sarcoma: Frequency of Nonaggressive MR Characteristics
Blacksin MF, Siegel JR, Benevenia J, et al (Univ of Medicine and Dentistry of New Jersey, Newark)
J Comput Assist Tomogr 21:785–789, 1997   13–29

Objective.—About 10% of all soft tissue sarcomas are synovial sarcomas. These tumors must be resected with wide margins, and careful surgical planning is needed to avoid amputation. The outcome is better for younger patients, for patients with tumors smaller than 5 cm, and for patients with tumors located in the distal extremity. In the authors' experience, many synovial sarcomas are initially interpreted as being nonaggressive or probably benign soft tissue masses. The MRI characteristics of synovial sarcomas were analyzed, including the frequency of a nonaggressive imaging appearance.

Methods.—The retrospective study included 15 patients with histologically confirmed synovial sarcoma who had undergone previous MRI evaluation. The MRI scans were assessed by an experienced musculoskeletal radiologist, who considered the type of margin, internal architecture, presence of cortical or medullary invasion, T1-weighted and T2-weighted signal characteristics, and homogeneity.

Results.—One third of the lesions, average size 4.8 cm, had MRI characteristics of benign lesions. They were well-circumscribed, homogeneous lesions that were isointense or greater in signal intensity than muscle on T1-weighted images. On T2-weighted images, they were of signal intensity equal to or greater than fat. Four synovial sarcomas showed inhomogeneous enhancement on contrast administration, whereas a ganglion or synovial cyst would be expected to be left unenhanced. The remaining 10 synovial sarcomas had mildly inhomogeneous to complex signal characteristics, with a mean size of 11 cm.

Conclusions.—About one third of synovial sarcomas may have a benign appearance on MRI. These are small lesions with well-circumscribed margins and homogeneous signal intensity. If they are mistaken for benign lesions, they may be subject to inappropriate surgical interventions, such as excisional biopsy via transverse incision, thus complicating future surgery. Other synovial sarcomas appeared larger and of more heterogeneous signal intensity.

▶ This is an important article for radiologists as well as orthopedic surgeons. It emphasizes the rather innocuous and benign appearance that high-grade sarcomas can display. Some radiologists believe and have published reports that the magnetic scan can differentiate between benign and malignant neoplasms. For those patients with indeterminate or somewhat suspicious lesions, the use of contrast material is mandatory. It is extremely important for the orthopedic surgeon to be aware of this need. It is also important to remember that malignant lesions can look "benign."

C.P. Beauchamp, M.D.

MR Imaging of Soft Tissues Adjacent to Orthopaedic Hardware: Techniques to Minimize Susceptibility Artefact

Eustace S, Goldberg R, Williamson D, et al (Boston Med Ctr)
Clin Radiol 52:589–594, 1997   13–30

Introduction.—Although MRI is used routinely for the preoperative assessment of orthopedic disorders, the metal screws and plates used in fixation become magnetized when placed within a superconducting magnet, reducing the utility of postoperative images. A number of simple techniques can minimize magnetic susceptibility artefact and allow visualization of adjacent soft tissues.

Definition.—Contributing to susceptibility artefact are induced magnetism in the ferromagnetic component itself and induced magnetism in protons adjacent to the component. The first results in a fixed field distortion, and the second results in an expanding field, gradual diffusions of protons into adjacent soft tissues, and dephasing of spins adjacent to the metal component.

The Orthopedic Component and Susceptibility Artefact.—Compared with both cobalt chrome and steel, titanium alloys are less ferromagnetic, induce less susceptibility artefact, and result in less marked image degradation (Fig 1). In each of these metals, induced magnetism is greater when placed in higher field strength systems. This results in associated greater field distortion or susceptibility artefact. Before an orthopedic component is imaged, it is crucial to select planes in which slice select gradients will have the least distortion. Imaging with frequency gradients in 1 direction, then re-imaging with frequency gradients in the opposite perpendicular axis may yield optimal results. Manipulation of matrix size does not appear to significantly decrease observed artefact.

Early acquisition of induced signal and manipulation of excitatory pulse sequences used to generate signal may limit susceptibility blooming secondary to proton diffusion and dephasing spins. Images acquired with gradient-echo sequences are more markedly degraded by metal-induced susceptibility. Two features of the fast spin-echo sequence—the echo train length and the echo spacing—may be modified to reduce artefact.

Conclusion.—Susceptibility artefact in tissues adjacent to orthopedic hardware may be reduced in a number of ways. Improved imaging is

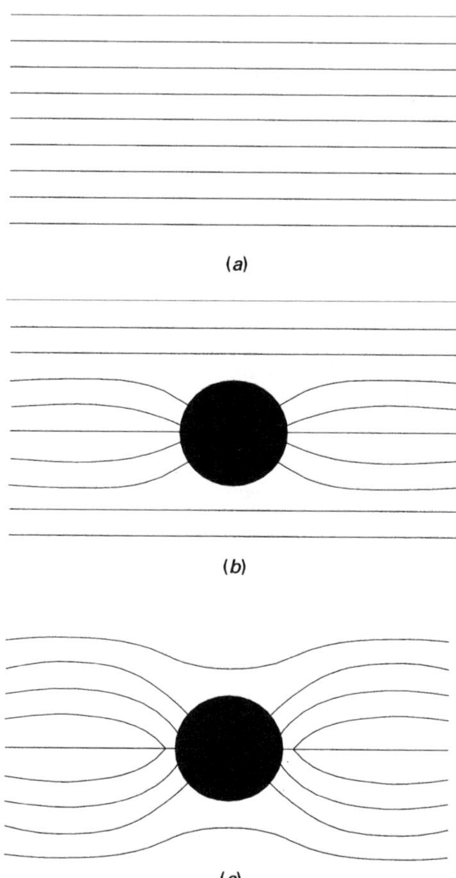

FIGURE 1.—Diagrammatic representations of (**A**) homogeneous (uniform) magnetic field, (**B**) field distortion secondary to the presence of titanium, and (**C**) marked field distortion secondary to steel. (Courtesy of Eustace S, Goldberg R, Williamson D, et al: MR imaging of soft tissues adjacent to orthopedic hardware: Techniques to minimize susceptibility artefact. *Clin Radiol* 52:589–594, 1997.)

achieved by use of a low–field-strength system, selection of an imaging plane to minimize the amount of metal in sections, selection of frequency encoding gradient to orientate axis of susceptibility artefact, and manipulation of fast spin-echo sequences.

▶ The authors outline a number of techniques and procedures that are effective in reducing susceptibility artefact in tissues adjacent to orthopedic hardware. This has significant implications for those who manage neoplastic disorders. Although we have very effective methods of reconstructing skeletal defects, it is quite difficult to follow patients for local recurrences or to evaluate patients seen with suspicious masses after resection of these lesions. It is extremely important that MR radiologists understand that there are techniques available for optimizing susceptibility blooming.

C.P. Beauchamp, M.D.

Osteogenic Sarcoma: Noninvasive In Vivo Assessment of Tumor Necrosis With Diffusion-weighted MR Imaging

Lang P, Wendland MF, Saeed M, et al (Stanford Univ, Calif; Univ of California, San Francisco)

Radiology 206:227–235, 1998   13–31

Objective.—Conventional MRI is limited in providing information about the response of osteogenic sarcoma to treatment. Some contrasting agents can diffuse into necrotic tissue obscuring tissue necrosis, and other agents that may be more accurate are expensive. Diffusion-weighted MRI can detect necrosis through increased membrane permeability and cellular breakdown. The differences in molecular diffusion between viable and necrotic tumor were explored using diffusion-weighted MRI in the rat.

Methods.—Cells from the rat osteogenic sarcoma cell line UMR 104 were implanted into the left hind legs of 12 skeletally immature, homozygous, nude, athymic rats. Magnetic resonance imaging was performed on a 2.0-T small-bore magnet. All imaging sequences were performed by using 4 signals acquired. T1-weighted spin-echo images with a thickness of 3 mm in the axial plane were acquired with a repetition time of 400 msec and an echo time of 12 msec. T2-weighted spin-echo images were acquired with 2500/40 and 80. Diffusion-weighted spin-echo images were acquired with 2500/80 with a diffusion-sensitizing gradient pulse of 20 msec. Gadopentetate dimeglumine (0.1 mmol/kg) was then administered IV and T1-weighted sequences were repeated. The tumors were examined histologically and compared with MR images.

Results.—Whereas viable tumor tissue showed high signal intensities on diffusion-weighted images, necrotic tumor with and without hemorrhage showed low signal intensities. The differences were significant. Viable tumor and necrotic tumor with and without hemorrhage showed increased signal intensity on contrast-enhanced T1-weighted images. There was some signal intensity overlap between edematous connective tissue and necrotic tumor with and without hemorrhage on diffusion-weighted images. Edematous connective tissue was located at the periphery of the lesion, whereas necrotic tumor was normally found in the center of the lesion.

Conclusion.—Diffusion-weighted MRI is a noninvasive way to differentiate between viable and necrotic tumor tissue and can be used to monitor the effects of chemotherapy.

▶ Assessment of the response to preoperative radiation therapy is extremely important. This, largely, has a predictive value for prognosis. It is well accepted that patients having 90% or greater necrosis at the time of definitive resection have a significantly better prognosis. We use a variety of parameters before surgery to determine whether a patient is a good "responder". These include radiographic evolution of the lesion, diminution of symptoms, and decreasing size.

It is becoming even more important to have this knowledge before surgery as the actual surgical procedure might be altered depending on the chemotherapeutic response. Patients who have an excellent response preoperatively may require less surgery with closer margins. Diffusion-weighted MRI has the advantage that it can provide a quantitative measure of actual tumor necrosis. Further study needs to be done on humans with osteosarcomas, and correlation with histologic material is needed.

C.P. Beauchamp, M.D.

Usefulness of Radiography in Differentiating Enchondroma From Central Grade I Chondrosarcoma

Geirnaerdt MJA, Hermans J, Bloem JL, et al (Leiden Univ, The Netherlands; Bowman Gray School of Medicine, Winston-Salem, NC)
AJR 169:1097–1104, 1997   13–32

Introduction.—In large series of primary bone tumors, central (medullary) grade 1 chondrosarcomas and enchondromas comprise up to 17% of tumors. Because enchondromas are clinically silent, many may be underreported. The usefulness of radiographic criteria used to differentiate enchondromas from grade 1 chondrosarcomas is doubtful. Surgical resection is the only curative treatment for chondrosarcoma. The risk for local recurrence and metastases is increased with intralesional treatment of grade 1 chondrosarcoma. It is difficult to differentiate between enchondromas and central grade 1 chondrosarcoma. The interobserver variability in assessing radiographic criteria of well-differentiated cartilaginous tumors was determined, as well as whether selected radiographic criteria can be used to discriminate central grade 1 chondrosarcomas from enchondromas.

Methods.—In 35 enchondromas and 43 central grade 1 chondrosarcomas, clinical symptoms, location, and size were evaluated. Three observers independently assessed radiographic features. Features with discriminating strength were identified with the chi-square test and linear discriminant analysis. To validate the consistency of observations among observers, Kappa values were calculated. The standard was a consensus diagnosis made by histologic findings and long-term follow-up.

Results.—Clinical symptoms and the benign or malignant nature of the neoplasms showed no statistically significant correlation. The axial skeleton and flat bones were most likely to be the locations of grade 1 chondrosarcomas. Enchondromas were significantly smaller than chondrosarcomas. Significant discrimination was found only with ill-defined margins and lobulated contours. There was still a 10% to 90% probability of malignancy with an optimal combination of 4 radiographic features in 72 of the 78 lesions, indicating poor discriminating power. Poor-to-fair agreement was found with Kappa values.

Conclusions.—The most reliable predictors of central grade 1 chondrosarcoma were location in the axial skeleton and size greater than 5 cm. The ability to differentiate between enchondromas and central grade 1 chondrosarcomas are not improved with morphologic features seen on radiographs and clinical symptoms. For enchondroma, intralesional treatment or an expectative approach is justified. Adequate en bloc resection is the curative treatment of grade 1 chondrosarcoma.

▶ The authors very nicely demonstrate the tremendous clinical and radiographic difficulty we have in sorting out patients who have low-grade malignant chondrosarcomas or benign enchondromas. Indeed, the pathologic diagnosis of a borderline lesion also underscores the diagnostic difficulties these patients present. Observation in this group of patients, I believe, is an important tool to assist in the decision-making process. The difficult patient, however, is the patient that has a painful lesion. A recent study presented at the 1998 Academy Meeting by Yaskow et al.[1] notes favorable results with intralesional curettage of low-grade chondrosarcomas. Of 40 patients, only 3 had a local recurrence and none developed distant metastases. This approach has some attractive advantages and needs to be evaluated further.

C.P. Beauchamp, M.D.

Reference

1. Yaskow A, et al: Low grade chondrosarcoma of the long bones: Leg results of curettage versus wide excision. Presented at the American Academy of Orthopaedic Surgeons 65th Annual Meeting, New Orleans, La. Paper No. 154.

Reconstruction

Effects of Ionizing Radiation on the Mechanical Properties of Human Bone
Currey JD, Foreman J, Laketić I, et al (Univ of York, England; East Anglian Tissue Bank, Cambridge, England)
J Orthop Res 15:111–117, 1997   13–33

Introduction.—Preventing transmission of infection is the primary concern in the preparation of allogeneic bone tissue for grafting. Any treatment of bone must be effective in preventing transmission of bacteria and virus infections and still retain the mechanical properties necessary for graft function. Ionizing radiation is effective in sterilizing human bone, but it is not known whether this process affects the mechanical properties of bone. Effective doses of radiation for sterilizing medical equipment, poliovirus, and HIV are 25, 48, and 60 kGy, respectively. Literature on the effects of large dose radiation on the mechanical properties of bone is limited and conflicting. The effects of ionizing radiation on quasistatic and impact mechanical properties of human bone were assessed.

TABLE 1.—Data Concerning the Donors and the Levels of Radiation to Which the Femora Were Exposed

	Donor 1	Donor 2	Donor 3	Donor 4
Age (yrs)	21	21	29	49
Sex	Female	Female	Female	Male
Cause of death	Head injury	Primary brain tumour	Amniotic fluid embolus	Drowning
Right femur: proximal	17 kGy (6)	Control (6)	94.7 kGy (10)	Control (9)
Left femur: proximal	Control (6)	17 kGy (6)	Control (10)	94.7 kGy (9)
Right femur: distal	Control (6)	17 kGy (6)	Control (11)	29.5 kGy (9)
Left femur: distal	17 kGy (6)	Control (6)	29.5 kGy (11)	Control (9)

Note: The numbers in parentheses are the number of specimens machined from each segment.

(Courtesy of Currey JD, Foreman J, Laketić I, et al: Effects of ionizing radiation on the mechanical properties of human bone. *J Orthop Res* 15:111–117, 1997.)

Methods.—Cadaver bone specimens from 4 paired femora of 4 donors underwent doses of 29.5 kGy (the standard commonly used by tissue banks), 94.7 kGy (high dose), or 17 kGy (low dose) ionizing radiation (Table 1). Mechanical tests performed on radiated bone specimens were Young's modulus, bending strength, work to fracture, and impact energy.

Results.—The impact of radiation on mechanical properties is shown in Table 2. Young's modulus was not changed by any level of radiation, but bending strength, work to fracture, and impact energy absorption were significantly decreased, with the severity of effect increasing with increasing radiation doses. Work to fracture was particularly diminished. Bone specimens irradiated with high doses absorbed only 5% of energy, compared to control specimens. On laser scanning confocal microscopy, control specimens had very extensive microcracking. Microcracking is associated with toughness, whereas little or no microcracking is associated with brittle behavior. Specimens that received 29.5 kGy had much less microcracking than controls. Specimens that received 94.7 kGy had hardly any microcracking.

Conclusion.—Young's modulus was not affected by any of the 3 levels of ionizing radiation, but the highest dose had severe effects on fracture properties. It is not possible to apply an effective viricidal dose of gamma irradiation without severely compromising the bone mechanically.

▶ Bacterial sterilization of bone with radiation is effective. Procurement of bone is often obtained under less than perfect conditions. The risk of bacterial contamination can be significant and procedures to ensure the grafts are not contaminated are rigorous and expensive. The security that radiation affords after procurement is indeed attractive. The main concerns for tissue banks are bacteria and viruses, the latter requiring significantly high doses of radiation therapy to effect sterility. The authors have demonstrated that with high levels of radiation therapy, those necessary to effect viral sterility, greatly affects the mechanical properties of bone. I believe their conclusions are certainly justified by the results of their study, although the numbers are small.

TABLE 2.—Mechanical Results

Property	Donor	N	Controls Mean	SD	Irradiated Mean	SD	Level	%	P	Lumped P
Young's modulus (GPa)	1	5	14.4	1.2	14.7	0.8	L	103	NS	
	2	6	9.1	0.7	9.5	1.0	L	104	NS	NS
	3	5	13.0	0.2	12.3	0.3	S	94	*	
	4	5	11.4	2.2	12.8	1.6	S	112	NS	NS
	3	4	12.4	1.3	12.6	0.7	H	102	NS	
	4	5	13.6	2.1	12.7	1.2	H	93	NS	NS
	3	*5*	*12.4*	*1.1*	*12.2*	*1.2*	*H*	*98*	*NS*	
Bending strength (MPa)	1	5	170	14	151	9	L	89	*	
	2	6	142	5	125	5	L	88	†	‡
	3	5	147	6	111	12	S	75	†	
	4	5	147	22	120	10	S	82	*	‡
	3	4	148	14	54	5	H	37	†	
	4	5	162	25	53	3	H	33	‡	‡
	3	*5*	*145*	*14*	*68*	*31*	*H*	*48*	*†*	
Work to fracture (J/m²)	1	5	9,570	2,990	4,880	1,340	L	51	*	
	2	6	9,520	3,180	5,600	1,860	L	59	*	‡
	3	5	7,130	1,640	2,690	610	S	38	†	
	4	5	12,600	3,320	2,980	310	S	24	†	§
	3	4	7,210	1,720	460	50	H	6.4	†	
	4	5	12,140	4,630	430	30	H	3.5	†	‡
	3	*5*	*6,750*	*1,810*	*1,750*	*2,880*	*H*	*26*	*NS*	
Impact energy (J/m²)	1	7	14,950	7,560	1,320	5,040	L	87	NS	
	2	6	26,460	8,650	14,780	4,120	L	56	†	*
	3	6	9,900	2,280	6,950	1,290	S	70	*	
	4	4	15,050	6,230	9,410	1,930	S	63	NS	*
	3	5	8,200	2,740	3,580	1,250	H	44	*	
	4	4	17,960	5,970	4,400	1,330	H	25	*	†

Note: The mean values of the various control and experimental specimens for each pair of bones are given. The statistical analysis, however, used paired *t* tests to compare the differences between homologous specimens from left and right femora. A standard *t* test was used to compare the sets of differences between irradiated and unirradiated specimens from different donors receiving the same amount of radiation. If the sets of differences were not themselves significantly different, they were lumped to increase the power of the paired comparison *t* test. *Lumped P* indicates probability resulting from such a paired comparison *t* test. Rows in italics in this table refer to the high-irradiation experiment in which values from the anomalous specimen and its pair have been retained.

*P < 0.05.
†P < 0.01.
‡P < 0.001.
§The comparison combining the values from the two donors could not be used here because the sets of differences were themselves shown to be different.

Abbreviations: N, number of pairs of specimens; *Level*, level of radiation on the experimental bones; *L*, low; *S*, standard; *H*, high; %, the mean value of the irradiated specimens expressed as a percentage of the mean value of the controls; P, probability resulting from a paired comparison *t* test on the differences between the paired specimens; *NS*, not significant.
(Courtesy of Currey JD, Foreman J, Laketic I, et al: Effects of ionizing radiation on the mechanical properties of human bone. *J Orthop Res* 15:111–117, 1997.)

Radiation osteitis (pathologic changes in bone that are seen with therapeutic levels of radiation therapy) has fairly characteristic histologic features. The bone, which is often necrotic, histologically demonstrates delamination of the lamellar bone. These splits and cracks in the bone that are observed histologically translate into altered mechanical properties. It is, therefore, extremely important for orthopedists using bone from tissue banks to be aware of the methods of harvesting, quality control, and how the bone is sterilized.

C.P. Beauchamp, M.D.

The Vertically Based Deep Fascia Turnover Flap of the Leg: Anatomic Studies and Clinical Applications

Worseg AP, Kuzbari R, Alt A, et al (Wilhelminenhospital, Vienna; Ludwig-Boltzmann-Inst for Endoscopic Plastic Surgery, Vienna; Univ of Vienna)
Plast Reconstr Surg 100:1746–1761, 1997   13–34

Background.—Fasciocutaneous turnover flaps are technically straightforward and quickly raised, but they are underused for covering smaller and medium-sized defects of the lower leg. Reconstructive surgeons are concerned about the lack of criteria for flap design and the risk of donor site problems. After anatomic studies were performed to evaluate the pattern of vessels supplying the deep fascia, a vertically based paratibial or parafibular deep fascia turnover flap was applied in 6 patients.

Methods.—Anatomical studies used 36 lower limbs amputated from 18 fresh female and male cadavers 12 to 48 hours after death. The deep fascia was dissected and mobilized medially from a longitudinal incision in the posterior midline to where it became contiguous with the deep transverse fascial septum and reflected over the tibial border. Fascial dissection was carried laterally to the point at which the fascia fused with the posterior peroneal intermuscular septum. Once the septum was cut, dissection continued to the anterior peroneal intermuscular septum. The fascia was then reflected laterally, together with the superficial peroneal nerve. The anterior peroneal intermuscular septum was then transected and the fascia mobilized to the lateral tibial border.

Results.—Findings in 33 evaluable limbs confirmed that the subfascial and epifascial vascular networks worked well, indicating adequate patency of the vasculature. A mean of 79.2 vessels supplied the fascia, with musculofascial, septofascial, and periosteofascial branches contributing to a richly anastomosing vascular network. The fascia is supplied by segmental vessels in a clearly defined pattern. Six patients with soft-tissue defects of the leg underwent surgery to cover defects with the vertically based deep fascia turnover flap. All had exposed bone but no signs of osteomyelitis or severe local soft-tissue infection. Surgery was successful in 5 cases; the remaining patient lost the graft to partial flap necrosis, but healing was achieved after regrafting with meshed split-thickness skin.

Conclusion.—Anatomical studies and clinical experience support the use of vertically based turnover flaps obtained from deep fascia of the leg. Even in patients with sizable flaps or an extremely thin skin, adequate perfusion is achieved because the transversely oriented deep turnover flap keeps its subcutaneous layer with its intact vascular plexus.

▶ Although the clinical numbers are small in this paper, the authors have made a fine presentation of the vascular anatomy of the deep fascia of the lower extremity. We are, thus, offered another option in the always difficult region of the lower extremity in terms of soft-tissue coverage. This may have a wider use in defects created for soft-tissue and bone tumors rather than in traumatic situations. This study is worth reviewing for those involved in difficult lower extremity soft-tissue problems.

C.P. Beauchamp, M.D.

Allograft Reconstruction of the Acetabulum After Resection of Stage-IIB Sarcoma: Intermediate-term Results
Bell RS, Davis AM, Wunder JS, et al (Mount Sinai Hosp, Toronto; Univ of Toronto)
J Bone Joint Surg Am 79-A:1663–1674, 1997   13–35

Introduction.—Hindquarter amputation, the alternative to limb-salvage resection of a periacetabular tumor, is cosmetically and functionally unacceptable if a safe alternative is available. Seventeen consecutive patients underwent allograft reconstruction after resection of a stage-IIB sarcoma of the periacetabular region.

Methods.—Patients ranged in age from 16 to 64 years at diagnosis. Initial diagnoses were chondrosarcoma in 9 cases, osteosarcoma in 6, Ewing's sarcoma in 1, and leiomyosarcoma in 1. Preoperative and postoperative chemotherapy was administered to all patients with osteosarcoma or Ewing's sarcoma; no patient had radiation treatment. Tumors were resected through either an ilioinguinal or an iliofemoral approach. The former approach was used when the proximal part of the femur was to be removed en bloc with the pelvis, and the latter when only the pelvis was to be resected. After evaluation of the margins, the osseous defect was reconstructed using irradiated allograft bone. Fifteen patients were managed with an allograft–total hip prosthesis composite. Cancellous-bone screws were inserted through the allograft into the bodies of the first and second sacral vertebrae when the resection had to be performed through the sacral ala or the sacro-iliac joint (Fig 2). Interfragmentary compression screws were inserted through an acetabular roof ring when the size of the allograft acetabulum allowed this device to be used. When a femoral allograft was used, the component was cemented into the graft before implantation; this composite was then press-fit (Fig 4) into the host femoral canal.

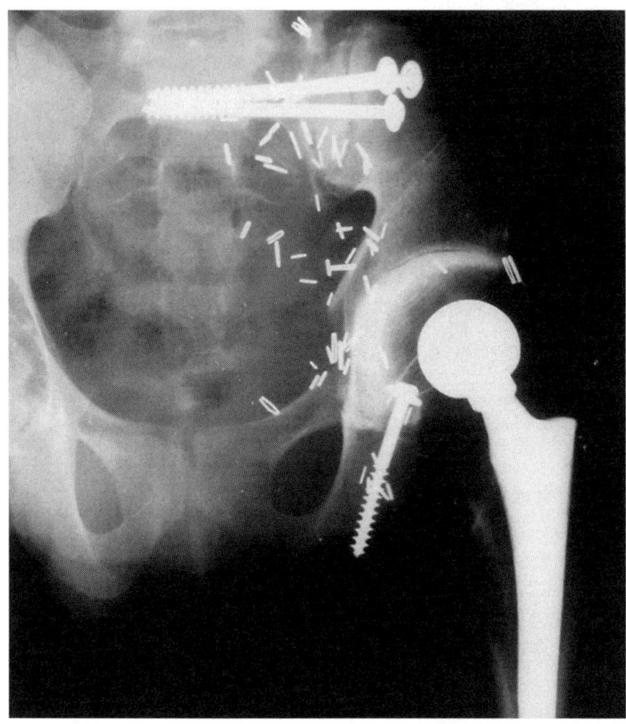

FIGURE 2.—Radiograph made 18 months postoperatively, showing fixation of the allograft to the sacral ala. In most patients, standard bone-ingrowth femoral prostheses were used to complete the total hip reconstruction. (Courtesy of Bell RS, Davis AM, Wunder JS, et al: Allograft reconstruction of the acetabulum after reconstruction of stage-IIB sarcoma: Intermediate-term results. *J Bone Joint Surg Am* 79-A:1663–1674, 1997.)

Results.—All 17 patients had a high-grade (stage-IIB) bone sarcoma extending into the periacetabular soft tissues. None had evidence of metastatic disease. Margins of resection were negative in 15 patients and positive in 2; both of the latter subsequently underwent hindquarter resection. Four patients died at 5, 8, and 24 months after operation. All had an intact reconstruction at the time of death. Causes of death were metastatic disease in 3 and complications of chemotherapy in 1. Two patients who experienced problems with wound healing in the early postoperative period had to have the graft removed. The status of the abductor muscles after resection and reconstruction appeared to be the most important factor in functional outcome.

Conclusion.—Carefully selected patients with a bone sarcoma involving the acetabulum may have the limb preserved with allograft reconstruction, but the risk of local recurrence or infection is high. Within 5 years of the index operation, 9 of the 17 patients in this series had died, had an amputation, or required removal of the graft.

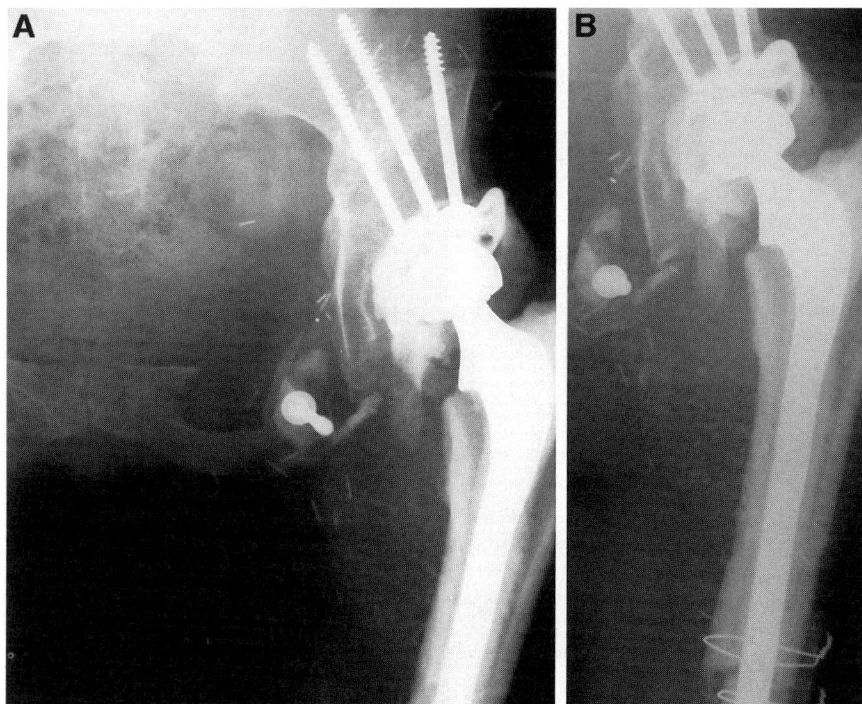

FIGURE 4.—Radiographs made 6 years after reconstruction of the pelvis and femur with an allograft-implant composite, performed after resection of an acetabular osteosarcoma that extended to the femur. **A,** insertion of interfragmentary screws through a roof reconstruction ring is the preferred method of reconstruction after resection through the ilium. Neutralization plates are generally avoided, when possible, to limit the number of holes in the allograft. **B,** the femur was reconstructed with a long-stem prosthesis that was cemented into the allograft and press-fit into the distal host femoral canal. (Courtesy of Bell RS, Davis AM, Wunder JS, et al: Allograft reconstruction of the acetabulum after reconstruction of stage-IIB sarcoma: Intermediate-term results. *J Bone Joint Surg Am* 79-A:1663–1674, 1997.)

Prognostic Factors for Patients With Sarcomas of the Pelvic Bones

Kawai A, Healey JH, Boland PJ, et al (Mem Sloan-Kettering Cancer Ctr, New York)

Cancer 82:851–859, 1998   13–36

Purpose.—The treatment of malignant tumors of the pelvis poses very difficult problems. It can be difficult to achieve excision with wide surgical margins, and local and systemic failures are common. These tumors are rare, so there are few data on the factors affecting patient outcome. Variables affecting local and systemic control of pelvic sarcomas were analyzed.

Patients.—A total of 102 patients undergoing surgical excision of localized pelvic sarcomas were studied. Sixty-five patients had tumors located in the ilium, 21 in the pubis, 8 in the ischium, and 8 in the sacrum. Chondrosarcoma was diagnosed in 49 patients, osteosarcoma in 26, Ewing's sarcoma in 20, malignant fibrous histiocytoma in 3, fibrosarcoma in 2, and unclassified sarcoma in 2 patients. Sixteen patients had secondary chondrosarcomas developing in preexisting cartilaginous lesions, whereas 8 had radiation-induced sarcomas. Mean tumor size, measured in the largest dimension in the surgical specimen, was 12 cm. As classified by the Musculoskeletal Tumor Society Classification, there were 18 stage IB and 84 stage IIB tumors.

Treatment and Outcomes.—Limb-sparing surgery was performed in 81% of patients, and hemipelvectomy was performed in 19%. Of the patients undergoing limb-sparing surgery, 58 had pelvic resection with disruption of the pelvic ring. Patients whose tumors were 20 cm or larger or who had symptoms related to tumor encroachment of the sciatic nerve and/or visceral organs were less likely to have limb-sparing surgery. Surgery achieved a wide margin in 54% of patients, a marginal margin in 20%, and an intralesional margin in 26%, with no significant difference for patients undergoing limb-sparing surgery vs. hemipelvectomy. A wide margin was achieved in only 15% of patients with tumors involving the sacrum.

Thirty-four percent of patients had local recurrences at a median of 7 months. On multivariate analysis, the only independent prognostic factor for local recurrence was the surgical margin. At 5 years, local recurrence-free survival was 82% for patients with a wide margin, 60% for those with a marginal margin, and 27% for those with a lesional margin. The local recurrence rate was higher for patients undergoing curettage and cryosurgery vs. en bloc excision. At last follow-up, 46% of patients were alive and free of disease. Overall survival was 88% at 1 year and 55% at 5 years. Five-year survival was 65% for patients with chondrosarcoma, 47% for those with osteosarcoma, 52% for those with Ewing's sarcoma, and 29% for those with other sarcoma. On multivariate analysis, significant prognostic factors for survival were type of surgery and surgical margin. Survival was 4 times lower for patients undergoing hemipelvectomy vs. limb-sparing surgery, and 3 times lower for those undergoing intralesional tumor excision vs. wide surgical excision.

Conclusions.—The only factor independently related to an increased risk of local recurrence of pelvic sarcoma is an inadequate surgical margin. Surgical stage is an independent prognostic factor for distant metastasis. Survival is lower for patients undergoing hemipelvectomy and those with an inadequate surgical margin.

▶ The article by Bell et al. (Abstract 13–35) is a study of a relatively large group of patients with extremely difficult tumors managed by a highly skilled orthopedic oncology team. The authors have critically reviewed their experience over a 12-year period. They have reported, as expected, a high complication rate for this very challenging problem. A number of important points can be emphasized. First, complications in this group of patients should be expected. The magnitude of the surgery, the significant loss of bone and soft tissue, the significant postoperative risk, wound complications, instability, and neurologic injury make a complication an expectation.

Other very experienced surgeons who are well skilled in this surgical procedure report similar complication rates.

Second, the local recurrence rate for this procedure is quite high. The authors have identified 2 difficult areas in which surgical margins are, indeed, troublesome. These areas remain difficult even if an ablated procedure is performed. There does not seem to be an advantage to amputation over limb-sparing procedures regarding the issue of local control. Although the authors believe that a local relapse rate of 17% is high, it is unlikely that this can be significantly improved upon.

Third, the paper has confirmed previous observations that in the absence of significant complication, patients actually do function quite well, considering the magnitude of resection. Finally, the authors noted only 1 nonunion in the entire series. One patient had a fracture that healed rapidly, confirming a good predictable union rate for this type of reconstruction. This is particularly important in that all of the graft had been treated with 25,000 Gy.

Kawai et al. (Abstract 13–36) note improved survival in patients undergoing limb-sparing procedures. These patients are more likely to have a more favorable lesion. Patients undergoing hemipelvectomy have more extensive disease. The authors report the importance of surgical margins on local recurrence.

C.P. Beauchamp, M.D.

Reconstruction of the Hemipelvis After the Excision of Malignant Tumours: Complications and Functional Outcome of Prostheses

Abudu A, Grimer RJ, Cannon SR, et al (Royal Orthopaedic Hosp, Birmingham, England; Royal Natl Orthopaedic Hosp, Stanmore, England)
J Bone Joint Surg Br 79-B:773–779, 1997   13–37

Objective.—Excision of malignant periacetabular tumors with limb salvage requires anatomical reconstruction. Results of an evaluation of mechanical reconstruction of the defect with custom-made prosthetic implants, the surgical and technical complications, and the functional outcome after excision of malignant periacetabular tumors were presented.

Methods.—Between 1971 and 1994, 35 patients (15 males), age 13–66, underwent reconstruction of the hemipelvis. Patients were followed for an average of 49 months. Function was assessed using the Musculoskeletal Tumor Society system.

> *Technique.*—An Ollier and an ilioinguinoperineal approach were used. The ilium was divided and the tumor removed. In a 1-stage ($n = 18$) or 2-stage ($n = 17$) procedure, the custom-made endoprosthesis with a 32 mm-head was cemented to the ilium, and a total hip replacement was performed. After bed rest for 2 weeks, the patients were allowed partial weight-bearing, and at 6 weeks, they began intensive physiotherapy.

Results.—At an average follow-up of 84 months, 15 patients (43%) were alive and disease free. Six were alive with metastatic disease at an average of 26 months. Twelve (34%) had died of their disease, and 2 (6%) died of other causes. Three patients had a local recurrence requiring a later hemipelvectomy. There were serious complications in 21 patients, including deep infection in 9 patients (26%) which required excision arthroplasty in 3 and secondary hindquarter amputation in 2. Recurrent dislocation in 6 patients was treated by physiotherapy and hydrotherapy and required replacement of a worn polyethylene acetabular cap in 1 patient. Bladder injury in 2 patients was managed conservatively. Other complications were as follows: thromboembolism in 1 treated by anticoagulation, loosening in 2 as a result of nonprogressive subsidence and tilt, aseptic loosening in 1 requiring revision, back pain in 1, incisional hernia in 1, and additional operations in 14. Functional scores in 13 patients tested were 70% of premorbid function.

Conclusion.—Whereas reconstruction of the hemipelvis provides satisfactory functional and oncologic outcomes, it carries a high incidence of serious complications.

▶ The authors have had a fairly extensive experience in treating primary malignant bone tumors of the periacetabular area by resection and prosthetic reconstruction. The complication and local recurrence rate with these procedures is high and, as the authors recommend, should only be carried out at centers specializing in orthopedic oncologic surgery.

T.C. Shives, M.D.

The Cost-effectiveness of Limb Salvage for Bone Tumour

Grimer RJ, Carter SR, Pynsent PB (Royal Orthopaedic Hosp, Birmingham, England)
J Bone Joint Surg Br 79-B:558–561, 1997   13–38

Background.—Limb salvage surgery has become very common among patients with primary bone tumors. Patients with primary bone sarcomas of the long bones require definitive reconstruction with allografts, rotationplasty, or endoprostheses. Research has shown that limb salvage surgery does not reduce survival, function, or quality of life, compared with amputation. The cost-effectiveness of limb salvage with an endoprosthesis was assessed and compared with that of amputation.

Methods.—Cost modeling for amputation was fairly simple, including the inpatient stay plus the provision and maintenance of an exoprosthesis. For limb salvage with an endoprosthesis, cost modeling started with the cost of the original procedure, which is affected by length of stay, the price of the implant, the complexity of the surgery, and rehabilitation. Other costs included follow-up, maintenance, and replacement of the endoprosthesis.

Findings.—Based on British National Health Service (NHS) data, the average cost of above-knee amputation was estimated at \$9,442. Estimated costs for a prosthesis and maintenance of the device for a young patient were \$7,716, recurring. Thus the actual cost for an NHS purchaser was estimated as \$9,442 + \$7,716y, where y is the number of years since amputation. Costs would be higher if the limb was provided in the private sector: \$9,442 + \$16,033y. The cost of endoprosthetic replacement—including inpatient care, outpatient care, servicing, and revision—was estimated at \$21,002 + \$1,419 per year. This figure included a 3% yearly risk of rebushing and a 4% yearly risk of revision.

Conclusions.—These calculations demonstrate the cost-effectiveness of limb salvage with an endoprosthesis in patients with bone tumors. For an average patient during a 20-year period, the cost savings produced by endoprostheses will be about 6 times the cost of the original procedure. Amputation is a surprisingly expensive option, and these costs are likely to increase as artificial limbs become more complex.

▶ There is no question that the expense of caring for patients with malignant tumors of the musculoskeletal system is substantial. This study carefully evaluates the cost-effectiveness of endoprosthetic replacement vs. amputation. Using data from the United Kingdom, it has been clearly shown that a limb-sparing procedure is cost effective, and in the long run, a more financially attractive procedure than amputation. This is particularly important information because the one-time cost of the actual implant is impressive and certainly attracts attention from payers for use of these devices. I think extrapolating the values to the United States is defendable because the relative values between the 2 procedures remains the same.

C.P. Beauchamp, M.D.

Revisions of Endoprosthetic Reconstructions After Limb Salvage in Musculoskeletal Oncology
Renard AJS, Veth RPH, Schreuder HWB, et al (Nijmegen Univ Hosp, The Netherlands; Groningen Univ Hosp, The Netherlands; Waldemar Link GmbH, Hamburg, Germany)
Arch Orthop Trauma Surg 117:125–131, 1998   13–39

Introduction.—A widely accepted mode of treatment of malignant bone and soft-tissue tumors is limb-saving surgery. Survival and local recurrence rates after limb salvage are similar to those after amputation, with better functional results than after amputation. However, the incidence of immediate and delayed complications after limb-saving surgery are higher than after amputation. Revision operations may be expected because limb-salvage procedures are performed predominantly in young individuals, and their long-term survival rates have increased considerably. The causes of and functional outcomes in 26 revision operations were reviewed.

Methods.—There were 91 limb-saving procedures using prosthetic reconstructions in a 20-year period, and of these, 26 revisions were performed in 16 patients. In 9 patients revision was due to polyethylene wear, in 9 it was due to aseptic loosening, 3 were due to recurrent hip dislocation, 2 were due to prosthetic stem fracture, 2 to infection, 1 to leg length discrepancy, and 1 to traumatic dislocation of a saddle prosthesis. There was a follow-up of 1.5–22 years with a medial of 13.5 years.

Results.—The functional results had deteriorated compared with after the primary operation in 5 patients after a follow-up period of 0.5–12 years after the revision operation. There was improvement in 2 patients. The results did not change in the remaining patients.

Conclusions.—Aseptic loosening was the major late complication after limb-salvage endoprosthetic replacement. There was an increase in prosthetic-associated complications in proximal femoral implants, distal femoral implants, and proximal tibial implants. There was a higher incidence of loosening in active, young individuals, in heavy patients, and in patients in whom more bone was removed. There was bone resorption present, but it was not extensive. Wear of the polyethylene components, often resulting in joint instability, was another frequent complication.. The functional results did not deteriorate in any of the 9 patients who had revisions because of polyethylene wear. Dislocation was managed satisfactorily after revision of the bipolar head of the acetabular cup. After endoprosthetic replacement, infection is the worst complication. The development of new materials and prosthetic designs that will survive longer are necessary for maintaining a large endoprosthetic replacement in an active, young individual.

▶ The consequences of complex reconstructions for limb salvage are now becoming a larger portion of the orthopedic oncologists' practice. More patients will have problems in the long-term with these complex reconstructions because long-term survival is increasing secondary to chemotherapy, complication rates from infection and local recurrence are decreasing, and improved soft tissue and skeletal reconstructions are allowing greater functional levels. It is reassuring that Renard et al. and other authors have shown very acceptable long-term survival rates for prosthetic function in this group of patients. In particular, this study is reassuring for patients who do have failure of the reconstruction; subsequent salvage surgery carries a predictable positive result.

C.P. Beauchamp, M.D.

Reimplantation of Autoclaved Tumour Bone in Limb Salvage Surgery
Sanjay BKS, Moreau PG, Younge DA (King Faisal Specialist Hosp and Research Centre, Riyadh, Saudi Arabia)
Int Orthop 21:291–297, 1997   13–40

Introduction.—The reconstruction of a residual defect in patients who have undergone wide resection of a malignant bone tumor is a significant problem in limb salvage surgery. A large amount of bone is needed to reconstruct the extensive defect, so autografting is limited. Allografting has its own problems with procurement, storage, immunological responses, and possible HIV infection. Use of autoclaved bone graft after complete ablation of the tumor provides immediate and anatomically correct filling of the defect. It is a technically and financially viable solution to the aforementioned problems. Surgical technique and outcome are reported for 7 patients with malignant bone tumors who were treated with resection of the tumor then reconstruction by reimplantation of the resected autoclaved tumor bone.

Surgical Technique.—The site of the proposed bone resection was determined by CT, MRI, and bone scans preoperatively. The tumor was removed en bloc with a wide margin. The rectus femoris muscle was able to be saved for lesions at the distal femur, but the menisci and the cruciate ligaments had to be removed from their tibial attachment. When the tumor involved the proximal tibia, these structures were removed from their femoral attachment. Before making the posterior dissection around the knee, the medial head of the gastrocnemius was cut to expose the neurovascular bundle. The posterior femur was then resected en bloc and the capsule and ligamentum teres were divided at the acetabulum. The tumor was resected, then the medullary canal of the distal femur was curetted to provide frozen section examination to rule out the presence of tumor. After removal of cartilage and soft tissue from the resected bone segment, the tumor bone segment was cleaned and irrigated with normal saline, then autoclaved for 5 minutes at 132°C at 29 pounds per square inch pressure. The bone segment was placed in the defect and fixed with a suitable implant, usually using an intramedullary nail. In the absence of an interlocking nail, the graft was fixed at the knee joint with additional staples to avoid rotation.

Results.—At an average follow-up of 20 months, 6 patients had no evidence of disease and 1 patient had a lung metastasis. One patient who underwent below-knee amputation after popliteal artery spasm was excluded. Four, 1, and 1 patients, respectively, had solid bone union, delayed union, and nonunion. There was no local recurrence of tumors. Lack of long locking nails caused inadequate fixation and implant failure in 2 patients. The original implants were removed and fixation was performed using appropriate long locking nails. Bone union was achieved in 1 patient, and the other patient had delayed union at the proximal host graft junction. There was histological evidence of bone ingrowth at the host graft junctions in specimens from patients who underwent repeat operations.

Conclusion.—Tumor recurrence was not observed in this cohort or in patient series from earlier reports of reimplantation of autoclaved tumor bone. Autoclaved bone does not require sophisticated instrumentation or a bone bank and avoids blood transmitted diseases and graft rejection problems. However, these grafts lack adequate mechanical strength in lytic type tumors. Autoclaved bone grafts may be used as an intercalary graft, a resection graft arthrodesis, or a composite graft with a long stem prosthesis. These grafts are useful in developing countries where resources for allograft of tumor prosthesis are sparse.

▶ The use of autoclaved tumor bone is a technique that has been in use for a number of years. It has not enjoyed widespread popularity because of the marked improvement in other reconstructive techniques over the years. The group from Riyadh, Saudi Arabia, rekindles the advantages of this technique particularly in areas where sophisticated and expensive prosthetic reconstructions are simply not an option. The use of autoclaved bone provides a fairly dependable way of reconstructing skeletal defects. The authors emphasize satisfactory rigid internal fixation as a requisite to insure graft host union. It remains an option in the reconstructive armamentarium of oncologic surgeons.

C.P. Beauchamp, M.D.

Limb Salvage Surgery and Adjuvant Radiotherapy for Soft Tissue Sarcomas of the Forearm and Hand

Bray PW, Bell RS, Bowen CVA, et al (Univ of Toronto)
J Hand Surg (Am) 22A:495–503, 1997   13–41

Introduction.—Simple local excision of soft tissue sarcoma of the extremities results in local recurrence rates as high as 50% to 90%. Limb salvage surgery with wide surgical margins combined with adjuvant irradiation is now considered optimal treatment for soft-tissue sarcoma of the extremities. Limb-preserving treatment of the forearm and hand is especially important in maintaining activities of daily living (ADL). The complex anatomy and limited tissue volumes of the hand and forearm make irradiation and surgery challenging. Treatment outcomes of 25 patients with distal upper-extremity soft-tissue sarcoma were reviewed.

Methods.—All patients underwent complete local and systemic staging before treatment. Patients with tumors close to neurovascular structures or tumors that would require significant postoperative radiation volumes underwent preoperative irradiation treatment. Postoperative treatment was administered after the surgical wound was healed. Important neural structures were usually preserved if they had minimal tumor involvement. Vascular structures were resected and reconstructed. Grossly involved nerves and vessels underwent resection. Reconstructive surgery was performed when it was necessary to restore integrity of soft tissue, bone, neurovascular, and musculotendinous structures. Functional assessments were performed before surgery and at 3, 6, 12, and 18 months after surgery and every 12 months thereafter. Patients were also assessed for changes related to irradiation; toxicity to skin, subcutaneous tissue, bone, and joints; limb edema; and sensory changes.

Results.—The 25 patients with soft-tissue sarcomas of the hand and forearm represent about 6% of all treated sarcomas in the same time period. Sarcomas were located in these places: 16 in the forearm, 1 in the wrist, and 8 in the hand. Seventeen patients received initial treatment elsewhere. Five patients had margins positive for microscopic disease. Of these 5, 3 had local recurrence from earlier excised tumors and 2 had not been treated elsewhere. Six patients underwent split-thickness skin grafts, and 4 underwent pedicled radial forearm fasciocutaneous flap when primary skin closure was not possible. Of 8 patients not undergoing functional assessment at follow-up 1 died of stroke, 1 died of heart attack, 4 underwent above- or below-elbow amputations, and 2 were lost to follow-up. Fifteen of 17 patients available for follow-up had returned to their previous occupations and levels of ADL. Two patients with significant functional limitations needed to modify their employment or activities in some way. Six patients had evidence of radiation-induced damage.

Conclusion.—The fact that most patients in this series had undergone prior treatment elsewhere complicated adequate oncological management, pathologic confirmation of margin status, and histologic identification of sarcoma within scar tissue. It is tempting to spare important functional structures with tumor involvement, but adjuvant therapy does not eliminate residual disease. All 3 local recurrences happened in patients who received adjuvant radiotherapy. Most patients did not experience radiation-induced injury. Most patients required soft tissue reconstruction. Treatment and management of patients with soft tissue sarcomas of the forearm can be challenging and should ideally take place at a musculoskeletal oncology treatment facility with the necessary multidisciplinary personnel.

▶ This study emphasizes the need for a multi-disciplinary sub-specialized approach to the patients with soft-tissue sarcomas. It was particularly distressing to note that two thirds of the patients ultimately referred to this oncologic group had an inappropriate surgical procedure prior to referral. This represents an ongoing continual problem that has a deleterious effect on patient care. It is certainly exemplified by the fact that these patients have a significantly higher risk of local recurrence. Excluding patients who were inappropriately managed prior to definitive surgery revealed a 100% local control rate. This is an outstanding result.

Eighty percent of these patients received radiation therapy, and the resultant morbidity associated with this was certainly acceptable. Of note, 80%

of patients were able to return to an excellent level of function with minimal or no limitations.

C.P. Beauchamp, M.D.

Limb Salvage Using Distraction Osteogenesis: A Classification of the Technique

Tsuchiya H, Tomita K, Minematsu K, et al (Kanazawa Univ, Japan)
J Bone Joint Surg Br 79-B:403–411, 1997   13–42

Objective.—Long-lasting survival and function of the limb with reconstruction after excision of skeletal tumors is enhanced with vascularized bone transfer. The results of distraction osteogenesis (callotasis) for the reconstruction of extensive defects after excision of skeletal tumors in limbs was reported.

Methods.—Bone transport, shortening-distraction, or both combined with the use of an intramedullary nail were used to reconstruct limbs in 19 patients (9 males), aged 10 to 72 years. Tumor types included osteosarcoma (10 patients), giant-cell tumor (5 patients), chondrosarcoma (2 patients), Ewing's sarcoma (1 patient), and malignant fibrous histiocytoma (1 patient). Two patients had failed previous treatment, 1 with an autoclaved bone graft and 1 with a vascularized fibular graft. Group 1 patients (5 with osteosarcoma and 5 with giant-cell tumor) had bone transport; group 2 patients (2 with osteosarcoma and 1 with Ewing's sarcoma) had shortening-distraction; and group 3 patients (3 with osteosarcoma, 2 with chondrosarcoma, and 1 with histiocytoma) had bone transport or shortening-distraction combined with an intramedullary nail. Seven to 14 days after surgery, distraction was begun at 0.5 mm twice daily or 0.25 mm 4 times daily. An external fixation index, a distraction index, and a maturation index were calculated and used to evaluate results.

Results.—The length of the average defect was 8.4 cm. The average external fixation index was 39.5 days/cm in group 1, 34.1 days/cm in group 2, and 24.0 days/cm in group 3. Overall functional results were excellent in 12 patients, good in 5, and fair in 2. There were 10 complications in 9 patients including skin invagination in 2 patients, pes equinus in 2, premature consolidation in 1, fracture in 2, subluxation of the fibular head in 1, skin necrosis in 1, and deep infection in 1. All were treated successfully. Reconstructions were classified as diaphyseal, metaphyseal, epiphyseal, subarticular, or arthrodesis.

Conclusion.—Distraction osteogenesis provides good results, particularly for patients with a good long-term prognosis and growing children. It provides early improvement in function.

▶ There exist a large number of options for the reconstruction of defects after excision for neoplasia. Each method of reconstruction carries with it advantages and disadvantages. It is important for the oncologist to have a variety of different reconstructive techniques available, dependent upon the patient, the tumor, the location, and the prognosis. The authors have had extensive experience in using distraction osteogenesis for the reconstructive of extensive defects. One of the goals of reconstructive surgery is to restore function as rapidly as possible and to maintain it for as long as possible. Distraction osteogenesis is a technique aimed at results in the long term. The price one pays for that is a very lengthy reconstructive period. This is therefore not an attractive choice for patients who have high-grade sarcomas of bone.

Patients who have benign neoplastic conditions present a different situation in that, in those individuals, it may be appropriate to perform reconstructive techniques that may be better in the long run but take longer to achieve. The skeletally immature child also presents a continual problem, and distraction osteogenesis may provide some flexibility in the reconstructive options for these patients as we are often limited to ablative surgery because of loss of the growth potential.

C.P. Beauchamp, M.D.

Distal Upper Extremity Function Following Proximal Humeral Resection and Reconstruction for Tumors: Contralateral Comparison
Damron TA, Rock MG, O'Connor MI, et al (State Univ of New York, Syracuse; Mayo Clinic and Found, Rochester, Minn; Mayo Clinic, Jacksonville, Fla)
Ann Surg Oncol 4:237–246, 1997   13–43

Objective.—Analysis of upper limb salvage methods for musculoskeletal tumors have generally assumed that the function of the distal upper extremity is largely unaffected. Upper extremity strength distal to the shoulder, as well as the functional capability of the reconstructed upper extremity after oncologic procedures that include resection of the proximal humerus, was examined prospectively.

Methods.—Between 1976 and 1992, 32 patients, aged 11 to 74 years at evaluation, with bone tumors of the proximal humerus or scapula were treated by resection of the shoulder joint and proximal humerus. Patients had dexterity and functional activity scores measured by a physical therapist using the Musculoskeletal Tumor Society functional assessment system. Patients were followed for an average of 42.3 months. There were 5 Tikhoff-Linberg resections, 9 modified Tikhoff-Linberg resections, 14 limited proximal humeral resections, and 4 extended proximal humeral resections. Osteoarticular proximal humeral allografts were used in 9 reconstructions, allograft-prosthetic composite in 1, arthrodesis in 7, and custom prosthesis in 15.

Results.—Grip strength, supination strength, pronation strength, elbow extension strength, and elbow flexion strength were significantly lower on the affected side than on the uninvolved side. The strength of the proximal musculature was most affected. Involved side grip strength and forearm pronation strength were significantly less in the Tikhoff-Linberg group. Supination strength on the involved side was significantly less in the modified Tikhoff-Linberg and limited proximal humeral resection groups. Differences were significant between sides in all groups for elbow extension and almost all elbow flexion measures. Grip strength on the involved side was significantly less in the fusion group, pronation strength in the prosthetic reconstruction group, and supination strength in the fusion and prosthetic reconstruction groups.

Allograft arthrodesis significantly diminished supination strength on the involved side. Elbow flexion and extension strength was significantly less on the involved side in the osteoarticular allograft, fusion, and prostheses groups. Elbow extension strength was significantly lower on the involved side in the osteoarticular allograft, fusion, allograft fusion, and prosthetic reconstruction groups. Self-assessed dexterity scores averaged 4.2 on a scale of 0 to 5, and more than one third of patients scored dexterity at 5. Functional activity scores averaged 2.3 on a 0 to 5 scale.

Conclusion.—Whereas a relatively high degree of distal function, particularly grip strength and forearm pronation strength, is maintained after limb salvage procedures, elbow flexion and extension strengths were lower in most groups. Proximal musculature strength was most affected.

▶ This is a large study of patients undergoing resections about the shoulder for tumor. The authors quite rightly point out a widely held belief by oncologic surgeons that the remnant of the extremity that is preserved will essentially be normal. They have noted a significant drop-off in measurable function in the affected limb. A large part of this functional loss has occurred around the elbow. We do realize that as more of the humerus is resected, the greater the impact it has on the humerus because of loss of the proximal humeral fulcrum. The basic principal of reconstruction of the shoulder is to at least restore the fulcrum of the humerus at the previous site of the shoulder whenever possible. The information that should be passed on to our patients should be that the hand, wrist, and forearm will not function normally and that the elbow function will be impaired.

C.P. Beauchamp, M.D.

Function After Subtotal Scapulectomy for Neoplasm of Bone and Soft Tissue
Gibbons CLMH, Bell RS, Wunder JS, et al (Nuffield Orthopaedic Center, Oxford, England; Mount Sinai Hosp, Toronto; Princess Margaret Comprehensive Cancer Ctr, Toronto)
J Bone Joint Surg Br 80-B:38–42, 1998   13–44

Objective.—Scapulectomy followed by irradiation and chemotherapy is the treatment of choice for tumors of bone and soft tissue. Little attention has been paid to outcome after reconstruction. The effect of a subtotal scapulectomy on subjective upper limb function in relation to bone and muscle resection and the method of reconstruction was assessed.

Methods.—Records were reviewed of 14 patients (7 men) undergoing subtotal scapulectomy for chondrosarcoma (8 patients), Ewing's sarcoma (2), aggressive fibromatosis, (3) and soft-tissue sarcoma (3) treated between 1989 and 1996. Patients were followed for an average of 52 months. Range of motion and strength were assessed using the Medical Research Council grading scale and the Musculoskeletal Tumour Society (MSTS) functional rating system. Patients completed a detailed evaluation of upper limb function.

Results.—All patients were alive at last follow-up, although 2 had evidence of recurrence. Nine patients had 80% or more of the scapula resected, and the remaining 5 had 50% to 80% resected. Eleven patients had primary reconstruction of soft tissue with remnants of the rotator cuff brought together and reattached to the residual scapula. In these patients, the serratus anterior was attached to the remnants of the latissimus dorsi and rhomboids, and the posterior deltoid was attached to the acromion and trapezius. The other 3 patients had muscle, soft-tissue, and skin reconstruction using the latissimus dorsi and pectoralis major muscle flaps. Two patients with positive margins had additional surgery or radiotherapy. Three patients had chemotherapy, and 5 were treated with irradiation. There was 1 wound infection in a patient receiving extensive radiation therapy. Functionally, 5 patients had pain after surgery: 3 had minor pain, and 2 had discomfort when lying down. Eight had full flexion, 2 had 90 degrees flexion, 3 had 60 degrees flexion, and 1 had minimal active movement. The mean MSTS score was 71.6 out of 100, and hand deficits occurred in 6 patients. Patients' subjective assessment averaged 79.9 out of 100. Twelve patients returned to presurgery activity levels.

Conclusion.—Subtotal scapulectomy provides an excellent functional result, even if the rotator cuff is excised, as long as the glenohumeral joint is preserved and the deltoid is reattached to the remains of the scapula and to the trapezius.

Clinical Significance.—Subtotal scapulectomy with preservation of the glenohumeral joint does not significantly affect outcome.

▶ In this review of the functional results of subtotal scapulectomy for sarcoma, the authors emphasize the importance of preserving as much of the glenoid humeral joint as possible. There is a significant difference between this and total scapulectomy in terms of functional loss.

C.P. Beauchamp, M.D.

Surgical Treatment for Myeloma of the Bone: A Retrospective Analysis of 22 Cases
Dürr HR, Kühne J-H, Hagena F-W, et al (Ludwig-Maximilians-Universität, München, Germany)
Arch Orthop Trauma Surg 116:463–469, 1997   13–45

Introduction.—A significant number of patients with myeloma, the most common primary malignant bone tumor, require surgery during the course of their disease. A retrospective study reviewed symptoms, diagnostic investigations, complications, and survival time in patients who underwent surgical treatment for myeloma of the bone.

Methods.—The 22 patients were treated surgically for solitary or multiple myeloma between 1980 and 1993. All patients were older than 40 years; 12 died during the observation period. Radiologic investigations performed included x-ray studies, isotope bone scans, CT, MRI, and angiography. Routine blood analyses were performed in all cases; iliac bone marrow aspiration was carried out in 16 cases and immune serum and urine electrophoresis in 21.

Results.—All patients reported pain at the time of evaluation for surgery. Fractures were present in 7 patients (32%) and neurologic symptoms in 3 (14%). The median duration of symptoms was 141 days. Most lesions were localized in the spine, pelvis, or proximal extremities. Pathologic changes were seen in 86% of patients with immune serum electrophoresis and in 35% of those with immune urine electrophoresis. Surgical treatment consisted of biopsy in 4 patients, curettage and cemented osteosynthetic stabilization in 3, and resection combined with decompression by laminectomy and a stabilizing vertebral osteosynthesis in 2. Vertebral prostheses were implanted after tumor resection in 7 patients. Five patients had reconstruction of resectional defects in the extremities by endoprostheses. A conventional prosthesis was used in 1 patient, together with partial tumor resection, osteosynthetic reconstruction, and a cemented acetabulum. Early mobilization was achieved in all cases. All patients underwent postoperative radiation, chemotherapy, or both. The 5-year survival rate was 48%.

Conclusion.—Surgery is usually performed in patients with multiple myeloma to prevent or treat fractures and neurologic symptoms. Full recovery is not always possible, but sufficient pain-free mobilization is often achieved. Immediate surgical decompression is recommended in cases of tumor-induced neurologic symptoms. Early fixation followed by radiotherapy should be carried out when weight-bearing bones are affected.

▶ The authors review their experience with surgical management of patients with myeloma. It is apparent that recent advances in surgical techniques have improved the orthopedic management of these patients. Internal fixation or prosthetic replacement are used as necessary to prevent and treat fractures. The advantages of modern orthopedic treatment of these patients is clear. It is particularly clear in the case of a solitary plasmacytoma because of the more entalant nature of the disease and the improved overall survival. This approach requires a team effort with close cooperation among various disciplines. Careful clinical evaluation is necessary because of the multisystem nature of the disease with its hematologic manifestations, hypercalcemia, renal impairment, susceptibility to infection, and bleeding defects.

F.G. Sim, M.D.

Soft Tissue Sarcoma

Oncological Outcomes of Operative Treatment of Subcutaneous Soft-Tissue Sarcomas of the Extremities

Gibbs CP, Peabody TD, Mundt AJ, et al (Univ of Chicago)
J Bone Joint Surg Am 79-A:888–897, 1997   13–46

Background.—Many soft-tissue sarcomas of the extremities are confined to the subcutaneous tissues. These sarcomas are often diagnosed only after excision of the subcutaneous lesion, at which time the patient is referred to a tertiary care center. It has been suggested that such patients should undergo reexcision, because most are found to have gross or microscopic residual tumor. Survival, local recurrence rate, and the effects of tumor and treatment-related variables were assessed retrospectively in patients with subcutaneous sarcoma.

Methods.—A total of 62 consecutive patients treated for subcutaneous sarcoma of an extremity were studied. The patients were 37 males and 25 females, with a median age of 47 years. The survivors were followed up for a median of 56 months. Forty-eight percent of the patients had malignant fibrous histiocytoma, 13% had liposarcoma, 8% each had fibrosarcoma and synovial sarcoma, and the rest had other diagnoses. On referral, only 3 of the patients had not previously been operated on. Forty-three had a previous excisional biopsy, 3 had an incisional biopsy, and 13 had a palpable local recurrence after a previous excision. Four patients required wide amputation because of the anatomical location of their recurrence. Forty-one of 43 patients with previous excisional biopsy were treated with attempted wide repeat excision; 49% of the surgical specimens showed residual tumor foci. Decisions about adjuvant therapy varied over time: 40% of patients received adjuvant radiation after surgery, whereas 2 received radiation as their initial therapy after referral.

Results.—At 5 years, cause-specific survival was 87% and disease-free survival 85%. At last follow-up, 81% of patients had been continuously disease free. Median survival for 8 patients who had died of disease was 29 months. Five of these patients had had stage IIIB disease. A large tumor was an unfavorable prognostic factor for disease-free survival but not for local recurrence. Both disease-free and cause-specific survival were worse for patients with stage IIIB vs. IIIA disease. Age, sex, previous surgery, residual disease, and local recurrence at referral were not significant prognostic factors.

Conclusions.—For patients with subcutaneous sarcoma, a careful wide excision produces excellent survival with a low local recurrence rate. The most important prognostic factors are the quality of this operation and the size of the tumor. Patients who have had a previous marginal excision of an unsuspected sarcoma should undergo wide repeat excision. The previous operative field must be excised en bloc, including the deep fascia, the area of hematoma, and the overlying skin. Most patients will need split-thickness skin grafting. Adjuvant radiation therapy may or may not be helpful—this must be determined in randomized trials.

▶ This retrospective study of 62 patients with subcutaneous malignancies provides valuable information regarding this small subset of patients with soft tissue sarcomas. The authors note a very satisfactory survival rate for these patients. They rightly point out that it is most likely related to tumor size because the more superficial the lesion is, the earlier it is picked up and diagnosed.

The disturbing part of this paper, again, is the problem related to inappropriate initial treatment. Many of these lesions are presumed to be benign, most likely lipomas, and are casually removed. It needs to be emphasized that a subcutaneous mass may indeed be a lipoma. A lipoma, however, has a very characteristic clinical feature associated with it. Lipomas need to be removed for cosmetic reasons only, not to find out what they are. If in the course of removing a lipoma it does not have the typical characteristic appearances of benign-appearing fat, an incisional biopsy frozen section should be obtained and the procedure stopped at that point if it is evident that this indeed is not a lipoma.

The importance of wound reexcision for these patients also cannot be underestimated. It has been shown by numerous authors in other studies that the incidence of residual disease and local recurrence is extremely high in these patients.

C.P. Beauchamp, M.D.

Skeletal Metastases From Soft-Tissue Sarcomas: Incidence, Patterns, and Radiological Features
Yoshikawa H, Ueda T, Mori S, et al (Osaka Univ, Japan)
J Bone Joint Surg Br 79-B:548–552, 1997   13–47

Introduction.—Recurrence of soft-tissue sarcomas with distant metastases is common. Rather than by lymphatics, they spread via the bloodstream. Metastases to the lung are most common and most life-threatening. There is less often involvement of bone, lymph nodes, liver, brain, and subcutaneous tissue. Intractable pain, pathologic fractures, and pareses may be involved in bony metastases. It is important to deal with skeletal metastases effectively to improve well-being and quality of life because of the increased survival rate of patients with soft-tissue sarcomas. Few reports have described the clinical characteristics and metastatic pattern in the skeleton of skeletal metastases from soft-tissue sarcoma. The characteristics of skeletal metastases from soft-tissue sarcoma were identified. The site of the primary tumor was correlated with the bones involved.

Methods.—There were 277 patients with soft-tissue sarcoma treated in a 20-year period. The incidence, distribution, time of appearance, and radiologic findings of skeletal metastases were reviewed.

Results.—Within a mean period of 18.6 months after admission, 28 (10.1%) had metastases. There was a varied incidence of skeletal metastases among the histologic subtypes of sarcoma. Higher incidences were seen with alveolar soft-part sarcoma, dedifferentiated liposarcoma, angiosarcoma, and rhabdomyosarcoma. In 13 of 28 patients (46.4%), the regional bones close to the primary tumor were affected. In 18 patients (64.3%), the axial bones were affected. Osteolytic changes were predominantly seen radiologically in the metastatic bony lesions. In 21 of 44 lesions, there were pathologic fractures.

Conclusions.—An osteolytic destruction with a permeative or moth-eaten pattern was seen in metastatic lesions from soft-tissue sarcomas. Pain caused by pathological fracture, impending fracture, or instability of spine may rapidly follow seeding to the bone, because these patterns indicate rapid destruction of bone. Pathologic fractures occurred in almost half of the metastatic bony lesions. For soft-tissue sarcoma metastases, surgical intervention may be more often required than for metastases with an osteoblastic or mixed pattern such as prostatic or breast carcinomas.

▶ Bony metastases from soft-tissue sarcomas, although rare, do indeed occur. It is important to know that this event can occur and that patients who have a history of a soft-tissue sarcoma and who have complaints of skeletal pain need to be evaluated with this clinical entity in mind. The lesions, once present, tend to behave in an aggressive manner, are destructive, and can cause pathologic fractures. The patients in this study were closely followed up, and nearly 50% had a pathologic fracture, emphasizing the need for early investigations in patients with potential metastatic bone disease from soft-tissue sarcomas.

C.P. Beauchamp, M.D.

Subject Index

A

Abuse
  substance, and rehabilitation for
    work-related upper extremity
    disorders, 195
Acetabulum
  component in total hip arthroplasty (*see
    under* Arthroplasty, hip, total)
  fracture, operations for, effect of
    indomethacin on heterotopic bone
    formation after, 71
  insufficient
    bone grafting in total hip arthroplasty
      for, 218
    replacement with Burch-Schneider
      cages, 221
  liner, elevated-rim, effect on loosening
    after total hip arthroplasty, 274
  reconstruction of, allograft, after
    resection of stage-IIB sarcoma,
    intermediate-term results, 403
Achilles tendon
  rupture
    bracing for, functional, 285
    early neglected, primary repair
      without augmentation for, 286
Actinomycin-D
  in Ewing's sarcoma
    femur, 361
    radiotherapy and, 362
Adipogenesis
  steroid-induced, in pluripotential cell
    line from bone marrow, 13
Administrative
  databases, quality of data regarding
    diagnoses of spinal disorders in,
    316
α-Adrenergic
  blocking drugs in reflex sympathetic
    dystrophy of upper extremity, 158
Adriamycin (*see* Doxorubicin)
Age
  combination Chevron plus Akin
    osteotomy for hallux valgus and,
    310
Aging
  detrimental effect on endurance of bone
    cement (in rabbit), 72
Aircast Cryo/Cuff
  after total knee replacement, 238
Aircast Sport Stirrup
  effect on functional performance after
    recurrent lateral ankle sprains, 279

Akin osteotomy
  combined with Chevron osteotomy for
    hallux valgus, and age, 310
Alcohol
  consumption and hip fracture in elderly
    men, 69
Allograft
  of intervertebral disc material to sciatic
    nerve, role of phospholipase A_2 and
    nitric oxide in pain-related
    behavior produced by (in rat), 341
  osteochondral, fresh, for posttraumatic
    osteochondral defects of knee, 252
  reconstruction of acetabulum after
    resection of stage-IIB sarcoma,
    intermediate-term results, 403
Allografting
  bone, in acetabular revisions, long-term
    follow-up, 219
  femoral impaction, cement mantle in
    Exeter, 212
    in hip arthroplasty, total, comparison
      of three systems, 215
Alloy
  particulate cobalt, chromium and
    cobalt-chromium, in vitro effects
    on osteoblast-like cells in, 1
Alpha-adrenergic
  blocking drugs in reflex sympathetic
    dystrophy of upper extremity, 158
Alveolar
  soft-part sarcoma, skeletal metastases
    from, 421
cAMP
  -mediated signaling mechanisms, role in
    modulation of cytokine production
    in titanium-stimulated peripheral
    blood monocytes by
    pharmacological agents, 3
Amputation
  level in ischemic limbs, determination
    of, 83
  limb, lower
    grade of surgeon and, 78
    seasonal variations in, 82
    stump and phantom pain prevention
      in, epidural bupivacaine and
      morphine in, 80
  risk due to infected puncture wounds in
    diabetics, and surgical morbidity,
    81
  for shoulder girdle tumors, malignant
    bone and soft tissue, 390
  surgery, 78

Amputees
transtibial, performance of ICEROSS
prostheses in, 85
veteran, British, phantom pain and
sensation among, 79
Amyoplasia
clubfoot deformity in, management of,
35
Analgesic
effect of intraarticular morphine and
clonidine alone or in combination,
59
Analgesics
for phantom limb pain, 80
Anaphylaxis
latex, intraoperative, in children, 48
Anatomic
basis for degree of displacement of
distal Chevron osteotomy in hallux
valgus, 301
considerations in arthroscopic capsule
release for stiff shoulder, 189
evaluation of atlantoaxial transarticular
screw fixation technique, 332
factors in snapping of medial head of
triceps and recurrent dislocation of
ulnar nerve, 172
feasibility of cervical pedicle screws *vs.*
lateral mass screws, 330
studies in vertically based deep fascial
turnover flap of leg, 402
Anatomy
of interosseous nerve, posterior, in
relation to fixation of radial head,
145
Anchor
suture
in rotator cuff repair, biomechanical
evaluation of, 183
technique of arthroscopic Bankart
reconstruction, long-term
follow-up, 187
Anesthesia
spinal, epidural, or propofol, for
outpatient knee arthroscopy, 245
Aneurysmal
bone cysts, primary, cementation of,
381
Angiosarcoma
skeletal metastases from, 421
Ankle
arthritis, 292
arthrodesis, stress fracture of tibia after,
288
fracture, acute, intermittent pneumatic
pedal compression and edema
resolution after, 309

hip-knee-ankle-foot orthoses,
conventional, *vs.* reciprocating-gait
orthoses for children with
high-level paraparesis, 40
impingement, anterior, arthroscopic
treatment of, 294
prognostic factors concerning
outcome of, 292
instability, lateral, acute repair and
delayed reconstruction for, 20-year
follow-up, 283
ligament injuries, 279
loading characteristics, tenodeses do not
fully restore, 280
normal, valgus stress radiography in,
282
orthoses, effect on functional
performance after recurrent lateral
ankle sprains, 279
osseous injuries, 288
revision, 301
sprains, recurrent lateral, effect of ankle
orthoses on functional performance
after, 279
tendon injuries, 284
Anteromedial
approach, open reduction through, for
congenital hip dislocation,
long-term outcome, 33
Antibiotic(s)
implant, biodegradable, in osteomyelitis
(in rabbit), 263
in surgical management of upper limb
lacerations, 64
Anti-inflammatory
drugs
nonsteroidal, for phantom limb pain,
80
nonsteroidal, in prevention of
heterotopic ossification after total
hip replacement, 225
in subacromial impingement
syndrome, 178
Anxiety
disorders and rehabilitation for
work-related upper extremity
disorders, 195
AO
classification of proximal humeral
fractures, poor reproducibility of,
197
AO/ASIF
fracture classification for distal tibia, 86
AOFAS Ankle-Hindfoot Scale score
after subtalar distraction bone block
fusion, 296

Arm
  motor performance decrease in,
      bilateral, in chronic tennis elbow
      patients, 162
Artery
  humeral, circumflex, in arthroscopic
      capsular release for stiff shoulder,
      189
Arthritis
  ankle, 292
  degenerative, distal interphalangeal
      joint, silicone interpositional
      arthroplasty for, 152
  foot, 292
  juvenile, chronic, survivorship of
      Charnley total hip arthroplasty in,
      46
  knee, 251
  osteoarthritis (*see* Osteoarthritis)
  posttraumatic, subtalar arthrodesis with
      internal compression for, 297
  rheumatoid
    cervical myelopathy due to, outcomes
        after surgical treatment, 339
    elbow, synovectomy for, arthroscopic,
        166
    elbow, synovectomy for, with radial
        head excision, 164
    hip, Charnley arthroplasty for,
        long-term results in young patients,
        203
    knee, arthroplasty for, total, infection
        after, results of 2-stage
        reimplantation for, 239
    spine, cervical, pedicle screw fixation
        for, 329
    wrist, arthroscopic synovectomy for,
        long-term follow-up, 142
  septic, effect of *Hemophilus influenzae*
      type b vaccination on incidence of,
      52
Arthrodesis
  (*See also* Fusion)
  ankle, stress fracture of tibia after, 288
  hindfoot, stress fracture of tibia after,
      288
  metatarsophalangeal, of first ray, in
      hallux valgus, in elderly, 303
  tibiotalar, salvage of pseudoarthrosis
      after, 300
Arthrofibrosis
  after reconstruction of anterior and
      posterior cruciate ligaments after
      knee dislocation, use of early
      protected postoperative motion to
      decrease, 246

Arthrography
  magnetic resonance, of wrist,
      scapholunate interosseous ligament
      in, 122
Arthrometer
  KT-1000 (*see* KT-1000 arthrometer
      score)
Arthroplasty
  basal joint, ligament reconstruction
      without tendon interposition, 146
  -derived macrophages differentiate into
      osteoclastic bone resorbing cells, 8
  elbow, total, for distal humeral
      fractures, in elderly, 170
  era of, role of shoulder fusion in, 193
  hip, total
    acetabular component in,
        uncemented, with cemented
        femoral component, long-term
        results, 209
    acetabular component in, uncemented
        stable, treatment of pelvic
        osteolysis associated with, 216
    for acetabular insufficiency, bone
        grafting in, 218
    acetabulum in, deficient, replacement
        with Burch-Schneider cages, 221
    blood salvage after, 66
    cement mantle in femoral impaction
        allografting in, comparison of three
        systems, 215
    cement mantle in femoral impaction
        allografting in, Exeter, 212
    Charnley, fixation failure after,
        aseptic, factors affecting, 205
    Charnley, long-term results in young
        patients with congenital
        dislocation, degenerative
        osteoarthritis, or rheumatoid
        arthritis, 203
    Charnley, survivorship in juvenile
        chronic arthritis, 46
    complications, 222
    conversion of intertrochanteric
        osteotomy to, coexistence of
        dissimilar metals after, 73
    dislocation after, prognosis of, 269
    femoral component in, cemented,
        forged cobalt-chromium-
        molybdenum, fatigue fracture
        of, 276
    femoral component in, cemented,
        with uncemented acetabular
        component, long-term results, 209
    femoral component in, uncemented,
        tapered design for, 208
    femoral component in, uncemented,
        10-year follow-up, 207

hybrid, long-term follow-up, 211
infections after, low-grade, 63
loosening after, effect of elevated-rim
  acetabular liner on, 274
in myeloma, 370
myocardial ischemia after, addition of
  continuous IV infusion of ketorolac
  to patient-controlled morphine
  reduces, 270
necrosis and, avascular, 227
nerve palsy associated with, 223
ossification after, heterotopic,
  irradiation *vs.* NSAIDs in
  prevention of, 225
primary, 203
quality of life after, health-related,
  233
reimplantation, outcome of
  reinfection after, 261
resection, for infected prosthesis, 262
revision, acetabular component, 216
revision, acetabular component, with
  allograft bone to repair bone
  defects, long-term follow-up, 219
revision, femoral component, 212
revision, impaction bone grafting
  before insertion of femoral stem
  with cement in, follow-up, 213
revision, isolated revision
  acetabuloplasty with porous-coated
  cementless acetabular component
  in, follow-up, 217
venous blood flow after, effect of
  active movement of foot on, 222
volume performed by providers
  related to postoperative
  complications, 267
knee
  medial compartment, St. Georg sledge
    for, 234
  quality of life after, health-related,
    231
knee, total, 234
  bilateral, concomitant, complications
    after, in elderly, 265
  bilateral, sequential, blood loss in,
    236
  blood salvage after, 66
  complications, 239
  dressings after, cold compression, 238
  infected, results of 2-stage
    reimplantation for, 239
  motion after, continuous passive, 237
  myocardial ischemia after, addition of
    continuous IV infusion of ketorolac
    to patient-controlled morphine
    reduces, 270

tibial component in, performance of,
  effect of shelf life and in vivo
  duration on, 240
silicone interpositional, distal
  interphalangeal joint, 152
Arthroscopy
ankle impingement treatment by,
  anterior, 294
  prognostic factors concerning
    outcome of, 292
Bankart reconstruction using suture
  anchor technique by, long-term
  follow-up, 187
capsular release by
  postoperative shoulder, 191
  for stiff shoulder, 189
in diagnosis of intraarticular soft tissue
  injuries with distal radial fractures,
  127
knee, 242
  analgesic effect of intraarticular
    morphine and clonidine in, 59
  in evaluation of accuracy of clinical
    examination, 242
  meniscal tears extending into
    avascular zone repaired by, 244
  outpatient, spinal, epidural or
    propofol anesthesia for, 245
labral repairs by, failed anterior, findings
  at open surgery, 188
rotator cuff repair by, technique and
  long-term results, 181
for subscapularis tendon tears,
  traumatic, 179
synovectomy by
  elbow, for rheumatoid arthritis, 166
  for rheumatoid wrist, long-term
    follow-up, 142
Arthrosis
subtalar, outcome of subtalar distraction
  bone block fusion for, 296
Arthrotomy
for subscapularis tendon tears,
  traumatic, 179
Articular
(*See also* Intraarticular)
cartilage effects of hyaluronan after
  partial meniscectomy (in rabbit),
  251
transarticular screw fixation,
  atlantoaxial
  technique, radiological and
    anatomical evaluation of, 332
  unilateral posterior, 335
Aseptic
failure of fixation after Charnley total
  hip arthroplasty, factors affecting,
  205

Athletes
  ankle sprains in, recurrent lateral, effect
      of ankle orthoses on functional
      performance after, 279
  recreational, Achilles tendon rupture in,
      early neglected, primary repair
      without augmentation for, 286
Athletic
  competition, return to, after anterior
      cruciate ligament reconstruction
      with autogenous patellar tendon
      graft followed by accelerated
      rehabilitation, 250
Atlantoaxial
  transarticular screw fixation
      technique, radiological and
          anatomical evaluation of, 332
      unilateral posterior, 335
Autoclaved
  tumor bone in limb salvage surgery,
      reimplantation of, 411
Autotransfusion
  intraoperative, quality assessment of, 65
Avascular
  necrosis of hip, 227
  zone, arthroscopic repair of meniscal
      tears extending into, 244
Axillary
  nerve
      in arthroscopic capsular release for
          stiff shoulder, 189
      injuries, combined with suprascapular
          nerve injuries, results of nerve
          grafting for, 201
Axis I disorders
  rehabilitation for work-related upper
      extremity disorders and, 195

B

Bankart procedure
  arthroscopic
      failed, findings at open surgery after,
          188
      suture anchor technique in, long-term
          follow-up, 187
      for shoulder instability, anterior,
          long-term outcome, 185
Basal
  joint arthroplasty, ligament
      reconstruction, without tendon
      interposition, 146
Behavior
  pain-related, produced by allograft of
      intervertebral disc material to
      sciatic nerve, role of phospholipase
      A_2 and nitric oxide in (in rat), 341

Benzalkonium
  chloride as disinfecting irrigation
      solution, 88
Betamethasone
  /lidocaine injection in trochanteric
      bursitis, evaluation of, 12
Bioabsorbable pin
  fixation of Chevron bunionectomy, 301
Biocoral
  /collagen carrier as bone graft substitute
      for lumbar spinal fusion (in rabbit),
      313
Biofeedback
  in reflex sympathetic dystrophy of
      upper extremity, 158
Biomechanical
  analysis
      of bone–pin interface in
          hydroxyapatite coated *vs.* uncoated
          pins (in sheep), 89
      of hip screw augmentation with
          calcium phosphate cement, in vitro,
          101
      of stress in fifth metatarsal, 292
  comparison of pedicle screws *vs.* lateral
      mass screws, 330
  evaluation of suture anchors in rotator
      cuff repair, 183
  investigation of fibular fixation in
      combined fractures of tibia and
      fibula, 114
Bladder
  injury after reconstruction of hemipelvis
      after excision of malignant tumors,
      408
Bleomycin
  in osteosarcoma, operable, 352
Block
  bone block fusion, subtalar distraction,
      outcome of, 296
  IV regional, in reflex sympathetic
      dystrophy of upper extremity, 158
  stellate ganglion, in reflex sympathetic
      dystrophy of upper extremity, 158
Blood
  flow
      resting, in diagnosis of reflex
          sympathetic dystrophy of upper
          extremity, 158
      venous, after total hip replacement,
          effect of active movement of foot
          on, 222
  loss
      in knee arthroplasty, sequential
          bilateral, 236
      postoperative, after pediatric scoliosis
          surgery, IV Premarin to decrease,
          29

peripheral blood monocytes,
    titanium-stimulated, modulation of
    cytokine production by
    pharmacological agents in, 3
salvage
    after arthroplasty, total hip and total
      knee, 66
    intraoperative, quality assessment of,
      65
Bone
    allografting in acetabular revisions,
      long-term follow-up, 219
    block fusion, subtalar distraction,
      outcome of, 296
    cement, endurance of, detrimental effect
      of aging on (in rabbit), 72
    chondrosarcoma of, myxoid, 382
    cysts
      aneurysmal, primary, cementation of,
        381
      simple, incomplete healing after
        steroid injections, in children, 50
    disease, disappearing, pathology of, 386
    formation, heterotopic (*see* Ossification,
      heterotopic)
    graft (*see* Graft, bone)
    histiocytoma (*see* Histiocytoma, bone,
      malignant fibrous)
    infections attributable to *Hemophilus*
      influenzae type b, decline in, 52
    injuries of ankle and foot, 288
    marrow, steroid-induced adipogenesis in
      pluripotential cell line from, 13
    mechanical properties, effects of
      ionizing radiation on, 399
    metastases
      painful, ^{153}Sm-EDTMP in, 368
      radiotherapy for, pain relief and
        quality of life after radiotherapy
        for, 363
    myeloma, surgical treatment for, 418
    -patella tendon-bone reconstruction of
      anterior cruciate ligament, 249
    pelvic, sarcoma of, prognostic factors,
      405
    -pin interface in hydroxyapatite coated
      vs. uncoated pins, biomechanical,
      scanning electron microscopy, and
      microhardness analyses of (in
      sheep), 89
    resorbing cells, osteoblastic,
      arthroplasty-derived macrophages
      differentiate into, 8
    scan, 3-phase, in reflex sympathetic
      dystrophy of upper extremity, 158
    tubular, subperiosteal origin of osteoid
      osteomas in, CT and MRI of, 376
    tumors

giant cell, pulmonary metastases
    from, long-term follow-up, 366
giant cell, pulmonary metastases
    from, prognosis and treatment, 365
limb salvage for, cost-effectiveness of,
    408
malignant, of shoulder girdle, 390
reimplantation of autoclaved tumor
    bone in limb salvage surgery, 411
scapulectomy for, subtotal, function
    after, 416
Bracing
    functional, for Achilles tendon rupture,
      285
    for scoliosis, efficacy of, 26
    for tibia vara, early infantile, 53
    valgus, joint loading with, in varus
      gonarthrosis, 254
Bridge
    plating osteosynthesis of comminuted
      femoral fractures, 105
Broberg and Morrey elbow scoring system
    validity of, 174
Bunionectomy
    Chevron, distal, fixation with
      bioabsorbable pins in, 301
Bupivacaine
    epidural, in prevention of stump and
      phantom pain in lower limb
      amputation, 80
Burch-Schneider cages
    replacement of deficient acetabulum
      with, 221
Bursitis
    trochanteric, evaluation of
      glucocorticosteroid injection in, 12

C

Cages
    Burch-Schneider, replacement of
      deficient acetabulum with, 221
    titanium, threaded, for lumbar
      interbody fusions, 328
Calcaneus
    fracture (*see* Fracture, calcaneus)
Calcium
    channel blockers in reflex sympathetic
      dystrophy of upper extremity, 158
    phosphate cement, hip screw
      augmentation with, in vitro
      biomechanical analysis of, 101
cAMP
    -mediated signaling mechanisms, role in
      modulation of cytokine production
      in titanium-stimulated peripheral
      blood monocytes by
      pharmacological agents, 3

Cancer
  childhood
    first, radiation and genetic factors in
      risk of second malignant neoplasms
      after, 358
    late mortality of long-term survivors
      of, 351
Capsular
  release, arthroscopic
    for postoperative shoulder
      contracture, 191
    for stiff shoulder, 189
Cardiovascular
  complications after concomitant
    bilateral total knee arthroplasty, in
    elderly, 265
Carpal
  tunnel syndrome, role of epineurotomy
    in operative treatment of, 159
Cartilage
  articular, effects of hyaluronan after
    partial meniscectomy on (in rabbit),
    251
Casting
  serial, in clubfoot deformity in
    amyoplasia, 35
  for tibial shaft fractures, closed, 108
Cell(s)
  giant cell tumor (*see* Giant cell tumor)
  Langerhans' cell histiocytosis in adults,
    clinical and therapeutic analysis,
    379
  line, pluripotential, from bone marrow,
    steroid-induced adipogenesis from,
    13
  osteoblastic bone resorbing,
    arthroplasty-derived macrophages
    differentiate into, 8
  osteoblast-like, in vitro effects of
    particulate cobalt, chromium and
    cobalt-chromium alloy on, 1
  retroviral producer, transplantation of,
    genetic correction of dystrophin
    deficiency and skeletal muscle
    remodeling via (in mice), 42
Cement
  bone, endurance of, detrimental effect
    of aging on (in rabbit), 72
  calcium phosphate, hip screw
    augmentation with, in vitro
    biomechanical analysis of, 101
  mantle in femoral impaction
    allografting
    comparison of three systems, 215
    Exeter, 212
Cementation
  of aneurysmal bone cysts, primary, 381

Cemented
  femoral component in total hip
    arthroplasty
    forged cobalt-chromium-
      molybdenum, fatigue fracture
      of, 276
    with uncemented acetabular
      component, long-term results, 209
  femoral stem in revision total hip
    arthroplasty, impaction bone
    grafting before, follow-up, 213
Centralization
  of hand on ulna for radial club hand,
    long-term follow-up, 34
Ceramic
  vs. titanium threaded cup in total hip
    arthroplasty for insufficient
    acetabulum, 218
Cerebral
  palsy patients, alterations in surgical
    decision making based on
    three-dimensional gait analysis in,
    41
Cervical
  discectomy and arthrodesis, failed
    anterior, analysis and treatment of,
    322
  lesions, nontraumatic, pedicle screw
    fixation for, 329
  myelopathy, rheumatoid, outcomes after
    surgical treatment, 339
  screw, lateral mass, *vs.* pedicle screws,
    330
Cesarean section
  rate increase after pelvic fracture, 100
Charcot foot deformity
  neuropathic ulcerations plantar to
    lateral column and, 306
Charnley total hip arthroplasty
  aseptic failure of fixation after, factors
    affecting, 205
  dislocation after, prognosis, 269
  survivorship in juvenile chronic
    arthritis, 46
  in young patients with congenital
    dislocation, degenerative
    osteoarthritis, or rheumatoid
    arthritis, long-term results, 203
Cheilectomy
  in hallux rigidus, 302
Chemotherapy, 348
  cisplatin, effect on extracortical tissue
    formation in diaphyseal segmental
    replacement (in dog), 359
  combination, in Langerhans' cell
    histiocytosis in adults, 380
  in Ewing's sarcoma of femur, 361

neoadjuvant, for high grade malignant
fibrous histiocytoma of bone, 348
in osteosarcoma
operable, two regimens, 352
P-glycoprotein expression as critical
determinant in response to, 349
of pulmonary metastases from giant cell
tumor of bone, 366, 367
/radiotherapy in Ewing's sarcoma,
long-term results, 362
Chevron bunionectomy
distal, fixation with bioabsorbable pins
in, 301
Chevron osteotomy
combined with Akin osteotomy for
hallux valgus, and age, 310
distal, for hallux valgus, anatomical
basis for degree of displacement of,
301
Children
arthritis in, chronic juvenile,
survivorship of Charnley total hip
arthroplasty in, 46
bone infections attributable to
Hemophilus influenzae type b in,
decline in, 52
cancer in
first, radiation and genetic factors in
risk of second malignant neoplasms
after, 358
late mortality of long-term survivors
after, 351
cerebral palsy in, alterations in surgical
decision making based on
three-dimensional gait analysis in,
41
clubfoot deformity in amyoplasia in,
management of, 35
coxa vara in, surgical outcomes for
valgus osteotomies for, 31
cruciate ligament tears in, anterior,
operative *vs.* nonoperative
treatment of, 45
fibromas in, nonossifying, pathologic
fractures through, 385
foot disorders in, congenital, 34
fracture in, 17
femoral shaft, external fixation or
flexible intramedullary nailing for,
17
forearm, unstable, intramedullary
nailing *vs.* plate fixation for, 18
humerus, epiphyseal, severely
displaced proximal, follow-up, 22
humerus, supracondylar, management
of pulseless pink hand in, 20
physeal, chronic, in myelodysplasia,
23

gait in
analysis of, 37
effect of limb-length discrepancy on,
37
genetic disorders in, 42
hand disorders in, congenital, 34
hip dislocation in, congenital
open reduction through anteromedial
approach for, long-term outcome,
33
Severin classification system for
evaluation of results of operative
treatment of, 32
hip disorders in, 31
infant
sternocleidomastoid tumor of, and
congenital muscular torticollis, 49
tibia vara in, early, brace treatment
of, 53
joint infections attributable to
Hemophilus influenzae type b in,
decline in, 52
latex anaphylaxis in, intraoperative, 48
limb salvage using distraction
osteogenesis in, 414
of orthopedic surgeons, effect of
surgeons' exposure to ionizing
radiation on, 6
osteogenesis imperfecta in, IV
pamidronate in, 44
paraparesis in, high-level, conventional
hip-knee-ankle-foot orthoses *vs.*
reciprocating-gait orthoses for, 40
scoliosis in (*see* Scoliosis)
shoulder fusion in, 194
spinal deformity in, anterior release and
fusion in, 28
Chondroblastoma
phenol instillation in, 383
Chondrosarcoma
acetabular, allograft reconstruction after
resection of, intermediate-term
results, 403
central grade I, radiographic
differentiation from enchondroma,
398
limb salvage using distraction
osteogenesis for, 414
myxoid, of bone, 382
pelvic bone, prognostic factors, 405
scapulectomy for, subtotal, function
after, 417
Chordoma
of spine above sacrum, treatment and
outcome, 389
Choroid
sarcoma of bone, 382

Chromium
  alloy, particulate, effects on
     osteoblast-like cells in vitro, 1
  -cobalt-molybdenum femoral
     component, forged, inserted with
     cement, fatigue fracture of, 276
Cigarette
  smoking (*see* Smoking)
Circumflex
  humeral artery in arthroscopic capsular
     release for stiff shoulder, 189
Cisplatin
  effect on extracortical tissue formation
     in diaphyseal segmental
     replacement (in dog), 359
  in two chemotherapy regimens in
     operable osteosarcoma, 352
Clinical
  prediction rule for prolonged nursing
     home residence after hip fracture,
     development and validation of, 70
Clonidine
  intraarticular, alone or combined with
     morphine, analgesic effect of, 59
Cloward arthrodesis
  cervical, complications after, 323
Club
  hand, radial, operative correction of,
     long-term follow-up, 34
Clubfoot
  deformity in amyoplasia, management
     of, 35
Co-amoxiclav
  in surgical management of upper limb
     lacerations, 64
Cobalt
  alloy, particulate, effects on
     osteoblast-like cells in vitro, 1
  -chromium-molybdenum femoral
     component, forged, inserted with
     cement, fatigue fracture of, 276
Coding
  spinal disorders and, 315
Cold
  compression dressings after total knee
     replacement, 238
  -stress testing in reflex sympathetic
     dystrophy of upper extremity, 158
Collagen
  /biocoral carrier as bone graft substitute
     for lumbar spinal fusion (in rabbit),
     313
Compartment
  syndrome, 93
    exertional, chronic, MRI in, 74
    fasciotomy for, early *vs.* late, 93

Composite
  resorbable osteoinductive, as graft
     substitute for lumbar spinal fusion
     (in rabbit), 313
Compression
  dressings, cold, after total knee
     replacement, 238
  internal, subtalar arthrodesis with, for
     posttraumatic arthritis, 297
  pedal, intermittent pneumatic, for
     edema after acute ankle fracture,
     309
  screw, parallel cannulated, figure-eight
     wiring through, for displaced
     transverse patella fractures, 119
Computed tomography
  evaluation of intraarticular fractures of
     calcaneus, preoperative and
     postoperative, 290
  impact on treatment plan and fracture
     classification of tibial plateau
     fractures, 256
  no value in reproducibility of
     classification of proximal humeral
     fractures, 197
  of skeletal muscle necrosis, idiopathic,
     in diabetics, 379
  of subperiosteal origin of osteoid
     osteomas in tubular bones, 376
Contracture
  shoulder capsular, postoperative,
     arthroscopic release of, 191
Corticosteroids (*see* Steroids)
Cost(s)
  of anesthesia, spinal, epidural, and
     propofol, for outpatient knee
     arthroscopy, 245
  -effectiveness of limb salvage for bone
     tumor, 408
  of thoracoscopic *vs.* open thoracotomy
     approach to anterior release and
     fusion in pediatric spinal deformity,
     28
Cotrel-Dubousset device
  decompression and stabilization for
     spinal metastases with, 374
Coventry high tibial valgization osteotomy
  time-dependent clinical and
     roentgenographic results of, 255
Coxa
  vara, surgical outcomes of valgus
     osteotomies for, 31
CPT impaction allografting system
  cement mantle in, 215
C-reactive protein
  in hip infections, periprosthetic
     low-grade, 63

Cruciate ligament
  anterior, 246
    reconstruction, after knee dislocation, 246
    reconstruction, bone-patella tendon-bone *vs.* semitendinosus anatomic, 249
    reconstruction, in patients older than 40 years, long-term follow-up and outcome, 247
    reconstruction, with autogenous patellar tendon graft and accelerated rehabilitation, long-term follow-up, 250
    tears, operative *vs.* nonoperative treatment, in children, 45
  posterior, reconstruction after knee dislocation, 246
Cryo/Cuff
  Aircast, after total knee replacement, 238
CT (*see* Computed tomography)
Cultures
  efficacy in management of open fractures, 92
Curettage
  and cementation for primary aneurysmal bone cysts, 381
  prophylactic, for pathologic fractures through nonossifying fibromas, 385
Cyclophosphamide
  in Ewing's sarcoma
    femur, 361
    radiotherapy and, 362
  in osteosarcoma, operable, 352
Cyst
  bone
    aneurysmal, primary, cementation of, 381
    simple, incomplete healing after steroid injections, in children, 50
Cytokine
  production in titanium-stimulated peripheral blood monocytes modulated by pharmacologic agents, 3

D

Dactinomycin
  in osteosarcoma, operable, 352
Databases
  administrative, quality of data regarding diagnoses of spinal disorders in, 316
Débridement
  surgical

  in osteomyelitis, followed by implantation of bioerodable polyanhydride-gentamicin beads (in rabbit), 272
  in rotator cuff tears, massive irreparable, results of, 182
Decision making
  errors in use of interlocking tibial nails, 110
  surgical, alterations in cerebral palsy patients based on three-dimensional gait analysis, 41
Decompression
  arthrodesis and, with and without spinal instrumentation, for degenerative lumbar spondylolisthesis with spinal stenosis, 319
  posterior
    with single-level posterolateral arthrodesis for isthmic spondylolisthesis in adults, 336
    stabilization and, for spinal metastases, 374
  subacromial, for massive irreparable rotator cuff tears, results of, 182
  in tarsal tunnel syndrome, 308
  outcome of, 308
Deformity
  Charcot foot, and neuropathic ulcerations plantar to lateral column, 306
  clubfoot, in amyoplasia, management of, 35
  planovalgus, acquired adult, subtalar fusion for, 284
  spinal, pediatric, anterior release and fusion in, 28
Degenerative
  lumbar spondylolisthesis with spinal stenosis, decompressive laminectomy and arthrodesis with and without spinal instrumentation for, 319
  osteoarthritis of hip, Charnley arthroplasty for, long-term results in young patients, 203
  spinal conditions, 319
11-Dehydrothromboxane B_2
  excretion, urinary, induction by fat embolism (in pig), 94
Delirium
  acute, after concomitant bilateral total knee arthroplasty, in elderly, 266
Depression
  major, and rehabilitation for work-related upper extremity disorders, 195

Dexamethasone
  -induced adipogenesis in pluripotential
    cell line from bone marrow, 13
Diabetes mellitus
  amputation in, seasonal variations in,
    82
  foot infections in, deep, clinical
    characteristics and outcome, 304
  necrosis of skeletal muscle in,
    idiopathic, 378
  puncture wounds in, infected, surgical
    morbidity and risk of amputation
    due to, 81
Diagnoses
  of spinal disorders in administrative
    databases, quality of data
    regarding, 316
Diaphyseal
  fracture of tibia, unstable, with distal
    intraarticular involvement,
    intramedullary nailing of, 109
  segmental replacement, effect of
    cisplatin on extracortical tissue
    formation in (in dog), 359
2,3-Dinor-6-ketoprostaglandin $F_{1\alpha}$
  excretion, urinary, induction by fat
    embolism (in pig), 94
Disability
  shoulder, related to occupational
    factors, 196
Disappearing bone disease
  pathology of, 386
Disc
  intervertebral, allograft of material
    from, to sciatic nerve, role of
    phospholipase A_2 and nitric oxide
    in pain-related behavior produced
    by (in rat), 341
Discectomy
  cervical, and arthrodesis, failed anterior,
    analysis and treatment of, 322
Disinfecting
  irrigation solution, potential,
    benzalkonium chloride as, 88
Dislocation
  fracture-dislocation of elbow,
    transolecranon, 168
  hip
    after arthroplasty, total hip, prognosis
      of, 269
    congenital, arthroplasty for, Charnley,
      long-term results in young patients,
      203
    congenital, open reduction through
      anteromedial approach for,
      long-term outcome, 33

  congenital, operative treatment
    results, Severin classification system
    for evaluation of, 32
  knee, reconstruction of anterior and
    posterior cruciate ligaments after,
    246
  patella
    primary, operative *vs.* closed
      treatment of, 258
    recurrence after, 257
  recurrent, after reconstruction of
    hemipelvis after excision of
    malignant tumors, 408
  shoulder, anterior, in elderly, 186
  ulnar nerve, recurrent, and snapping of
    medial head of triceps, 172
Distraction
  bone block fusion, subtalar, outcome of,
    296
  external, for unstable distal radius
    fractures, 128
  osteogenesis in limb salvage, 414
Distractor
  radiolucent, for indirect reduction and
    intramedullary nailing, 106
Documentation
  spinal disorders and, 315
DonJoy Ankle Ligament Protector
  effect on functional performance after
    recurrent lateral ankle sprains, 279
Doppler
  monitoring of intraoperative
    intravascular volume optimization
    after repair of proximal femoral
    fracture, 103
Doxorubicin
  in Ewing's sarcoma
    femur, 361
    radiotherapy and, 362
  in osteosarcoma, operable, 352
Dressings
  cold compression, after total knee
    replacement, 238
Drugs
  α-adrenergic blocking, in reflex
    sympathetic dystrophy of upper
    extremity, 158
  anti-inflammatory (*see*
    Anti-inflammatory, drugs)
  modulation of cytokine production in
    titanium-stimulated peripheral
    blood monocytes by, 3
  mood elevating, in reflex sympathetic
    dystrophy of upper extremity, 158
  neuropathic, for painful neuroma, 154

Dystrophin
    deficiency, genetic correction via
        transplantation of retroviral
        producer cells (in mice), 42
Dystrophy
    reflex sympathetic, in upper extremity,
        156

E

Edema
    after ankle fracture, acute, intermittent
        pneumatic pedal compression for,
        309
EDTMP
    ^{153}Sm-, for painful bone metastases, 368
Elavil
    for painful neuroma, 154
Elbow
    arthroplasty, total, for distal humeral
        fractures, in elderly, 170
    fracture, radial head/neck, reliability of
        fat-pad sign in, 118
    fracture-dislocation of, transolecranon,
        168
    ligamentomuscular protective reflex in
        (in cat), 171
    ossification about, heterotopic, early
        excision followed by radiation
        therapy for, 271
    pain, function, and disability, validity of
        observer-based aggregate scoring
        systems as descriptors of, 174
    synovectomy (see Synovectomy, elbow)
    tennis, 161
        chronic, motor performance in arms
            in, bilaterally decreased, 162
        lateral, salvage surgery for, 163
    trauma, 168
Elderly
    chordoma of spine above sacrum in,
        treatment and outcome, 389
    fracture in
        femur, proximal, intraoperative
            intravascular optimization and
            length of hospital stay after repair
            of, 103
        hip, mortality and rehabilitation after,
            67
        hip, nursing home residence after,
            prolonged, development and
            validation of clinical prediction rule
            for, 70
        hip, prognostic factors and outcomes,
            in men, 69
        humerus, distal, total elbow
            arthroplasty for, 170

hallux valgus in, metatarsophalangeal
    arthrodesis of first ray in, 303
knee arthroplasty in, total
    bilateral, concomitant, complications
        after, in elderly, 265
    health-related quality of life after, 231
orthopedic surgery in, major, and
    relation between mortality rates
    and hospital patient volume, 267
shoulder dislocation in, anterior, 186
Electrical
    nerve stimulation, transcutaneous
        for phantom limb pain, 80
        in reflex sympathetic dystrophy of
            upper extremity, 158
    surface stimulation, lateral, for scoliosis,
        efficacy of, 26
Electroacpuncture
    in reflex sympathetic dystrophy of
        upper extremity, 158
Electrocautery
    in arthroscopic capsular release for stiff
        shoulder, 189
Electron
    microscopy
        analysis of bone–pin interface in
            hydroxyapatite coated $vs.$ uncoated
            pins (in sheep), 89
        in sternocleidomastoid pseudotumor
            of infants and congenital muscular
            torticollis, 49
Embolism
    fat
        after fracture fixation with plate $vs.$
            intramedullary nailing (in dog), 95
        urine 2,3-dinor-6-ketoprostaglandin
            $F_{1\alpha}$ and 11-dehydrothromboxane B_2
            excretion induced by (in pig), 94
Enchondroma
    phenol instillation in, 383
    radiographic differentiation from central
        grade I chondrosarcoma, 398
Endoprosthetic
    reconstructions after limb salvage in
        musculoskeletal oncology, revisions
        of, 409
Epicondylitis
    medial, steroid injection for, 161
Epidural
    anesthesia for outpatient knee
        arthroscopy, 245
    bupivacaine and morphine in prevention
        of stump and phantom pain in
        lower limb amputation, 80
    corticosteroid injections for sciatica due
        to herniated nucleus pulposus, 321

Epineurotomy
  role in operative treatment of carpal
    tunnel syndrome, 159
Epiphyseal
  fractures, severely displaced proximal
    humeral, follow-up, in children, 22
Erythrocyte
  sedimentation rate
    in hip infections, periprosthetic
      low-grade, 63
    in osteomyelitis, pyogenic vertebral,
      325
Ethylenediaminetetramethylenephosphonate
  ^{153}Sm-, for painful bone metastases, 368
Etoposide
  in Ewing's sarcoma of femur, 361
  /methylprednisolone in Langerhans' cell
    histiocytosis in adults, 380
EVAIA
  chemotherapy in Ewing's sarcoma of
    femur, 361
Evans procedure
  for lateral ankle instability, 20-year
    follow-up, 283
Ewald et al. elbow scoring system
  validity of, 174
Ewing's sarcoma (*see* Sarcoma, Ewing's)
Ewing's Tumor Study
  first UKCCSG, long-term results from,
    362
Examination
  clinical, of knee, accuracy evaluated by
    knee arthroscopy, 242
Excision
  early, of heterotopic ossification about
    elbow, radiation therapy after, 271
  en bloc, of chordoma of spine above
    sacrum, 389
  of periacetabular malignant tumors,
    reconstruction of hemipelvis after,
    407
  radial head, with elbow synovectomy in
    rheumatoid arthritis, 164
Exercise
  isotonic, for shoulder impingement
    syndrome, 178
  in reflex sympathetic dystrophy of
    upper extremity, 158
Exertional
  compartment syndrome, chronic, MRI
    in, 74
Exeter impaction allografting technique
  cement mantle in, 212
    comparison study, 215
Extensor
  tendon injuries, early active
    mobilization for, 149

Extracortical
  tissue formation in diaphyseal segmental
    replacement, effect of cisplatin on
    (in dog), 359
Extremity
  (*See also* Limb)
  lower
    amputation (*see* Amputation, limb,
      lower)
    flap of leg, vertically based deep
      fascia turnover, 402
  sarcoma, subcutaneous soft tissue,
    oncological outcomes of operative
    treatment of, 419
  trauma, early *vs.* late fasciotomy in, 93
  upper
    disorders, work-related, rehabilitation
      for, and psychosocial factors, 194
    distal, function after proximal
      humeral resection and
      reconstruction for tumors, 415
    function after subtotal scapulectomy
      for neoplasm of bone and soft
      tissue, 416
    lacerations, antibiotics in surgical
      management of, 64
    motor performance decrease in arm,
      bilateral, in chronic tennis elbow
      patients, 162
    reflex sympathetic dystrophy in, 156

F

Fascia
  turnover flap of leg, deep, vertically
    based, 402
Fasciotomy
  early *vs.* late, in extremity trauma, 93
Fat
  embolism
    after fracture fixation with plate *vs.*
      intramedullary nailing (in dog), 95
    induces urine
      2,3-dinor-6-ketoprostaglandin $F_{1\alpha}$
      and 11-dehydrothromboxane B_2
      excretion (in pig), 94
  -pad sign in radial head/neck fractures
    of elbow, reliability of, 118
Fatigue
  fracture of femoral component, forged
    cobalt-chromium-molybdenum,
    inserted with cement, 276
Feedback
  practice pattern, effects on primary care
    physicians' use of lumbar spine
    imaging tests, 343

Femur, 104
  component in hip arthroplasty (*see under* Arthroplasty, hip, total)
  distal, osteosarcoma, MRI-based strategies in limb salvage surgery for, 391
  fracture (*see* Fracture, femur)
  head osteonecrosis
    osteotomies for, rotation, 229
    trapdoor procedure for, 227
  impaction allografting, cement mantle in
    comparison of three systems, 215
    Exeter, 212
  impaction grafting, massive early subsidence after, 275
  lengthening over intramedullary nail, 61
  nailing
    reamed, in patients with multiple injuries, 98
    thigh pain after, proximal, 104
  osteoma in, osteoid, 377
  proximal, disappearing bone disease of, pathology of, 386
  sarcoma of, Ewing's, prognosis, 360
  surgery, major, mortality rate related to hospital patient volume in Medicare patients undergoing, 267
Fibrocartilage
  complex, triangular, of wrist, high-resolution MRI in, 125
Fibromas
  nonossifying, pathologic fractures through, 385
Fibromatosis
  aggressive, function after subtotal scapulectomy for, 417
Fibrosarcoma
  of extremities, oncological outcomes of operative treatment of, 419
  pelvic, prognostic factors, 406
Fibrous
  histiocytoma (*see* Histiocytoma, of bone, malignant fibrous)
Fibula
  fixation, role in combined fractures of tibia and fibula, 114
  fracture
    combined with tibial fracture, role of fibular fixation in, 114
    stress, after arthrodesis of ankle or hindfoot, 289
Figure-eight
  wiring through parallel cannulated compression screws for displaced transverse patella fractures, 119

Fixation
  of arthroplasty, Charnley total hip, factors affecting aseptic failure of, 205
  with bioabsorbable pins in Chevron bunionectomy, 301
  external, for femoral shaft fracture, in children, 17
  fibular, role in combined fractures of tibia and fibula, 114
  fracture, with plate *vs.* intramedullary nailing, pulmonary effects of (in dog), 95
  internal
    of calcaneus fractures, from medial side, 291
    of elbow fracture-dislocation, 169
    of patella fractures, displaced transverse, with figure-eight wiring through parallel cannulated compression screws, 119
    of tibial shaft fractures, closed, 108
  plate
    dorsal, of distal radius fractures, 131
    vs. intramedullary nailing for unstable forearm fractures in children, 18
  radial head, anatomy of posterior interosseous nerve in relation to, 145
  screw (*see* Screw)
Flap
  of leg, vertically based deep fascia turnover, 402
Fluoroscopy
  radiation exposure to orthopedic surgical team during, 10
Foot
  arthritis, 292
  clubfoot deformity in amyoplasia, management of, 35
  compression, intermittent pneumatic, for edema after acute ankle fracture, 309
  deformity, Charcot, and neuropathic ulcerations plantar to lateral column, 306
  disorders, congenital, 34
  hindfoot arthrodesis, stress fracture of tibia after, 288
  hip-knee-ankle-foot orthoses, conventional, *vs.* reciprocating-gait orthoses for children with high-level paraparesis, 40
  infections, deep, in diabetics, clinical characteristics and outcome, 304
  ligament injuries, 279

movement, active, effect on venous
blood flow after total hip
replacement, 222
osseous injuries, 288
revision, 301
tendon injuries, 284
wounds, infected diabetic puncture,
surgical morbidity and risk of
amputation due to, 81
Forces
ground-reaction, after functional
bracing for Achilles tendon rupture,
285
Forearm
fracture, unstable, intramedullary
nailing *vs.* plate fixation for, in
children, 18
interosseous membrane, reconstruction
of, 143
sarcoma, soft tissue, limb salvage
surgery and adjuvant radiotherapy
for, 412
Fracture
acetabular, operations for, effect of
indomethacin on heterotopic bone
formation after, 71
ankle, acute, intermittent pneumatic
pedal compression and edema
resolution after, 309
calcaneus
arthritis after, subtalar, subtalar
arthrodesis with internal
compression for, 297
intraarticular, preoperative and
postoperative CT evaluation of,
290
treatment with open reduction and
internal fixation from medial side,
291
classification, 85
AO/ASIF, for distal tibia, 86
reliability in, critical assessment of
factors influencing, 85
-dislocation of elbow, transolecranon,
168
elbow, radial head/neck, reliability of
fat-pad sign in, 118
fatigue, of femoral component, forged
cobalt-chromium-molybdenum,
inserted with cement, 276
femur
comminuted, bridge plating
osteosynthesis of, 105
proximal, repair, intraoperative
intravascular volume optimization
and length of stay after, 102

shaft, external fixation or flexible
intramedullary nailing for, in
children, 17
fibula
combined with tibial fracture, role of
fibular fixation in, 114
stress, after arthrodesis of ankle or
hindfoot, 289
fixation with plate *vs.* intramedullary
nailing, pulmonary effects of (in
dog), 95
forearm, unstable, intramedullary
nailing *vs.* plate fixation for, in
children, 18
hip, 101
mortality and rehabilitation after, in
elderly, 67
nursing home residence after,
prolonged, development and
validation of clinical prediction rule
for, 70
prognostic factors and outcomes, in
elderly men, 69
humerus
distal, total elbow arthroplasty for, in
elderly, 170
epiphyseal, severely displaced
proximal, follow-up, in children,
22
proximal, poor reproducibility of
classification of, 197
supracondylar, management of
pulseless pink hand in, in children,
20
open, 88
cultures in management of, efficacy
of, 92
patella, displaced transverse, open
reduction and internal fixation with
figure-eight wiring through parallel
cannulated compression screws,
119
pathologic
in myeloma, prosthetic hip
replacement for, 370
through fibromas, nonossifying, 385
pediatric, 17
pelvic, 99
effect on female genitourinary, sexual,
and reproductive function, 100
ring, posterior, early complications of
percutaneous iliosacral screw
fixation of, 99
physeal, chronic, in myelodysplasia, 23
radius
distal, healing, acceleration in patients
who smoke, 109

distal, intraarticular soft tissue
injuries with, arthroscopic
diagnosis of, 127
distal, malunited, volarly displaced,
corrective osteotomy for, 136
distal, plate for dorsal fixation of,
131
distal, unstable, treatment of, 128
head, of elbow, reliability of fat-pad
sign in, 118
neck, of elbow, reliability of fat-pad
sign in, 118
scaphoid, acute, repeat screw
stabilization with bone grafting
after failed Herbert screw fixation
for, 138
tibia
combined with fibular fracture, role
of fibular fixation in, 114
diaphyseal, unstable, with distal
intraarticular involvement,
intramedullary nailing of, 109
healing, acceleration in patients who
smoke, 109
nail in, interlocking, decision making
errors in use of, 110
nailing of, intramedullary, knee pain
after, 115
plafond, classification of, critical
assessment of factors influencing
reliability of, 85
plateau, impact of CT scan on
treatment plan and fracture
classification of, 256
proximal third, technique of
intramedullary nailing of, 112
shaft, closed, three treatment
methods, 108
stress, after arthrodesis of ankle or
hindfoot, 288
Function
extremity, distal upper, after proximal
humeral resection and
reconstruction for tumor, 415
after scapulectomy, subtotal, for bone
and soft tissue tumors, 416
Functional
outcome after surgery for tarsal tunnel
syndrome, 307
performance after recurrent lateral
ankle sprains, effect of ankle
orthoses on, 279
Fusion
(*See also* Arthrodesis)
shoulder, role in era of arthroplasty, 193
spinal
cervical, failed anterior, analysis and
treatment of, 322

laminectomy and, with and without
spinal instrumentation, for
degenerative lumbar
spondylolisthesis with spinal
stenosis, 319
lumbar, graft substitute for,
resorbable osteoinductive
composite as (in rabbit), 313
lumbar, interbody, threaded titanium
cages for, 328
for pediatric spinal deformity, 28
single-level posterolateral, for isthmic
spondylolisthesis in adults, 336
subtalar
distraction bone block, outcome of,
296
with internal compression for
posttraumatic arthritis, 297
for planovalgus deformities, acquired
adult, 284

G

Gadolinium
-enhanced MRI of chronic physeal
fractures in myelodysplasia, 25
Gait
analysis
in children, 37
three-dimensional, alterations in
surgical decision making in cerebral
palsy patients based on, 41
effect of limb-length discrepancy on, in
children, 37
reciprocating-gait orthoses *vs.*
conventional hip-knee-ankle-foot
orthoses for children with
high-level paraparesis, 40
Ganglion
blocks, stellate, in reflex sympathetic
dystrophy of upper extremity, 158
Genetic
correction of dystrophin deficiency via
transplantation of retroviral
producer cells (in mice), 42
disorders, 42
factors in risk of second malignant
neoplasms after first childhood
cancer, 358
Genitourinary
function, female, effect of trauma and
pelvic fracture on, 100
Gentamicin
-polyanhydride beads, bioerodable,
implantation in osteomyelitis (in
rabbit), 272
Giant cell tumor
bone

limb salvage using distraction
osteogenesis for, 414
pulmonary metastases from,
long-term follow-up, 366
pulmonary metastases from,
prognosis and treatment, 365
spine, clinical outcome study of, 287
Glenohumeral
joint steroid injections, accuracy of
placement for shoulder symptoms,
and clinical outcome, 200
Glenoid
labrum repairs, failed arthroscopic
anterior, findings at open surgery,
188
Glucocorticosteroid
injection in trochanteric bursitis,
evaluation of, 12
Glycoprotein
P-, expression as critical determinant in
response to osteosarcoma
chemotherapy, 349
Gonarthrosis
varus, joint loading with valgus bracing
in, 254
Graft
allograft (*see* Allograft)
bone
autogenous cortical and cancellous, in
trapdoor procedure for
osteonecrosis of femoral head, 227
in hip arthroplasty, total, for
insufficient acetabulum, 218
impaction, before insertion of
cemented femoral stem in revision
total hip arthroplasty, follow-up,
213
for pathologic fractures through
nonossifying fibromas, 385
procurement from iliac crest, 57
screw stabilization with, repeat, after
failed Herbert screw fixation for
acute scaphoid fractures and
nonunion, 138
substitute, for lumbar spinal fusion,
resorbable osteoinductive
composite as (in rabbit), 313
substitutes, in spine, 313
femoral impaction, massive early
subsidence after, 275
nerve, results for injuries of axillary and
suprascapular nerves, 201
tendon, autogenous patellar, in anterior
cruciate ligament reconstruction,
long-term follow-up, 250
Grosse-Kempf nail
for femoral shaft fractures, proximal
thigh pain after, 104

for tibial fracture, knee pain after, 115
Ground
-reaction forces after functional bracing
for Achilles tendon rupture, 285
Guidelines
practice
effects on primary care physicians'
use of lumbar spine imaging tests,
343
for spinal disorders, 343
Gunshot
wounds
impact on orthopedic surgical service
in urban trauma center, 91
through knee, intraarticular findings
after, 90

H

Hallux
arthrodesis, metatarsophalangeal, for
hallux valgus in elderly, 303
rigidus, cheilectomy in, 302
valgus
in elderly, metatarsophalangeal
arthrodesis of first ray in, 303
osteotomy for, Chevron, combined
with Akin osteotomy, and age, 310
osteotomy for, Chevron, distal,
anatomical basis for degree of
displacement of, 301
Hand
club, radial, operative correction of,
long-term follow-up, 34
disorders, congenital, 34
pulseless pink, management in pediatric
supracondylar fractures of
humerus, 20
sarcoma, soft tissue, limb salvage
surgery and adjuvant radiotherapy
for, 412
Hardware
orthopedic, MRI of soft tissues adjacent
to, 395
Harrison Precoat impaction allografting
cement mantle in, 215
Healing
fracture, tibial and distal radius,
acceleration in patients who smoke,
109
incomplete, of simple bone cysts, after
steroid injections, in children, 50
Health
-related quality of life
after elective surgery, 232
after knee replacement, 231

Heart
  failure, congestive, after concomitant
    bilateral total knee arthroplasty, in
    elderly, 265
Hematogenous
  osteomyelitis, effect of *Hemophilus
    influenzae* type b vaccination on
    incidence of, 52
Hemipelvectomy
  for sarcomas of pelvic bones, 406
Hemipelvis
  reconstruction after excision of
    malignant tumors, 407
Hemodialysis
  long-term, causing destructive cervical
    spondyloarthropathy, pedicle screw
    fixation for, 329–330
Hemophilus influenzae
  type b, decline of bone and joint
    infections attributable to, 52
Herbert screw
  fixation for acute scaphoid fractures
    and nonunions, failed, repeat screw
    stabilization with bone grafting
    after, 138
Herniation
  nucleus pulposus, causing sciatica,
    epidural corticosteroid injections
    for, 321
Heterotopic
  bone formation (*see* Ossification,
    heterotopic)
  ossification (*see* Ossification,
    heterotopic)
Hindfoot
  arthrodesis, stress fracture of tibia after,
    288
Hip
  arthroplasty (*see* Arthroplasty, hip)
  dislocation (*see* Dislocation, hip)
  disorders, congenital, 31
  fracture (*see* Fracture, hip)
  infections, periprosthetic low-grade, 63
  -knee-ankle-foot orthoses, conventional,
    vs. reciprocating-gait orthoses for
    children with high-level
    paraparesis, 40
  replacement (*see* Arthroplasty, hip)
  screw augmentation with calcium
    phosphate cement, in vitro
    biomechanical analysis of, 101
  surgery, major, mortality rate related to
    hospital patient volume in
    Medicare patients undergoing, 267
Histiocytoma
  of bone, malignant fibrous
    extremity, oncological outcomes of
    operative treatment of, 419

  high grade, neoadjuvant
    chemotherapy for, 348
  limb salvage using distraction
    osteogenesis for, 414
  pelvic, prognostic factors, 406
Histiocytosis
  Langerhans' cell, in adults, clinical and
    therapeutic analysis, 379
Holmium
  :YAG laser, tissue shrinkage with (in
    rabbit), 60
Home
  nursing home residence, prolonged,
    after hip fracture, development and
    validation of clinical prediction rule
    for, 70
Hospital
  length of stay after repair of proximal
    femur fracture, 102
  patient volume related to mortality rates
    for Medicare patients undergoing
    major orthopedic surgery, 267
  for Special Surgery scale scores after
    reconstruction of anterior cruciate
    ligament in patients older than 40
    years, 248
  volume of total hip replacements related
    to postoperative complications, 267
Humeral
  artery, circumflex, in arthroscopic
    capsular release for stiff shoulder,
    189
Humerus
  fracture (*see* Fracture, humerus)
  osteoma in, osteoid, 377
  proximal, resection and reconstruction
    for tumors, distal upper extremity
    function after, 415
Hyaluronan
  effects on meniscus and articular
    cartilage after partial meniscectomy
    (in rabbit), 251
Hyaluronidase
  -digested nucleus pulposus, effects on
    nerve root structure and function
    (in pig), 340
Hydroxyapatite
  -coated pins, bone–pin interface in,
    biomechanical, scanning electron
    microscopy, and microhardness
    analyses of (in sheep), 89
  -coated titanium cages for lumbar
    interbody fusions, 328

I

ICEROSS prostheses
  performance in transtibial amputees, 85

Ifosfamide
  in Ewing's sarcoma of femur, 361
Iliac
  crest, procurement of bone graft from,
    57
Iliosacral
  screw fixation, early complications of
    percutaneous technique, 99
Ilium
  sarcoma of, prognostic factors, 405
Ilizarov
  femoral lengthening *vs.* lengthening over
    intramedullary nail, 61
Imaging
  magnetic resonance (*see* Magnetic
    resonance imaging)
  tests, lumbar spine, primary care
    physicians' use of, 343
Immunohistochemical
  study of disappearing bone disease, 386
Impingement
  ankle, anterior, arthroscopic treatment
    of, 294
    prognostic factors concerning
      outcome of, 292
  subacromial, syndrome, nonoperative
    treatment of, 177
Implant
  antibiotic, biodegradable, in
    osteomyelitis (in rabbit), 263
  polyanhydride-gentamicin bead,
    bioerodable, in osteomyelitis (in
    rabbit), 272
Inclinometric
  measurement of spinal range of motion,
    accuracy and sources of error with,
    315
Indomethacin
  effect on heterotopic bone formation
    after operation for acetabular
    fracture, 71
  in prevention of heterotopic ossification
    after total hip replacement, 225
Infant
  sternocleidomastoid tumor of, and
    congenital muscular torticollis, 49
  tibia vara in, early, brace treatment of,
    53
Infection
  arthroplasty, total
    hip, reinfection outcome after
      reimplantation for, 261
    knee, results of 2-stage reimplantation
      for, 239
  bone, attributable to *Hemophilus
    influenzae* type b, decline in, 52

deep, after reconstruction of hemipelvis
  after excision of malignant tumors,
  408
foot, deep, in diabetics, clinical
  characteristics and outcome, 304
hip, periprosthetic low-grade, 63
joint, attributable to *Hemophilus
  influenzae* type b, decline in, 52
spinal, 324
Infectious
  spondylitis, cervical, pedicle screw
    fixation for, 330
Injury (*see* Trauma)
Instrumentation
  spinal, 328
    decompressive laminectomy and
      arthrodesis with, for degenerative
      lumbar spondylolisthesis with
      spinal stenosis, 319
Insulin
  -dependent diabetes mellitus, idiopathic
    necrosis of skeletal muscle in, 378
Interferon
  in Langerhans' cell histiocytosis in
    adults, 380
Interleukin
  -6 production in titanium-stimulated
    peripheral blood monocytes
    modulated by pharmacological
    agents, 3
International Knee Ligament Standard
  Evaluation Form
  results after reconstruction of anterior
    cruciate ligament in patients older
    than 40 years, 247
Interosseous
  ligament, scapholunate, in MR
    arthrography of wrist, 122
  membrane of forearm, reconstruction
    of, 143
  nerve, posterior, anatomy in relation to
    fixation of radial head, 145
Interphalangeal joint
  distal, arthroplasty, silicone
    interpositional, 152
Intertrochanteric
  osteotomy conversion to total hip
    arthroplasty, coexistence of
    dissimilar metals after, 73
Intervertebral
  disc material allograft to sciatic nerve,
    role of phospholipase A_2 and nitric
    oxide in pain-related behavior
    produced by (in rat), 341
Intraarticular
  findings after gunshot wounds through
    knee, 90

fracture, calcaneal, preoperative and postoperative CT evaluation of, 290

involvement, distal, unstable diaphyseal fractures of tibia with, intramedullary nailing of, 109

morphine and clonidine alone or in combination, analgesic effect of, 59

soft tissue injuries with distal radial fractures, arthroscopic diagnosis of, 127

surgical reconstruction for anterior cruciate ligament tears in children, 45

Intramedullary

nail, femoral lengthening over, 61

nailing (*see* Nailing, intramedullary)

Intraoperative

blood salvage and autotransfusion, quality assessment of, 65

latex anaphylaxis, in children, 48

Intravascular

volume optimization after repair of proximal femur fracture, 102

Irradiation (*see* Radiation)

Irrigation

solution, disinfecting, potential, benzalkonium chloride as, 88

Ischemia

limb, determination of amputation level in, 83

myocardial, postoperative, after total hip or knee arthroplasty, addition of continuous IV infusion of ketorolac to patient-controlled morphine reduces, 270

Ischium

sarcoma of, prognostic factors, 405

Isotonic

exercises for shoulder impingement syndrome, 178

Isthmic

spondylolisthesis in adults, single-level posterolateral arthrodesis for, 336

J

Joint

basal joint arthroplasty, ligament reconstruction, without tendon interposition, 146

glenohumeral, steroid injections, accuracy of placement for shoulder symptoms, and clinical outcome, 200

infections attributable to *Hemophilus influenzae* type b, decline in, 52

interphalangeal, distal, silicone interposition arthroplasty of, 152

loading with valgus bracing in varus gonarthrosis, 254

replacement (*see* Arthroplasty)

Juvenile (*see* Children)

K

Kempf rotation osteotomy

for osteonecrosis of femoral head, 230

Ketorolac

infusion, continuous, addition to patient-controlled morphine reduces postoperative myocardial ischemia after total hip or knee arthroplasty, 270

Kienböck's disease

osteotomy for, radial recession, 140

Kirschner wire

placement in distal radius, risks of, 134

Knee

arthritis, 251

arthroplasty (*see* Arthroplasty, knee)

arthroscopy (*see* Arthroscopy, knee)

dislocation, reconstruction of anterior and posterior cruciate ligaments after, 246

examination, clinical, accuracy evaluated by knee arthroscopy, 242

gunshot wounds through, intaarticular findings after, 90

hip-knee-ankle-foot orthoses, conventional, *vs.* reciprocating-gait orthoses for children with high-level paraparesis, 40

injuries, acute, radiography in, implementation of Ottawa Knee Rule for use of, 117

osteoarthritis, total arthroplasty for infection after, results of 2-stage reimplantation for, 239

sequential bilateral, blood loss in, 236

osteoarthrosis, unicompartmental, Coventry high tibial valgization osteotomy for, 255

osteochondral defects of, posttraumatic, fresh osteochondral allografts for, 252

pain after intramedullary tibial nailing, 115

prosthesis, congruent meniscal, reduction of polyethylene in, 235

replacement (*see* Arthroplasty, knee)

Rule, Ottawa, implementation for use of radiography in acute knee injuries, 117

surgery, major, mortality rate related to
hospital patient volume in
Medicare patients undergoing, 267
KT-1000 arthrometer score
after cruciate ligament reconstruction,
anterior
bone-patella tendon-bone *vs.*
semitendinosus anatomic, 249
with patellar tendon graft,
autogenous, and accelerated
rehabilitation, 250
in patients older than 40 years, 247
K-wire
risks of placement in distal radius, 134
Kyphosis
anterior release and fusion in, in
children, 28

L

Labral
repairs, failed arthroscopic anterior,
findings at open surgery, 188
Laceration
limb, upper, antibiotics in surgical
management of, 64
Laminectomy
decompressive, and arthrodesis with
and without spinal instrumentation
for degenerative lumbar
spondylolisthesis with spinal
stenosis, 319
Langerhans' cell
histocytosis, in adults, clinical and
therapeutic analysis, 379
Laser
holmium:YAG, tissue shrinkage with (in
rabbit), 60
Latex
anaphylaxis, intraoperative, in children,
48
Leg
flap of, vertically based deep fascia
turnover, 402
Leiomyosarcoma
acetabular, allograft reconstruction after
resection of, intermediate-term
results, 403
Length of stay
after repair of proximal femur fracture,
102
Lengthening
femoral, over intramedullary nail, 61
Leukemia
childhood, late mortality of long-term
survivors of, 351

Lidocaine
/betamethasone injection in trochanteric
bursitis, evaluation of, 12
/methylprednisolone injection in medial
epicondylitis, 161
Ligament
ankle, injuries, 279
cruciate (*see* Cruciate ligament)
foot, injuries, 279
longitudinal, posterior, ossification of,
pedicle screw fixation for, 329
Protector, DonJoy Ankle, effect on
functional performance after
recurrent lateral ankle sprains, 279
reconstruction basal joint arthroplasty
without tendon interposition, 146
scapholunate interosseous, in MR
arthrography of wrist, 122
Ligamentomuscular
protective reflex in elbow (in cat), 171
Light
microscopy in sternocleidomastoid
pseudotumor of infants and
congenital muscular torticollis, 49
Limb
(*See also* Extremity)
ischemia, determination of amputation
level in, 83
-length discrepancy, effect on gait, in
children, 37
salvage
for bone tumor, cost-effectiveness of,
408
distraction osteogenesis in, 414
in musculoskeletal oncology, revisions
of endoprosthetic reconstructions
after, 409
for neuropathic ulcerations plantar to
lateral column in Charcot foot
deformity, 306
surgery, for osteosarcoma of distal
femur, MRI-based strategies in, 391
surgery, reimplantation of autoclaved
tumor bone in, 411
surgery, with adjuvant radiotherapy
for soft tissue sarcomas of forearm
and hand, 412
-sparing procedures for malignant bone
and soft tissue tumors of shoulder
girdle, 390
-sparing surgery for sarcomas of pelvic
bones, 406
Liner
acetabular, elevated-rim, effect on
loosening after total hip
arthroplasty, 274

Liposarcoma
dedifferentiated, skeletal metastases
from, 421
of extremities, oncological outcomes of
operative treatment of, 419
Longitudinal ligament
posterior, ossification of, pedicle screw
fixation for, 329
Lumbar
fusion
graft substitute for, resorbable
osteoinductive composite as (in
rabbit), 313
interbody, threaded titanium cages
for, 328
imaging tests, primary care physicians'
use of, 343
range of motion, inclinometric
measurement, accuracy and sources
of error with, 315
spondylolisthesis, degenerative, with
spinal stenosis, decompressive
laminectomy and arthrodesis with
and without spinal instrumentation
for, 319
Lung (*see* Pulmonary)
Lymphoma
childhood, late mortality of long-term
survivors of, 351
Lysholm and Gillquist scale
scores after reconstruction of anterior
cruciate ligament in patients older
than 40 years, 248

M

McReynolds medial approach
modified, for open reduction and
internal fixation of calcaneus
fractures, 291
Macrophages
arthroplasty-derived, differentiation into
osteoclastic bone resorbing cells, 8
Magnetic resonance arthrography
of wrist, scapholunate interosseous
ligament in, 122
Magnetic resonance imaging
-based strategies in limb salvage surgery
for osteosarcoma of distal femur,
391
characteristics of synovial sarcoma, 394
in compartment syndrome, chronic
exertional, 74
diffusion-weighted, of osteogenic
sarcoma (in rat), 397
high-resolution, of triangular
fibrocartilage complex of wrist, 125
in osteomyelitis, pyogenic vertebral, 326

of physeal fractures, chronic, in
myelodysplasia, 23
of skeletal muscle necrosis, idiopathic,
in diabetics, 379
of soft tissues adjacent to orthopedic
hardware, 395
of subperiosteal origin of osteoid
osteomas in tubular bones, 376
of subscapularis tendon tears,
traumatic, 179
in tarsal tunnel syndrome, 308
Malunion
radius fracture, volarly displaced distal,
corrective osteotomy for, 136
Marrow
steroid-induced adipogenesis in
pluripotential cell line from, 13
Mayo elbow-performance index
validity of, 174
Medicare
patients undergoing major orthopedic
surgery, mortality rates related to
hospital patient volume for, 267
Membrane
interosseous, of forearm, reconstruction
of, 143
Meniscal
effects of hyaluronan after partial
meniscectomy (in rabbit), 251
knee prosthesis, congruent, reduction of
polyethylene in, 235
tears extending into avascular zone,
arthroscopic repair of, 244
Meniscectomy
partial, effects of hyaluronan on
meniscus and articular cartilage
after (in rabbit), 251
Metals
dissimilar, coexistence after conversion
of intertrochanteric osteotomy to
total hip arthroplasty, 73
Metastases
bone
painful, [153]Sm-EDTMP in, 368
radiotherapy for, pain relief and
quality of life after radiotherapy
for, 363
pelvic, surgical treatment of, 372
pulmonary, from giant cell tumor of
bone
long-term follow-up, 366
prognosis and treatment, 365
skeletal, from soft tissue sarcoma, 420
spinal, posterior decompression and
stabilization for, 374
Metastatic
disease, 363

Metatarsal
  fifth, stress in, biomechanical study of, 292
Metatarsophalangeal
  arthrodesis of first ray in hallux valgus, in elderly, 303
Methicillin
  -resistant *Staphylococcus aureus* infection after total knee arthroplasty, results of 2-stage reimplantation for, 240
Methotrexate
  in osteosarcoma, operable, 352
Methylprednisolone
  injection
    in epicondylitis, medial, 161
    epidural, for sciatica due to herniated nucleus pulposus, 321
    healing of simple bone cysts after, incomplete, in children, 50
  in spinal cord injury, acute, 344
  /vinblastine in Langerhans' cell histiocytosis in adults, 380
Microhardness
  analysis of bone–pin interface in hydroxyapatite coated *vs.* uncoated pins (in sheep), 89
Microscopy
  electron
    analysis of bone–pin interface in hydroxyapatite coated *vs.* uncoated pins (in sheep), 89
    in sternocleidomastoid pseudotumor of infants and congenital muscular torticollis, 49
  light, in sternocleidomastoid pseudotumor of infants and congenital muscular torticollis, 49
Milwaukee brace
  for scoliosis, 27
Mitek suture anchor technique
  of arthroscopic Bankart reconstruction, long-term follow-up, 187
Mobilization
  active, early, for extensor tendon injuries, 149
Molybdenum
  -cobalt-chromium femoral component, forged, inserted with cement, fatigue fracture of, 276
Monocytes
  peripheral blood, titanium-stimulated, modulation of cytokine production by pharmacological agents in, 3
Mood
  elevating drugs in reflex sympathetic dystrophy of upper extremity, 158

Morbidity
  decreased, procurement of bone graft from iliac crest with, 57
  surgical, of amputation due to infected puncture wounds in diabetics, 81
Morphine
  epidural, in prevention of stump and phantom pain in lower limb amputation, 80
  intraarticular, alone or combined with clonidine, analgesic effect of, 59
  patient-controlled, continuous IV infusion of ketorolac added to, effect on postoperative myocardial ischemia after total hip or knee arthroplasty, 270
Mortality
  of hip fracture, in elderly, 67
    in men, 69
  late, of long-term survivors of childhood cancer, 351
  rates related to hospital patient volume for Medicare patients undergoing major orthopedic surgery, 267
Motion
  passive, continuous, after total knee arthroplasty, 237
  postoperative, early protected, to decrease arthrofibrosis after reconstruction of anterior and posterior cruciate ligaments after knee dislocation, 246
  shoulder, range in swimmers, 198
  spinal, range of, inclinometric measurement, accuracy and sources of error with, 315
Motor
  performance of arms in chronic tennis elbow patients, bilaterally decreased, 162
MRI (*see* Magnetic resonance imaging)
Muscle
  skeletal
    necrosis, idiopathic, in diabetics, 378
    remodeling, and genetic correction of dystrophin deficiency via transplantation of retroviral producer cells (in mice), 42
    temperature in diagnosis of reflex sympathetic dystrophy of upper extremity, 158
  torticollis, congenital, and sternocleidomastoid pseudotumor of infants, 49
Musculoskeletal
  oncology, revisions of endoprosthetic reconstructions after limb salvage in, 409

trauma, 85
Myelodysplasia
  physeal fractures in, chronic, 23
Myeloma
  bone, surgical treatment for, 418
  hip replacement in, prosthetic, 370
Myelopathy
  rheumatoid cervical, outcomes after
    surgical treatment, 339
Myocardial
  ischemia, postoperative, after total hip
    or knee arthroplasty, addition of
    continuous IV infusion of ketorolac
    to patient-controlled morphine
    reduces, 270
Myxoid
  chondrosarcoma of bone, 382

N

Nail(s)
  intramedullary, femoral lengthening
    over, 61
  tibial, interlocking, decision making
    errors in use of, 110
Nailing
  femoral
    reamed, in multiply injured patients,
      98
    thigh pain after, proximal, 104
  intramedullary
    flexible, for femoral shaft fracture, in
      children, 17
    pulmonary effects of (in dog), 95
    radiolucent distractor for, 106
    tibial, knee pain after, 115
    of tibial fractures, proximal third,
      technique, 112
    of tibial fractures, unstable
      diaphyseal, with distal
      intraarticular involvement, 109
    vs. plate fixation for unstable forearm
      fractures in children, 18
Necrosis
  avascular, of hip, 227
  idiopathic, of skeletal muscle in
    diabetics, 378
  tumor, in osteogenic sarcoma,
    diffusion-weighted MRI of (in rat),
    397
Neer classification
  of humeral fractures, proximal, poor
    reproducibility of, 197
Neoplasm (*see* Tumor)
Nerve
  axillary
    in arthroscopic capsular release for
      stiff shoulder, 189
    injuries, combined with suprascapular
      nerve injuries, results of nerve
      grafting for, 201
  grafting results for injuries of axillary
    and suprascapular nerves, 201
  interosseous, posterior, anatomy in
    relation to fixation of radial head,
    145
  palsy associated with total hip
    replacement, 223
  root structure and function, effects of
    normal, frozen, and
    hyaluronidase-digested nucleus
    pulposus on (in pig), 340
  sciatic, allograft of intervertebral disc
    material to, role of phospholipase
    A_2 and nitric oxide in pain-related
    behavior produced by (in rat), 341
  stimulation, transcutaneous electrical
    for phantom limb pain, 80
    in reflex sympathetic dystrophy of
      upper extremity, 158
  suprascapular, injuries, combined with
    axillary nerve injuries, results of
    nerve grafting for, 201
  ulnar, recurrent dislocation, and
    snapping of medial head of triceps,
    172
Neurologic
  complications after concomitant
    bilateral total knee arthroplasty, in
    elderly, 266
Neuroma
  painful, evaluation and treatment of,
    154
Neurontin
  for painful neuroma, 154
Neuropathic
  drugs for painful neuroma, 154
  ulcerations plantar to lateral column
    and Charcot foot deformity, 306
Night
  splinting in clubfoot deformity in
    amyoplasia, 35
Nitric oxide
  role in pain-related behavior produced
    by allograft of intervertebral disc
    material to sciatic nerve (in rat),
    341
Nonunion
  scaphoid, repeat screw stabilization
    with bone grafting after failed
    Herbert screw fixation for, 138
Norwich regime
  for extensor tendon injuries, 149

NSAIDs (*see* Anti-inflammatory, drugs, nonsteroidal)

Nucleus pulposus
herniated, causing sciatica, epidural corticosteroid injections for, 321
normal, frozen, and hyaluronidase-digested, effects on nerve root structure and function (in pig), 340

Nursing
home residence, prolonged, after hip fracture, development and validation of clinical prediction rule for, 70

O

Occupational
factors related to shoulder pain and disability, 196

Olerud posterior fixator
for spinal metastases, 374

Oncological
outcomes of operative treatment of subcutaneous soft tissue sarcomas of extremities, 419

Oncology
musculoskeletal, revisions of endoprosthetic reconstructions after limb salvage in, 409

ORIF
vs. external distraction-ORIF neutralization in unstable distal radius fractures, 128

Orthopedic
hardware, MRI of soft tissues adjacent to, 395
surgeons' offspring, effect of surgeons' exposure to ionizing radiation on, 6
surgery
major, mortality rates related to hospital patient volume for Medicare patients undergoing, 267
service in urban trauma center, impact of gunshot wounds on, 91
team exposure to radiation during fluoroscopy, 10

Orthosis
ankle, effect on functional performance after recurrent lateral ankle sprains, 279
hip-knee-ankle-foot, conventional, *vs.* reciprocating-gait orthosis, for children with high-level paraparesis, 40

Osseous (*see* Bone)

Ossification
heterotopic
about elbow, early excision followed by radiation therapy for, 271
after hip arthroplasty, total, irradiation *vs.* NSAIDs in prevention of, 225
after operation for acetabular fracture, effect of indomethacin on, 71
posterior longitudinal ligament, pedicle screw fixation for, 329

Osteoarthritis
degenerative, of hip, Charnley arthroplasty for, long-term results in young patients, 203
knee, arthroplasty for, total
infection after, results of 2-stage reimplantation for, 239
sequential bilateral, blood loss in, 236

Osteoarthrosis
knee, unicompartmental, Coventry high tibial valgization osteotomy for, 255

Osteoblast
-like cells, in vitro effects of particulate cobalt, chromium and cobalt-chromium alloy on, 1

Osteochondral
allografts, fresh, for posttraumatic osteochondral defects of knee, 252

Osteoclastic
bone resorbing cells, arthroplasty-derived macrophages differentiate into, 8

Osteoclastoma
phenol instillation in, 383

Osteogenesis
distraction, in limb salvage, 414
imperfecta, IV pamidronate in, 44

Osteogenic
sarcoma, diffusion-weighted MRI of (in rat), 397

Osteoid
osteoma, subperiosteal
radiographic and pathologic manifestations of, 377
in tubular bones, CT and MRI of, 376

Osteoinductive
composite, resorbable, as graft substitute for lumbar spinal fusion (in rabbit), 313

Osteolysis
pelvic, associated with stable uncemented acetabular component in total hip replacement, treatment of, 216
Osteoma
osteoid, subperiosteal
radiographic and pathologic manifestations of, 377
in tubular bones, CT and MRI of, 376
Osteomyelitis
antibiotic implant for, biodegradable (in rabbit), 263
hematogenous, effect of *Hemophilus influenzae* type b vaccination on incidence of, 52
treatment by surgical débridement and implantation of bioerodable polyanhydride-gentamicin beads (in rabbit), 272
vertebral, pyogenic, 324
erythrocyte sedimentation rate in, 325
MRI in, 326
Osteonecrosis
femoral head
osteotomies for, rotation, 229
trapdoor procedure for, 227
Osteoporosis
risk factors after hip fracture in elderly men, 69
Osteosarcoma
acetabular, allograft reconstruction after resection of, intermediate-term results, 403
chemotherapy, P-glycoprotein expression as critical determinant in response to, 349
femur, distal, MRI-based strategies in limb salvage surgery for, 391
limb salvage using distraction osteogenesis for, 414
operable, two regimens of chemotherapy in, 352
pelvic bone, prognostic factors, 405
shoulder girdle, 390
Osteosynthesis
bridge plating, of comminuted femoral fractures, 105
Osteotomy
Akin, combined with Chevron osteotomy for hallux valgus, and age, 310
Chevron
combined with Akin osteotomy for hallux valgus, and age, 310
distal, for hallux valgus, anatomical basis for degree of displacement after, 301
corrective, for malunited, volarly displaced fractures of distal radius, 136
Coventry high tibial valgization, time-dependent clinical and roentgenographic results of, 255
intertrochanteric, conversion to total hip arthroplasty, coexistence of dissimilar metals after, 73
radial recession, for Kienböck's disease, 140
rotation, for osteonecrosis of femoral head, 229
valgus, for coxa vara, surgical outcomes, 31
Ottawa Knee Rule
implementation for use of radiography in acute knee injuries, 117
Oxygen
transcutaneous partial pressure of, in determination of amputation level in ischemic limbs, 83

P

Pain
elbow, validity of observer-based aggregate scoring systems descriptor of, 174
knee, after intramedullary tibial nailing, 115
phantom
among British veteran amputees, 79
after lower limb amputation, epidural bupivacaine and morphine in prevention of, 80
postoperative, after spinal, epidural, or propofol anesthesia for outpatient knee arthroscopy, 245
-related behavior produced by allograft of intervertebral disc material to sciatic nerve, role of phospholipase A$_2$ and nitric oxide in (in rat), 341
relief after radiotherapy for bone metastases, 363
shoulder, related to occupational factors, 196
stump, in lower limb amputation, epidural bupivacaine and morphine in prevention of, 80
thigh, proximal, after femoral nailing, 104
Painful
bone metastases, [153]Sm-EDTMP in, 368

neuroma, evaluation and treatment of,
154
Palsy
cerebral palsy patients, alterations in
surgical decision making based on
three-dimensional gait analysis in,
41
nerve, associated with total hip
replacement, 223
Pamidronate
IV, in osteogenesis imperfecta, 44
Paraparesis
high-level, conventional
hip-knee-ankle-foot orthoses *vs.*
reciprocating-gait orthoses for, 40
Particulate
cobalt, chromium, and
cobalt-chromium, effects on
osteoblast-like cells in vitro, 1
Patella, 257
bone-patella tendon-bone reconstruction
of anterior cruciate ligament, 249
dislocation
primary, operative *vs.* closed
treatment of, 258
recurrence after, 257
fracture, displaced transverse, open
reduction and internal fixation with
figure-eight wiring through parallel
cannulated compression screws,
119
Patellar
tendon graft, autogenous, in anterior
cruciate ligament reconstruction,
long-term follow-up, 250
Pathologic
fracture
in myeloma, prosthetic hip
replacement for, 370
through fibromas, nonossifying, 385
manifestations of subperiosteal osteoid
osteoma, 377
Pathology
of disappearing bone disease, 386
Patient
-controlled morphine, continuous IV
infusion of ketorolac added to,
effect on postoperative myocardial
ischemia after total hip or knee
arthroplasty, 270
volume, hospital, related to mortality
rates for Medicare patients
undergoing major orthopedic
surgery, 267
Pedal (*see* Foot)
Pediatric (*see* Children)
Pedicle
screw

cervical, *vs.* lateral mass screws, 330
fixation for nontraumatic lesions of
cervical spine, 329
Pelvic
bone sarcoma, prognostic factors, 405
fracture (*see* Fracture, pelvic)
metastases, surgical treatment of, 372
osteolysis associated with stable
uncemented acetabular component
in total hip replacement, 216
trauma, effect on female genitourinary,
sexual, and reproductive function,
100
Percutaneous
placement of iliosacral screws, early
complications of, 99
Periacetabular
tumors, malignant, reconstruction of
hemipelvis after excision of, 407
Periprosthetic
hip infections, low-grade, 63
P-glycoprotein
expression as critical determinant in
response to osteosarcoma
chemotherapy, 349
Phantom pain
among amputees, British veteran, 79
in lower limb amputation, epidural
bupivacaine and morphine in
prevention of, 80
Phantom sensation
among amputees, British veteran, 79
Pharmacologic
agents (*see* Drugs)
Phenol
characteristics of, 383
Phospholipase
A_2, role in pain-related behavior
produced by allograft of
intervertebral disc material to
sciatic nerve (in rat), 341
Physeal
fractures, chronic, in myelodysplasia, 23
Physical
therapy
alone or with continuous passive
motion after total knee
arthroplasty, 237
after Bankart repair for anterior
shoulder instability, 185
supervised, for subacromial
impingement syndrome, 178
Physicians
primary care, use of lumbar spine
imaging tests by, 343

Physiotherapy (*see* Physical, therapy)
Pin(s)
bioabsorbable, fixation of Chevron
bunionectomy with, 301
hydroxyapatite coated *vs.* uncoated,
bone–pin interface in,
biomechanical, scanning electron
microscopy, and microhardness
analyses of (in sheep), 89
Pink
hand, pulseless, management in
pediatric supracondylar fractures of
humerus, 20
Pivot-shift test
results after reconstruction of anterior
cruciate ligament in patients older
than 40 years, 247
Planovalgus
deformities, acquired adult, subtalar
fusion for, 284
Plate
fixation
dorsal, of distal radius fractures, 131
of elbow fracture-dislocation, 169
of fracture, pulmonary effects of (in
dog), 95
vs. intramedullary nailing for unstable
forearm fractures in children, 18
Plating
bridge, for comminuted femoral
fractures, 105
Pluripotential
cell line from bone marrow,
steroid-induced adipogenesis from,
13
Pneumatic
pedal compression, intermittent, for
edema after acute ankle fracture,
309
Poly (DL-lactide):co-glycolide
in biodegradable antibiotic implant in
osteomyelitis (in rabbit), 263
Polyanhydride
-gentamicin beads, bioerodable,
implantation in osteomyelitis (in
rabbit), 272
Polyethylene
reduction in congruent meniscal knee
prosthesis, 235
tibial bearings, impacts of shelf life and
in vivo duration on performance
of, 240
Polylactic acid
in biodegradable antibiotic implant in
osteomyelitis (in rabbit), 263
Polymethylmethacrylate
antibiotic containing beads in
osteomyelitis (in rabbit), 263

Porous
-coated acetabular component in
isolated revision acetabuloplasty,
follow-up, 217
Postoperative
blood loss after pediatric scoliosis
surgery, IV Premarin to decrease,
29
complications after total hip
replacements related to volume
performed by providers, 267
motion, early protected, to decrease
arthrofibrosis after reconstruction
of anterior and posterior cruciate
ligaments after knee dislocation,
246
pain after spinal, epidural, or propofol
anesthesia for outpatient knee
arthroscopy, 245
shoulder capsular contracture,
arthroscopic release of, 191
Practice
guidelines
effects on primary care physicians'
use of lumbar spine imaging tests,
343
for spinal disorders, 343
pattern feedback, effects on primary
care physicians' use of lumbar
spine imaging tests, 343
Prediction
rule, clinical, for prolonged nursing
home residence after hip fracture,
development and validation of, 70
Premarin
IV, to decrease postoperative blood loss
after pediatric scoliosis surgery, 29
Primary care
physicians' use of lumbar spine imaging
tests, 343
Pritchard elbow scoring system
validity of, 174
Propofol
anesthesia for outpatient knee
arthroscopy, 245
Prosthesis
diaphyseal segmental replacement, effect
of cisplatin on extracortical tissue
formation in (in dog), 359
ICEROSS, performance in transtibial
amputees, 85
knee, congruent meniscal, reduction of
polyethylene in, 235
Protein
C-reactive, in periprosthetic low-grade
hip infections, 63
Pseudoarthrosis
salvage after tibiotalar arthrodesis, 300

Pseudotumor
   sternocleidomastoid, of infants, and
      congenital muscular torticollis, 49
Psychosocial
   factors and rehabilitation for chronic
      work-related upper extremity
      disorders, 194
Pubis
   sarcoma of, prognostic factors, 405
Pulmonary
   effects of fracture fixation with plate *vs.*
      intramedullary nailing (in dog), 95
   metastases from giant cell tumor of
      bone
      long-term follow-up, 366
      prognosis and treatment, 365
Puncture
   wounds in diabetics, infected, surgical
      morbidity and risk of amputation
      due to, 81
Pyogenic
   osteomyelitis, vertebral (*see*
      Osteomyelitis, vertebral, pyogenic)

Q

Quality
   assessment of intraoperative blood
      salvage and autotransfusion, 65
   of life
      health-related, after elective surgery,
       232
      health-related, after knee replacement,
       231
      after radiotherapy for bone
       metastases, 363
      after surgical treatment of pelvic
       metastases, 372

R

Radial
   club hand, operative correction of,
      long-term follow-up, 34
   recession osteotomy for Kienböck's
      disease, 140
Radiation
   diagnostic (*see* Radiography)
   exposure to orthopedic surgical team
      during fluoroscopy, 10
   ionizing
      are orthopedic surgeons' offspring at
       risk? 6
      effects on mechanical properties of
       bone, 399
   therapeutic (*see* Radiotherapy)

Radiographic
   manifestations of subperiosteal osteoid
      osteoma, 377
Radiography
   enchondroma differentiated from
      central grade I chondrosarcoma by,
      398
   in knee injuries, acute, implementation
      of Ottawa Knee Rule for use of,
      117
   results of Coventry tibial valgization
      osteotomy, 255
   valgus stress, in normal ankles, 282
Radiological
   evaluation of atlantoaxial transarticular
      screw fixation technique, 332
   features of skeletal metastases from soft
      tissue sarcomas, 420
Radiology
   of orthopedic oncology, 391
Radiolucent
   distractor for indirect reduction and
      intramedullary nailing, 106
Radiotherapy
   adjuvant, with limb salvage surgery for
      soft tissue sarcomas of forearm and
      hand, 412
   for bone metastases, pain relief and
      quality of life after, 363
   /chemotherapy in Ewing's sarcoma,
      long-term results, 362
   in childhood cancer, first, risk of second
      malignant neoplasms after, 358
   of chordoma of spine above sacrum,
      389
   after excision of heterotopic ossification
      about elbow, early, 271
   postoperative, in prevention of
      heterotopic ossification after total
      hip replacement, 225
   of pulmonary metastases from giant cell
      tumor of bone, 366, 367
   in sarcoma, Ewing's, of femur, 361
Radius
   distal, risks of Kirschner wire placement
      in, 134
   fracture (*see* Fracture, radius)
   head
      excision with elbow synovectomy in
       rheumatoid arthritis, 164
      fixation of, anatomy of posterior
       interosseous nerve in relation to,
       145
Range of motion
   shoulder, in swimmers, 198
   spinal, inclinometric measurement,
      accuracy and sources of error with,
      315

452 / Subject Index

Ray-titanium fusion cage
    for lumbar interbody fusions, 328
Reconstruction
    acute, for lateral ankle instability,
        20-year follow-up, 283
    allograft, of acetabulum after resection
        of stage-IIB sarcoma,
        intermediate-term results, 403
    Bankart (*see* Bankart procedure)
    cruciate ligament
        anterior (*see* Cruciate ligament,
            anterior, reconstruction)
        posterior, after knee dislocation, 246
    delayed, for lateral ankle instability,
        20-year follow-up, 283
    endoprosthetic, revisions after limb
        salvage in musculoskeletal
        oncology, 409
    hemipelvis, after excision of malignant
        tumors, 407
    humerus, proximal, for tumors, distal
        upper extremity function after, 415
    of interosseous membrane of forearm,
        143
    intraarticular surgical, for anterior
        cruciate ligament tears in children,
        45
    ligament reconstruction basal joint
        arthroplasty without tendon
        interposition, 146
    sagittal band, 152
Reduction
    indirect, radiolucent distractor for, 106
    open
        of elbow fracture-dislocation, 169
        and internal fixation from medial
            side, of calcaneus fractures, 291
        of patella fractures, displaced
            transverse, and fixation with
            figure-eight wiring through parallel
            cannulated compression screws,
            119
        through anteromedial approach for
            congenital hip dislocation,
            long-term outcome, 33
        of tibial shaft fractures, closed, 108
Reflex
    ligamentomuscular protective, in elbow
        (in cat), 171
    sympathetic dystrophy in upper
        extremity, 156
Rehabilitation
    after hip fracture, in elderly, 67
    program, accelerated, after anterior
        cruciate ligament reconstruction
        with autogenous patellar tendon
        graft, 250

for work-related upper extremity
    disorders, chronic, and
    psychosocial factors, 194
Reimplantation
    arthroplasty, total
        hip, outcome of reinfection after, 261
        knee, infected, two-stage procedure,
            239
    of autoclaved tumor bone in limb
        salvage surgery, 411
Reinfection
    outcome after reimplantation hip
        arthroplasty, 261
Reproductive
    function, female, effect of trauma and
        pelvic fracture on, 100
Respiratory
    distress syndrome, adult, 94
Retroviral
    producer cells, transplantation of,
        genetic correction of dystrophin
        deficiency and skeletal muscle
        remodeling via (in mice), 42
Rhabdomyosarcoma
    skeletal metastases from, 421
Rheumatoid
    arthritis (*see* Arthritis, rheumatoid)
Robinson-type arthrodesis
    cervical, multilevel, anterior migration
        with, 323
Rotaglide knee prosthesis
    polyethylene reduction in, 235
Rotation
    osteotomies for osteonecrosis of femoral
        head, 229
Rotator cuff, 177
    tears
        massive irreparable, results of
            operative débridement and
            subacromial decompression for,
            182
        repair of, arthroscopic, technique and
            long-term results, 181
        repair of, suture anchors in,
            biomechanical evaluation of, 183
        shoulder dislocation and, anterior, in
            elderly, 186
Rule
    Ottawa Knee, implementation for use of
        radiography in acute knee injuries,
        117
Rupture
    (*See also* Tears)
    Achilles tendon
        bracing for, functional, 285
        early neglected, primary repair
            without augmentation for, 286

S

Sacrum
  chordoma of spine above, treatment
      and outcome, 389
  sarcoma of, prognostic factors, 405
Sagittal
  band reconstruction, 152
St. Georg sledge
  for medial compartment knee
      replacement, 234
Sarcoma
  bone
    pelvic, prognostic factors in, 405
    of shoulder girdle, 390
  choroid, of bone, 382
  Ewing's, 360
    acetabular, allograft reconstruction
        after resection of, intermediate-term
        results, 403
    chemotherapy/radiotherapy in,
        long-term results, 362
    femur, prognosis, 360
    limb salvage using distraction
        osteogenesis for, 414
    pelvic bone, prognostic factors,
        405–406
    scapulectomy for, subtotal, function
        after, 417
    shoulder girdle, 390
  osteogenic, diffusion-weighted MRI of
      (in rat), 397
  soft tissue, 419
    forearm and hand, limb salvage
        surgery and adjuvant radiotherapy
        for, 412
    metastases from, skeletal, 420
    scapulectomy for, subtotal, function
        after, 417
    of shoulder girdle, 390
    subcutaneous, of extremities,
        oncological outcomes of operative
        treatment of, 419
  stage-IIB, resection of, allograft
      reconstruction of acetabulum after,
      intermediate-term results, 403
  synovial
    of extremities, oncological outcomes
        of operative treatment of, 419
    MRI characteristics of, 394
Scan
  bone, 3-phase, in reflex sympathetic
      dystrophy of upper extremity, 158
Scaphoid
  acute fracture and nonunion, repeat
      screw stabilization with bone
      grafting after failed Herbert screw
      fixation for, 138
Scapholunate
  interosseous ligament in MR
      arthrography of wrist, 122
Scapulectomy
  subtotal, for neoplasm of bone and soft
      tissue, function after, 416
Sciatic
  nerve, allograft of intervertebral disc
      material to, role of phospholipase
      A$_2$ and nitric oxide in pain-related
      behavior produced by (in rat), 341
  nerve palsy associated with total hip
      replacement, 223
Sciatica
  herniated nucleus pulposus due to,
      epidural corticosteroid injections
      for, 321
  pathophysiology of, 340
Scoliosis, 26
  anterior release and fusion in, 28
  idiopathic, efficacy of non-operative
      treatments for, 26
  surgery, pediatric, IV Premarin to
      decrease postoperative blood loss
      after, 29
Scoring
  systems, observer-based aggregate,
      validity as descriptors of elbow
      pain, function, and disability, 174
Screw(s)
  augmentation, hip, with calcium
      phosphate cement, in vitro
      biomechanical analysis of, 101
  cervical, lateral mass, *vs.* pedicle screws,
      330
  compression
    parallel cannulated, figure-eight
        wiring through, for displaced
        transverse patella fractures, 119
    in subtalar arthrodesis for
        posttraumatic arthritis, 297
  fixation
    atlantoaxial transarticular, technique,
        radiological and anatomical
        evaluation of, 332
    atlantoaxial transarticular, unilateral
        posterior, 335
    of elbow fracture-dislocation, 169
    iliosacral, early complications of
        percutaneous technique, 99
    pedicle, for cervical spine lesions,
        nontraumatic, 329
    pedicle, cervical, *vs.* lateral mass screws,
        330
    stabilization, repeat, with bone grafting
        after failed Herbert screw fixation
        for acute scaphoid fractures and
        nonunion, 138

Seasonal
  variations in lower extremity
    amputation, 82
Semitendinosus
  anatomic reconstruction of anterior
    cruciate ligament, 249
Sensation
  phantom, among British veteran
    amputees, 79
Septic
  arthritis, effect of *Hemophilus
    influenzae* type b vaccination on
    incidence of, 52
Severin classification system
  for evaluation of results of operative
    treatment for congenital hip
    dislocation, 32
Sexual
  function, female, effect of trauma and
    pelvic fracture on, 100
SF-36 health survey
  for health-related quality of life after
    elective surgery, 232
Shelf life
  of tibial bearings, effect on
    performance, 240
Short Form Health Survey
  36-item for health-related quality of life
    after elective surgery, 232
Shoulder
  capsule contracture, postoperative,
    arthroscopic release of, 191
  disability related to occupational
    factors, 196
  dislocation, anterior, in elderly, 186
  fusion, role in era of arthroplasty, 193
  girdle, malignant bone and soft tissue
    tumors of, 390
  instability, 185
    anterior, Bankart repair for, long-term
      outcome, 185
  pain related to occupational factors,
    196
  range of motion in swimmers, 198
  stiff, arthroscopic capsular release for,
    189
  strength in swimmers, 198
  symptoms, accuracy of steroid
    placement and clinical outcome
    with, 199
Silicone
  arthroplasty, distal interphalangeal joint
    interpositional, 152
Skeletal
  metastases from soft tissue sarcoma,
    420
  muscle
    necrosis, idiopathic, in diabetics, 378

remodeling and genetic correction of
  dystrophin deficiency via
  transplantation of retroviral
  producer cells (in mice), 42
^{153}Sm-EDTMP
  for painful bone metastases, 368
Smoking
  arthrodesis for isthmic spondylolisthesis
    in adults and, single-level posterior
    lateral, 336
  fracture healing and, tibial and distal
    radius, acceleration of healing, 109
  hip fracture and, in elderly men, 69
Snapping
  of triceps head, medial, and recurrent
    dislocation of ulnar nerve, 172
Soft tissue
  adjacent to orthopedic hardware, MRI
    of, 395
  injuries, intraarticular, with distal radial
    fractures, arthroscopic diagnosis of,
    127
  sarcoma (*see* Sarcoma, soft tissue)
  tumor
    malignant, of shoulder girdle, 390
    scapulectomy for, subtotal, function
      after, 416
Solid tumors
  childhood, late mortality of long-term
    survivors of, 351
Spinal
  anesthesia for outpatient knee
    arthroscopy, 245
Spine
  bone graft substitutes, 313
  cervical (*see* Cervical)
  chordoma of, above sacrum, treatment
    and outcome, 389
  cord
    injury, 344
    injury, acute, methylprednisolone or
      tirilazad in, 344
    tumor, pedicle screw fixation for, 329
  deformity, anterior release and fusion
    in, in children, 28
  disorders
    in administrative databases, quality of
      data regarding diagnoses of, 316
    coding and documentation and, 315
    degenerative, 319
    practice guidelines for, 343
    surgical management, outcomes of,
      336
  fusion (*see* Fusion, spinal)
  infection, 324
  instrumentation, 328

decompressive laminectomy and
arthrodesis with, for degenerative
lumbar spondylolisthesis with
spinal stenosis, 319
lumbar (*see* Lumbar)
metastases, posterior decompression and
stabilization for, 374
range of motion, 315
stenosis, degenerative lumbar
spondylolisthesis with,
decompressive laminectomy and
arthrodesis with and without spinal
instrumentation for, 319
surgery, major, mortality rate related to
hospital patient volume in
Medicare patients undergoing, 267
tumors, system for surgical staging and
management of, 387
Splinting
night, in clubfoot deformity in
amyoplasia, 35
static, for reflex sympathetic dystrophy
of upper extremity, 158
Spondylitis
infectious, cervical, pedicle screw
fixation for, 330
Spondyloarthropathy
destructive cervical, due to long-term
hemodialysis, pedicle screw fixation
for, 329–330
Spondylolisthesis
isthmic, in adults, single-level
posterolateral arthrodesis for, 336
lumbar, degenerative, with spinal
stenosis, decompressive
laminectomy and arthrodesis with
and without spinal instrumentation
for, 319
Spondylosis
cervical, pedicle screw fixation for, 329
Sports
injury, in children, 45
Sprains
ankle, recurrent lateral, effect of ankle
orthoses on functional performance
after, 279
Stabilization
posterior decompression and, for spinal
metastases, 374
Staphylococcus
aureus causing pyogenic vertebral
osteomyelitis, 325, 326
epidermidis causing pyogenic vertebral
osteomyelitis, 325
infection after total knee arthroplasty,
results of 2-stage reimplantation
for, 239

reinfection after reimplantation hip
arthroplasty, 262
Stellate
ganglion blocks in reflex sympathetic
dystrophy of upper extremity, 158
Stenosis
spinal, degenerative lumbar
spondylolisthesis with,
decompressive laminectomy and
arthrodesis with and without spinal
instrumentation for, 319
Sternocleidomastoid
pseudotumor of infants and congenital
muscular torticollis, 49
Steroid(s)
effect on survivorship of Charnley total
hip arthroplasty in juvenile chronic
arthritis, 46
-induced adipogenesis in pluripotential
cell line from bone marrow, 13
injections
accuracy of placement for shoulder
symptoms, and clinical outcome,
199
in epicondylitis, medial, 161
epidural, for sciatica due to herniated
nucleus pulposus, 321
incomplete healing of simple bone
cysts after, in children, 50
Stiff shoulder
arthroscopic capsular release for, 189
Strength
shoulder, in swimmers, 198
Streptococcus
infection after total knee arthroplasty,
results of 2-stage reimplantation
for, 239
viridans causing pyogenic vertebral
osteomyelitis, 325
Stress
fracture
fibula, after arthrodesis of ankle or
hindfoot, 289
tibia, after arthrodesis of ankle or
hindfoot, 288
in metatarsal, fifth, biomechanical study
of, 292
radiography, valgus, in normal ankles,
282
Stump
pain in lower limb amputation, epidural
bupivacaine and morphine in
prevention of, 80
Subacromial
decompression for massive irreparable
rotator cuff tears, results of, 182
impingement syndrome, nonoperative
treatment of, 177

steroid injections, accuracy of placement for shoulder symptoms, and clinical outcome, 200

Subcutaneous
soft tissue sarcoma of extremities, oncological outcomes of operative treatment of, 419

Subperiosteal
origin of osteoid osteomas in tubular bones, CT and MRI of, 376
osteoid osteoma, radiographic and pathologic manifestations of, 377

Subscapularis
tendon, traumatic tears of, 179

Subsidence
massive early, after femoral impaction grafting, 275

Substance
abuse and rehabilitation for work-related upper extremity disorders, 195

Subtalar
arthritis, posttraumatic, subtalar arthrodesis with internal compression for, 297
fusion (*see* Fusion, subtalar)

Sugioka rotation osteotomy
for osteonecrosis of femoral head, 229

Supracondylar
fractures of humerus, management of pulseless pink hand in, in children, 20

Suprascapular
nerve injuries combined with axillary nerve injuries, results of nerve grafting for, 201

Surgeons
grade of, and lower limb amputation, 78
orthopedic, effect of exposure to ionizing radiation on offspring of, 6
volume and postoperative complications after total hip replacements, 267

Surgery
elective, health-related quality of life after, 232
orthopedic, major, mortality rates related to hospital patient volume for Medicare patients undergoing, 267

Surgical
service, orthopedic, in urban trauma center, impact of gunshot wounds on, 91
team, orthopedic, radiation exposure during fluoroscopy to, 10

Suture
anchor
in rotator cuff repair, biomechanical evaluation of, 183
technique of arthroscopic Bankart reconstruction, long-term follow-up, 187
repair of rotator cuff, arthroscopic, technique and long-term results, 181

Swimmers
shoulder strength and range of motion in, 198

Sympathetic
dystrophy, reflex, in upper extremity, 156

Synovectomy
arthroscopic, of rheumatoid wrist, long-term follow-up, 142
elbow, 164
arthroscopic, for rheumatoid arthritis, 166
with radial head excision in rheumatoid arthritis, 164

Synovial
sarcoma
of extremities, oncological outcomes of operative treatment of, 419
MRI characteristics of, 394

T

Taperloc femoral component
in hip arthroplasty, total, 10-year follow-up, 207

Tarsal
tunnel syndrome
diagnosis, surgical technique, and functional outcome, 307
surgery in, outcome of, 308

TcPO$_2$
measurement in determination of amputation level in ischemic limbs, 83

Tears
(*See also* Rupture)
cruciate ligament, anterior, operative *vs.* nonoperative treatment of, 45
meniscal, extending into avascular zone, arthroscopic repair of, 244
rotator cuff (*see* Rotator cuff, tears)
subscapularis tendon, traumatic, 179
triangular fibrocartilage complex of wrist, high-resolution MRI of, 125

Tegretol
for painful neuroma, 154

Temperature
  muscle, in diagnosis of reflex
    sympathetic dystrophy of upper
    extremity, 158
Tendon
  Achilles, rupture
    bracing for, functional, 285
    early neglected, primary repair
      without augmentation for, 286
  ankle, injuries, 284
  extensor, injuries, early active
    mobilization for, 149
  foot, injuries, 284
  patellar, autogenous graft, in anterior
    cruciate ligament reconstruction,
    long-term follow-up, 250
  subscapularis, traumatic tears of, 179
Tennis
  elbow (*see* Elbow, tennis)
Tenodeses
  do not fully restore ankle loading
    characteristics, 280
TENS
  for phantom limb pain, 80
The Hospital for Special Surgery
  elbow scoring system, validity of, 174
Thermography
  in reflex sympathetic dystrophy of
    upper extremity, 158
Thigh
  pain, proximal, after femoral nailing,
    104
Thoracoscopic
  vs. open thoracotomy approach to
    anterior release and fusion in
    pediatric spinal deformity, 28
Thoracotomy
  open, *vs.* thoracoscopic approach to
    anterior release and fusion in
    pediatric spinal deformity, 28
Thromboembolism
  after reconstruction of hemipelvis after
    excision of malignant tumors, 408
Tibia, 108
  bearings, performance of, impacts of
    shelf life and in vivo duration on,
    240
  distal, AO/ASIF fracture classification
    for, 86
  fracture (*see* Fracture, tibia)
  nails, interlocking, decision making
    errors in use of, 110
  osteoma in, osteoid, 377
  transtibial amputees, performance of
    ICEROSS prostheses in, 85
  valgization osteotomy, Coventry high,
    time-dependent clinical and
    roentgenographic results of, 255

vara, early infantile, brace treatment of,
  53
Tibiotalar
  arthrodesis, salvage of pseudoarthrosis
    after, 300
Tirilazad
  in spinal cord injury, acute, 344
Tissue
  formation, extracortical, in diaphyseal
    segmental replacement, effect of
    cisplatin chemotherapy on (in dog),
    359
  shrinkage with holmium:YAG laser (in
    rabbit), 60
  soft (*see* Soft tissue)
Titanium
  cages, threaded, for lumbar interbody
    fusions, 328
  -stimulated peripheral blood monocytes,
    modulation of cytokine production
    by pharmacological agents in, 3
  vs. ceramic threaded cup in total hip
    arthroplasty for insufficient
    acetabulum, 218
Toe
  great (*see* Hallux)
Tomography
  computed (*see* Computed tomography)
Torticollis
  muscular, congenital, and
    sternocleidomastoid pseudotumor
    of infants, 49
Tourniquet
  use with reamed femoral nailing in
    multiply injured patients, 98
Transarticular
  screw fixation, atlantoaxial
    technique, radiological and
    anatomical evaluation of, 332
    unilateral posterior, 335
Transcutaneous
  electrical nerve stimulation
    for phantom limb pain, 80
    in reflex sympathetic dystrophy of
      upper extremity, 158
  partial pressure of oxygen in
    determination of amputation level
    in ischemic limbs, 83
Transfusion
  autotransfusion, intraoperative, quality
    assessment of, 65
Transolecranon
  fracture-dislocation of elbow, 168
Transplantation
  of retroviral producer cells, genetic
    correction of dystrophin deficiency
    and skeletal muscle remodeling via
    (in mice), 42

458 / Subject Index

Transtibial
amputees, performance of ICEROSS
prostheses in, 85
Trapdoor
procedure for osteonecrosis of femoral
head, 227
Trauma
arthritis after, subtalar arthrodesis with
internal compression for, 297
center, urban, impact of gunshot
wounds on orthopedic surgical
service in, 91
elbow, 168
extremity, early *vs.* late fasciotomy in,
93
knee, acute, radiography in,
implementation of Ottawa Knee
Rule for use of, 117
ligament
ankle, 279
foot, 279
multiple, reamed femoral nailing in
patients with, 98
musculoskeletal, 85
nerve, combined axillary and
suprascapular, results of nerve
grafting for, 201
osseous, of ankle and foot, 288
osteochondral defects of knee after,
fresh osteochondral allografts for,
252
pelvic, effect on female genitourinary,
sexual, and reproductive function,
100
soft tissue, intraarticular, with distal
radial fractures, arthroscopic
diagnosis of, 127
spinal cord, 344
acute, methylprednisolone or tirilazad
in, 344
sports, in children, 45
tendon
ankle, 284
extensor, early active mobilization for,
149
foot, 284
subscapularis, 179
Triangular
fibrocartilage complex of wrist,
high-resolution MRI in, 125
Triceps
head, medial, snapping of, and
recurrent dislocation of ulnar
nerve, 172
Trochanteric
bursitis, evaluation of
glucocorticosteroid injection in, 12

Tubular
bones, subperiosteal origin of osteoid
osteomas in, CT and MRI of, 376
Tumor(s)
bone (*see* Bone, tumors)
Ewing's Tumor Study, first UKCCSG,
long-term results from, 362
giant cell (*see* Giant cell tumor)
humeral resection and reconstruction
for, proximal, distal upper
extremity function after, 415
necrosis factor-α production in
titanium-stimulated peripheral
blood monocytes modulated by
pharmacological agents, 3
necrosis in osteogenic sarcoma,
diffusion-weighted MRI assessment
of (in rat), 397
periacetabular, malignant, excision of,
reconstruction of hemipelvis after,
407
second malignant, after first childhood
cancer, radiation and genetic
factors in risk of, 358
soft tissue, function after subtotal
scapulectomy for, 416
solid, childhood, late mortality of
long-term survivors of, 351
spine
cord, pedicle screw fixation for, 329
system for surgical staging and
management of, 387
vertebra, cervical, pedicle screw fixation
for, 329
Tunnel
carpal tunnel syndrome, role of
epineurotomy in operative
treatment of, 159
tarsal tunnel syndrome
diagnosis, surgical technique, and
functional outcome, 307
surgery in, outcome of, 308

U

Ulcerations
neuropathic, plantar to lateral column,
and Charcot foot deformity, 306
Ulna
centralization of hand on, for radial
club hand, long-term follow-up, 34
Ulnar
nerve dislocation, recurrent, and
snapping of medial head of triceps,
172

Ultrasound
  device to accelerate tibia and distal
      radius fracture healing in patients
      who smoke, 109
  Doppler, monitoring, of intraoperative
      intravascular volume optimization
      after repair of proximal femoral
      fracture, 103
Urban
  trauma center, impact of gunshot
      wounds on orthopedic surgical
      service in, 91
Urine
  excretion of
      2,3-dinor-6-ketoprostaglandin $F_{1\alpha}$
      and 11-dehydrothromboxane B_2
      induced by fat embolism (in pig),
      94

V

VACA
  chemotherapy in Ewing's sarcoma of
      femur, 361
Vaccination
  Hemophilus influenzae type b, decline
      of bone and joint infections after,
      52
Valgization
  osteotomy, Coventry high tibial,
      time-dependent clinical and
      roentgenographic results of, 255
Valgus
  bracing, joint loading with, in varus
      gonarthrosis, 254
  deformity, hallux (*see* Hallux, valgus)
  osteotomies for coxa vara, surgical
      outcomes, 31
  stress radiography in normal ankles,
      282
Vancomycin
  systemic, with biodegradable antibiotic
      implant in osteomyelitis (in rabbit),
      263
Varus
  gonarthrosis, joint loading with valgus
      bracing in, 254
Vein
  blood flow after total hip replacement,
      effect of active movement of foot
      on, 222
Vertebra
  cervical, tumors, pedicle screw fixation
      for, 329
  osteomyelitis, pyogenic (*see*
      Osteomyelitis, vertebral, pyogenic)

Vertical
  translocation in rheumatoid arthritis
      patients, surgical outcomes, 339
Veteran
  amputees, British, phantom pain and
      sensation among, 79
Vinblastine
  /methylprednisolone in Langerhans' cell
      histiocytosis in adults, 380
Vincristine
  in Ewing's sarcoma
      femur, 361
      radiotherapy and, 362
  in osteosarcoma, operable, 352
Volume
  optimization, intraoperative
      intravascular, after repair of
      proximal femur fracture, 102

W

Watson-Jones procedure
  for lateral ankle instability, 20-year
      follow-up, 283
Weinstein-Boriani-Biagini system
  for classification of spinal tumors, 387
Wiberg-Baumgartl unstable patellar type
      dislocation
  recurrence of, 257
Wire
  Kirschner, risks of placement in distal
      radius, 134
Wiring
  figure-eight, through parallel cannulated
      compression screws for displaced
      transverse patella fractures, 119
Women
  effect of trauma and pelvic fracture on
      genitourinary, sexual, and
      reproductive function in, 100
Work
  -related upper extremity disorders,
      rehabilitation for, and psychosocial
      factors, 194
Workplace
  performance of ICEROSS prostheses in
      transtibial amputees in, 85
Wounds
  gunshot
      impact on orthopedic surgical service
          in urban trauma center, 91
      through knee, intraarticular findings
          after, 90
  puncture, infected, in diabetics, surgical
      morbidity and risk of amputation
      due to, 81

Wrist
    arthrography of, MR, scapholunate
        interosseous ligament in, 122
    rheumatoid, arthroscopic synovectomy
        for, long-term follow-up, 142
    triangular fibrocartilage complex of,
        high-resolution MRI in, 125

Y

YAG
    holmium:YAG laser, tissue shrinkage
        with (in rabbit), 60

Author Index

A

Abudu A, 407
Abumi K, 329
Ackroyd CE, 234
Adams GL, 85
Adolfsson L, 142
Allen AA, 191
Allen MJ, 1
Alt A, 402
Altchek DW, 179
Amis AA, 183
Amstutz HC, 223
Andriacchi TP, 254
Andrini L, 386
Anglen JO, 88
Ansari S, 234
Apelqvist J, 304
Arangio GA, 292
Armstrong DG, 81, 82
Arnoczky SP, 60
Asnis-Ernberg L, 125
Avci S, 219
Axon JMC, 164

B

Bacci G, 348
Badwey TM, 301
Bailie DS, 307
Bak K, 198
Balian G, 13
Barber-Westin SD, 244, 246
Bar-On E, 17
Barthel T, 225
Battistella F, 98
Bauer HCF, 374
Baxter DE, 310
Beals SB, 315
Beals TC, 296
Beaton DE, 174
Beattie WS, 270
Beauchamp RD, 20
Bednar DA, 57
Bednarz PA, 296
Bell RS, 403, 412, 416
Beltran J, 377
Bembi B, 44
Benevenia J, 394
Bennett JD, 127
Berg EE, 119
Bergamini TM, 65
Beringer DC, 22
Bernstein SM, 26

Bertsch C, 280
Bettin D, 255
Biagini R, 387
Bickels J, 390
Bilderback KK, 29
Blacksin MF, 394
Blaine TA, 3
Bloem JL, 391, 398
Blyth M, 302
Bobyn JD, 276
Boden SD, 313
Boland PJ, 405
Bonar SK, 86
Bonato M, 386
Bono C, 145
Boriani S, 387, 389
Bosse MJ, 100
Bottega M, 44
Bould M, 236
Bounameaux H, 83
Bowen CVA, 412
Bowerman SG, 52
Boyett J, 351
Bracken MB, 344
Branca A, 294
Bray PW, 412
Brennwald J, 131
Briggs KK, 247
Briggs TWR, 6
Brisby H, 340
Brophy DP, 199
Broste SK, 316
Brown TD, 91
Bucca C, 294
Buehler KC, 112
Burdeaux BD Jr, 291
Burton K, 194

C

Caja VL, 89
Calhoun JH, 263
Cannon SR, 407
Carette S, 321
Carr AJ, 164
Carragee EJ, 324, 325, 326, 336
Carroll K, 31
Carter SR, 408
Caruso R, 379
Casey ATH, 332, 339
Cassell OCS, 64
Ceroni D, 304
Chan HSL, 349
Chan PSH, 256

Chatal J-F, 368
Cheng JC, 365
Chevalley F, 389
Chompret A, 358
Chrisovitsinos JP, 105
Christensen JH, 80
Chrzan JS, 306
Ciarelli MJ, 60
Claes LE, 280
Clemence LM, 279
Cobb TK, 170, 274
Cole WG, 50
Coleman S, 31
Collier JP, 240
Colterjohn NR, 57
Connors N, 219
Cook SD, 109
Cooke EA, 222
Copeland CE, 100
Corcoran S, 237
Coumas JM, 301
Court-Brown CM, 115
Cox BD, 279
Coyte P, 231
Craft AW, 352, 362
Crane HS, 267
Crockard HA, 339
Croft PR, 196
Cui Q, 13
Currey JD, 399
Currier BH, 240
Currier JH, 240

D

Dahl V, 245
Dahm DL, 297
Dahners LE, 106
Dailiana Z, 66
Dainton JN, 104
Damron TA, 378, 415
Danisa OA, 217
Dasgupta AK, 85
Davis AM, 252, 403
Davis RB III, 41
DeHaven KE, 285
DeLuca PA, 41
Dennis DA, 267
Desai P, 377
Deutsch A, 179
de Vathaire F, 358
Deyo RA, 267
Di Palma L, 294
Diamond TH, 69
Dickman CA, 335

DiPasquale TG, 10
Dirschl DR, 85
Dobyns JH, 140
Dodenhoff RM, 104
Dolan LA, 33
Dormans JP, 48
Duncan CP, 212, 215
Dürr HR, 418
Dutkowsky JP, 301

E

Easley ME, 385
Eilertsen TB, 70
Einhorn TA, 227
Eldridge JDJ, 275
Eneroth M, 304
Erginousakis DA, 67
Eskelin MKK, 74
Etches R, 270
Eustace JA, 199
Eustace S, 395

F

Faciszewski T, 316
Fardon D, 316
Fassati A, 42
Feagin JA Jr, 249
Fernandez DL, 136
Feroussis JC, 211
Ferris LR, 288
Fischer MD, 128
Fischgrund JS, 319
Fleming LL, 284
Fleming SS, 284
Fletcher CDM, 382
Foreman J, 399
Fourastier J, 229
Frankenburg EP, 101
Freeborn DK, 343
Freeman BJC, 236
Frisén M, 142
Frogameni AD, 177
Fujikawa Y, 8

G

Gainor BJ, 88
Galanis EC, 370
Gartsman GM, 182
Gatchel RJ, 194
Gaze MN, 363
Gebhard F, 185
Geirnaerdt MJA, 398
Gellman H, 156

Gendi NST, 164
Gentili M, 59
Gerwin M, 146
Ghalambor N, 309
Ghazavi MT, 252
Gibbons CLMH, 416
Gibbs CP, 419
Gibney RP, 199
Gierløff C, 245
Gilbert MS, 193
Gill LH, 301
Gill TJ, 185
Giona F, 379
Giurea A, 372
Giurini JM, 306
Goldberg R, 395
Goldman L, 232
Goldner RD, 172
González-Díaz R, 193
Goulet JA, 101
Graves SC, 301
Gray T, 250
Green J, 112
Green NE, 52
Gregory RJH, 118
Greipp PR, 370
Griffith A, 146
Grimer RJ, 407, 408
Grogan TM, 349
Gross MT, 279
Grudziak JS, 32
Guidera PM, 152
Gullichsen E, 94
Gumina S, 186
Guntner P, 308
Güntner P, 197
Gustilo T, 115

H

Haddad G, 349
Hagena F-W, 418
Haghighi P, 376
Haideri N, 40
Hall R, 288
Halliday SE, 37
Hamann W, 79
Hammond NL III, 159
Hanssen AD, 261
Hantes K, 218
Harrington RM, 114
Harris WH, 209
Hart RA, 387
Harwood FL, 251
Hashemi-Nejad A, 50
Hashizume H, 341
Hawker G, 231
Head WC, 208

Healey JH, 405
Heller JG, 330
Henley MB, 114
Herkowitz HN, 319
Hermans J, 398
Herzenberg JE, 61
Herzwurm P, 216
Hewett TE, 254
Hickmon SG, 272
Hierner R, 122
Hillman A, 360
Hillmann A, 381
Hirakawa K, 239
Hoag RH, 117
Hochwald NL, 134, 145
Hockman DE, 88
Hoffmann C, 360
Houssel P, 59
Hubble MJ, 275
Hudson MM, 351
Hughes SS, 322
Huhtala H, 257
Hui RC, 90
Hutchins PM, 104
Hutton WC, 313

I

Ilkjaer S, 80
Ilstrup DM, 265, 274
Inoue G, 138
Inwards CY, 382
Ioannidis TT, 72
Ion L, 64
Irshad F, 118
Ivory JP, 238

J

Jain R, 95
James S, 102
Jaramillo D, 23
Jarvis JG, 45
Johnston JO, 365
Jones D, 351
Jones EL, 330
Joshi A, 269
Jupiter JB, 131, 136, 168

K

Kallio PE, 258
Kaneda K, 329
Kang CH, 290
Karatzas GD, 211

Karbowski A, 255
Katz DE, 40
Kaufman T, 161
Kauranen K, 162
Kautiainen H, 46
Kavadias C, 72
Kawai A, 405
Kawakami M, 341
Kayser F, 376
Keating EM, 213
Kelikian AS, 307
Kelly CG, 363
Kerr GR, 363
Kilpatrick SE, 382
Kim D, 325
Kitaoka HB, 283, 297
Klimkiewicz JJ, 256
Kneisl JS, 385
Knelles D, 225
Kobayashi S, 205
Koepsell T, 267
Kölbl O, 225
Kollender Y, 390
Kondraske G, 315
Konrath G, 109
Kony SJ, 358
Koss S, 187
Koukoubis T, 218
Kramer AM, 70
Kraushaar BS, 163
Kreder HJ, 267
Kroon HM, 391
Kubitzek C, 122
Kuhn JE, 189
Kühne J-H, 418
Kuwahata Y, 138
Kuzbari R, 402

L

Laketić I, 399
Lam WL, 34
Lamb DW, 34
Lambert KL, 249
Lang P, 397
Langlais F, 229
Lapoint JM, 188
Larson C, 110
Lavery LA, 81, 82
Leclaire R, 321
Lee BPH, 166
Lee CM, 269
Lee J, 92
Lee KR, 207
Lee MD, 283
Lehtimäki MY, 46
Lehto MUK, 46, 257
Leinberry CF, 159

Leith JM, 282
Letts RM, 45
Leuenberger A, 304
Levine R, 134
Levine SE, 300
Levinsohn EM, 378
Li D, 282
Lidor C, 288
Lindenfeld TN, 254
Lindner N, 381
Linscheid RL, 140
Littenberg B, 108
Little DG, 37
Liu Z, 49
Logan A, 149
Loizides AA, 67
Lombardi AV Jr, 208
Lötjönen JMP, 74
Lucas P, 299
Luchette FA, 93
Luchetti WT, 256
Lynch NM, 265

M

Mackay DC, 302
Mackay M, 319
Mackinnon SE, 154
Madawi AA, 332
Mader JT, 263
Mäenpää H, 257
Magnusson SP, 198
Malizos KN, 66
Mallory TH, 208
Maloney WJ, 216
Maltarello MC, 89
Mangione CM, 232
Mangone PG, 284
Mannarino FP, 286
Manoli A II, 296
Mäntysaari MJ, 74
Marcoux S, 321
Markovic L, 269
Marks PH, 191
Marsh JL, 86
Martin DF, 301
Martin JS, 86
Masri BA, 212, 215
Masterson EL, 212, 215
Matta JM, 71
Mayer TG, 315
McAuliffe JA, 271
McBride MT, 188
McCabe J, 109
McCall RE, 29
McCarren M, 108
McCarthy ML, 100
McCaul K, 237

McCluskie PJA, 85
McComis GP, 285
McConkey JP, 282
McElroy BJ, 183
McLaughlin JR, 207
McNally MA, 222
McQuail TM, 378
Meding JB, 213
Mehlman CT, 10
Meller I, 390
Mencio GA, 52
Mercuri M, 348
Meyer MD, 33
Michas P, 91
Micheli LJ, 185
Michet CJ Jr, 12
Mikami Y, 201
Milbauer JP, 276
Miller FB, 65
Millett PJ, 1
Mills WJ, 99
Min BW, 290
Minematsu K, 414
Moed BR, 109
Mollan RAB, 222
Mologne TS, 188
Mont MA, 227
Moore DC, 101
Morcuende JA, 33
Moreau PG, 411
Mori S, 420
Moroni A, 89
Moroz P, 18
Morrey BF, 166, 170, 274, 283
Morrison DS, 177
Mosca VS, 35
Moskal JT, 217
Movin T, 197
Mubarak SJ, 28
Müller G, 383
Müller RT, 383
Mullooly JP, 343
Mundt AJ, 419
Myer BJ, 1
Myerson MS, 300

N

Nagano A, 201
Nawoczenski DA, 285
Neale S, 8
Neitosvaara Y, 258
Nelson CL, 272
Newman JH, 234
Newton PO, 28
Nichols D, 156
Niki H, 35

Nikku R, 258
Nikolajsen L, 80
Nirschl RP, 163
Noble JS, 22
Noordin S, 223
Noyes FR, 244, 246

O

Ochial N, 201
O'Connor MI, 415
O'Duffy JD, 12
Olmarker K, 340
Omland E, 245
Orav EJ, 232
Organ SW, 163
Osman M, 59
Otsuka NY, 18
Õunpuu S, 41
Ozaki T, 360, 381

P

Pagnano MW, 261
Paley D, 61
Palmer AK, 143
Papaconstantinou HT, 93
Papagelopoulos PJ, 370
Papakostides KG, 105
Papapolychroniou T, 73
Paprosky W, 216
Paremain G, 61
Park H-J, 242
Parma A, 44
Patel VS, 85
Pazzaglia UE, 386
Peabody TD, 419
Pecking A, 368
Perlman M, 309
Petrie S, 171
Petsatodes G, 221
Pettey J, 98
Petty W, 219
Phillips D, 171
Picci P, 348
Pienimäki TT, 162
Plancher KD, 247
Polatin PB, 194
Pollak AN, 98
Pollice PF, 3
Polyzoides AJ, 235
Pope DP, 196
Pope RO, 237
Porat S, 17
Porter DA, 286
Porter ML, 203
Postacchini F, 186

Potter HG, 125
Pournaros J, 221
Pressman AE, 45
Pritchard CM, 196
Pritzker KP, 252
Pullyblank A, 236
Putnam MD, 128
Pynsent PB, 408

Q

Quan X, 49
Quebedeaux TL, 81
Quenzer DE, 140
Quint U, 383

R

Rah J-H, 242
Rautanen M, 94
Ray CD, 328
Renard AJS, 409
Resche I, 368
Resnick D, 376
Rhymaszewski LA, 302
Richards RR, 174
Richards RS, 127
Richmond JC, 187
Riddick MF, 26
Riew KD, 322
Ring D, 131, 168
Ritschl P, 372
Ritter MA, 213
Riutta A, 94
Rivero-Melián C, 308
Rock MG, 359, 366, 415
Rodgers WB, 23
Rodríguez-Merchán EC, 193
Rosenbaum D, 280
Rosenblum BI, 306
Rosier RN, 3
Rossouw DJ, 183
Roth JH, 127
Routt MLC Jr, 99
Rowe DE, 26
Rubman MH, 244
Ryaby JP, 109

S

Sabharwal S, 20
Sabokbar A, 8
Sadri H, 304
Saeed M, 397
Sagiv S, 17

Saito N, 205
Salathe EP, 292
Sanders RW, 168
Sanjay BKS, 411
Sanzén L, 63
Sarafis KA, 211
Saragaglia D, 303
Schaefer SL, 60
Scheck RJ, 122
Schemitsch EH, 95
Schimandle JH, 313
Schmalzried TP, 223
Schreiner MS, 48
Schreuder HWB, 409
Schwend RM, 23
Schwering L, 255
Scott H, 34
Sdrenias C, 72
Sekel R, 69
Sgro Serpente PA, 42
Shaffrey CI, 217
Shankman S, 377
Shaw AD, 115
Shaw NJ, 118
Shaw Wilgis EF, 152
Shbeeb MI, 12
Shea K, 136
Shean CJ, 53
Shelbourne KD, 250
Shih L-Y, 359
Shye D, 343
Siebenrock KA, 366
Siegel JR, 394
Siegfried JW, 159
Sienbenrock KA, 71
Silcox DH, 330
Simonian PT, 99
Sinclair S, 102
Singer M, 102
Sjödén GOJ, 197
Skahen JR III, 143
Skinner RA, 272
Smith EJ, 275
Smith SE, 209
Snead D, 286
Sochart DH, 203
Solanki GA, 332
Solomonow M, 171
Song GS, 335
Song K, 40
Song KM, 37
Song KS, 290
Sonoda M, 251
Souhami RL, 352
Spain DA, 65
Spinner RJ, 172
Sponseller PD, 227
Staheli LT, 35
Stahl S, 161

Stavrou ZP, 67
Steadman JR, 247
Steiner JF, 70
Stenström A, 304
Stevens J, 339
Stevens PM, 31
Stiell IG, 117
Stulberg BN, 239
Sundberg M, 63
Sylaidis P, 149
Symeonides P, 221

T

Takaoka K, 205
Tamaki T, 341
Tang S, 49
Tauro JC, 181
Taylor HD, 267
Templeman D, 110
Templeton J, 48
Testi AM, 379
Theodore N, 335
Thompson MM, 78
Thordarson DB, 309
Thornley SW, 69
Tol JL, 292
Tollison ME, 310
Tomita K, 414
Tornetta P III, 90, 134, 145
Tourné Y, 303
Tredwell SJ, 20
Trousdale RT, 261, 265
Tsakonas AC, 235
Tsuchiya H, 414
Turan I, 308
Turchin DC, 95, 174

U

Ueda T, 420
Unni KK, 366

V

Vafiadis J, 73
Van der Eijken JW, 352
Van der Reis WL, 18
van der Vlugt T, 325
van Dijk CN, 292
van Houtum WH, 82
van Trommel MF, 391
Vanharanta H, 162
Varecka T, 110
Veltri DM, 179
Verheyen CCPM, 292
Veth RPH, 409
Vogt M, 32

W

Wada Y, 251
Wang G-J, 13
Ward WT, 32
Warner JJP, 191
Warriner CB, 270
Wartan SW, 79
Watson HK, 152
Watson JT, 109
Webb JM, 238
Weber TG, 114
Wedley JR, 79
Weiland AJ, 125, 146
Weiner DS, 22
Weinstein JN, 389
Weinstein LP, 108
Weinzweig J, 152
Wells DJ, 42
Wells GA, 117
Wendland MF, 397
Wenger DR, 28
Werner FW, 143
White SA, 78
Wilde AH, 239
Williams AB, 93
Williams D, 238

Williams RE, 91
Williamson D, 395
Wills RP, 249
Windhager R, 372
Wolfson AH, 271
Woll TS, 112
Woodward JS Jr, 187
Woodworth P, 177
Woolson ST, 276
Worseg AP, 402
Wright J, 231
Wunder JS, 403, 416
Wütschert R, 83

X

Xenakis T, 105, 218
Xenakis TA, 66
Xiao D, 292

Y

Yabuki S, 340
Yoon Y-S, 242
Yoshikawa H, 420
Youatt M, 149
Young DR, 359
Younge DA, 411

Z

Zacharopoiulos K, 73
Zadeh HG, 6
Zanotti RM, 189
Zattara A, 303
Zdeblick TA, 322
Zickerman AM, 78
Zionts LE, 53